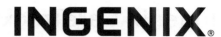
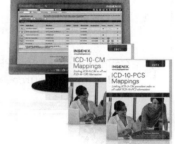
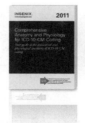 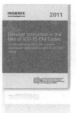 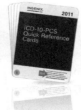 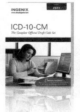 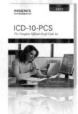

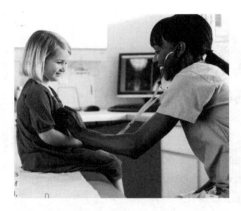

INGENIX®
*e*solutions

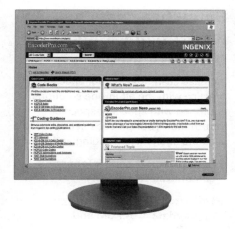

Electronic coding, billing and reimbursement products.

Ingenix provides a robust suite of eSolutions to solve a wide variety of coding, billing and reimbursement issues. As the industry moves to electronic products, you can rely on Ingenix to help support you through the transition.

← **Web-based applications for all markets**

← **Dedicated support**

← **Environmentally responsible**

Key Features and Benefits

Using eSolutions is a step in the right direction when it comes to streamlining your coding, billing and reimbursement practices. Ingenix eSolutions can help you save time and increase your efficiency with accurate and on-time content.

- **Simplify ICD-10 transition.** ICD-10 mapping tools provide crosswalks between ICD-9-CM and ICD-10 codes quickly and easily

- **Save time and money.** Ingenix eSolutions combine the content of over 37 code books and data files

- **Increase accuracy.** Electronic solutions are updated regularly so you know you're always working with the most current content available

- **Get the training and support you need.** Convenient, monthly webinars and customized training programs are available to meet your specific needs

- **Rely on a leader in health care.** Ingenix has been producing quality coding products for over 26 years. All of the expert content that goes into our books goes into our electronic resources

- **Get Started.** Visit **shopingenix.com/ eSolutions** for product listing

---

Ingenix | Information is the Lifeblood of Health Care | Call toll-free 1.800.INGENIX (464.3649), option 1.

100% Money Back Guarantee If our merchandise ever fails to meet your expectations, please contact our Customer Service Department toll-free at 1.800.INGENIX (464.3649), option 1, for an immediate response. Software: Credit will be granted for unopened packages only.

Also available from your medical bookstore or distributor.

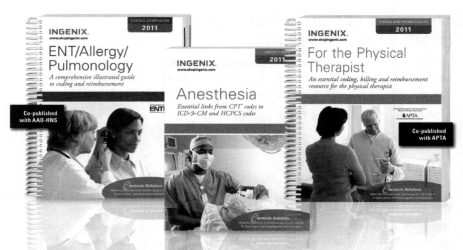

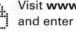
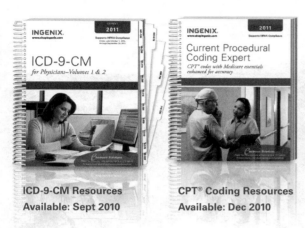
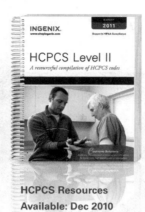

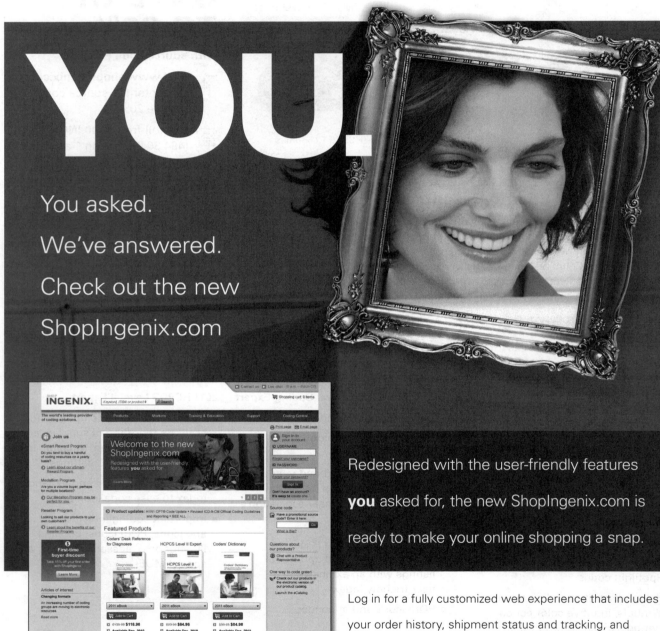

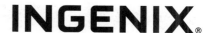

INGENIX®

March 2011

Dear Ingenix Customer:

This is your 2011 draft for the *ICD-10-PCS: The Complete Official Draft Code Set*.

The Centers for Medicare and Medicaid Services (CMS) is the agency charged with maintaining and updating the International Classification of Diseases 10th Revision Procedure Classification System (ICD-10-PCS). This 2011 draft represents the most current changes to the ICD-10-PCS as released by CMS.

Remember, the codes in ICD-10-PCS are not currently valid for any documentation or reporting of health care services. It is anticipated that CMS will make several updates and revisions to the draft prior to implementation of ICD-10-PCS; however, the basic structure will remain the same.

The Department of Health and Human Services (HHS) published the final rule regarding the adoption of both ICD-10-CM and ICD-10-PCS in the January 16, 2009, *Federal Register* (45 CFR part 162 [CMS—0013—F]). The compliance date for implementation of ICD-10-CM and ICD-10-PCS as a replacement for ICD-9-CM is October 1, 2013.

ICD-10-PCS would replace ICD-9-CM Volume 3, including the official coding guidelines, for the following procedures or other actions taken for diseases, injuries, and impairments on **hospital inpatients reported by hospitals**: prevention, diagnosis, treatment, and management.

We appreciate your choosing Ingenix to meet your ICD-10-PCS conversion preparation and coding training needs. If you have any questions or comments concerning your draft *ICD-10-PCS: The Complete Official Draft Code Set*, please do not hesitate to call out customer service department. The toll-free number is 1-800-INGENIX (464-3649), option 1.

INGENIX®

ICD-10-PCS
The Complete Official Draft
Code Set

DRAFT

2011

Notice

ICD-10-PCS: The Complete Official Draft Code Set is designed to be an accurate and authoritative source regarding coding and every reasonable effort has been made to ensure accuracy and completeness of the content. However, Ingenix makes no guarantee, warranty, or representation that this publication is accurate, complete, or without errors. It is understood that Ingenix is not rendering any legal or other professional services or advice in this publication and that Ingenix bears no liability for any results or consequences that may arise from the use of this book. Please address all correspondence to:

Ingenix
2525 Lake Park Blvd
Salt Lake City, UT 84120

Our Commitment to Accuracy

Ingenix is committed to producing accurate and reliable materials. To report corrections, please visit www.ingenixonline.com/accuracy or email accuracy@ingenix.com. You can also reach customer service by calling 1.800.INGENIX (464.3649), option 1.

Copyright

Acknowledgments

Anita C. Hart, RHIA, CCS, CCS-P, *Product Manager*
Karen Schmidt, BSN, *Technical Director*
Stacy Perry, *Manager, Desktop Publishing*
Tracy Betzler, *Desktop Publishing Specialist*
Hope M. Dunn, *Desktop Publishing Specialist*
Kate Holden, *Editor*

Anita C. Hart, RHIA, CCS, CCS-P

Ms. Hart's experience includes conducting and publishing research in clinical medicine and human genetics for Yale University, Massachusetts General Hospital, and Massachusetts Institute of Technology. In addition, Ms. Hart has supervised medical records management, health information management, coding and reimbursement, and worker's compensation issues as the office manager for a physical therapy rehabilitation clinic. Ms. Hart is an expert in physician and facility coding, reimbursement systems, and compliance issues. Ms. Hart developed the *ICD-9-CM Changes: An Insider's View*. She has served as technical consultant for numerous other publications for hospital and physician practices. Currrently, Ms. Hart is the Product Manager for the ICD-9-CM and ICD-10-CM/PCS product lines.

Beth Ford, RHIT, CCS

Ms. Ford is a clinical/technical editor for Ingenix. She has extensive background in both physician and facility ICD-9-CM and CPT/HCPCS coding. Ms. Ford has served as a coding specialist, coding manager, coding trainer/educator, and coding consultant, as well as a health information management director. She is an active member of the American Heath Information Management Association (AHIMA).

Melinda Stegman, MBA, CCS

Ms. Stegman has more than 25 years of experience in the HIM profession and has been responsible for the update and maintenance of the ICD-9-CM, ICD-10, DRG resources and some cross coder products for Ingenix. In the past, she also managed the clinical aspects of the HSS/Ingenix HIM Consulting practice in the Washington, DC area office. Her areas of specialization include training on inpatient and DRG coding, outpatient coding, and Ambulatory Payment Classifications (APCs) for HIM professionals, software developers, and other clients; developing an outpatient billing/coding compliance tool for a major accounting firm; and managing HIM consulting practices. Ms. Stegman is a regular contributing author for *Advance for Health Information Management Professionals* and for the *Journal of Health Care Compliance*. She has performed coding assessments and educational sessions throughout the country. Ms. Stegman is credentialed by the American Health Information Management Association (AHIMA) as a Certified Coding Specialist (CCS) and holds a Master of Business Administration degree with a concentration in health care management from the University of New Mexico – Albuquerque.

Contents

Preface

This draft of the International Classification of Diseases, 10th Revision, Procedure Classification System (ICD-10-PCS) has been developed as a replacement for volume 3 of the International Classification of Diseases, Ninth Revision (ICD-9-CM). The development of ICD-10-PCS was funded by the U.S. Centers for Medicare and Medicaid Services under contract nos. 90-138, 91-22300 500-95-0005 and HHSM-550-2004-00011C to 3M Health Information Systems. ICD-10-PCS has a multi-axial, seven-character, alphanumeric code structure that provides a unique code for all substantially different procedures and allows new procedures to be easily incorporated as new codes. The initial draft was formally tested and evaluated by an independent contractor; the final version was released in 1998, with annual updates since the final release.

What's New for 2011

The Centers for Medicare and Medicaid Services is the agency charged with maintaining and updating the ICD-10-PCS. The most current revisions were released by CMS in December 2010. A summary of the changes may be found on the CMS website at: http://www.cms.hhs.gov/ICD10/Downloads/pcs_whats_new_2011.pdf

The CMS website that contains all information and files related to both ICD-10-PCS and ICD-10-CM is: http://www.cms.gov/ICD10/01_Overview.asp#TopOfPage

Due to the unique structure of ICD-10-PCS, a change in a character value may affect many individual codes and several Code Tables.

Change Summary Table

2009 Table	2010 New Codes	2010 Revised Codes	2010 Deleted Codes	2010 Total
71,957	446	302	322	72,081

ICD-10-PCS Code 2010 Total, By Section

Medical and Surgical	62,022
Obstetrics	300
Placement	864
Administration	1,438
Measurement and Monitoring	327
Extracorporeal Assistance and Performance	41
Extracorporeal Therapies	42
Osteopathic	100
Other Procedures	60
Chiropractic	90
Imaging	2,934
Nuclear Medicine	463
Radiation Oncology	1,929
Rehabilitation and Diagnostic Audiology	1,382
Mental Health	30
Substance Abuse Treatment	59
Total	72,081

ICD-10-PCS Code Changes

The code revisions for 2011:

- Codes were added and deleted in parallel with new ICD-9-CM codes that were valid October 1, 2010

- Individual codes were added, revised, or deleted

  — In response to public input, including

    – New qualifier **Humeral Surface**, which was added to shoulder joint body part to specify partial shoulder replacement

    – Device values that were streamlined for interbody spinal fusion devices

  — Based on internal review for clarity and ease of use, including

    – Added body part **Hemorrhoidal Plexus** to root operation tables Ø65 Destruction and Ø6B Excision

    – Revised transplant compatibility qualifier values in table ØUY to match all other transplant compatibility qualifier values in the Medical & Surgical section

ICD-10-PCS Draft Guidelines Revised, Updated, and Posted As a Separate Document

- Comprehensive review, revision, and updates by the Cooperating Parties based on industry feedback

- Posted as a stand-alone document and also included in the ICD-10-PCS Reference Manual, appendix B

New ICD-10-PCS Files

- **General Equivalence Mappings (GEM) Technical FAQs**

  — Downloadable PDF format

  — Comprehensive definitions of GEMs inclusion criteria with examples of each for diagnosis and procedure codes

  — Other frequently asked questions based on public input

Updated ICD-10-PCS Files

- **ICD-10-PCS long descriptions**

  — Text file format

  — 2011 version of ICD-10-PCS

  — Accompanying readme file in PDF format

- **ICD-10-PCS table descriptions**

  — Machine readable text file for developers

  — 2011 version of ICD-10-PCS

  — Accompanying readme file in PDF format

- **ICD-10-PCS 2011 Final Addenda**

  — New code titles for 2011 in ICD-10-PCS standard tables (PDF format)

    – List of revised code titles for 2011

  — Invalid 2010 code titles in ICD-10-PCS standard tables (PDF format)

    – List of original 2010 code titles revised, for comparison with 2011 list

  — Comprehensive file of new, revised, and invalid code titles in machine readable text format for developers

    – Accompanying readme file in PDF format

- **ICD-10-PCS Reference Manual**

  — Downloadable PDF format

  — 2011 version of ICD-10-PCS

  — New coding practice examples added in response to public input

- — Appendix A:
    - – PCS explanation and body part key entries revised
        - - In response to public input
        - - Based on internal review for clarity and completeness
- — Appendix B:
    - – Draft guidelines updated, based on a comprehensive review and revisions by the Cooperating Parties based on industry feedback

- **ICD-10-PCS slide presentation**
    - — Reference slides available in PDF format

- **ICD-10-PCS and ICD-9-CM General Equivalence Mappings (GEM)**
    - — Text file format
    - — Individual GEM entries added, revised, or deleted based on:
        - – ICD-10-PCS official coding guidelines
        - – Public input from GEM users
        - – Comprehensive review of ICD-9-CM GEMs to ensure they meet criteria as defined in GEMs Technical FAQs

- — 2011 version of ICD-10-PCS and ICD-9-CM
    - – ICD-10-PCS to ICD-9-CM GEM
    - – ICD-9-CM to ICD-10-PCS GEM
- — Procedure Code Set GEM Documentation and User's Guide (PDF format)
    - – Examples updated based on public input
    - – Glossary and file format information updated

- **ICD-10 Reimbursement Mappings**
    - — Text file format
    - — ICD-10-PCS to ICD-9-CM, 2011 version
        - – Applied procedure mapping for reimbursement purposes
        - – Derived based on inpatient hospital data
    - — ICD-10-CM to ICD-9-CM, 2011 version
        - – Applied diagnosis mapping for reimbursement purposes
        - – Derived based on inpatient hospital data
    - — Updated documentation and users' guide in PDF format
        - – Rule set posted in response to public comment

Introduction

Volume 3 of the International Classification of Diseases Ninth Revision Clinical Modification (ICD-9-CM) has been used in the United States for reporting inpatient procedures since 1979. The structure of volume 3 of ICD-9-CM has not allowed new procedures associated with rapidly changing technology to be effectively incorporated as new codes. As a result, in 1992 the U.S. Centers for Medicare and Medicaid Services funded a project to design a replacement for volume 3 of ICD-9-CM. In 1995 CMS awarded 3M Health Information Systems a three-year contract to complete development of the replacement system. The new system is the ICD-10 Procedure Coding System (ICD-10-PCS).

History of ICD-10-PCS

The World Health Organization has maintained the International Classification of Diseases (ICD) for recording cause of death since 1893. It has updated the ICD periodically to reflect new discoveries in epidemiology and changes in medical understanding of disease.

The International Classification of Diseases Tenth Revision (ICD-10), published in 1992, is the latest revision of the ICD. The WHO authorized the National Center for Health Statistics (NCHS) to develop a clinical modification of ICD-10 for use in the United States. This version, called ICD-10-CM, is intended to replace the previous U.S. clinical modification, ICD-9-CM, that has been in use since 1979. ICD-9-CM contains a procedure classification; ICD-10-CM does not.

CMS, the agency responsible for maintaining the inpatient procedure code set in the United States, contracted with 3M Health Information Systems in 1993 to design and then develop a procedure classification system to replace volume 3 of ICD-9-CM.

The result, ICD-10-PCS, was initially completed in 1998. The code set has been updated annually since that time to ensure that ICD-10-PCS includes classifications for new procedures, devices, and technologies.

The development of ICD-10-PCS had as its goal the incorporation of the following major attributes:

- **Completeness:** There should be a unique code for all substantially different procedures. In volume 3 of ICD-9-CM, procedures on different body parts, with different approaches, or of different types are sometimes assigned to the same code.

- **Unique definitions:** Because ICD-10-PCS codes are constructed of individual values rather than lists of fixed codes and text descriptions, the unique, stable definition of a code in the system is retained. New values may be added to the system to represent a specific new approach or device or qualifier, but whole codes by design cannot be given new meanings and reused.

- **Expandability:** As new procedures are developed, the structure of ICD-10-PCS should allow them to be easily incorporated as unique codes.

- **Multi-axial codes:** ICD-10-PCS codes should consist of independent characters, with each individual component retaining its meaning across broad ranges of codes to the extent possible.

- **Standardized terminology:** ICD-10-PCS should include definitions of the terminology used. While the meaning of specific words varies in common usage, ICD-10-PCS should not include multiple meanings for the same term, and each term must be assigned a specific meaning. There are no eponyms or common procedure terms in ICD-10-PCS.

- **Structural integrity:** ICD-10-PCS can be easily expanded without disrupting the structure of the system. ICD-10-PCS allows unique new codes to be added to the system because values for the seven characters that make up a code can be combined as needed. The system can evolve as medical technology and clinical practice evolve, without disrupting the ICD-10-PCS structure.

In the development of ICD-10-PCS, several additional general characteristics were added:

- **Diagnostic information is not included in procedure description:** When procedures are performed for specific diseases or disorders, the disease or disorder is not contained in the procedure code. The diagnosis codes, not the procedure codes, specify the disease or disorder.

- **Explicit not otherwise specified (NOS) options are restricted:** Explicit "not otherwise specified," (NOS) options are restricted in ICD-10-PCS. A minimal level of specificity is required for each component of the procedure.

- **Limited use of not elsewhere classified (NEC) option:** Because all significant components of a procedure are specified in ICD-10-PCS, there is generally no need for a "not elsewhere classified" (NEC) code option. However, limited NEC options are incorporated into ICD-10-PCS where necessary. For example, new devices are frequently developed, and therefore it is necessary to provide an "other device" option for use until the new device can be explicitly added to the coding system.

- **Level of specificity:** All procedures currently performed can be specified in ICD-10-PCS. The frequency with which a procedure is performed was not a consideration in the development of the system. A unique code is available for variations of a procedure that can be performed.

ICD-10-PCS code structure results in qualities that optimize the performance of the system in electronic applications, and maximize the usefulness of the coded healthcare data. These qualities include:

- Optimal search capability

- Consistent character definitions

- Consistent values wherever possible

- Code readability

- **Optimal search capability:** ICD-10-PCS is designed for maximum versatility in the ability to aggregate coded data. Values belonging to the same character as defined in a section or sections can be easily compared, since they occupy the same position in a code. This provides a high degree of flexibility and functionality for data mining.

- **Consistent characters and values:** Stability of characters and values across vast ranges of codes provides the maximum degree of functionality and flexibility for the collection and analysis of data. Because the character definition is consistent, and only the individual values assigned to that character differ as needed, meaningful comparisons of data over time can be conducted across a virtually infinite range of procedures.

- **Code readability:** ICD-1Ø-PCS resembles a language in the sense that it is made up of semi-independent values combined by following the rules of the system, much the way a sentence is formed by combining words and following the rules of grammar and syntax. As with words in their context, the meaning of any single value is a combination of its position in the code and any preceding values on which it may be dependent.

ICD-1Ø-PCS Code Structure

ICD-1Ø-PCS has a seven-character alphanumeric code structure. Each character contains up to 34 possible values. Each value represents a specific option for the general character definition. The 1Ø digits Ø–9 and the 24 letters A–H, J–N, and P–Z may be used in each character. The letters O and I are not used so as to avoid confusion with the digits Ø and 1. An ICD-1Ø-PCS code is the result of a process rather than as a single fixed set of digits or alphabetic characters. The process consists of combining semi-independent values from among a selection of values, according to the rules governing the construction of codes.

	Section	Body System	Root Operation	Body Part	Approach	Device	Qualifier
Characters:	1	2	3	4	5	6	7

A code is derived by choosing a specific value for each of the seven characters. Based on details about the procedure performed, values for each character specifying the section, body system, root operation, body part, approach, device, and qualifier are assigned. Because the definition of each character is also a function of its physical position in the code, the same letter or number placed in a different position in the code has different meaning.

The seven characters that make up a complete code have specific meanings that vary for each of the 16 sections of the manual. (The resource section of this manual lists character meanings for each section along with body-part definitions.)

Procedures are then divided into sections that identify the general type of procedure (e.g., Medical and Surgical, Obstetrics, Imaging). The first character of the procedure code always specifies the section. The second through seventh characters have the same meaning within each section, but may mean different things in other sections. In all sections, the third character specifies the general type of procedure performed (e.g., Resection, Transfusion, Fluoroscopy), while the other characters give additional information such as the body part and approach.

In ICD-1Ø-PCS, the term *procedure* refers to the complete specification of the seven characters.

Number of Codes in ICD-1Ø-PCS

At the time of this publication, there are 72,Ø81 codes in the 2Ø11 ICD-1Ø-PCS. This is a substantial increase over the number of ICD-9-CM procedure codes. However, many codes have been eliminated from ICD-1Ø-PCS from the Medical and Surgical section as part of a planned streamlining and refinement initiated in 2ØØ6. This code reduction has also included the deletion of certain body system values specified as "other" in order to facilitate more selective body part and system values. For 2Ø11, 446 new codes were added to the system, combined with the deletion of 322 codes, resulting in a total of 72,Ø81 ICD-1Ø-PCS codes.

The table structure of ICD-1Ø-PCS permits the specification of a large number of codes on a single page.

ICD-1Ø-PCS Manual

Index

Codes may be found in the index based on the general type of procedure (e.g., resection, transfusion, fluoroscopy), or a more commonly used term (e.g., appendectomy). For example, the code for percutaneous intraluminal dilation of the coronary arteries with an intraluminal device can be found in the Index under *Dilation*, or a synonym of *Dilation* (e.g., angioplasty). The Index then specifies the first three or four values of the code or directs the user to see another term.

Example:

Dilation
    Artery
        Coronary
            One Site Ø27Ø

Based on the first three values of the code provided in the Index, the corresponding table can be located. In the example above, the first three values indicate table Ø27 is to be referenced for code completion.

The tables and characters are arranged first by number and then by letter for each character (tables for ØØ-, Ø1-, Ø2-, etc., are followed by those for ØB-, ØC-, ØD-, etc., followed by ØB1, ØB2, etc., followed by ØBB, ØBC, ØBD, etc.).

Note: The Tables section must be used to construct a complete and valid code by specifying the last three or four values.

Tables

The Tables section is organized differently from ICD-9-CM. Each page in the section is composed of rows that specify the valid combinations of code values. In most sections of the system, the upper portion of each table contains a description of the first three characters of the procedure code. In the Medical and Surgical section, for example, the first three characters contain the name of the section, the body system, and the root operation performed.

For instance, the values *Ø27* specify the section *Medical and Surgical* (Ø), the body system *Heart and Great Vessels* (2) and the root operation *Dilation* (7). As shown in table Ø27, the root operation (*Dilation*) is accompanied by its definition.

The lower portion of the table specifies all the valid combinations of characters 4 through 7. The four columns in the table specify the last four characters. In the Medical and Surgical section they are labeled body part, approach, device and qualifier, respectively. Each row in the table specifies the valid combination of values for characters 4 through 7.

0 Medical and Surgical
2 Heart and Great Vessels
7 Dilation   Expanding an orifice or the lumen of a tubular body part

Body Part Character 4	Approach Character 5	Device Character 6	Qualifier Character 7
0 Coronary Artery, One Site **1** Coronary Artery, Two Sites **2** Coronary Artery, Three Sites **3** Coronary Artery, Four or More Sites	**0** Open **3** Percutaneous **4** Percutaneous Endoscopic	**4** Drug-eluting Intraluminal Device **D** Intraluminal Device **T** Radioactive Intraluminal Device **Z** No Device	**6** Bifurcation **Z** No Qualifier
F Aortic Valve **G** Mitral Valve **H** Pulmonary Valve **J** Tricuspid Valve **K** Ventricle, Right **P** Pulmonary Trunk **Q** Pulmonary Artery, Right **S** Pulmonary Vein, Right **T** Pulmonary Vein, Left **V** Superior Vena Cava **W** Thoracic Aorta	**0** Open **3** Percutaneous **4** Percutaneous Endoscopic	**4** Drug-eluting Intraluminal Device **D** Intraluminal Device **Z** No Device	**Z** No Qualifier
R Pulmonary Artery, Left	**0** Open **3** Percutaneous **4** Percutaneous Endoscopic	**4** Drug-eluting Intraluminal Device **D** Intraluminal Device **Z** No Device	**T** Ductus Arteriosus **Z** No Qualifier

The rows of this table can be used to construct 213 unique procedure codes. For example, code 02703DZ specifies the procedure for dilation of one coronary artery using an intraluminal device via percutaneous approach (i.e., percutaneous transluminal coronary angioplasty with stent).

Following are the 24 valid combinations of characters 5 through 7 for the Medical and Surgical procedure dilation of the heart and great vessels coronary artery, one site (0270):

0270046	Dilation of Coronary Artery, One Site, Bifurcation, with Drug-eluting Intraluminal Device, Open Approach
027004Z	Dilation of Coronary Artery, One Site with Drug-eluting Intraluminal Device, Open Approach
02700D6	Dilation of Coronary Artery, One Site, Bifurcation, with Intraluminal Device, Open Approach
02700DZ	Dilation of Coronary Artery, One Site with Intraluminal Device, Open Approach
02700T6	Dilation of Coronary Artery, One Site, Bifurcation, with Radioactive Intraluminal Device, Open Approach
02700TZ	Dilation of Coronary Artery, One Site with Radioactive Intraluminal Device, Open Approach
02700Z6	Dilation of Coronary Artery, One Site, Bifurcation, Open Approach
02700ZZ	Dilation of Coronary Artery, One Site, Open Approach
0270346	Dilation of Coronary Artery, One Site, Bifurcation, with Drug-eluting Intraluminal Device, Percutaneous Approach
027034Z	Dilation of Coronary Artery, One Site with Drug-eluting Intraluminal Device, Percutaneous Approach
02703D6	Dilation of Coronary Artery, One Site, Bifurcation, with Intraluminal Device, Percutaneous Approach
02703DZ	Dilation of Coronary Artery, One Site with Intraluminal Device, Percutaneous Approach
02703T6	Dilation of Coronary Artery, One Site, Bifurcation, with Radioactive Intraluminal Device, Percutaneous Approach
02703TZ	Dilation of Coronary Artery, One Site with Radioactive Intraluminal Device, Percutaneous Approach
02703Z6	Dilation of Coronary Artery, One Site, Bifurcation, Percutaneous Approach
02703ZZ	Dilation of Coronary Artery, One Site, Percutaneous Approach
0270446	Dilation of Coronary Artery, One Site, Bifurcation, with Drug-eluting Intraluminal Device, Percutaneous Endoscopic Approach
027044Z	Dilation of Coronary Artery, One Site with Drug-eluting Intraluminal Device, Percutaneous Endoscopic Approach
02704D6	Dilation of Coronary Artery, One Site, Bifurcation, with Intraluminal Device, Percutaneous Endoscopic Approach
02704DZ	Dilation of Coronary Artery, One Site with Intraluminal Device, Percutaneous Endoscopic Approach
02704T6	Dilation of Coronary Artery, One Site, Bifurcation, with Radioactive Intraluminal Device, Percutaneous Endoscopic Approach
02704TZ	Dilation of Coronary Artery, One Site with Radioactive Intraluminal Device, Percutaneous Endoscopic Approach
02704Z6	Dilation of Coronary Artery, One Site, Bifurcation, Percutaneous Endoscopic Approach
02704ZZ	Dilation of Coronary Artery, One Site, Percutaneous Endoscopic Approach

Each table contains only those combinations of values that make up a valid procedure code. In some instances, the tables are split, indicating that there is a restriction in the combination of character choices. In table 027 above, character 7, qualifier 6 Bifurcation can be used only with coronary artery body part characters 0–3. Character 7, qualifier T Ductus Arteriosus can be used only with body part character R Pulmonary Artery, Left.

The lower portion of table 001, shown below, is split into two sections; values of characters must be selected from within the same section (row) of the table.

Ø   **Medical and Surgical**
Ø   **Central Nervous System**
1   **Bypass**   Altering the route of passage of the contents of a tubular body part

Body Part Character 4	Approach Character 5	Device Character 6	Qualifier Character 7
6 Cerebral Ventricle	**Ø** Open	**7** Autologous Tissue Substitute **J** Synthetic Substitute **K** Nonautologous Tissue Substitute	**Ø** Nasopharynx **1** Mastoid Sinus **2** Atrium **3** Blood Vessel **4** Pleural Cavity **5** Intestine **6** Peritoneal Cavity **7** Urinary Tract **8** Bone Marrow **B** Cerebral Cisterns
U Spinal Canal	**Ø** Open	**7** Autologous Tissue Substitute **J** Synthetic Substitute **K** Nonautologous Tissue Substitute	**4** Pleural Cavity **6** Peritoneal Cavity **7** Urinary Tract **9** Fallopian Tube

Body part value *6* may be in combination with device values *7, J,* or *K.* Body part (character 4) value *U* may be used only in combination with qualifier (character 7) values of 4, 6, 7, and 9. In other words, code ØØ1UØ73 is invalid since the qualifier character appears above the line separating the two sections of the table.

Note: In this manual, there are instances in which some tables due to length must be continued on the next page. Each section must be used separately and value selection must be made within the same section (row) of the table.

Character Meanings

In each section each character has a specific meaning. Within a section all character meanings remain constant. The resource section of this manual lists character meanings for each section.

Sections

Procedures are divided into sections that identify the general type of procedure (e.g., Medical and Surgical, Obstetrics, Imaging). The first character of the procedure code always specifies the section.

The sections are listed below:

Ø   Medical and Surgical

1   Obstetrics

2   Placement

3   Administration

4   Measurement and Monitoring

5   Extracorporeal Assistance and Performance

6   Extracorporeal Therapies

7   Osteopathic

8   Other Procedures

9   Chiropractic

B   Imaging

C   Nuclear Medicine

D   Radiation Oncology

F   Physical Rehabilitation and Diagnostic Audiology

G   Mental Health

H   Substance Abuse Treatment

Medical and Surgical Section (Ø)

Character Meaning

The seven characters for Medical and Surgical procedures have the following meaning:

Character	Meaning
1	Section
2	Body System
3	Root Operation
4	Body Part
5	Approach
6	Device
7	Qualifier

The Medical and Surgical section constitutes the vast majority of procedures reported in an inpatient setting. Medical and Surgical procedure codes all have a first-character value of Ø. The second character indicates the general body system (e.g., Mouth and Throat, Gastrointestinal). The third character indicates the root operation, or specific objective, of the procedure (e.g., Excision). The fourth character indicates the specific body part on which the procedure was performed (e.g., Tonsils, Duodenum). The fifth character indicates the approach used to reach the procedure site (e.g., Open). The sixth character indicates whether a device was used in the procedure (e.g., Synthetic Substitute). The seventh character is qualifier, which has a specific meaning for each root operation. For example, the qualifier can be used to identify the destination site of a *Bypass*. The first through fifth characters are always assigned a specific value, but the device (sixth character) and the qualifier (seventh character) are not applicable to all procedures. The value *Z* is used for the sixth and seventh characters to indicate that a specific device or qualifier does not apply to the procedure.

Section (Character 1)

Medical and Surgical procedure codes all have a first-character value of Ø.

Body Systems (Character 2)

Body systems for Medical and Surgical section codes are specified in the second character.

Body Systems

0	Central Nervous System
1	Peripheral Nervous System
2	Heart and Great Vessels
3	Upper Arteries
4	Lower Arteries
5	Upper Veins
6	Lower Veins
7	Lymphatic and Hemic Systems
8	Eye
9	Ear, Nose, Sinus
B	Respiratory System
C	Mouth and Throat
D	Gastrointestinal System
F	Hepatobiliary System and Pancreas
G	Endocrine System
H	Skin and Breast
J	Subcutaneous Tissue and Fascia
K	Muscles
L	Tendons
M	Bursae and Ligaments
N	Head and Facial Bones
P	Upper Bones
Q	Lower Bones
R	Upper Joints
S	Lower Joints
T	Urinary System
U	Female Reproductive System
V	Male Reproductive System
W	Anatomical Regions, General
X	Anatomical Regions, Upper Extremities
Y	Anatomical Regions, Lower Extremities

Root Operations (Character 3)

The root operation is specified in the third character. In the Medical and Surgical section there are 31 different root operations. The root operation identifies the objective of the procedure. Each root operation has a precise definition.

- *Alteration:* Modifying the natural anatomic structure of a body part without affecting the function of the body part

- *Bypass:* Altering the route of passage of the contents of a tubular body part

- *Change:* Taking out or off a device from a body part and putting back an identical or similar device in or on the same body part without cutting or puncturing the skin or a mucous membrane

- *Control:* Stopping, or attempting to stop, postprocedural bleeding

- *Creation:* Making a new genital structure that does not physically take the place of a body part

- *Destruction:* Physical eradication of all or a portion of a body part by the direct use of energy, force, or a destructive agent

- *Detachment:* Cutting off all or a portion of the upper or lower extremities

- *Dilation:* Expanding an orifice or the lumen of a tubular body part

- *Division:* Cutting into a body part without draining fluids and/or gases from the body part in order to separate or transect a body part

- *Drainage:* Taking or letting out fluids and/or gases from a body part

- *Excision:* Cutting out or off, without replacement, a portion of a body part

- *Extirpation:* Taking or cutting out solid matter from a body part

- *Extraction:* Pulling or stripping out or off all or a portion of a body part by the use of force

- *Fragmentation:* Breaking solid matter in a body part into pieces

- *Fusion:* Joining together portions of an articular body part rendering the articular body part immobile

- *Insertion:* Putting in a nonbiological appliance that monitors, assists, performs, or prevents a physiological function but does not physically take the place of a body part

- *Inspection:* Visually and/or manually exploring a body part

- *Map:* Locating the route of passage of electrical impulses and/or locating functional areas in a body part

- *Occlusion:* Completely closing an orifice or lumen of a tubular body part

- *Reattachment:* Putting back in or on all or a portion of a separated body part to its normal location or other suitable location

- *Release:* Freeing a body part from an abnormal physical constraint by cutting or by use of force

- *Removal:* Taking out or off a device from a body part

- *Repair:* Restoring, to the extent possible, a body part to its normal anatomic structure and function

- *Replacement:* Putting in or on biological or synthetic material that physically takes the place and/or function of all or a portion of a body part

- *Reposition:* Moving to its normal location or other suitable location all or a portion of a body part

- *Resection:* Cutting out or off, without replacement, all of a body part

- *Restriction:* Partially closing an orifice or lumen of a tubular body part

- *Revision:* Correcting, to the extent possible, a malfunctioning or displaced device

- *Supplement:* Putting in or on biological or synthetic material that physically reinforces and/or augments the function of a portion of a body part

- *Transfer:* Moving, without taking out, all or a portion of a body part to another location to take over the function of all or a portion of a body part

- *Transplantation:* Putting in or on all or a portion of a living body part taken from another individual or animal to physically take the place and/or function of all or a portion of a similar body part

The above definitions of root operation illustrate the precision of code values defined in the system. There is a clear distinction between each root operation.

A root operation specifies the objective of the procedure. The term *anastomosis* is not a root operation, because it is a means of joining and is always an integral part of another procedure (e.g., Bypass, Resection) with a specific objective. Similarly, *incision* is not a root operation, since it is always part of the objective of another procedure (e.g., Division, Drainage). The root operation *Repair* in the Medical and Surgical section functions as a "not elsewhere classified" option. *Repair* is used when the procedure performed is not one of the other specific root operations.

Appendix A provides additional explanation and representative examples of the Medical and Surgical root operations. Appendix B groups all root operations in the Medical and Surgical section into subcategories and provides an example of each root operation.

Body Part (Character 4)
The body part is specified in the fourth character. The body part indicates the specific part of the body system on which the procedure was performed (e.g., Duodenum). Tubular body parts are defined in ICD-10-PCS as those hollow body parts that provide a route of passage for solids, liquids, or gases. They include the cardiovascular system and body parts such as those contained in the gastrointestinal tract, genitourinary tract, biliary tract, and respiratory tract.

Approach (Character 5)
The technique used to reach the site of the procedure is specified in the fifth character. There are seven different approaches:

- *Open*: Cutting through the skin or mucous membrane and any other body layers necessary to expose the site of the procedure

- *Percutaneous*: Entry, by puncture or minor incision, of instrumentation through the skin or mucous membrane and any other body layers necessary to reach the site of the procedure

- *Percutaneous Endoscopic*: Entry, by puncture or minor incision, of instrumentation through the skin or mucous membrane and any other body layers necessary to reach and visualize the site of the procedure

- *Via Natural or Artificial Opening*: Entry of instrumentation through a natural or artificial external opening to reach the site of the procedure

- *Via Natural or Artificial Opening Endoscopic*: Entry of instrumentation through a natural or artificial external opening to reach and visualize the site of the procedure

- *Via Natural or Artificial Opening with Percutaneous Endoscopic Assistance:* Entry of instrumentation through a natural or artificial external opening and entry, by puncture or minor incision, of instrumentation through the skin or mucous membrane and any other body layers necessary to aid in the performance of the procedure

- *External*: Procedures performed directly on the skin or mucous membrane and procedures performed indirectly by the application of external force through the skin or mucous membrane

The approach comprises three components: the access location, method, and type of instrumentation.

Access location: For procedures performed on an internal body part, the access location specifies the external site through which the site of the procedure is reached. There are two general types of access locations: skin or mucous membranes, and external orifices. Every approach value except external includes one of these two access locations. The skin or mucous membrane can be cut or punctured to reach the procedure site. All open and percutaneous approach values use this access location. The site of a procedure can also be reached through an external opening. External openings can be natural (e.g., mouth) or artificial (e.g., colostomy stoma).

Method: For procedures performed on an internal body part, the method specifies how the external access location is entered. An open method specifies cutting through the skin or mucous membrane and any other intervening body layers necessary to expose the site of the procedure. An instrumentation method specifies the entry of instrumentation through the access location to the internal procedure site. Instrumentation can be introduced by puncture or minor incision, or through an external opening. The puncture or minor incision does not constitute an open approach because it does not expose the site of the procedure. An approach can define multiple methods. For example, *Via Natural or Artificial Opening with Percutaneous Endoscopic Assistance* includes both the initial entry of instrumentation to reach the site of the procedure, and the placement of additional percutaneous instrumentation into the body part to visualize and assist in the performance of the procedure.

Type of instrumentation: For procedures performed on an internal body part, instrumentation means that specialized equipment is used to perform the procedure. Instrumentation is used in all internal approaches other than the basic open approach. Instrumentation may or may not include the capacity to visualize the procedure site. For example, the instrumentation used to perform a sigmoidoscopy permits the internal site of the procedure to be visualized, while the instrumentation used to perform a needle biopsy of the liver does not. The term "endoscopic" as used in approach values refers to instrumentation that permits a site to be visualized.

Procedures performed directly on the skin or mucous membrane are identified by the external approach (e.g., skin excision). Procedures performed indirectly by the application of external force are also identified by the external approach (e.g., closed reduction of fracture).

Appendix E compares the components (access location, method, and type of instrumentation) of each approach and provides an example of each approach.

Device (Character 6)
The device is specified in the sixth character and is used only to specify devices that remain after the procedure is completed. There are four general types of devices:

- Biological or synthetic material that takes the place of all or a portion of a body part (e.g., skin graft and joint prosthesis)

- Biological or synthetic material that assists or prevents a physiological function (e.g., IUD)

- Therapeutic material that is not absorbed by, eliminated by, or incorporated into a body part (e.g., radioactive implant)

- Mechanical or electronic appliances used to assist, monitor, take the place of, or prevent a physiological function (e.g., cardiac pacemaker, orthopaedic pin)

While all devices can be removed, some cannot be removed without putting in another nonbiological appliance or body-part substitute. Specific device values may be coded with the root operations *Alteration, Bypass, Creation, Dilation, Drainage, Fusion, Occlusion, Reposition,* and *Restriction*. Specific device values must be coded with the root operations *Change, Insertion, Removal, Replacement,* and *Revision.* Instruments used to visualize the procedure site are specified in the approach, not the device, value.

If the objective of the procedure is to put in the device, then the root operation is *Insertion.* If the device is put in to meet an objective other than *Insertion,* then the root operation defining the underlying objective of the procedure is used, with the device specified in the device character. For example, if a procedure to replace the hip joint is performed, the root operation *Replacement* is coded, and the prosthetic device is specified in the device character. Materials that are incidental to a procedure such as clips, ligatures, and sutures are not specified in the device character. Because new devices can be developed, the value *Other Device* is provided as a temporary option for use until a specific device value is added to the system.

Qualifier (Character 7)

The qualifier is specified in the seventh character. The qualifier contains unique values for individual procedures. For example, the qualifier can be used to identify the destination site in a *Bypass.*

Medical and Surgical Section Principles

In developing the Medical and Surgical procedure codes, several specific principles were followed.

Composite Terms Are Not Root Operations

Composite terms such as colonoscopy, sigmoidectomy, or appendectomy do not describe root operations, but they do specify multiple components of a specific root operation. In ICD-10-PCS, the components of a procedure are defined separately by the characters making up the complete code. And the only component of a procedure specified in the root operation is the objective of the procedure. With each complete code the underlying objective of the procedure is specified by the root operation (third character), the precise part is specified by the body part (fourth character), and the method used to reach and visualize the procedure site is specified by the approach (fifth character). While colonoscopy, sigmoidectomy, and appendectomy are included in the Index, they do not constitute root operations in the Tables section. The objective of colonoscopy is the visualization of the colon and the root operation (character 3) is *Inspection.* Character 4 specifies the body part, which in this case is part of the colon. These composite terms, like colonoscopy or appendectomy, are included as cross-reference only. The index provides the correct root operation reference. Examples of other types of composite terms not representative of root operations are *partial* sigmoidectomy, *total* hysterectomy, and *partial* hip replacement. Always refer to the correct root operation in the Index and Tables section.

Root Operation Based on Objective of Procedure

The root operation is based on the objective of the procedure, such as *Resection* of transverse colon or *Dilation* of an artery. The assignment of the root operation is based on the procedure actually performed, which may or may not have been the intended procedure. If the intended procedure is modified or discontinued (e.g., excision instead of resection is performed), the root operation is determined by the procedure actually performed. If the desired result is not attained after completing the procedure (i.e., the artery does not remain expanded after the dilation procedure), the root operation is still determined by the procedure actually performed.

Examples:

- Dilating the urethra is coded as *Dilation* since the objective of the procedure is to dilate the urethra. If dilation of the urethra includes putting in an intraluminal stent, the root operation remains

Dilation and not *Insertion* of the intraluminal device because the underlying objective of the procedure is dilation of the urethra. The stent is identified by the intraluminal device value in the sixth character of the dilation procedure code.

- If the objective is solely to put a radioactive element in the urethra, then the procedure is coded to the root operation *Insertion,* with the radioactive element identified in the sixth character of the code.

- If the objective of the procedure is to correct a malfunctioning or displaced device, then the procedure is coded to the root operation *Revision.* In the root operation *Revision,* the original device being revised is identified in the device character. *Revision* is typically performed on mechanical appliances (e.g., pacemaker) or materials used in replacement procedures (e.g., synthetic substitute). Typical revision procedures include adjustment of pacemaker position and correction of malfunctioning knee prosthesis.

Combination Procedures Are Coded Separately

If multiple procedures as defined by distinct objectives are performed during an operative episode, then multiple codes are used. For example, obtaining the vein graft used for coronary bypass surgery is coded as a separate procedure from the bypass itself.

Redo of Procedures

The complete or partial redo of the original procedure is coded to the root operation that identifies the procedure performed rather than *Revision.*

Example:

A complete redo of a hip replacement procedure that requires putting in a new prosthesis is coded to the root operation *Replacement* rather than *Revision.*

The correction of complications arising from the original procedure, other than device complications, is coded to the procedure performed. Correction of a malfunctioning or displaced device would be coded to the root operation *Revision.*

Example:

A procedure to control hemorrhage arising from the original procedure is coded to *Control* rather than *Revision.*

Examples of Procedures Coded in the Medical Surgical Section

The following are examples of procedures from the Medical and Surgical section, coded in ICD-10-PCS.

- Suture of skin laceration, left lower arm: ØHQEXZZ

  Medical and Surgical section (Ø), body system *Skin and Breast* (H), root operation *Repair* (Q), body part *Skin, Left Lower Arm* (E), *External* Approach (X) *No device* (Z), and *No qualifier* (Z).

- Laparoscopic appendectomy: ØDTJ4ZZ

  Medical and surgical section (Ø), body system *Gastrointestinal* (D), root operation *Resection* (T), body part *Appendix* (J), *Percutaneous Endoscopic* approach (4), No *Device* (Z), and No qualifier (Z).

- Sigmoidoscopy with biopsy: ØDBN8ZX

  Medical and Surgical section (Ø), body system *Gastrointestinal* (D), root operation *Excision* (B), body part *Sigmoid Colon* (N), *Via Natural or Artificial Opening Endoscopic* approach (8), *No Device* (Z), and with qualifier *Diagnostic* (X).

- Tracheostomy with tracheostomy tube: ØB11ØF4

  Medical and Surgical section (Ø), body system *Respiratory* (B), root operation *Bypass* (1), body part *Trachea* (1), *Open* approach (Ø), with *Tracheostomy Device* (F), and qualifier *Cutaneous* (4).

Obstetrics Section

Character Meanings
The seven characters in the Obstetrics section have the same meaning as in the Medical and Surgical section.

Character	Meaning
1	Section
2	Body System
3	Root Operation
4	Body Part
5	Approach
6	Device
7	Qualifier

The Obstetrics section includes procedures performed on the products of conception only. Procedures on the pregnant female are coded in the Medical and Surgical section (e.g., episiotomy). The term "products of conception" refers to all physical components of a pregnancy, including the fetus, amnion, umbilical cord, and placenta. There is no differentiation of the products of conception based on gestational age. Thus, the specification of the products of conception as a zygote, embryo or fetus, or the trimester of the pregnancy is not part of the procedure code but can be found in the diagnosis code.

Section (Character 1)
Obstetrics procedure codes have a first-character value of *1*.

Body System (Character 2)
The second-character value for body system is *Pregnancy*.

Root Operation (Character 3)
The root operations *Change, Drainage, Extraction, Insertion, Inspection, Removal, Repair, Reposition, Resection,* and *Transplantation* are used in the obstetrics section and have the same meaning as in the Medical and Surgical section.

The Obstetrics section also includes two additional root operations, *Abortion* and *Delivery*, defined below:

- *Abortion*: Artificially terminating a pregnancy
- *Delivery*: Assisting the passage of the products of conception from the genital canal

A cesarean section is not a separate root operation because the underlying objective is *Extraction* (i.e., pulling out all or a portion of a body part).

Body Part (Character 4)
The body-part values in the obstetrics section are:

- *Products of conception*
- *Products of conception, retained*
- *Products of conception, ectopic*

Approach (Character 5)
The fifth character specifies approaches and is defined as are those in the Medical and Surgical section. In the case of an abortion procedure that uses a laminaria or an abortifacient, the approach is *Via Natural or Artificial Opening*.

Device (Character 6)
The sixth character is used for devices such as fetal monitoring electrodes.

Qualifier (Character 7)
Qualifier values are specific to the root operation and are used to specify the type of extraction (e.g., low forceps, high forceps, etc.), the type of cesarean section (e.g., classical, low cervical, etc.), or the type of fluid taken out during a drainage procedure (e.g., amniotic fluid, fetal blood, etc.).

Placement Section

Character Meanings
The seven characters in the Placement section have the following meaning:

Character	Meaning
1	Section
2	Anatomical Region
3	Root Operation
4	Body Region/Orifice
5	Approach
6	Device
7	Qualifier

Placement section codes represent procedures for putting a device in or on a body region for the purpose of protection, immobilization, stretching, compression, or packing.

Section (Character 1)
Placement procedure codes have a first-character value of *2*.

Body System (Character 2)
The second character contains two values specifying either *Anatomical Regions* or *Anatomical Orifices*.

Root Operation (Character 3)
The root operations in the Placement section include only those procedures that are performed without making an incision or a puncture. The root operations *Change* and *Removal* are in the Placement section and have the same meaning as in the Medical and Surgical section.

The Placement section also includes five additional root operations, defined as follows:

- *Compression*: Putting pressure on a body region
- *Dressing*: Putting material on a body region for protection
- *Immobilization*: Limiting or preventing motion of an external body region

- *Packing*: Putting material in a body region or orifice
- *Traction*: Exerting a pulling force on a body region in a distal direction

Body Region (Character 4)

The fourth-character values are either body regions (e.g., *Upper Leg*) or natural orifices (e.g., *Ear*).

Approach (Character 5)

Since all placement procedures are performed directly on the skin or mucous membrane, or performed indirectly by applying external force through the skin or mucous membrane, the approach value is always *External*.

Device (Character 6)

The device character is always specified (except in the case of manual traction) and indicates the device placed during the procedure (e.g., cast, splint, bandage, etc.). Except for casts for fractures and dislocations, devices in the Placement section are off the shelf and do not require any extensive design, fabrication, or fitting. Placement of devices that require extensive design, fabrication, or fitting are coded in the Rehabilitation section.

Qualifier (Character 7)

The qualifier character is not specified in the Placement section; the qualifier value is always *No Qualifier*.

Administration Section

Character Meanings

The seven characters in the Administration section have the following meaning:

Character	Meaning
1	Section
2	Physiological System and Anatomical Region
3	Root Operation
4	Body System/Region
5	Approach
6	Substance
7	Qualifier

Administration section codes represent procedures for putting in or on a therapeutic, prophylactic, protective, diagnostic, nutritional, or physiological substance. The section includes transfusions, infusions, and injections, along with other similar services such as irrigation and tattooing.

Section (Character 1)

Administration procedure codes have a first-character value of *3*.

Body System (Character 2)

The body-system character contains only three values: *Indwelling Device, Physiological Systems and Anatomical Regions,* or *Circulatory System*. The *Circulatory System* is used for transfusion procedures.

Root Operation (Character 3)

There are three root operations in the Administration section.

- *Introduction*: Putting in or on a therapeutic, diagnostic, nutritional, physiological, or prophylactic substance except blood or blood products
- *Irrigation*: Putting in or on a cleansing substance
- *Transfusion*: Putting in blood or blood products

Body/System Region (Character 4)

The fourth character specifies the body system/region. The fourth character identifies the site where the substance is administered, not the site where the substance administered takes effect. Sites include *Skin and Mucous Membrane, Subcutaneous Tissue* and *Muscle*. These differentiate intradermal, subcutaneous, and intramuscular injections, respectively. Other sites include *Eye, Respiratory Tract, Peritoneal Cavity,* and *Epidural Space*.

The body systems/regions for arteries and veins are *Peripheral Artery, Central Artery, Peripheral Vein,* and *Central Vein*. The *Peripheral Artery* or *Vein* is typically used when a substance is introduced locally into an artery or vein. For example, chemotherapy is the introduction of an antineoplastic substance into a peripheral artery or vein by a percutaneous approach. In general, the substance introduced into a peripheral artery or vein has a systemic effect.

The *Central Artery* or *Vein* is typically used when the site where the substance is introduced is distant from the point of entry into the artery or vein. For example, the introduction of a substance directly at the site of a clot within an artery or vein using a catheter is coded as an introduction of a thrombolytic substance into a central artery or vein by a percutaneous approach. In general, the substance introduced into a central artery or vein has a local effect.

Approach (Character 5)

The fifth character specifies approaches as defined in the Medical and Surgical section. The approach for intradermal, subcutaneous, and intramuscular introductions (i.e., injections) is *Percutaneous*. If a catheter is placed to introduce a substance into an internal site within the circulatory system, then the approach is also *Percutaneous*. For example, if a catheter is used to introduce contrast directly into the heart for angiography, then the procedure would be coded as a percutaneous introduction of contrast into the heart.

Substance (Character 6)

The sixth character specifies the substance being introduced. Broad categories of substances are defined, such as anesthetic, contrast, dialysate, and blood products such as platelets.

Qualifier (Character 7)

The seventh character is a qualifier and is used to indicate whether the substance is *Autologous* or *Nonautologous*, or to further specify the substance.

Measurement and Monitoring Section

Character Meanings

The seven characters in the Measurement and Monitoring section have the following meaning:

Character	Meaning
1	Section
2	Physiological System
3	Root Operation
4	Body System
5	Approach
6	Function/Device
7	Qualifier

Measurement and Monitoring section codes represent procedures for determining the level of a physiological or physical function.

Section (Character 1)

Measurement and Monitoring procedure codes have a first-character value of *4*.

Body System (Character 2)

The second-character values for body system are A, *Physiological Systems* or B, *Physiological Devices*.

Root Operation (Character 3)

There are two root operations in the Measurement and Monitoring section, as defined below:

- *Measurement*: Determining the level of a physiological or physical function at a point in time

- *Monitoring*: Determining the level of a physiological or physical function repetitively over a period of time

Body System (Character 4)

The fourth character specifies the specific body system measured or monitored.

Approach (Character 5)

The fifth character specifies approaches as defined in the Medical and Surgical section.

Function/Device (Character 6)

The sixth character specifies the physiological or physical function being measured or monitored. Examples of physiological or physical functions are *Conductivity, Metabolism, Pulse, Temperature,* and *Volume*. If a device used to perform the measurement or monitoring is inserted and left in, then insertion of the device is coded as a separate Medical and Surgical procedure.

Qualifier (Character 7)

The seventh-character qualifier contains specific values as needed to further specify the body part (e.g., central, portal, pulmonary) or a variation of the procedure performed (e.g., ambulatory, stress). Examples of typical procedures coded in this section are EKG, EEG, and cardiac catheterization. An EKG is the measurement of cardiac electrical activity, while an EEG is the measurement of electrical activity of the central nervous system. A cardiac catheterization performed to measure the pressure in the heart is coded as the measurement of cardiac pressure by percutaneous approach.

Extracorporeal Assistance and Performance Section

Character Meanings

The seven characters in the Extracorporeal Assistance and Performance section have the following meaning:

Character	Meaning
1	Section
2	Physiological System
3	Root Operation
4	Body System
5	Duration
6	Function
7	Qualifier

In Extracorporeal Assistance and Performance procedures, equipment outside the body is used to assist or perform a physiological function. The section includes procedures performed in a critical care setting, such as mechanical ventilation and cardioversion; it also includes other services such as hyperbaric oxygen treatment and hemodialysis.

Section (Character 1)

Extracorporeal Assistance and Performance procedure codes have a first-character value of *5*.

Body System (Character 2)

The second-character value for body system is A, *Physiological Systems*.

Root Operation (Character 3)

There are three root operations in the Extracorporeal Assistance and Performance section, as defined below.

- *Assistance*: Taking over a portion of a physiological function by extracorporeal means

- *Performance*: Completely taking over a physiological function by extracorporeal means

- *Restoration*: Returning, or attempting to return, a physiological function to its natural state by extracorporeal means

The root operation *Restoration* contains a single procedure code that identifies extracorporeal cardioversion.

Body System (Character 4)

The fourth character specifies the body system (e.g., cardiac, respiratory) to which extracorporeal assistance or performance is applied.

Duration (Character 5)

The fifth character specifies the duration of the procedure—*Single, Intermittent*, or *Continuous*. For respiratory ventilation assistance or performance, the duration is specified in hours— *< 24 Consecutive Hours, 24–96 Consecutive Hours*, or *> 96 Consecutive Hours*. Value 6, *Multiple* identifies serial procedure treatment.

Function (Character 6)

The sixth character specifies the physiological function assisted or performed (e.g., oxygenation, ventilation) during the procedure.

Qualifier (Character 7)
The seventh-character qualifier specifies the type of equipment used, if any.

Extracorporeal Therapies Section

Character Meanings
The seven characters in the Extracorporeal Therapies section have the following meaning:

Character	Meaning
1	Section
2	Physiological Systems
3	Root Operation
4	Body System
5	Duration
6	Qualifier
7	Qualifier

In extracorporeal therapy, equipment outside the body is used for a therapeutic purpose that does not involve the assistance or performance of a physiological function.

Section (Character 1)
Extracorporeal Therapy procedure codes have a first-character value of 6.

Body System (Character 2)
The second-character value for body system is *Physiological Systems*.

Root Operation (Character 3)
There are 10 root operations in the Extracorporeal Therapy section, as defined below.

- *Atmospheric Control*: Extracorporeal control of atmospheric pressure and composition
- *Decompression*: Extracorporeal elimination of undissolved gas from body fluids

  Coding note: The root operation *Decompression* involves only one type of procedure: treatment for decompression sickness (the bends) in a hyperbaric chamber.
- *Electromagnetic Therapy*: Extracorporeal treatment by electromagnetic rays
- *Hyperthermia*: Extracorporeal raising of body temperature

  Coding note: The term hyperthermia is used to describe both a temperature imbalance treatment and also as an adjunct radiation treatment for cancer. When treating the temperature imbalance, it is coded to this section; for the cancer treatment, it is coded in section *D Radiation Oncology*.
- *Hypothermia*: Extracorporeal lowering of body temperature
- *Pheresis*: Extracorporeal separation of blood products

  Coding note: Pheresis may be used for two main purposes: to treat diseases when too much of a blood component is produced (e.g., leukemia) and to remove a blood product such as platelets from a donor, for transfusion into another patient.
- *Phototherapy*: Extracorporeal treatment by light rays

  Coding note: Phototherapy involves using a machine that exposes the blood to light rays outside the body, recirculates it, and then returns it to the body.
- *Shock Wave Therapy*: Extracorporeal treatment by shock waves
- *Ultrasound Therapy*: Extracorporeal treatment by ultrasound
- *Ultraviolet Light Therapy*: Extracorporeal treatment by ultraviolet light

Body System (Character 4)
The fourth character specifies the body system on which the extracorporeal therapy is performed (e.g., skin, circulatory).

Duration (Character 5)
The fifth character specifies the duration of the procedure (e.g., single or intermittent).

Qualifier (Character 6)
The sixth character is not specified for Extracorporeal Therapies and always has the value *No Qualifier*.

Qualifier (Character 7)
The seventh-character qualifier is used in the root operation *Pheresis* to specify the blood component on which pheresis is performed and in the root operation *Ultrasound Therapy* to specify site of treatment.

Osteopathic Section

Character Meanings
The seven characters in the Osteopathic section have the following meaning:

Character	Meaning
1	Section
2	Anatomical Region
3	Root Operation
4	Body Region
5	Approach
6	Method
7	Qualifier

Section (Character 1)
Osteopathic procedure codes have a first-character value of *7*.

Body System (Character 2)
The body-system character contains the value *Anatomical Regions*.

Root Operation (Character 3)
There is only one root operation in the Osteopathic section.

- *Treatment*: Manual treatment to eliminate or alleviate somatic dysfunction and related disorders

Body Region (Character 4)
The fourth character specifies the body region on which the osteopathic treatment is performed.

Approach (Character 5)
The approach for osteopathic treatment is always *External*.

Method (Character 6)

The sixth character specifies the method by which the treatment is accomplished.

Qualifier (Character 7)

The seventh character is not specified in the Osteopathic section and always has the value *None*.

Other Procedures Section

Character Meanings

The seven characters in the Other Procedures section have the following meaning:

Character	Meaning
1	Section
2	Body System
3	Root Operation
4	Body Region
5	Approach
6	Method
7	Qualifier

The Other Procedures section includes acupuncture, suture removal, and in vitro fertilization.

Section (Character 1)

Other Procedure section codes have a first-character value of *8*.

Body System (Character 2)

The second-character value for body system is *Physiological Systems and Anatomical Regions*.

Root Operation (Character 3)

The Other Procedures section has only one root operation, defined as follows:

- *Other Procedures*: Methodologies that attempt to remediate or cure a disorder or disease.

Body Region (Character 4)

The fourth character contains specified body-region values, and also the body-region value *None* for Extracorporeal Procedures.

Approach (Character 5)

The fifth character specifies approaches as defined in the Medical and Surgical section.

Method (Character 6)

The sixth character specifies the method (e.g., *Acupuncture, Therapeutic Massage*).

Qualifier (Character 7)

The seventh character is a qualifier and contains specific values as needed.

Chiropractic Section

Character Meanings

The seven characters in the Chiropractic section have the following meaning:

Character	Meaning
1	Section
2	Anatomical Regions
3	Root Operation
4	Body Region
5	Approach
6	Method
7	Qualifier

Section (Character 1)

Chiropractic section procedure codes have a first-character value of *9*.

Body System (Character 2)

The second-character value for body system is *Anatomical Regions*.

Root Operation (Character 3)

There is only one root operation in the *Chiropractic* section.

- *Manipulation:* Manual procedure that involves a directed thrust to move a joint past the physiological range of motion, without exceeding the anatomical limit.

Body Region (Character 4)

The fourth character specifies the body region on which the chiropractic manipulation is performed.

Approach (Character 5)

The approach for chiropractic manipulation is always *External*.

Method (Character 6)

The sixth character is the method by which the manipulation is accomplished.

Qualifier (Character 7)

The seventh character is not specified in the Chiropractic section and always has the value *None*.

Imaging Section

Character Meanings

The seven characters in Imaging procedures have the following meaning:

Character	Meaning
1	Section
2	Body System
3	Root Type
4	Body Part
5	Contrast
6	Qualifier
7	Qualifier

Imaging procedures include plain radiography, fluoroscopy, CT, MRI, and ultrasound. Nuclear medicine procedures, including PET, uptakes, and scans, are in the nuclear medicine section. Therapeutic radiation procedure codes are in a separate radiation oncology section.

Section (Character 1)
Imaging procedure codes have a first-character value of *B*.

Body System (Character 2)
In the Imaging section, the second character defines the body system, such as *Heart* or *Gastrointestinal System*.

Root Type (Character 3)
The third character defines the type of imaging procedure (e.g., MRI, ultrasound). The following list includes all types in the *Imaging* section with a definition of each type:

- *Computerized Tomography (CT Scan)* : Computer-reformatted digital display of multiplanar images developed from the capture of multiple exposures of external ionizing radiation

- *Fluoroscopy*: Single plane or bi-plane real-time display of an image developed from the capture of external ionizing radiation on fluorescent screen. The image may also be stored by either digital or analog means

- *Magnetic Resonance Imaging (MRI)* : Computer reformatted digital display of multiplanar images developed from the capture of radiofrequency signals emitted by nuclei in a body site excited within a magnetic field

- *Plain Radiography*: Planar display of an image developed from the capture of external ionizing radiation on photographic or photoconductive plate

- *Ultrasonography*: Real-time display of images of anatomy or flow information developed from the capture of reflected and attenuated high-frequency sound waves

Body Part(Character 4)
The fourth character defines the body part with different values for each body system (character 2) value.

Contrast (Character 5)
The fifth character specifies whether the contrast material used in the imaging procedure is *High* or *Low Osmolar*, when applicable.

Qualifier (Character 6)
The sixth character qualifier provides further detail as needed, such as *Unenhanced and Enhanced*.

Qualifier (Character 7)
The seventh character is a qualifier and specifies whether the procedure was performed intraoperatively or using densitometry.

Nuclear Medicine Section

Character Meanings
The seven characters in the Nuclear Medicine section have the following meaning:

Character	Meaning
1	Section
2	Body System
3	Root Type
4	Body Part
5	Radionuclide
6	Qualifier
7	Qualifier

Nuclear Medicine is the introduction of radioactive material into the body to create an image, to diagnose and treat pathologic conditions, or to assess metabolic functions. The Nuclear Medicine section does not include the introduction of encapsulated radioactive material for the treatment of cancer. These procedures are included in the Radiation Oncology section.

Section (Character 1)
Nuclear Medicine procedure codes have a first-character value of *C*.

Body System (Character 2)
The second character specifies the body system on which the nuclear medicine procedure is performed.

Root Type (Character 3)
The third character indicates the type of nuclear medicine procedure (e.g., planar imaging or nonimaging uptake). The following list includes the types of nuclear medicine procedures with a definition of each type.

- *Nonimaging Uptake:* Introduction of radioactive materials into the body for measurements of organ function, from the detection of radioactive emissions

- *Nonimaging Probe:* Introduction of radioactive materials into the body for the study of distribution and fate of certain substances by the detection of radioactive emissions; or alternatively, measurement of absorption of radioactive emissions from an external source

- *Nonimaging Assay:* Introduction of radioactive materials into the body for the study of body fluids and blood elements, by the detection of radioactive emissions

- *Planar Imaging:* Introduction of radioactive materials into the body for single-plane display of images developed from the capture of radioactive emissions

- *Positron Emission Tomography (PET):* Introduction of radioactive materials into the body for three-dimensional display of images developed from the simultaneous capture, 180 degrees apart, of radioactive emissions

- *Systemic Therapy:* Introduction of unsealed radioactive materials into the body for treatment

- *Tomographic (Tomo) Imaging:* Introduction of radioactive materials into the body for three dimensional display of images developed from the capture of radioactive emissions

Body Part (Character 4)

The fourth character indicates the body part or body region studied. *Regional* (e.g., lower extremity veins) and *Combination* (e.g., liver and spleen) body parts are commonly used in this section.

Radionuclide (Character 5)

The fifth character specifies the radionuclide, the radiation source. The option *Other Radionuclide* is provided in the nuclear medicine section for newly approved radionuclides until they can be added to the coding system. If more than one radiopharmaceutical is given to perform the procedure, then more than one code is used.

Qualifier (Character 6 and 7)

The sixth and seventh characters are qualifiers but are not specified in the *Nuclear Medicine* section; the value is always *None*.

Radiation Oncology Section

Character Meanings

The seven characters in the Radiation Oncology section have the following meaning:

Character	Meaning
1	Section
2	Body System
3	Root Type
4	Treatment Site
5	Modality Qualifier
6	Isotope
7	Qualifier

Section (Character 1)

Radiation oncology procedure codes have a first-character value of *D*.

Body System (Character 2)

The second character specifies the body system (e.g., central nervous system, musculoskeletal) irradiated.

Root Type (Character 3)

The third character specifies the general modality used (e.g., beam radiation).

Treatment Site (Character 4)

The fourth character specifies the body part that is the focus of the radiation therapy.

Modality Qualifier (Character 5)

The fifth character further specifies the radiation modality used (e.g., photons, electrons).

Isotope (Character 6)

The sixth character specifies the isotopes introduced into the body, if applicable.

Qualifier (Character 7)

The seventh character may specify whether the procedure was performed intraoperatively.

Physical Rehabilitation and Diagnostic Audiology Section

Character Meanings

The seven characters in the Physical Rehabilitation and Diagnostic Audiology section have the following meaning:

Character	Meaning
1	Section
2	Section Qualifier
3	Root Type
4	Body System & Region
5	Type Qualifier
6	Equipment
7	Qualifier

Physical rehabilitation procedures include physical therapy, occupational therapy, and speech-language pathology. Osteopathic procedures and chiropractic procedures are in separate sections.

Section (Character 1)

Physical Rehabilitation and Diagnostic Audiology procedure codes have a first-character value of *F*.

Section Qualifier (Character 2)

The section qualifier *Rehabilitation* or *Diagnostic Audiology* is specified in the second character.

Root Type (Character 3)

The third character specifies the root type. There are 14 different root type values, which can be classified into four basic types of rehabilitation and diagnostic audiology procedures, defined as follows:

- *Assessment*: Includes a determination of the patient's diagnosis when appropriate, need for treatment, planning for treatment, periodic assessment, and documentation related to these activities

- *Caregiver Training*: Educating caregiver with the skills and knowledge used to interact with and assist the patient

- *Fitting(s)*: Design, fabrication, modification, selection, and/or application of splint, orthosis, prosthesis, hearing aids, and/or other rehabilitation device

- *Treatment*: Use of specific activities or methods to develop, improve, and/or restore the performance of necessary functions, compensate for dysfunction and/or minimize debilitation

The type of treatment includes training as well as activities that restore function.

Body System & Region (Character 4)

The fourth character specifies the body region and/or system on which the procedure is performed.

Type Qualifier (Character 5)

The fifth character is a type qualifier that further specifies the procedure performed. Examples include therapy to improve the range of motion and training for bathing techniques. Refer to appendix D for definitions of these types of procedures.

Equipment (Character 6)

The sixth character specifies the equipment used. Specific equipment is not defined in the equipment value. Instead, broad categories of equipment are specified (e.g., aerobic endurance and conditioning, assistive/adaptive/supportive, etc.)

Qualifier (Character 7)

The seventh character is not specified in the Physical Rehabilitation and Diagnostic Audiology section and always has the value *None*.

Mental Health Section

Character Meanings

The seven characters in the Mental Health section have the following meaning:

Character	Meaning
1	Section
2	Body System
3	Root Type
4	Type Qualifier
5	Qualifier
6	Qualifier
7	Qualifier

Section (Character 1)

Mental health procedure codes have a first-character value of *G*.

Body System (Character 2)

The second character is used to identify the body system elsewhere in ICD-10-PCS. In this section it always has the value *None*.

Root Type (Character 3)

The third character specifies the procedure type, such as crisis intervention or counseling. There are 12 types of mental health procedures, some of which are defined below.

Psychological Tests:

- Developmental: Age-normed developmental status of cognitive, social, and adaptive behavior skills

- Intellectual and Psychoeducational: Intellectual abilities, academic achievement, and learning capabilities (including behavior and emotional factors affecting learning)

- Neurobehavioral and Cognitive Status: Includes neurobehavioral status exam, interview(s), and observation for the clinical assessment of thinking, reasoning, and judgment, acquired knowledge, attention, memory, visual spatial abilities, language functions, and planning

- Neuropsychological: Thinking, reasoning and judgment, acquired knowledge, attention, memory, visual spatial abilities, language functions, planning

- Personality and Behavioral: Mood, emotion, behavior, social functioning, psychopathological conditions, personality traits, and characteristics

Crisis intervention: Includes defusing, debriefing, counseling, psychotherapy, and/or coordination of care with other providers or agencies

Individual Psychotherapy:

- Behavior: Primarily to modify behavior. Includes modeling and role playing, positive reinforcement of target behaviors, response cost, and training of self-management skills

- Cognitive/behavioral: Combining cognitive and behavioral treatment strategies to improve functioning. Maladaptive responses are examined to determine how cognitions relate to behavior patterns in response to an event. Uses learning principles and information-processing models

- Cognitive: Primarily to correct cognitive distortions and errors

- Interactive: Uses primarily physical aids and other forms of nonoral interaction with a patient who is physically, psychologically, or developmentally unable to use ordinary language for communication (e.g., the use of toys in symbolic play)

- Interpersonal: Helps an individual make changes in interpersonal behaviors to reduce psychological dysfunction. Includes exploratory techniques, encouragement of affective expression, clarification of patient statements, analysis of communication patterns, use of therapy relationship, and behavior change techniques.

- Psychoanalysis: Methods of obtaining a detailed account of past and present mental and emotional experiences to determine the source and eliminate or diminish the undesirable effects of unconscious conflicts by making the individual aware of their existence, origin, and inappropriate expression in emotions and behavior.

- Psychodynamic: Exploration of past and present emotional experiences to understand motives and drives using insight-oriented techniques (e.g., empathetic listening, clarifying self-defeating behavior patterns, and exploring adaptive alternatives) to reduce the undesirable effects of internal conflicts on emotions and behavior

- Psychophysiological: Monitoring and alternation of physiological processes to help the individual associate physiological reactions combined with cognitive and behavioral strategies to gain improved control of these processes to help the individual cope more effectively

- Supportive: Formation of therapeutic relationship primarily for providing emotional support to prevent further deterioration in functioning during periods of particular stress. Often used in conjunction with other therapeutic approaches

Counseling:

- Vocational: Exploration of vocational interest, aptitudes, and required adaptive behavior skills to develop and carry out a plan for achieving a successful vocational placement, enhancing work-related adjustment, and/or pursuing viable options in training education or preparation

Family Psychotherapy:

- Remediation of emotional or behavioral problems presented by one or more family members when psychotherapy with more than one family member is indicated

Electroconvulsive Therapy: Includes appropriate sedation and other preparation of the individual

Biofeedback: Includes electroencephalogram (EEG), blood pressure, skin temperature or peripheral blood flow, electrocardiogram (ECG), electrooculogram, electromyogram (EMG), respirometry or capnometry, galvanic skin response (GSR) or electrodermal response (EDR), perineometry to monitor and regulate bowel or bladder activity, and electrogastrogram to monitor and regulate gastric motility

Other Mental Health procedures include *Hypnosis, Narcosynthesis, Group Psychotherapy, Light Therapy* and *Medication Management.* There are no ICD-10-PCS definitions of these procedures at this time.

Type Qualifier (Character 4)
The fourth character is a type qualifier (e.g., to indicate that counseling was educational or vocational).

Qualifier (Character 5, 6 and 7)
The fifth, sixth, and seventh characters are not specified and always have the value *None*.

Substance Abuse Treatment Section

Character Meanings
The seven characters in the Substance Abuse Treatment section have the following meaning:

Character	Meaning
1	Section
2	Body System
3	Root Type
4	Type Qualifier
5	Qualifier
6	Qualifier
7	Qualifier

Section (Character 1)
Substance Abuse Treatment codes have a first-character value of *H*.

Body System (Character 2)
The second character is used to identify the body system elsewhere in ICD-10-PCS. In this section, it always has the value *None*.

Root Type (Character 3)
The third character specifies the procedure. There are seven root type values classified in this section, as listed below:

- *Detoxification Services:* Not a treatment modality but helps the patient stabilize physically and psychologically until the body becomes free of drugs and the effects of alcohol

- *Individual Counseling:* Comprising several techniques, which apply various strategies to address drug addiction

- *Group Counseling:* Provides structured group counseling sessions and healing power through the connection with others

- *Family Counseling:* Provides support and education for family members of addicted individuals. Family member participation seen as critical to substance abuse treatment

- Other root type values in this section include *Individual Psychotherapy, Medication Management,* and *Pharmacotherapy*; there are no ICD-10-PCS definitions of these procedures at this time.

Type Qualifier (Character 4)
The fourth character further specifies the procedure type. Type Qualifier values vary dependent upon the Root Type procedure (Character 3). Root type 2, *Detoxification Services* contains only the value Z, *None* and Root type 6, *Family Counseling* contains only the value 3, *Other Family Counseling* , whereas the remainder Root Type procedures include nine to twelve total possible values.

Qualifier (Character 5, 6 and 7)
The fifth through seventh characters are designated as qualifiers but are never specified, so they always have the value *None*.

Comparison of ICD-10-PCS and ICD-9-CM
In 1993, the National Committee on Vital and Health Statistics (NCVHS) issued a report specifying recommendations for a new procedure classification system. NCVHS identified the essential characteristics that a procedure classification system should possess. Those characteristics include hierarchical structure, expandability, comprehensive, nonoverlapping, ease of use, setting and provider neutrality, multi-axial structure, and limited to classification of procedures.

ICD-10-PCS meets virtually all NCVHS characteristics, while ICD-9-CM fails to meet many NCVHS characteristics. In addition to the NCVHS characteristics, there are several other attributes of a procedure coding system that should be taken into consideration when comparing systems.

Completeness and Accuracy of Codes
The procedures coded in ICD-10-PCS provided a much more complete and accurate description of the procedure performed. The specification of the procedures performed not only affects payment, but is integral to internal management systems, external performance comparisons, and the assessment of quality of care. The detail and completeness of ICD-10-PCS is essential in today's health care environment.

General Equivalence Mappings
Due to the complexities of ICD-10-PCS and the drastic structural differences between the two coding systems, a direct code crosswalk is not possible. However, a general "mapping" of similar code choices has been developed. This network of relationships between the two code sets may be referred to as general equivalence mappings (GEMs). The purpose of these mappings, from ICD-9-CM to ICD-10-PCS, and vice versa, is to attempt to find corresponding procedure codes in lieu of a direct translation. For example:

- The ICD-9-CM to ICD-10-PCS GEM may help with analyzing or comparing data coded using the ICD-9-CM system to facilitate "forward mapping" to ICD-10-PCS.

- The ICD-10-PCS to ICD-9-CM GEM may help in comparing coded data using the ICD-10-PCS system to facilitate "backward mapping" to ICD-9-CM.

The 2011 ICD-10-PCS update includes data mapping files which are posted on the CMS website at the URL below: http://www.cms.gov/ICD10/llb_2011_ICD10PCS.asp#TopOfPage.

Communications with Physicians
ICD-9-CM procedure codes often poorly describe the precise procedure performed. Physicians or others reviewing or analyzing data coded in ICD-9-CM may have difficulty developing clinical pathways, evaluating the coding for possible fraud and abuse, or conducting research. The

ICD-1Ø-PCS codes provide more clinically relevant procedure descriptions that can be more readily understood and used by physicians.

Independent evaluation of ICD-1Ø-PCS demonstrated that there is a learning curve associated with ICD-1Ø-PCS. Because of the additional specificity in ICD-1Ø-PCS, it probably takes longer to attain a minimum level of coding proficiency for ICD-1Ø-PCS than for ICD-9-CM. However, it should take less time to become *highly* proficient with ICD-1Ø-PCS than with ICD-9-CM. ICD-9-CM lacks clear definitions, and many substantially different procedures are coded with the same code. Therefore, identifying the correct code requires extensive knowledge of the American Hospital Association's *Coding Clinic for ICD-9-CM* and other coding guidelines. Becoming completely familiar with all the conventions associated with ICD-9-CM requires extensive and continued effort. As a result, becoming highly proficient in ICD-9-CM can take a long time.

Conclusion

ICD-1Ø-PCS has been developed as a replacement for volume 3 of ICD-9-CM. The system has evolved during its development based on extensive input from many segments of the health care industry. The multi-axial structure of the system, combined with its detailed definition of terminology, permits a precise specification of procedures for use in health services research, epidemiology, statistical analysis, and administrative areas. ICD-1Ø-PCS will also allow health information coders to assign accurate procedure codes with minimal effort.

Sources

All material contained in this manual is derived from the ICD-1Ø-PCS Coding System and Training Manual and related files revised and distributed by the Centers for Medicare and Medicaid Services, January 2Ø11.

ICD-10-PCS Draft Coding Guidelines

Conventions

A1. ICD-10-PCS codes are composed of seven characters. Each character is an axis of classification that specifies information about the procedure performed. Within a defined code range, a character specifies the same type of information in that axis of classification.

Example: The fifth axis of classification specifies the approach in sections Ø through 4 and 7 through 9 of the system.

A2. One of 34 possible values can be assigned to each axis of classification in the seven-character code: they are the numbers Ø through 9 and the alphabet (except I and O because they are easily confused with the numbers 1 and Ø). The number of unique values used in an axis of classification differs as needed.

Example: Where the fifth axis of classification specifies the approach, seven different approach values are currently used to specify the approach.

A3. The valid values for an axis of classification can be added to as needed.

Example: If a significantly distinct type of device is used in a new procedure, a new device value can be added to the system.

A4. As with words in their context, the meaning of any single value is a combination of its axis of classification and any preceding values on which it may be dependent.

Example: The meaning of a body part value in the Medical and Surgical section is always dependent on the body system value. The body part value Ø in the Central Nervous body system specifies Brain and the body part value Ø in the Peripheral Nervous body system specifies Cervical Plexus.

A5. As the system is expanded to become increasingly detailed, over time more values will depend on preceding values for their meaning.

Example: In the Lower Joints body system, the device value 3 in the root operation Insertion specifies Infusion Device and the device value 3 in the root operation Fusion specifies Interbody Fusion Device.

A6. The purpose of the alphabetic index is to locate the appropriate table that contains all information necessary to construct a procedure code. The PCS Tables should always be consulted to find the most appropriate valid code.

A7. It is not required to consult the index first before proceeding to the tables to complete the code. A valid code may be chosen directly from the tables.

A8. All seven characters must be specified to be a valid code. If the documentation is incomplete for coding purposes, the physician should be queried for the necessary information.

A9. Within a PCS table, valid codes include all combinations of choices in characters 4 through 7 contained in the same row of the table. In the example below, ØJHT3VZ is a valid code, and ØJHW3VZ is not a valid code.

A10. "And," when used in a code description, means "and/or."

Example: Lower Arm and Wrist Muscle means lower arm and/or wrist muscle.

A11. Many of the terms used to construct PCS codes are defined within the system. It is the coder's responsibility to determine what the documentation in the medical record equates to in the PCS definitions. The physician is not expected to use the terms used in PCS code descriptions, nor is the coder required to query the physician when the correlation between the documentation and the defined PCS terms is clear.

Example: When the physician documents "partial resection" the coder can independently correlate "partial resection" to the root operation Excision without querying the physician for clarification.

Sample ICD-10-PCS Table

Ø   **Medical and Surgical**
J   **Subcutaneous Tissue and Fascia**
H   **Insertion**   Putting in a nonbiological appliance that monitors, assists, performs, or prevents a physiological function but does not physically take the place of a body part

Body Part Character 4	Approach Character 5	Device Character 6	Qualifier Character 7
S Subcutaneous Tissue and Fascia, Head and Neck **V** Subcutaneous Tissue and Fascia, Upper Extremity **W** Subcutaneous Tissue and Fascia, Lower Extremity	**Ø** Open **3** Percutaneous	**1** Radioactive Element **3** Infusion Device	**Z** No Qualifier
T Subcutaneous Tissue and Fascia, Trunk	**Ø** Open **3** Percutaneous	**1** Radioactive Element **3** Infusion Device **V** Infusion Pump	**Z** No Qualifier

Medical and Surgical Section Guidelines (section 0)

B2. Body System

General guidelines

B2.1a. The procedure codes in the general anatomical regions body systems should only be used when the procedure is performed on an anatomical region rather than a specific body part (e.g., root operations Control and Detachment, drainage of a body cavity) or on the rare occasion when no information is available to support assignment of a code to a specific body part.

Example: Control of postoperative hemorrhage is coded to the root operation Control found in the general anatomical regions body systems.

B2.1b. Body systems designated as upper or lower contain body parts located above or below the diaphragm respectively.

Example: Vein body parts above the diaphragm are found in the Upper Veins body system; vein body parts below the diaphragm are found in the Lower Veins body system.

B3. Root Operation

General guidelines

B3.1a. In order to determine the appropriate root operation, the full definition of the root operation as contained in the PCS Tables must be applied.

B3.1b. Components of a procedure specified in the root operation definition and explanation are not coded separately. Procedural steps necessary to reach the operative site and close the operative site are also not coded separately.

Example: Resection of a joint as part of a joint replacement procedure is included in the root operation definition of Replacement and is not coded separately. Laparotomy performed to reach the site of an open liver biopsy is not coded separately.

Multiple procedures

B3.2. During the same operative episode, multiple procedures are coded if:

a. The same root operation is performed on different body parts as defined by distinct values of the body part character.

   Example: Diagnostic excision of liver and pancreas are coded separately.

b. The same root operation is repeated at different body sites that are included in the same body part value.

   Example: Excision of the sartorius muscle and excision of the gracilis muscle are both included in the upper leg muscle body part value, and multiple procedures are coded.

c. Multiple root operations with distinct objectives are performed on the same body part.

   Example: Destruction of sigmoid lesion and bypass of sigmoid colon are coded separately.

d. The intended root operation is attempted using one approach, but is converted to a different approach.

   Example: Laparoscopic cholecystectomy converted to an open cholecystectomy is coded as percutaneous endoscopic Inspection and open Resection.

Discontinued procedures

B3.3. If the intended procedure is discontinued, code the procedure to the root operation performed. If a procedure is discontinued before any other root operation is performed, code the root operation Inspection of the body part or anatomical region inspected.

Example: A planned aortic valve replacement procedure is discontinued after the initial thoracotomy and before any incision is made in the heart muscle, when the patient becomes hemodynamically unstable. This procedure is coded as an open Inspection of the mediastinum.

Biopsy followed by more definitive treatment

B3.4. If a diagnostic Excision, Extraction, or Drainage procedure (biopsy) is followed by a more definitive procedure, such as Destruction, Excision or Resection at the same procedure site, both the biopsy and the more definitive treatment are coded.

Example: Biopsy of breast followed by partial mastectomy at the same procedure site, both the biopsy and the partial mastectomy procedure are coded.

Overlapping body layers

B3.5. If the root operations Excision, Repair or Inspection are performed on overlapping layers of the musculoskeletal system, the body part specifying the deepest layer is coded.

Example: Excisional debridement that includes skin and subcutaneous tissue and muscle is coded to the muscle body part.

Bypass procedures

B3.6a. Bypass procedures are coded by identifying the body part bypassed "from" and the body part bypassed "to." The fourth character body part specifies the body part bypassed from, and the qualifier specifies the body part bypassed to.

Example: Bypass from stomach to jejunum, stomach is the body part and jejunum is the qualifier.

B3.6b. Coronary arteries are classified by number of distinct sites treated, rather than number of coronary arteries or anatomic name of a coronary artery (e.g., left anterior descending). Coronary artery bypass procedures are coded differently than other bypass procedures as described in the previous guideline. Rather than identifying the body part bypassed from, the body part identifies the number of coronary artery sites bypassed to, and the qualifier specifies the vessel bypassed from.

Example: Aortocoronary artery bypass of one site on the left anterior descending coronary artery and one site on the obtuse marginal coronary artery is classified in the body part axis of classification as two coronary artery sites and the qualifier specifies the aorta as the body part bypassed from.

B3.6c. If multiple coronary artery sites are bypassed, a separate procedure is coded for each coronary artery site that uses a different device and/or qualifier.

Example: Aortocoronary artery bypass and internal mammary coronary artery bypass are coded separately.

Control vs. more definitive root operations

B3.7. The root operation Control is defined as, "Stopping, or attempting to stop, postprocedural bleeding." If an attempt to stop postprocedural bleeding is initially unsuccessful, and to stop the bleeding requires performing any of the definitive root operations Bypass, Detachment, Excision, Extraction, Reposition, Replacement, or Resection, then that root operation is coded instead of Control.

Example: Resection of spleen to stop postprocedural bleeding is coded to Resection instead of Control.

Excision vs. Resection

B3.8. PCS contains specific body parts for anatomical subdivisions of a body part, such as lobes of the lungs or liver and regions of the intestine. Resection of the specific body part is coded whenever all of the body part is cut out or off, rather than coding Excision of a less specific body part.

Example: Left upper lung lobectomy is coded to Resection of Upper Lung Lobe, Left rather than Excision of Lung, Left.

Excision for graft

B3.9. If an autograft is obtained from a different body part in order to complete the objective of the procedure, a separate procedure is coded.

Example: Coronary bypass with excision of saphenous vein graft, excision of saphenous vein is coded separately.

Fusion procedures of the spine

B3.10a. The body part coded for a spinal vertebral joint(s) rendered immobile by a spinal fusion procedure is classified by the level of the spine (e.g. thoracic). There are distinct body part values for a single vertebral joint and for multiple vertebral joints at each spinal level.

Example: Body part values specify Lumbar Vertebral Joint, Lumbar Vertebral Joints, 2 or More and Lumbosacral Vertebral Joint.

B3.10b. If multiple vertebral joints are fused, a separate procedure is coded for each vertebral joint that uses a different device and/or qualifier.

Example: Fusion of lumbar vertebral joint, posterior approach, anterior column and fusion of lumbar vertebral joint, posterior approach, posterior column are coded separately.

B3.10c. Combinations of devices and materials are often used on a vertebral joint to render the joint immobile. When combinations of devices are used on the same vertebral joint, the device value coded for the procedure is as follows:

- If an interbody fusion device is used to render the joint immobile (alone or containing other material like bone graft), the procedure is coded with the device value Interbody Fusion Device

- If internal fixation is used to render the joint immobile and an interbody fusion device is not used, the procedure is coded with the device value Internal Fixation Device

- If bone graft is the only device used to render the joint immobile, the procedure is coded with the device value Nonautologous Tissue Substitute or Autologous Tissue Substitute

- If a mixture of autologous and nonautologous bone graft (with or without biological or synthetic extenders or binders) is used to render the joint immobile, code the procedure with the device value Autologous Tissue Substitute

Examples: Fusion of a vertebral joint using a cage style interbody fusion device containing morsellized bone graft is coded to the device Interbody Fusion Device.

Fusion of a vertebral joint using a bone dowel interbody fusion device made of cadaver bone and packed with a mixture of local morsellized bone and demineralized bone matrix is coded to the device Interbody Fusion Device.

Fusion of a vertebral joint using rigid plates affixed with screws and reinforced with bone cement is coded to the device Internal Fixation Device.

Fusion of a vertebral joint using both autologous bone graft and bone bank bone graft is coded to the device Autologous Tissue Substitute.

Inspection procedures

B3.11a. Inspection of a body part(s) performed in order to achieve the objective of a procedure is not coded separately.

Example: Fiberoptic bronchoscopy performed for irrigation of bronchus, only the irrigation procedure is coded.

B3.11b. If multiple tubular body parts are inspected, the most distal body part inspected is coded. If multiple non-tubular body parts in a region are inspected, the body part that specifies the entire area inspected is coded.

Examples: Cystoureteroscopy with inspection of bladder and ureters is coded to the ureter body part value.

Exploratory laparotomy with general inspection of abdominal contents is coded to the peritoneal cavity body part value.

B3.11c. When both an Inspection procedure and another procedure are performed on the same body part during the same episode, if the Inspection procedure is performed using a different approach than the other procedure, the Inspection procedure is coded separately.

Example: Endoscopic Inspection of the duodenum is coded separately when open Excision of the duodenum is performed during the same procedural episode.

Occlusion vs. Restriction for vessel embolization procedures

B3.12. If the objective of an embolization procedure is to completely close a vessel, the root operation Occlusion is coded. If the objective of an embolization procedure is to narrow the lumen of a vessel, the root operation Restriction is coded.

Examples: Tumor embolization is coded to the root operation Occlusion, because the objective of the procedure is to cut off the blood supply to the vessel.

Embolization of a cerebral aneurysm is coded to the root operation Restriction, because the objective of the procedure is not to close off the vessel entirely, but to narrow the lumen of the vessel at the site of the aneurysm where it is abnormally wide.

Release procedures

B3.13. In the root operation Release, the body part value coded is the body part being freed and not the tissue being manipulated or cut to free the body part.

Example: Lysis of intestinal adhesions is coded to the specific intestine body part value.

Release vs. Division

B3.14. If the sole objective of the procedure is freeing a body part without cutting the body part, the root operation is Release. If the sole objective of the procedure is separating or transecting a body part, the root operation is Division.

Examples: Freeing a nerve root from surrounding scar tissue to relieve pain is coded to the root operation Release. Severing a nerve root to relieve pain is coded to the root operation Division.

Reposition for fracture treatment

B3.15. Reduction of a displaced fracture is coded to the root operation Reposition and the application of a cast or splint in conjunction with the Reposition procedure is not coded separately. Treatment of a nondisplaced fracture is coded to the procedure performed.

Examples: Putting a pin in a nondisplaced fracture is coded to the root operation Insertion.

Casting of a nondisplaced fracture is coded to the root operation Immobilization in the Placement section.

Transplantation vs. Administration

B3.16. Putting in a mature and functioning living body part taken from another individual or animal is coded to the root operation Transplantation. Putting in autologous or nonautologous cells is coded to the Administration section.

Example: Putting in autologous or nonautologous bone marrow, pancreatic islet cells or stem cells is coded to the Administration section.

B4. Body Part

General guidelines

B4.1a. If a procedure is performed on a portion of a body part that does not have a separate body part value, code the body part value corresponding to the whole body part.

Example: A procedure performed on the alveolar process of the mandible is coded to the mandible body part.

B4.1b. If the prefix "peri" is combined with a body part to identify the site of the procedure, the procedure is coded to the body part named.

Example: A procedure site identified as perirenal is coded to the kidney body part.

Branches of body parts

B4.2. Where a specific branch of a body part does not have its own body part value in PCS, the body part is coded to the closest proximal branch that has a specific body part value.

Example: A procedure performed on the mandibular branch of the trigeminal nerve is coded to the trigeminal nerve body part value

Bilateral body part values

B4.3. Bilateral body part values are available for a limited number of body parts. If the identical procedure is performed on contralateral body parts, and a bilateral body part value exists for that body part, a single procedure is coded using the bilateral body part value. If no bilateral body part value exists, each procedure is coded separately using the appropriate body part value.

Example: The identical procedure performed on both fallopian tubes is coded once using the body part value Fallopian Tube, Bilateral. The identical procedure performed on both knee joints is coded twice using the body part values Knee Joint, Right and Knee Joint, Left.

Coronary arteries

B4.4. The coronary arteries are classified as a single body part that is further specified by number of sites treated and not by name or number of arteries. Separate body part values are used to specify the number of sites treated when the same procedure is performed on multiple sites in the coronary arteries.

Examples: Angioplasty of two distinct sites in the left anterior descending coronary artery with placement of two stents is coded as Dilation of Coronary Arteries, Two Sites, with Intraluminal Device.

Angioplasty of two distinct sites in the left anterior descending coronary artery, one with stent placed and one without, is coded separately as Dilation of Coronary Artery, One Site with Intraluminal Device, and Dilation of Coronary Artery, One Site with no device.

Tendons, ligaments, bursae and fascia near a joint

B4.5. Procedures performed on tendons, ligaments, bursae and fascia supporting a joint are coded to the body part in the respective body system that is the focus of the procedure. Procedures performed on joint structures themselves are coded to the body part in the joint body systems.

Example: Repair of the anterior cruciate ligament of the knee is coded to the knee bursae and ligament body part in the bursae and ligaments body system. Knee arthroscopy with shaving of articular cartilage is coded to the knee joint body part in the Lower Joints body system.

Skin, subcutaneous tissue and fascia overlying a joint

B4.6. If a procedure is performed on the skin, subcutaneous tissue or fascia overlying a joint, the procedure is coded to the following body part:

- Shoulder is coded to Upper Arm
- Elbow is coded to Lower Arm
- Wrist is coded to Lower Arm
- Hip is coded to Upper Leg
- Knee is coded to Lower Leg
- Ankle is coded to Foot

Fingers and toes

B4.7. If a body system does not contain a separate body part value for fingers, procedures performed on the fingers are coded to the body part value for the hand. If a body system does not contain a separate body part value for toes, procedures performed on the toes are coded to the body part value for the foot.

Example: Excision of finger muscle is coded to one of the hand muscle body part values in the Muscles body system.

B5. Approach

Open approach with percutaneous endoscopic assistance

B5.2. Procedures performed using the open approach with percutaneous endoscopic assistance are coded to the approach Open.

Example: Laparoscopic-assisted sigmoidectomy is coded to the approach Open.

External approach

B5.3a. Procedures performed within an orifice on structures that are visible without the aid of any instrumentation are coded to the approach External.

Example: Resection of tonsils is coded to the approach External.

B5.3b. Procedures performed indirectly by the application of external force through the intervening body layers are coded to the approach External.

Example: Closed reduction of fracture is coded to the approach External.

Percutaneous procedure via device

B5.4. Procedures performed percutaneously via a device placed for the procedure are coded to the approach Percutaneous.

Example: Fragmentation of kidney stone performed via percutaneous nephrostomy is coded to the approach Percutaneous.

B6. Device

General guidelines

B6.1a. A device is coded only if a device remains after the procedure is completed. If no device remains, the device value No Device is coded.

B6.1b. Materials such as sutures, ligatures, radiological markers and temporary post-operative wound drains are considered integral to the performance of a procedure and are not coded as devices.

B6.1c. Procedures performed on a device only and not on a body part are specified in the root operations Change, Irrigation, Removal and Revision, and are coded to the procedure performed.

Example: Irrigation of percutaneous nephrostomy tube is coded to the root operation Irrigation of indwelling device in the Administration section.

Drainage device

B6.2. A separate procedure to put in a drainage device is coded to the root operation Drainage with the device value Drainage Device.

Obstetric Section Guidelines (section 1)

C. Obstetrics Section

Products of conception

C1. Procedures performed on the products of conception are coded to the Obstetrics section. Procedures performed on the pregnant female other than the products of conception are coded to the appropriate root operation in the Medical and Surgical section.

Example: Amniocentesis is coded to the products of conception body part in the Obstetrics section. Repair of obstetric urethral laceration is coded to the urethra body part in the Medical and Surgical section.

Procedures following delivery or abortion

C2. Procedures performed following a delivery or abortion for curettage of the endometrium or evacuation of retained products of conception are all coded in the Obstetrics section, to the root operation Extraction and the body part Products of Conception, Retained. Diagnostic or therapeutic dilation and curettage performed during times other than the postpartum or post-abortion period are all coded in the Medical and Surgical section, to the root operation Extraction and the body part Endometrium.

Coding Exercises

Using the ICD-10-PCS tables construct the code that accurately represents the procedure performed. Answers to these coding exercises may be found in appendix G.

Medical Surgical Section

Procedure	Code
Excision of malignant melanoma from skin of right ear	
Laparoscopy with excision of endometrial implant from left ovary	
Percutaneous needle core biopsy of right kidney	
EGD with gastric biopsy	
Open endarterectomy of left common carotid artery	
Excision of basal cell carcinoma of lower lip	
Open excision of tail of pancreas	
Percutaneous biopsy of right gastrocnemius muscle	
Sigmoidoscopy with sigmoid polypectomy	
Open excision of lesion from right Achilles tendon	
Open resection of cecum	
Total excision of pituitary gland, open	
Explantation of left failed kidney, open	
Open left axillary total lymphadenectomy	
Laparoscopic-assisted total vaginal hysterectomy	
Right total mastectomy, open	
Open resection of papillary muscle	
Radical retropubic prostatectomy, open	
Laparoscopic cholecystectomy	
Endoscopic bilateral total maxillary sinusectomy	
Amputation at right elbow level	
Right below-knee amputation, proximal tibia/fibula	
Fifth ray carpometacarpal joint amputation, left hand	
Right leg and hip amputation through ischium	
DIP joint amputation of right thumb	
Right wrist joint amputation	
Trans-metatarsal amputation of foot at left big toe	
Mid-shaft amputation, right humerus	
Left fourth toe amputation, mid-proximal phalanx	
Right above-knee amputation, distal femur	
Cryotherapy of wart on left hand	
Percutaneous radiofrequency ablation of right vocal cord lesion	

Medical Surgical Section (Continued)

Procedure	Code
Left heart catheterization with laser destruction of arrhythmogenic focus, A-V node	
Cautery of nosebleed	
Transurethral endoscopic laser ablation of prostate	
Cautery of oozing varicose vein, left calf	
Laparoscopy with destruction of endometriosis, bilateral ovaries	
Laser coagulation of right retinal vessel hemorrhage, percutaneous	
Talc injection pleurodesis, left side	
Sclerotherapy of brachial plexus lesion, alcohol injection	
Forceps total mouth extraction, upper and lower teeth	
Removal of left thumbnail	
Extraction of right intraocular lens without replacement, percutaneous	
Laparoscopy with needle aspiration of ova for in vitro fertilization	
Nonexcisional debridement of skin ulcer, right foot	
Open stripping of abdominal fascia, right side	
Hysteroscopy with D&C, diagnostic	
Liposuction for medical purposes, left upper arm	
Removal of tattered right ear drum fragments with tweezers	
Microincisional phlebectomy of spider veins, right lower leg	
Routine Foley catheter placement	
Incision and drainage of external perianal abscess	
Percutaneous drainage of ascites	
Laparoscopy with left ovarian cystotomy and drainage	
Laparotomy with hepatotomy and drain placement for liver abscess, right lobe	
Right knee arthrotomy with drain placement	
Thoracentesis of left pleural effusion	
Phlebotomy of left median cubital vein for polycythemia vera	
Percutaneous chest tube placement for right pneumothorax	
Endoscopic drainage of left ethmoid sinus	
Thoracentesis of left pleural effusion	
Arterial blood gas sample from right brachial artery line	
Percutaneous chest tube placement for right pneumothorax	

Medical Surgical Section (Continued)

Procedure	Code
Endoscopic drainage of left ethmoid sinus	
Removal of foreign body, right cornea	
Percutaneous mechanical thrombectomy, left brachial artery	
Esophagogastroscopy with removal of bezoar from stomach	
Foreign body removal, skin of left thumb	
Transurethral cystoscopy with removal of bladder stone	
Forceps removal of foreign body in right nostril	
Laparoscopy with excision of old suture from mesentery	
Incision and removal of right lacrimal duct stone	
Nonincisional removal of intraluminal foreign body from vagina	
Open excision of retained sliver, subcutaneous tissue of left foot	
Extracorporeal shock-wave lithotripsy (ESWL), bilateral ureters	
Endoscopic retrograde cholangiopancreatography (ERCP) with lithotripsy of common bile duct stone	
Thoracotomy with crushing of pericardial calcifications	
Transurethral cystoscopy with fragmentation of bladder calculus	
Hysteroscopy with intraluminal lithotripsy of left fallopian tube calcification	
Division of right foot tendon, percutaneous	
Left heart catheterization with division of bundle of HIS	
Open osteotomy of capitate, left hand	
EGD with esophagotomy of esophagogastric junction	
Sacral rhizotomy for pain control, percutaneous	
Laparotomy with exploration and adhesiolysis of right ureter	
Incision of scar contracture, right elbow	
Frenulotomy for treatment of tongue-tie syndrome	
Right shoulder arthroscopy with coracoacromial ligament release	
Mitral valvulotomy for release of fused leaflets, open approach	
Percutaneous left Achilles tendon release	
Laparoscopy with lysis of peritoneal adhesions	
Manual rupture of right shoulder joint adhesions under general anesthesia	
Open posterior tarsal tunnel release	
Laparoscopy with freeing of left ovary and fallopian tube	
Liver transplant with donor matched liver	
Orthotopic heart transplant using porcine heart	
Right lung transplant, open, using organ donor match	

Medical Surgical Section (Continued)

Procedure	Code
Left kidney/pancreas organ bank transplant	
Replantation of avulsed scalp	
Reattachment of severed right ear	
Reattachment of traumatic left gastrocnemius avulsion, open	
Closed replantation of three avulsed teeth, lower jaw	
Reattachment of severed left hand	
Right hand open palmaris longus tendon transfer	
Endoscopic radial to median nerve transfer	
Fasciocutaneous flap closure of left thigh, open	
Transfer left index finger to left thumb position, open	
Percutaneous fascia transfer to fill defect, anterior neck	
Trigeminal to facial nerve transfer, percutaneous endoscopic	
Endoscopic left leg flexor hallucis longus tendon transfer	
Right scalp advancement flap to right temple	
Bilateral TRAM pedicle flap reconstruction status post mastectomy, muscle only, open	
Skin transfer flap closure of complex open wound, left lower back	
Open fracture reduction, right tibia	
Laparoscopy with gastropexy for malrotation	
Left knee arthroscopy with reposition of anterior cruciate ligament	
Open transposition of ulnar nerve	
Closed reduction with percutaneous internal fixation of right femoral neck fracture	
Trans-vaginal intraluminal cervical cerclage	
Cervical cerclage using Shirodkar technique	
Thoracotomy with banding of left pulmonary artery using extraluminal device	
Restriction of thoracic duct with intraluminal stent, percutaneous	
Craniotomy with clipping of cerebral aneurysm	
Nonincisional, transnasal placement of restrictive stent in right lacrimal duct	
Percutaneous ligation of esophageal vein	
Percutaneous embolization of left internal carotid-cavernous fistula	
Laparoscopy with bilateral occlusion of fallopian tubes using Hulka extraluminal clips	
Open suture ligation of failed A-V graft, left brachial artery	
Percutaneous embolization of vascular supply, intracranial meningioma	
ERCP with balloon dilation of common bile duct	

Medical Surgical Section (Continued)

Procedure	Code
PTCA of two coronary arteries, LAD with stent placement, RCA with no stent	
Cystoscopy with intraluminal dilation of bladder neck stricture	
Open dilation of old anastomosis, left femoral artery	
Dilation of upper esophageal stricture, direct visualization, with Bougie sound	
PTA of right brachial artery stenosis	
Transnasal dilation and stent placement in right lacrimal duct	
Hysteroscopy with balloon dilation of bilateral fallopian tubes	
Tracheoscopy with intraluminal dilation of tracheal stenosis	
Cystoscopy with dilation of left ureteral stricture, with stent placement	
Open gastric bypass with Roux-en-Y limb to jejunum	
Right temporal artery to intracranial artery bypass using Gore-Tex graft, open	
Tracheostomy formation with tracheostomy tube placement, percutaneous	
PICVA (percutaneous in situ coronary venous arterialization) of single coronary artery	
Open left femoral-popliteal artery bypass using cadaver vein graft	
Shunting of intrathecal cerebrospinal fluid to peritoneal cavity using synthetic shunt	
Colostomy formation, open, transverse colon to abdominal wall	
Open urinary diversion, left ureter, using ileal conduit to skin	
CABG of LAD using left internal mammary artery, open off-bypass	
Open pleuroperitoneal shunt, right pleural cavity, using synthetic device	
End-of-life replacement of spinal neurostimulator generator, dual array, in lower abdomen	
Percutaneous insertion of spinal neurostimulator lead, lumbar spinal cord	
Percutaneous placement of pacemaker lead in left atrium	
Open placement of dual chamber pacemaker generator in chest wall	
Percutaneous placement of venous central line in right internal jugular	
Open insertion of multiple channel cochlear implant, left ear	
Percutaneous placement of Swan-Ganz catheter in superior vena cava	
Bronchoscopy with insertion of brachytherapy seeds, right main bronchus	
Placement of intrathecal infusion pump for pain management, percutaneous	

Medical Surgical Section (Continued)

Procedure	Code
Open insertion of interspinous process device into lumbar vertebral joint	
Open placement of bone growth stimulator, left femoral shaft	
Cystoscopy with placement of brachytherapy seeds in prostate gland	
Full-thickness skin graft to right lower arm, autograft (do not code graft harvest for this exercise)	
Excision of necrosed left femoral head with bone bank bone graft to fill the defect, open	
Penetrating keratoplasty of right cornea with donor matched cornea, percutaneous approach	
Bilateral mastectomy with concomitant saline breast implants, open	
Excision of abdominal aorta with Gore-Tex graft replacement, open	
Total right knee arthroplasty with insertion of total knee prosthesis	
Bilateral mastectomy with free TRAM flap reconstruction	
Tenonectomy with graft to right ankle using cadaver graft, open	
Mitral valve replacement using porcine valve, open	
Percutaneous phacoemulsification of right eye cataract with prosthetic lens insertion	
Aortic valve annuloplasty using ring, open	
Laparoscopic repair of left inguinal hernia with marlex plug	
Autograft nerve graft to right median nerve, percutaneous endoscopic (do not code graft harvest for this exercise)	
Exchange of liner in femoral component of previous left hip replacement, open approach	
Anterior colporrhaphy with polypropylene mesh reinforcement, open approach	
Implantation of CorCap cardiac support device, open approach	
Abdominal wall herniorrhaphy, open, using synthetic mesh	
Tendon graft to strengthen injured left shoulder using autograft, open (do not code graft harvest for this exercise)	
Onlay lamellar keratoplasty of left cornea using autograft, external approach	
Resurfacing procedure on right femoral head, open approach	
Exchange of drainage tube from right hip joint	
Tracheostomy tube exchange	
Change chest tube for left pneumothorax	
Exchange of cerebral ventriculostomy drainage tube	
Foley urinary catheter exchange	
Open removal of lumbar sympathetic neurostimulator lead	

Medical Surgical Section (Continued)

Procedure	Code
Nonincisional removal of Swan-Ganz catheter from right pulmonary artery	
Laparotomy with removal of pancreatic drain	
Extubation, endotracheal tube	
Nonincisional PEG tube removal	
Transvaginal removal of extraluminal cervical cerclage	
Incision with removal of K-wire fixation, right first metatarsal	
Cystoscopy with retrieval of left ureteral stent	
Removal of nasogastric drainage tube for decompression	
Removal of external fixator, left radial fracture	
Reposition of Swan-Ganz catheter insertion to superior vena cava	
Open revision of right hip replacement, with readjustment of prosthesis	
Adjustment of position, pacemaker lead in left ventricle, percutaneous	
External repositioning of Foley catheter to bladder	
Revision of VAD reservoir placement in chest wall, causing patient discomfort, open	
Thoracotomy with exploration of right pleural cavity	
Diagnostic laryngoscopy	
Exploratory arthrotomy of left knee	
Colposcopy with diagnostic hysteroscopy	
Digital rectal exam	
Diagnostic arthroscopy of right shoulder	
Endoscopy of bilateral maxillary sinus	
Laparotomy with palpation of liver	
Transurethral diagnostic cystoscopy	
Colonoscopy, abandoned at sigmoid colon	
Percutaneous mapping of basal ganglia	
Heart catheterization with cardiac mapping	
Intraoperative whole brain mapping via craniotomy	
Mapping of left cerebral hemisphere, percutaneous endoscopic	
Intraoperative cardiac mapping during open heart surgery	
Hysteroscopy with cautery of post-hysterectomy oozing and evacuation of clot	
Open exploration and ligation of post-op arterial bleeder, left forearm	
Control of postoperative retroperitoneal bleeding via laparotomy	
Reopening of thoracotomy site with drainage and control of post-op hemopericardium	
Arthroscopy with drainage of hemarthrosis at previous operative site, right knee	

Medical Surgical Section (Continued)

Procedure	Code
Radiocarpal fusion of left hand with internal fixation, open	
Posterior spinal fusion at L1–L3 level with BAK cage interbody fusion device, open	
Intercarpal fusion of right hand with bone bank bone graft, open	
Sacrococcygeal fusion with bone graft from same operative site, open	
Interphalangeal fusion of left great toe, percutaneous pin fixation	
Suture repair of left radial nerve laceration	
Laparotomy with suture repair of blunt force duodenal laceration	
Cosmetic face lift, open, no other information available	
Bilateral breast augmentation with silicone implants, open	
Cosmetic rhinoplasty with septal reduction and tip elevation using local tissue graft, open	
Abdominoplasty (tummy tuck), open	
Liposuction of bilateral thighs	
Creation of penis in female patient using tissue bank donor graft	
Creation of vagina in male patient using synthetic material	

Obstetrics

Procedure	Code
Abortion by dilation and evacuation following laminaria insertion	
Manually assisted spontaneous abortion	
Abortion by abortifacient insertion	
Bimanual pregnancy examination	
Extraperitoneal C-section, low transverse incision	
Fetal spinal tap, percutaneous	
Fetal kidney transplant, laparoscopic	
Open in utero repair of congenital diaphragmatic hernia	
Laparoscopy with total excision of tubal pregnancy	
Transvaginal removal of fetal monitoring electrode	

Placement

Procedure	Code
Placement of packing material, right ear	
Mechanical traction of entire left leg	
Removal of splint, right shoulder	
Placement of neck brace	
Change of vaginal packing	

Placement (Continued)

Procedure	Code
Packing of wound, chest wall	
Sterile dressing placement to left groin region	
Removal of packing material from pharynx	
Placement of intermittent pneumatic compression device, covering entire right arm	
Exchange of pressure dressing to left thigh	

Administration

Procedure	Code
Peritoneal dialysis via indwelling catheter	
Transvaginal artificial insemination	
Infusion of total parenteral nutrition via central venous catheter	
Esophagogastroscopy with Botox injection into esophageal sphincter	
Percutaneous irrigation of knee joint	
Epidural injection of mixed steroid and local anesthetic for pain control	
Chemical pleurodesis using injection of tetracycline	
Transfusion of antihemophilic factor, (nonautologous) via arterial central line	
Transabdominal in vitro fertilization, implantation of donor ovum	
Autologous bone marrow transplant via central venous line	

Measurement and Monitoring

Procedure	Code
Cardiac stress test, single measurement	
EGD with biliary flow measurement	
Temperature monitoring, rectal	
Peripheral venous pulse, external, single measurement	
Holter monitoring	
Respiratory rate, external, single measurement	
Fetal heart rate monitoring, transvaginal	
Visual mobility test, single measurement	
Pulmonary artery wedge pressure monitoring from Swan-Ganz catheter	
Olfactory acuity test, single measurement	

Extracorporeal Assistance and Performance

Procedure	Code
Mechanical ventilation, 16 hours	
Liver dialysis, single encounter	
Cardiac countershock with successful conversion to sinus rhythm	
IPPB (intermittent positive pressure breathing) for mobilization of secretions, 22 hours	
Measurement and monitoring of intracranial pressure, percutaneous approach	
Renal dialysis, series of encounters	
IABP (intra-aortic balloon pump) continuous	
Intra-operative cardiac pacing, continuous	
ECMO (extracorporeal membrane oxygenation), continuous	
Controlled mechanical ventilation (CMV), 45 hours	
Pulsatile compression boot with intermittent inflation	

Extracorporeal Therapies

Procedure	Code
Donor thrombocytapheresis, single encounter	
Bili-lite UV phototherapy, series treatment	
Whole body hypothermia, single treatment	
Circulatory phototherapy, single encounter	
Shock wave therapy of plantar fascia, single treatment	
Antigen-free air conditioning, series treatment	
TMS (transcranial magnetic stimulation), series treatment	
Therapeutic ultrasound of peripheral vessels, single treatment	
Plasmapheresis, series treatment	
Extracorporeal electromagnetic stimulation (EMS) for urinary incontinence, single treatment	

Osteopathic

Procedures	Code
Isotonic muscle energy treatment of right leg	
Low velocity-high amplitude osteopathic treatment of head	
Lymphatic pump osteopathic treatment of left axilla	
Indirect osteopathic treatment of sacrum	
Articulatory osteopathic treatment of cervical region	

Other Procedures

Procedure	Code
Near infrared spectroscopy of leg vessels	
CT computer assisted sinus surgery	
Suture removal, abdominal wall	
Isolation after infectious disease exposure	
Robotic assisted open prostatectomy	

Chiropractic

Procedure	Code
Chiropractic treatment of lumbar region using long lever specific contact	
Chiropractic manipulation of abdominal region, indirect visceral	
Chiropractic extra-articular treatment of hip region	
Chiropractic treatment of sacrum using long and short lever specific contact	
Mechanically-assisted chiropractic manipulation of head	

Imaging

Procedure	Code
Noncontrast CT of abdomen and pelvis	
Ultrasound guidance for catheter placement, left subclavian artery	
Chest x-ray, AP/PA and lateral views	
Endoluminal ultrasound of gallbladder and bile ducts	
MRI of thyroid gland, contrast unspecified	
Esophageal videofluoroscopy study with oral barium contrast	
Portable x-ray study of right radius/ulna shaft, standard series	
Routine fetal ultrasound, second trimester twin gestation	
CT scan of bilateral lungs, high osmolar contrast with densitometry	
Fluoroscopic guidance for percutaneous transluminal angioplasty (PTA) of left common femoral artery, low osmolar contrast	

Nuclear Medicine

Procedure	Code
Tomo scan of right and left heart, unspecified radiopharmaceutical, qualitative gated rest	
Technetium pentetate assay of kidneys, ureters, and bladder	
Uniplanar scan of spine using technetium oxidronate, with first-pass study	
Thallous chloride tomographic scan of bilateral breasts	
PET scan of myocardium using rubidium	
Gallium citrate scan of head and neck, single plane imaging	
Xenon gas nonimaging probe of brain	
Upper GI scan, radiopharmaceutical unspecified, for gastric emptying	
Carbon 11 PET scan of brain with quantification	
Iodinated albumin nuclear medicine assay, blood plasma volume study	

Radiation Oncology

Procedure	Code
Plaque radiation of left eye, single port	
8 MeV photon beam radiation to brain	
IORT of colon, 3 ports	
HDR brachytherapy of prostate using palladium-103	
Electron radiation treatment of right breast, with custom device	
Hyperthermia oncology treatment of pelvic region	
Contact radiation of tongue	
Heavy particle radiation treatment of pancreas, four risk sites	
LDR brachytherapy to spinal cord using iodine	
Whole body phosphorus-32 administration with risk to hematopoetic system	

Physical Rehabilitation and Diagnostic Audiology

Procedure	Code
Bekesy assessment using audiometer	
Individual fitting of left eye prosthesis	
Physical therapy for range of motion and mobility, patient right hip, no special equipment	
Bedside swallow assessment using assessment kit	
Caregiver training in airway clearance techniques	

Physical Rehabilitation and Diagnostic Audiology (Continued)

Procedure	Code
Application of short arm cast in rehabilitation setting	
Verbal assessment of patient's pain level	
Caregiver training in communication skills using manual communication board	
Group musculoskeletal balance training exercises, whole body, no special equipment	
Individual therapy for auditory processing using tape recorder	

Mental Health

Procedure	Code
Cognitive-behavioral psychotherapy, individual	
Narcosynthesis	
Light therapy	
ECT (electroconvulsive therapy), unilateral, multiple seizure	
Crisis intervention	
Neuropsychological testing	
Hypnosis	
Developmental testing	
Vocational counseling	
Family psychotherapy	

Substance Abuse Treatment

Procedure	Code
Naltrexone treatment for drug dependency	
Substance abuse treatment family counseling	
Medication monitoring of patient on methadone maintenance	
Individual interpersonal psychotherapy for drug abuse	
Patient in for alcohol detoxification treatment	
Group motivational counseling	
Individual 12-step psychotherapy for substance abuse	
Post-test infectious disease counseling for IV drug abuser	
Psychodynamic psychotherapy for drug-dependent patient	
Group cognitive-behavioral counseling for substance abuse	

A

Abdominal aortic plexus *use* Nerve, Abdominal Sympathetic
Abdominal esophagus *use* Esophagus, Lower
Abdominohysterectomy
  see Excision, Uterus ØUB9
  see Resection, Uterus ØUT9
Abdominoplasty
  see Alteration, Abdominal Wall ØWØF
  see Repair, Abdominal Wall ØWQF
  see Supplement, Abdominal Wall ØWUF
Abductor hallucis muscle
  use Muscle, Foot, Right
  use Muscle, Foot, Left
Ablation *see* Destruction
Abortion
  Products of Conception 10AØ
  Abortifacient 10AØ7ZX
  Laminaria 10AØ7ZW
  Vacuum 10AØ7Z6
Abrasion *see* Extraction
Accessory cephalic vein
  use Vein, Cephalic, Right
  use Vein, Cephalic, Left
Accessory obturator nerve *use* Nerve, Lumbar Plexus
Accessory phrenic nerve *use* Nerve, Phrenic
Accessory spleen *use* Spleen
Acetabulectomy
  see Excision, Lower Bones ØQB
  see Resection, Lower Bones ØQT
Acetabulofemoral joint
  use Joint, Hip, Right
  use Joint, Hip, Left
Acetabuloplasty
  see Repair, Lower Bones ØQQ
  see Replacement, Lower Bones ØQR
  see Supplement, Lower Bones ØQU
Achilles tendon
  use Tendon, Lower Leg, Left
  use Tendon, Lower Leg, Right
Achillorrhaphy *see* Repair, Tendons ØLQ
Achillotenotomy, achillotomy
  see Division, Tendons ØL8
  see Drainage, Tendons ØL9
Acromioclavicular ligament
  use Bursa and Ligament, Shoulder, Right
  use Bursa and Ligament, Shoulder, Left
Acromion (process)
  use Scapula, Left
  use Scapula, Right
Acromionectomy
  see Excision, Upper Joints ØRB
  see Resection, Upper Joints ØRT
Acromioplasty
  see Repair, Upper Joints ØRQ
  see Replacement, Upper Joints ØRR
  see Supplement, Upper Joints ØRU
Activities of Daily Living Assessment FØ2
Activities of Daily Living Treatment FØ8
Acupuncture
  Breast
    Anesthesia 8EØH300
    No Qualifier 8EØH30Z
  Integumentary System
    Anesthesia 8EØH300
    No Qualifier 8EØH30Z
Adductor brevis muscle
  use Muscle, Upper Leg, Left
  use Muscle, Upper Leg, Right
Adductor hallucis muscle
  use Muscle, Foot, Left
  use Muscle, Foot, Right
Adductor longus muscle
  use Muscle, Upper Leg, Right
  use Muscle, Upper Leg, Left
Adductor magnus muscle
  use Muscle, Upper Leg, Right
  use Muscle, Upper Leg, Left
Adenohypophysis *usee* Gland, Pituitary
Adenoidectomy
  see Excision, Adenoids ØCBQ
  see Resection, Adenoids ØCTQ

Adenoidotomy *see* Drainage, Adenoids ØC9Q
Adhesiolysis *see* Release
Administration
  Blood products *see* Transfusion
  Other substance *see* Introduction
Adrenalectomy
  see Excision, Endocrine System ØGB
  see Resection, Endocrine System ØGT
Adrenalorrhaphy *see* Repair, Endocrine System ØGQ
Adrenalotomy *see* Drainage, Endocrine System ØG9
Advancement
  see Reposition
  see Transfer
Airway
  Insertion of device in
    Esophagus ØDH5
    Mouth and Throat ØCHY
    Nasopharynx Ø9HN
  Removal of device from
    Esophagus ØDP5
    Mouth and Throat ØCPY
    Nose Ø9PK
  Revision of device in
    Esophagus ØDW5
    Mouth and Throat ØCWY
    Nose Ø9WK
Alar ligament of axis *use* Bursa and Ligament, Head and Neck
Alimentation *see* Introduction
Alteration
  Abdominal Wall ØWØF
  Ankle Region
    Left ØYØL
    Right ØYØK
  Arm
    Lower
      Left ØXØF
      Right ØXØD
    Upper
      Left ØXØ9
      Right ØXØ8
  Axilla
    Left ØXØ5
    Right ØXØ4
  Back
    Lower ØWØL
    Upper ØWØK
  Breast
    Bilateral ØHØV
    Left ØHØU
    Right ØHØT
  Buttock
    Left ØYØ1
    Right ØYØØ
  Chest Wall ØWØ8
  Ear
    Bilateral Ø9Ø2
    Left Ø9Ø1
    Right Ø9ØØ
  Elbow Region
    Left ØXØC
    Right ØXØB
  Extremity
    Lower
      Left ØYØB
      Right ØYØ9
    Upper
      Left ØXØ7
      Right ØXØ6
  Eyelid
    Lower
      Left Ø8ØR
      Right Ø8ØQ
    Upper
      Left Ø8ØP
      Right Ø8ØN
  Face ØWØ2
  Head ØWØØ
  Jaw
    Lower ØWØ5
    Upper ØWØ4

Alteration —*continued*
  Knee Region
    Left ØYØG
    Right ØYØF
  Leg
    Lower
      Left ØYØJ
      Right ØYØH
    Upper
      Left ØYØD
      Right ØYØC
  Lip
    Lower ØCØ1X
    Upper ØCØØX
  Neck ØWØ6
  Nose Ø9ØK
  Perineum
    Female ØWØN
    Male ØWØM
  Shoulder Region
    Left ØXØ3
    Right ØXØ2
  Subcutaneous Tissue and Fascia
    Abdomen ØJØ8
    Back ØJØ7
    Buttock ØJØ9
    Chest ØJØ6
    Face ØJØ1
    Lower Arm
      Left ØJØH
      Right ØJØG
    Lower Leg
      Left ØJØP
      Right ØJØN
    Neck
      Anterior ØJØ4
      Posterior ØJØ5
    Upper Arm
      Left ØJØF
      Right ØJØD
    Upper Leg
      Left ØJØM
      Right ØJØL
  Wrist Region
    Left ØXØH
    Right ØXØG
Alveolar process of mandible
  use Mandible, Left
  use Mandible, Right
Alveolar process of maxilla
  use Maxilla, Right
  use Maxilla, Left
Alveolectomy
  see Excision, Head and Facial Bones ØNB
  see Resection, Head and Facial Bones ØNT
Alveoloplasty
  see Repair, Head and Facial Bones ØNQ
  see Replacement, Head and Facial Bones ØNR
  see Supplement, Head and Facial Bones ØNU
Alveolotomy
  see Division, Head and Facial Bones ØN8
  see Drainage, Head and Facial Bones ØN9
Ambulatory cardiac monitoring 4A12X45
Amniocentesis *see* Drainage, Products of Conception 1Ø9Ø
Amnioinfusion *see* Introduction, Products of Conception 3EØE
Amnioscopy 1ØJØ8ZZ
Amniotomy *see* Drainage, Products of Conception 1Ø9Ø
Amputation *see* Detachment
Anal orifice *use* Anus
Analog radiography *see* Plain Radiography
Analog radiology *see* Plain Radiography
Anastomosis *see* Bypass
Anatomical snuffbox
  use Muscle, Lower Arm and Wrist, Left
  use Muscle, Lower Arm and Wrist, Right
Angiectomy
  see Excision, Heart and Great Vessels Ø2B
  see Excision, Upper Arteries Ø3B
  see Excision, Lower Arteries Ø4B
  see Excision, Upper Veins Ø5B

Angiectomy —continued
  see Excision, Lower Veins Ø6B
Angiocardiography
  Combined right and left heart see Plain
    Radiography, Heart, Right and Left B2Ø6
  Left Heart see Plain Radiography, Heart, Left B2Ø5
  Right Heart see Plain Radiography, Heart, Right B2Ø4
  SPY see Fluoroscopy, Heart B21
Angiography
  see Plain Radiography, Heart B2Ø
  see Fluoroscopy, Heart B21
Angioplasty
  see Dilation, Heart and Great Vessels Ø27
  see Repair, Heart and Great Vessels Ø2Q
  see Replacement, Heart and Great Vessels Ø2R
  see Dilation, Upper Arteries Ø37
  see Repair, Upper Arteries Ø3Q
  see Replacement, Upper Arteries Ø3R
  see Dilation, Lower Arteries Ø47
  see Repair, Lower Arteries Ø4Q
  see Replacement, Lower Arteries Ø4R
  see Supplement, Heart and Great Vessels Ø2U
  see Supplement, Upper Arteries Ø3U
  see Supplement, Lower Arteries Ø4U
Angiorrhaphy
  see Repair, Heart and Great Vessels Ø2Q
  see Repair, Upper Arteries Ø3Q
  see Repair, Lower Arteries Ø4Q
Angioscopy
  Great Vessel Ø2JY4ZZ
  Lower Artery Ø4JY4ZZ
  Upper Artery Ø3JY4ZZ
Angiotripsy
  see Occlusion, Upper Arteries Ø3L
  see Occlusion, Lower Arteries Ø4L
Angular artery use Artery, Face
Angular vein
  use Vein, Face, Left
  use Vein, Face, Right
Annular ligament
  use Bursa and Ligament, Elbow, Left
  use Bursa and Ligament, Elbow, Right
Annuloplasty
  see Repair, Heart and Great Vessels Ø2Q
  see Supplement, Heart and Great Vessels Ø2U
Anoplasty
  see Repair, Anus ØDQQ
  see Supplement, Anus ØDUQ
Anorectal junction use Rectum
Anoscopy ØDJD8ZZ
Ansa cervicalis use Nerve, Cervical Plexus
Antabuse therapy HZ93ZZZ
Antebrachial fascia
  use Subcutaneous Tissue and Fascia, Lower Arm, Left
  use Subcutaneous Tissue and Fascia, Lower Arm, Right
Anterior (pectoral) lymph node
  use Lymphatic, Axillary, Right
  use Lymphatic, Axillary, Left
Anterior cerebral artery use Artery, Intracranial
Anterior cerebral vein use Vein, Intracranial
Anterior choroidal artery use Artery, Intracranial
Anterior circumflex humeral artery
  use Artery, Axillary, Left
  use Artery, Axillary, Right
Anterior communicating artery use Artery, Intracranial
Anterior cruciate ligament (ACL)
  use Bursa and Ligament, Knee, Left
  use Bursa and Ligament, Knee, Right
Anterior crural nerve use Nerve, Femoral
Anterior facial vein
  use Vein, Face, Left
  use Vein, Face, Right
Anterior intercostal artery
  use Artery, Internal Mammary, Right
  use Artery, Internal Mammary, Left
Anterior interosseous nerve use Nerve, Median
Anterior lateral malleolar artery
  use Artery, Anterior Tibial, Right
  use Artery, Anterior Tibial, Left
Anterior lingual gland use Gland, Minor Salivary

Anterior medial malleolar artery
  use Artery, Anterior Tibial, Right
  use Artery, Anterior Tibial, Left
Anterior spinal artery
  use Artery, Vertebral, Right
  use Artery, Vertebral, Left
Anterior tibial recurrent artery
  use Artery, Anterior Tibial, Right
  use Artery, Anterior Tibial, Left
Anterior ulnar recurrent artery
  use Artery, Ulnar, Right
  use Artery, Ulnar, Left
Anterior vagal trunk use Nerve, Vagus
Anterior vertebral muscle
  use Muscle, Neck, Left
  use Muscle, Neck, Right
Antihelix
  use Ear, External, Right
  use Ear, External, Left
  use Ear, External, Bilateral
Antitragus
  use Ear, External, Bilateral
  use Ear, External, Right
  use Ear, External, Left
Antrostomy see Drainage, Ear, Nose, Sinus Ø99
Antrotomy see Drainage, Ear, Nose, Sinus Ø99
Antrum of Highmore
  use Sinus, Maxillary, Left
  use Sinus, Maxillary, Right
Aortic annulus use Valve, Aortic
Aortic arch use Aorta, Thoracic
Aortic intercostal artery use Aorta, Thoracic
Aortography
  see Plain Radiography, Upper Arteries B3Ø
  see Fluoroscopy, Upper Arteries B31
  see Plain Radiography, Lower Arteries B4Ø
  see Fluoroscopy, Lower Arteries B41
Aortoplasty
  see Repair, Aorta, Thoracic Ø2QW
  see Replacement, Aorta, Thoracic Ø2RW
  see Supplement, Aorta, Thoracic Ø2UW
  see Repair, Aorta, Abdominal Ø4QØ
  see Replacement, Aorta, Abdominal Ø4RØ
  see Supplement, Aorta, Abdominal Ø4UØ
Apical (subclavicular) lymph node
  use Lymphatic, Axillary, Left
  use Lymphatic, Axillary, Right
Apneustic center use Pons
Appendectomy
  see Excision, Appendix ØDBJ
  see Resection, Appendix ØDTJ
Appendicolysis see Release, Appendix ØDNJ
Appendicotomy see Drainage, Appendix ØD9J
Application see Introduction
Aquapheresis
  6A55ØZ3
Aqueduct of Sylvius use Cerebral Ventricle
Aqueous humour
  use Anterior Chamber, Right
  use Anterior Chamber, Left
Arachnoid mater
  use Spinal Meninges
  use Cerebral Meninges
Arcuate artery
  use Artery, Foot, Left
  use Artery, Foot, Right
Areola
  use Nipple, Left
  use Nipple, Right
AROM (artificial rupture of membranes)
  10907ZC
Arterial canal (duct) use Artery, Pulmonary, Left
Arterial pulse tracing see Measurement, Arterial 4AØ3
Arteriectomy
  see Excision, Heart and Great Vessels Ø2B
  see Excision, Upper Arteries Ø3B
  see Excision, Lower Arteries Ø4B
Arteriography
  see Plain Radiography, Heart B2Ø
  see Fluoroscopy, Heart B21
  see Plain Radiography, Upper Arteries B3Ø
  see Fluoroscopy, Upper Arteries B31
  see Plain Radiography, Lower Arteries B4Ø

Arteriography—continued
  see Fluoroscopy, Lower Arteries B41
Arterioplasty
  see Repair, Heart and Great Vessels Ø2Q
  see Replacement, Heart and Great Vessels Ø2R
  see Repair, Upper Arteries Ø3Q
  see Replacement, Upper Arteries Ø3R
  see Repair, Lower Arteries Ø4Q
  see Replacement, Lower Arteries Ø4R
  see Supplement, Upper Arteries Ø3U
  see Supplement, Lower Arteries Ø4U
  see Supplement, Heart and Great Vessels Ø2U
Arteriorrhaphy
  see Repair, Heart and Great Vessels Ø2Q
  see Repair, Upper Arteries Ø3Q
  see Repair, Lower Arteries Ø4Q
Arterioscopy
  Great Vessel Ø2JY4ZZ
  Lower Artery Ø4JY4ZZ
  Upper Artery Ø3JY4ZZ
Arthrectomy
  see Excision, Upper Joints ØRB
  see Resection, Upper Joints ØRT
  see Excision, Lower Joints ØSB
  see Resection, Lower Joints ØST
Arthrocentesis
  see Drainage, Upper Joints ØR9
  see Drainage, Lower Joints ØS9
Arthrodesis
  see Fusion, Upper Joints ØRG
  see Fusion, Lower Joints ØSG
Arthrography
  see Plain Radiography, Skull and Facial Bones BNØ
  see Plain Radiography, Non-Axial Upper Bones BPØ
  see Plain Radiography, Non-Axial Lower Bones BQØ
Arthrolysis
  see Release, Upper Joints ØRN
  see Release, Lower Joints ØSN
Arthropexy
  see Repair, Upper Joints ØRQ
  see Reposition, Upper Joints ØRS
  see Repair, Lower Joints ØSQ
  see Reposition, Lower Joints ØSS
Arthroplasty
  see Repair, Upper Joints ØRQ
  see Replacement, Upper Joints ØRR
  see Repair, Lower Joints ØSQ
  see Replacement, Lower Joints ØSR
  see Supplement, Lower Joints ØSU
  see Supplement, Upper Joints ØRU
Arthroscopy
  see Inspection, Upper Joints ØRJ
  see Inspection, Lower Joints ØSJ
Arthrotomy
  see Drainage, Upper Joints ØR9
  see Drainage, Lower Joints ØS9
Artificial Sphincter
  Insertion of device in
    Anus ØDHQ
    Bladder ØTHB
    Bladder Neck ØTHC
    Urethra ØTHD
  Removal of device from
    Anus ØDPQ
    Bladder ØTPB
    Urethra ØTPD
  Revision of device in
    Anus ØDWQ
    Bladder ØTWB
    Urethra ØTWD
Aryepiglottic fold use Larynx
Arytenoid cartilage use Larynx
Arytenoid muscle
  use Muscle, Neck, Left
  use Muscle, Neck, Right
Arytenoidectomy see Excision, Larynx ØCBS
Arytenoidopexy
  see Repair, Larynx ØCQS
  see Repair, Larynx ØCQS
Ascending aorta use Aorta, Thoracic
Ascending palatine artery use Artery, Face

Ascending pharyngeal artery
   use Artery, External Carotid, Left
   use Artery, External Carotid, Right
Aspiration *see* Drainage
Assessment
   Activities of daily living *see* Activities of Daily Living
      Assessment, Rehabilitation FØ2
   Hearing *see* Hearing Assessment, Diagnostic
      Audiology F13
   Hearing aid *see* Hearing Aid Assessment, Diagnostic
      Audiology F14
   Motor function *see* Motor Function Assessment,
      Rehabilitation FØ1
   Nerve function *see* Motor Function Assessment,
      Rehabilitation FØ1
   Speech *see* Speech Assessment, Rehabilitation FØØ
   Vestibular *see* Vestibular Assessment, Diagnostic
      Audiology F15
   Vocational *see* Activities of Daily Living Treatment,
      Rehabilitation FØ8
Assistance
   Cardiac
      Continuous
         Balloon Pump 5AØ221Ø
         Impeller Pump 5AØ221D
         Other Pump 5AØ2216
         Pulsatile Compression 5AØ2215
      Intermittent
         Balloon Pump 5AØ211Ø
         Impeller Pump 5AØ211D
         Other Pump 5AØ2116
         Pulsatile Compression 5AØ2115
   Circulatory
      Continuous
         Hyperbaric 5AØ5221
         Supersaturated 5AØ522C
      Intermittent
         Hyperbaric 5AØ5121
         Supersaturated 5AØ512C
   Respiratory
      24-96 Consecutive Hours
         Continuous Negative Airway Pressure
            5AØ9459
         Continuous Positive Airway Pressure 5AØ9457
         Intermittent Negative Airway Pressure
            5AØ945B
         Intermittent Positive Airway Pressure
            5AØ9458
         No Qualifier 5AØ945Z
      Greater than 96 Consecutive Hours
         Continuous Negative Airway Pressure
            5AØ9559
         Continuous Positive Airway Pressure 5AØ9557
         Intermittent Negative Airway Pressure
            5AØ955B
         Intermittent Positive Airway Pressure
            5AØ9558
         No Qualifier 5AØ955Z
      Less than 24 Consecutive Hours
         Continuous Negative Airway Pressure
            5AØ9359
         Continuous Positive Airway Pressure 5AØ9357
         Intermittent Negative Airway Pressure
            5AØ935B
         Intermittent Positive Airway Pressure
            5AØ9358
         No Qualifier 5AØ935Z
Atherectomy
   see Extirpation, Heart and Great Vessels Ø2C
   see Extirpation, Upper Arteries Ø3C
   see Extirpation, Lower Arteries Ø4C
Atlantoaxial joint *use* Joint, Cervical Vertebral
Atmospheric Control 6AØZ
Atrioseptoplasty
   see Repair, Heart and Great Vessels Ø2Q
   see Replacement, Heart and Great Vessels Ø2R
   see Supplement, Heart and Great Vessels Ø2U
Atrioventricular node *use* Conduction Mechanism
Atrium dextrum cordis *use* Atrium, Right
Atrium pulmonale *use* Atrium, Left
Audiology, diagnostic
   see Hearing Assessment, Diagnostic Audiology F13

Audiology, diagnostic—*continued*
   see Hearing Aid Assessment, Diagnostic Audiology
      F14
   see Vestibular Assessment, Diagnostic Audiology
      F15
Audiometry *see* Hearing Assessment, Diagnostic
   Audiology F13
Auditory tube
   use Eustachian Tube, Right
   use Eustachian Tube, Left
Auerbach's (myenteric) plexus *use* Nerve, Abdominal
   Sympathetic
Auricle
   use Ear, External, Left
   use Ear, External, Bilateral
   use Ear, External, Right
Auricularis muscle *use* Muscle, Head
Autotransfusion *see* Transfusion
Autotransplant
   Adrenal tissue *see* Reposition, Endocrine System ØGS
   Kidney *see* Reposition, Urinary System ØTS
   Pancreatic tissue *see* Reposition, Pancreas ØFSG
   Parathyroid tissue *see* Reposition, Endocrine System
      ØGS
   Thyroid tissue *see* Reposition, Endocrine System ØGS
   Tooth *see* Reattachment, Mouth and Throat ØCM
Avulsion *see* Extraction
Axillary fascia
   use Subcutaneous Tissue and Fascia, Upper Arm,
      Left
   use Subcutaneous Tissue and Fascia, Upper Arm,
      Right
Axillary nerve *use* Nerve, Brachial Plexus

B

Balanoplasty
   see Repair, Penis ØVQS
   see Supplement, Penis ØVUS
Balloon Pump
   Continuous, Output 5AØ221Ø
   Intermittent, Output 5AØ211Ø
Bandage, Elastic *see* Compression
Banding *see* Restriction
Barium swallow *see* Fluoroscopy, Gastrointestinal
   System BD1
Bartholin's (greater vestibular) gland *use* Gland,
   Vestibular
Basal (internal) cerebral vein *use* Vein, Intracranial
Basal metabolic rate (BMR) *see* Measurement,
   Physiological Systems 4AØZ
Basal nuclei *use* Basal Ganglia
Basilar artery *use* Artery, Intracranial
Basis pontis *use* Pons
Beam Radiation
   Abdomen DWØ3
      Intraoperative DWØ33ZØ
   Adrenal Gland DGØ2
      Intraoperative DGØ23ZØ
   Bile Ducts DFØ2
      Intraoperative DFØ23ZØ
   Bladder DTØ2
      Intraoperative DTØ23ZØ
   Bone
      Other DPØC
      Intraoperative DPØC3ZØ
   Bone Marrow D7ØØ
      Intraoperative D7ØØ3ZØ
   Brain DØØØ
      Intraoperative DØØØ3ZØ
   Brain Stem DØØ1
      Intraoperative DØØ13ZØ
   Breast
      Left DMØØ
         Intraoperative DMØØ3ZØ
      Right DMØ1
         Intraoperative DMØ13ZØ
   Bronchus DBØ1
      Intraoperative DBØ13ZØ
   Cervix DUØ1
      Intraoperative DUØ13ZØ

Beam Radiation —*continued*
   Chest DWØ2
      Intraoperative DWØ23ZØ
   Chest Wall DBØ7
      Intraoperative DBØ73ZØ
   Colon DDØ5
      Intraoperative DDØ53ZØ
   Diaphragm DBØ8
      Intraoperative DBØ83ZØ
   Duodenum DDØ2
      Intraoperative DDØ23ZØ
   Ear D9ØØ
      Intraoperative D9ØØ3ZØ
   Esophagus DDØØ
      Intraoperative DDØØ3ZØ
   Eye D8ØØ
      Intraoperative D8ØØ3ZØ
   Femur DPØ9
      Intraoperative DPØ93ZØ
   Fibula DPØB
      Intraoperative DPØB3ZØ
   Gallbladder DFØ1
      Intraoperative DFØ13ZØ
   Gland
      Adrenal DGØ2
         Intraoperative DGØ23ZØ
      Parathyroid DGØ4
         Intraoperative DGØ43ZØ
      Pituitary DGØØ
         Intraoperative DGØØ3ZØ
      Thyroid DGØ5
         Intraoperative DGØ53ZØ
   Glands
      Salivary D9Ø6
         Intraoperative D9Ø63ZØ
   Head and Neck DWØ1
      Intraoperative DWØ13ZØ
   Hemibody DWØ4
      Intraoperative DWØ43ZØ
   Humerus DPØ6
      Intraoperative DPØ63ZØ
   Hypopharynx D9Ø3
      Intraoperative D9Ø33ZØ
   Ileum DDØ4
      Intraoperative DDØ43ZØ
   Jejunum DDØ3
      Intraoperative DDØ33ZØ
   Kidney DTØØ
      Intraoperative DTØØ3ZØ
   Larynx D9ØB
      Intraoperative D9ØB3ZØ
   Liver DFØØ
      Intraoperative DFØØ3ZØ
   Lung DBØ2
      Intraoperative DBØ23ZØ
   Lymphatics
      Abdomen D7Ø6
         Intraoperative D7Ø63ZØ
      Axillary D7Ø4
         Intraoperative D7Ø43ZØ
      Inguinal D7Ø8
         Intraoperative D7Ø83ZØ
      Neck D7Ø3
         Intraoperative D7Ø33ZØ
      Pelvis D7Ø7
         Intraoperative D7Ø73ZØ
      Thorax D7Ø5
         Intraoperative D7Ø53ZØ
   Mandible DPØ3
      Intraoperative DPØ33ZØ
   Maxilla DPØ2
      Intraoperative DPØ23ZØ
   Mediastinum DBØ6
      Intraoperative DBØ63ZØ
   Mouth D9Ø4
      Intraoperative D9Ø43ZØ
   Nasopharynx D9ØD
      Intraoperative D9ØD3ZØ
   Neck and Head DWØ1
      Intraoperative DWØ13ZØ
   Nerve
      Peripheral DØØ7
         Intraoperative DØØ73ZØ

Beam Radiation—*continued*
 Nose D9Ø1
  Intraoperative D9Ø13ZØ
 Oropharynx D9ØF
  Intraoperative D9ØF3ZØ
 Ovary DUØØ
  Intraoperative DUØØ3ZØ
 Palate
  Hard D9Ø8
   Intraoperative D9Ø83ZØ
  Soft D9Ø9
   Intraoperative D9Ø93ZØ
 Pancreas DFØ3
  Intraoperative DFØ33ZØ
 Parathyroid Gland DGØ4
  Intraoperative DGØ43ZØ
 Pelvic Bones DPØ8
  Intraoperative DPØ83ZØ
 Pelvic Region DWØ6
  Intraoperative DWØ63ZØ
 Pineal Body DGØ1
  Intraoperative DGØ13ZØ
 Pituitary Gland DGØØ
  Intraoperative DGØØ3ZØ
 Pleura DBØ5
  Intraoperative DBØ53ZØ
 Prostate DVØØ
  Intraoperative DVØØ3ZØ
 Radius DPØ7
  Intraoperative DPØ73ZØ
 Rectum DDØ7
  Intraoperative DDØ73ZØ
 Rib DPØ5
  Intraoperative DPØ53ZØ
 Sinuses D9Ø7
  Intraoperative D9Ø73ZØ
 Skin
  Abdomen DHØ8
   Intraoperative DHØ83ZØ
  Arm DHØ4
   Intraoperative DHØ43ZØ
  Back DHØ7
   Intraoperative DHØ73ZØ
  Buttock DHØ9
   Intraoperative DHØ93ZØ
  Chest DHØ6
   Intraoperative DHØ63ZØ
  Face DHØ2
   Intraoperative DHØ23ZØ
  Leg DHØB
   Intraoperative DHØB3ZØ
  Neck DHØ3
   Intraoperative DHØ33ZØ
 Skull DPØØ
  Intraoperative DPØØ3ZØ
 Spinal Cord DØØ6
  Intraoperative DØØ63ZØ
 Spleen D7Ø2
  Intraoperative D7Ø23ZØ
 Sternum DPØ4
  Intraoperative DPØ43ZØ
 Stomach DDØ1
  Intraoperative DDØ13ZØ
 Testis DVØ1
  Intraoperative DVØ13ZØ
 Thymus D7Ø1
  Intraoperative D7Ø13ZØ
 Thyroid Gland DGØ5
  Intraoperative DGØ53ZØ
 Tibia DPØB
  Intraoperative DPØB3ZØ
 Tongue D9Ø5
  Intraoperative D9Ø53ZØ
 Trachea DBØØ
  Intraoperative DBØØ3ZØ
 Ulna DPØ7
  Intraoperative DPØ73ZØ
 Ureter DTØ1
  Intraoperative DTØ13ZØ
 Urethra DTØ3
  Intraoperative DTØ33ZØ
 Uterus DUØ2
  Intraoperative DUØ23ZØ

Beam Radiation—*continued*
 Whole Body DWØ5
  Intraoperative DWØ53ZØ
Biceps brachii muscle
 use Muscle, Upper Arm, Right
 use Muscle, Upper Arm, Left
Biceps femoris muscle
 use Muscle, Upper Leg, Right
 use Muscle, Upper Leg, Left
Bicipital aponeurosis
 use Subcutaneous Tissue and Fascia, Lower Arm, Left
 use Subcutaneous Tissue and Fascia, Lower Arm, Right
Bicuspid valve *use* Valve, Mitral
Bililite therapy *see* Ultraviolet Light Therapy, Skin 6A8Ø
Bioactive Intraluminal Device
 Occlusion
  Common Carotid
   Left Ø3LJ
   Right Ø3LH
  External Carotid
   Left Ø3LN
   Right Ø3LM
  Internal Carotid
   Left Ø3LL
   Right Ø3LK
  Intracranial Ø3LG
  Vertebral
   Left Ø3LQ
   Right Ø3LP
 Removal of device from, Artery, Upper Ø3PY
 Restriction
  Common Carotid
   Left Ø3VJ
   Right Ø3VH
  External Carotid
   Left Ø3VN
   Right Ø3VM
  Internal Carotid
   Left Ø3VL
   Right Ø3VK
  Intracranial Ø3VG
  Vertebral
   Left Ø3VQ
   Right Ø3VP
 Revision of device in, Artery, Upper Ø3WY
Biofeedback
 GZC9ZZZ
Biopsy
 see Drainage, Diagnostic
 see Excision, Diagnostic
BiPAP *see* Assistance, Respiratory 5AØ9
Bisection *see* Division
Blepharectomy
 see Excision, Eye Ø8B
 see Resection, Eye Ø8T
Blepharoplasty
 see Repair, Eye Ø8Q
 see Replacement, Eye Ø8R
 see Supplement, Eye Ø8U
 see Reposition, Eye Ø8S
Blepharorrhaphy *see* Repair, Eye Ø8Q
Blepharotomy *see* Drainage, Eye Ø89
Block, Nerve, anesthetic injection 3EØT3CZ
Blood pressure *see* Measurement, Arterial 4AØ3
BMR (basal metabolic rate) *see* Measurement, Physiological Systems 4AØZ
Body of femur
 use Femoral Shaft, Right
 use Femoral Shaft, Left
Body of fibula
 use Fibula, Right
 use Fibula, Left
Bone Growth Stimulator
 Insertion of device in
  Bone
   Facial ØNHW
   Lower ØQHY
   Nasal ØNHB
   Upper ØPHY
  Skull ØNHØ

Bone Growth Stimulator—*continued*
 Removal of device from
  Bone
   Facial ØNPW
   Lower ØQPY
   Nasal ØNPB
   Upper ØPPY
  Skull ØNPØ
 Revision of device in
  Bone
   Facial ØNWW
   Lower ØQWY
   Nasal ØNWB
   Upper ØPWY
  Skull ØNWØ
Bone marrow transplant *see* Transfusion
Bony labyrinth
 use Ear, Inner, Left
 use Ear, Inner, Right
Bony orbit
 use Orbit, Right
 use Orbit, Left
Bony vestibule
 use Ear, Inner, Right
 use Ear, Inner, Left
Botallo's duct *use* Artery, Pulmonary, Left
BP (blood pressure) *see* Measurement, Arterial 4AØ3
Brachial (lateral) lymph node
 use Lymphatic, Axillary, Left
 use Lymphatic, Axillary, Right
Brachialis muscle
 use Muscle, Upper Arm, Right
 use Muscle, Upper Arm, Left
Brachiocephalic artery *use* Artery, Innominate
Brachiocephalic trunk *use* Artery, Innominate
Brachiocephalic vein
 use Vein, Innominate, Right
 use Vein, Innominate, Left
Brachioradialis muscle
 use Muscle, Lower Arm and Wrist, Right
 use Muscle, Lower Arm and Wrist, Left
Brachytherapy
 Abdomen DW13
 Adrenal Gland DG12
 Bile Ducts DF12
 Bladder DT12
 Bone Marrow D71Ø
 Brain DØ1Ø
 Brain Stem DØ11
 Breast
  Left DM1Ø
  Right DM11
 Bronchus DB11
 Cervix DU11
 Chest DW12
 Chest Wall DB17
 Colon DD15
 Diaphragm DB18
 Duodenum DD12
 Ear D91Ø
 Esophagus DD1Ø
 Eye D81Ø
 Gallbladder DF11
 Gland
  Adrenal DG12
  Parathyroid DG14
  Pituitary DG1Ø
  Thyroid DG15
 Glands, Salivary D916
 Head and Neck DW11
 Hypopharynx D913
 Ileum DD14
 Jejunum DD13
 Kidney DT1Ø
 Larynx D91B
 Liver DF1Ø
 Lung DB12
 Lymphatics
  Abdomen D716
  Axillary D714
  Inguinal D718
  Neck D713
  Pelvis D717

Brachytherapy—*continued*
   Lymphatics—*continued*
     Thorax D715
   Mediastinum DB16
   Mouth D914
   Nasopharynx D91D
   Neck and Head DW11
   Nerve, Peripheral D017
   Nose D911
   Oropharynx D91F
   Ovary DU10
   Palate
     Hard D918
     Soft D919
   Pancreas DF13
   Parathyroid Gland DG14
   Pelvic Region DW16
   Pineal Body DG11
   Pituitary Gland DG10
   Pleura DB15
   Prostate DV10
   Rectum DD17
   Sinuses D917
   Spinal Cord D016
   Spleen D712
   Stomach DD11
   Testis DV11
   Thymus D711
   Thyroid Gland DG15
   Tongue D915
   Trachea DB10
   Ureter DT11
   Urethra DT13
   Uterus DU12
Broad ligament *use* Uterine Supporting Structure
Bronchial artery *use* Aorta, Thoracic
Bronchography
   see Plain Radiography, Respiratory System BB0
   see Fluoroscopy, Respiratory System BB1
Bronchoplasty
   see Repair, Respiratory System 0BQ
   see Supplement, Respiratory System 0BU
Bronchorrhaphy *see* Repair, Respiratory System 0BQ
Bronchoscopy 0BJ08ZZ
Bronchotomy *see* Drainage, Respiratory System 0B9
Buccal gland *use* Buccal Mucosa
Buccinator lymph node *use* Lymphatic, Head
Buccinator muscle *use* Muscle, Facial
Buckling, scleral with implant *see* Supplement, Eye 08U
Bulbospongiosus muscle *use* Muscle, Perineum
Bulbourethral (Cowper's) gland *use* Urethra
Bundle of His *use* Conduction Mechanism
Bundle of Kent *use* Conduction Mechanism
Bunionectomy *see* Excision, Lower Bones 0QB
Bursectomy
   see Excision, Bursae and Ligaments 0MB
   see Resection, Bursae and Ligaments 0MT
Bursocentesis *see* Drainage, Bursae and Ligaments 0M9
Bursography
   see Plain Radiography, Non-Axial Upper Bones BP0
   see Plain Radiography, Non-Axial Lower Bones BQ0
Bursotomy
   see Division, Bursae and Ligaments 0M8
   see Drainage, Bursae and Ligaments 0M9
Bypass
   Anterior Chamber
     Left 08133
     Right 08123
   Aorta
     Abdominal 0410
     Thoracic 021W
   Artery
     Axillary
       Left 03160
       Right 03150
     Brachial
       Left 03180
       Right 03170
     Common Carotid
       Left 031J0
       Right 031H0

Bypass—*continued*
   Artery—*continued*
     Common Iliac
       Left 041D
       Right 041C
     Coronary
       Four or More Sites 0213
       One Site 0210
       Three Sites 0212
       Two Sites 0211
     External Carotid
       Left 031N0
       Right 031M0
     External Iliac
       Left 041J
       Right 041H
     Femoral
       Left 041L
       Right 041K
     Innominate 03120
     Internal Carotid
       Left 031L0
       Right 031K0
     Internal Iliac
       Left 041F
       Right 041E
     Intracranial 031G0
     Popliteal
       Left 041N
       Right 041M
     Radial
       Left 031C0
       Right 031B0
     Splenic 0414
     Subclavian
       Left 03140
       Right 03130
     Temporal
       Left 031T0
       Right 031S0
     Ulnar
       Left 031A0
       Right 03190
   Atrium
     Left 0217
     Right 0216
   Bladder 0T1B
   Cavity, Cranial 0W110J
   Cecum 0D1H
   Cerebral Ventricle 00160
   Colon
     Ascending 0D1K
     Descending 0D1M
     Sigmoid 0D1N
     Transverse 0D1L
   Duct
     Common Bile 0F19
     Cystic 0F18
     Hepatic
       Left 0F16
       Right 0F15
     Lacrimal
       Left 081Y
       Right 081X
     Pancreatic 0F1D
       Accessory 0F1F
   Duodenum 0D19
   Ear
     Left 091E0
     Right 091D0
   Esophagus 0D15
     Lower 0D13
     Middle 0D12
     Upper 0D11
   Fallopian Tube
     Left 0U16
     Right 0U15
   Gallbladder 0F14
   Ileum 0D1B
   Jejunum 0D1A
   Kidney Pelvis
     Left 0T14
     Right 0T13

Bypass—*continued*
   Pancreas 0F1G
   Pelvic Cavity 0W1J
   Peritoneal Cavity 0W1G
   Pleural Cavity
     Left 0W1B
     Right 0W19
   Spinal Canal 001U0
   Stomach 0D16
   Trachea 0B11
   Ureter
     Left 0T17
     Right 0T16
   Ureters, Bilateral 0T18
   Vas Deferens
     Bilateral 0V1Q
     Left 0V1P
     Right 0V1N
   Vein
     Axillary
       Left 0518
       Right 0517
     Azygos 0510
     Basilic
       Left 051C
       Right 051B
     Brachial
       Left 051A
       Right 0519
     Cephalic
       Left 051F
       Right 051D
     Colic 0617
     Common Iliac
       Left 061D
       Right 061C
     Esophageal 0613
     External Iliac
       Left 061G
       Right 061F
     External Jugular
       Left 051Q
       Right 051P
     Face
       Left 051V
       Right 051T
     Femoral
       Left 061N
       Right 061M
     Foot
       Left 061V
       Right 061T
     Gastric 0612
     Greater Saphenous
       Left 061Q
       Right 061P
     Hand
       Left 051H
       Right 051G
     Hemiazygos 0511
     Hepatic 0614
     Hypogastric
       Left 061J
       Right 061H
     Inferior Mesenteric 0616
     Innominate
       Left 0514
       Right 0513
     Internal Jugular
       Left 051N
       Right 051M
     Intracranial 051L
     Lesser Saphenous
       Left 061S
       Right 061R
     Portal 0618
     Renal
       Left 061B
       Right 0619
     Splenic 0611
     Subclavian
       Left 0516
       Right 0515

Change device in—*continued*
Pleural Cavity
Left 0W2BX
Right 0W29X
Products of Conception 10207
Prostate and Seminal Vesicles 0V24X
Retroperitoneum 0W2HX
Scrotum and Tunica Vaginalis 0V28X
Sinus 092YX
Skin 0H2PX
Skull 0N20X
Spinal Canal 002UX
Spleen 072PX
Subcutaneous Tissue and Fascia
Head and Neck 0J2SX
Lower Extremity 0J2WX
Trunk 0J2TX
Upper Extremity 0J2VX
Tendon
Lower 0L2YX
Upper 0L2XX
Testis 0V2DX
Thymus 072MX
Thyroid Gland 0G2KX
Trachea 0B21
Tracheobronchial Tree 0B20X
Ureter 0T29X
Urethra 0T2DX
Uterus and Cervix 0U2DXHZ
Vagina and Cul-de-sac 0U2HXGZ
Vas Deferens 0V2RX
Vulva 0U2MX
Change device on or in
Abdominal Wall 2W03X
Anorectal 2Y03X5Z
Arm
Lower
Left 2W0DX
Right 2W0CX
Upper
Left 2W0BX
Right 2W0AX
Back 2W05X
Chest Wall 2W04X
Ear 2Y02X5Z
Extremity
Lower
Left 2W0MX
Right 2W0LX
Upper
Left 2W09X
Right 2W08X
Face 2W01X
Finger
Left 2W0KX
Right 2W0JX
Foot
Left 2W0TX
Right 2W0SX
Genital Tract, Female 2Y04X5Z
Hand
Left 2W0FX
Right 2W0EX
Head 2W00X
Inguinal Region
Left 2W07X
Right 2W06X
Leg
Lower
Left 2W0RX
Right 2W0QX
Upper
Left 2W0PX
Right 2W0NX
Mouth and Pharynx 2Y00X5Z
Nasal 2Y01X5Z
Neck 2W02X
Thumb
Left 2W0HX
Right 2W0GX
Toe
Left 2W0VX
Right 2W0UX

Change device on or in—*continued*
Urethra 2Y05X5Z
Chemoembolization *see* Introduction
Chemosurgery, Skin 3E00XTZ
Chemothalamectomy *see* Destruction, Thalamus 0059
Chemotherapy, Infusion for cancer *see* Introduction
Chest x-ray *see* Plain Radiography, Chest BW03
Chiropractic Manipulation
Abdomen 9WB9X
Cervical 9WB1X
Extremities
Lower 9WB6X
Upper 9WB7X
Head 9WB0X
Lumbar 9WB3X
Pelvis 9WB5X
Rib Cage 9WB8X
Sacrum 9WB4X
Thoracic 9WB2X
Choana *use* Nasopharynx
Cholangiogram
see Plain Radiography, Hepatobiliary System and Pancreas BF0
see Fluoroscopy, Hepatobiliary System and Pancreas BF1
Cholecystectomy
see Excision, Gallbladder 0FB4
see Resection, Gallbladder 0FT4
Cholecystojejunostomy
see Bypass, Hepatobiliary System and Pancreas 0F1
see Drainage, Hepatobiliary System and Pancreas 0F9
Cholecystopexy
see Repair, Gallbladder 0FQ4
see Reposition, Gallbladder 0FS4
Cholecystoscopy 0FJ44ZZ
Cholecystostomy
see Drainage, Gallbladder 0F94
see Bypass, Gallbladder 0F14
Cholecystotomy *see* Drainage, Gallbladder 0F94
Choledochectomy
see Excision, Hepatobiliary System and Pancreas 0FB
see Resection, Hepatobiliary System and Pancreas 0FT
Choledocholithotomy *see* Extirpation, Duct, Common Bile 0FC9
Choledochoplasty
see Repair, Hepatobiliary System and Pancreas 0FQ
see Replacement, Hepatobiliary System and Pancreas 0FR
see Supplement, Hepatobiliary System and Pancreas 0FU
Choledochoscopy 0FJB8ZZ
Choledochotomy *see* Drainage, Hepatobiliary System and Pancreas 0F9
Cholelithotomy *see* Extirpation, Hepatobiliary System and Pancreas 0FC
Chondrectomy
see Excision, Upper Joints 0RB
see Excision, Lower Joints 0SB
Knee *see* Excision, Lower Joints 0SB
Semilunar cartilage *see* Excision, Lower Joints 0SB
Chondroglossus muscle *use* Muscle, Tongue, Palate, Pharynx
Chorda tympani *use* Nerve, Facial
Chordotomy *see* Division, Central Nervous System 008
Choroid plexus *use* Cerebral Ventricle
Choroidectomy
see Excision, Eye 08B
see Resection, Eye 08T
Ciliary body
use Eye, Right
use Eye, Left
Ciliary ganglion *use* Nerve, Head and Neck Sympathetic
Circle of Willis *use* Artery, Intracranial
Circumflex iliac artery
use Artery, Femoral, Right
use Artery, Femoral, Left
Clamping *see* Occlusion
Claustrum *use* Basal Ganglia

Claviculectomy
see Excision, Upper Bones 0PB
see Resection, Upper Bones 0PT
Claviculotomy
see Division, Upper Bones 0P8
see Drainage, Upper Bones 0P9
Clipping, aneurysm *use* Restriction using Extraluminal Device
Clitorectomy, clitoridectomy
see Excision, Clitoris 0UBJ
see Resection, Clitoris 0UTJ
Closure
see Occlusion
see Repair
Clysis *see* Introduction
Coagulation *see* Destruction
Coccygeal body *use* Coccygeal Glomus
Coccygeus muscle
use Muscle, Trunk, Left
use Muscle, Trunk, Right
Cochlea
use Ear, Inner, Left
use Ear, Inner, Right
Cochlear Implant Treatment F0BZ0
Cochlear nerve *use* Nerve, Acoustic
Cochlear Prosthesis
Multiple channel
Left 09HE0S3
Right 09HD0S3
Single Channel
Left 09HE0S2
Right 09HD0S2
Colectomy
see Excision, Gastrointestinal System 0DB
see Resection, Gastrointestinal System 0DT
Collapse *see* Occlusion
Collection from
Breast, Breast Milk 8E0HX62
Indwelling Device
Circulatory System
Blood 8C02X6K
Other Fluid 8C02X6L
Nervous System
Cerebrospinal Fluid 8C01X6J
Other Fluid 8C01X6L
Integumentary System, Breast Milk 8E0HX62
Reproductive System, Male, Sperm 8E0VX63
Colocentesis *see* Drainage, Gastrointestinal System 0D9
Colofixation
see Repair, Gastrointestinal System 0DQ
see Reposition, Gastrointestinal System 0DS
Cololysis *see* Release, Gastrointestinal System 0DN
Colonoscopy 0DJD8ZZ
Colopexy
see Repair, Gastrointestinal System 0DQ
see Reposition, Gastrointestinal System 0DS
Coloplication *see* Restriction, Gastrointestinal System 0DV
Coloproctectomy
see Excision, Gastrointestinal System 0DB
see Resection, Gastrointestinal System 0DT
Coloproctostomy
see Bypass, Gastrointestinal System 0D1
see Drainage, Gastrointestinal System 0D9
Colopuncture *see* Drainage, Gastrointestinal System 0D9
Colorrhaphy *see* Repair, Gastrointestinal System 0DQ
Colostomy
see Bypass, Gastrointestinal System 0D1
see Drainage, Gastrointestinal System 0D9
Colpectomy
see Excision, Vagina 0UBG
see Resection, Vagina 0UTG
Colpocentesis *see* Drainage, Vagina 0U9G
Colpopexy
see Repair, Vagina 0UQG
see Reposition, Vagina 0USG
Colpoplasty
see Repair, Vagina 0UQG
see Supplement, Vagina 0UUG
Colporrhaphy *see* Repair, Vagina 0UQG
Colposcopy 0UJH8ZZ

Computerized Tomography (CT Scan)—*continued*
Leg
Left BQ2F
Right BQ2D
Liver BF25
Liver and Spleen BF26
Lung, Bilateral BB24
Mandible BN26
Nasopharynx B92F
Neck BW2F
Neck and Head BW29
Orbit, Bilateral BN23
Oropharynx B92F
Pancreas BF27
Patella
Left BQ2W
Right BQ2V
Pelvic Region BW2G
Pelvis BR2C
Chest and Abdomen BW25
Pelvis and Abdomen BW21
Pituitary Gland B029
Prostate BV23
Ribs
Left BP2Y
Right BP2X
Sacrum BR2F
Scapula
Left BP27
Right BP26
Sella Turcica B029
Shoulder
Left BP29
Right BP28
Sinus
Intracranial B522
Intravascular Optical Coherence B522Z2Z
Paranasal B922
Skull BN20
Spinal Cord B02B
Spine
Cervical BR20
Lumbar BR29
Thoracic BR27
Spleen and Liver BF26
Thorax BP2W
Tibia
Left BQ2C
Right BQ2B
Toe
Left BQ2Q
Right BQ2P
Trachea BB2F
Tracheobronchial Tree
Bilateral BB29
Left BB28
Right BB27
Vein
Pelvic (Iliac)
Left B52G
Intravascular Optical Coherence B52GZ2Z
Right B52F
Intravascular Optical Coherence B52FZ2Z
Pelvic (Iliac)
Bilateral B52H
Intravascular Optical Coherence B52HZ2Z
Portal B52T
Intravascular Optical Coherence B52TZ2Z
Pulmonary
Bilateral B52S
Intravascular Optical Coherence B52SZ2Z
Left B52R
Intravascular Optical Coherence B52RZ2Z
Right B52Q
Intravascular Optical Coherence B52QZ2Z
Renal
Bilateral B52L
Intravascular Optical Coherence B52LZ2Z
Left B52K
Intravascular Optical Coherence B52KZ2Z
Right B52J
Intravascular Optical Coherence B52JZ2Z

Computerized Tomography (CT Scan)—*continued*
Vein—*continued*
Splanchnic B52T
Intravascular Optical Coherence B52TZ2Z
Vena Cava
Inferior B529
Intravascular Optical Coherence B529Z2Z
Superior B528
Intravascular Optical Coherence B528Z2Z
Ventricle, Cerebral B028
Wrist
Left BP2M
Right BP2L
Condylectomy
see Excision, Head and Facial Bones 0NB
see Excision, Upper Bones 0PB
see Excision, Lower Bones 0QB
Condyloid process
use Mandible, Left
use Mandible, Right
Condylotomy
see Division, Head and Facial Bones 0N8
see Drainage, Head and Facial Bones 0N9
see Division, Upper Bones 0P8
see Drainage, Upper Bones 0P9
see Division, Lower Bones 0Q8
see Drainage, Lower Bones 0Q9
Condylysis
see Release, Head and Facial Bones 0NN
see Release, Upper Bones 0PN
see Release, Lower Bones 0QN
Conization, cervix *see* Excision, Uterus 0UB9
Conjunctivoplasty
see Repair, Eye 08Q
see Replacement, Eye 08R
Construction
Auricle, ear *see* Replacement, Ear, Nose, Sinus 09R
Ileal conduit *see* Bypass, Urinary System 0T1
Contact Radiation
Abdomen DWY37ZZ
Adrenal Gland DGY27ZZ
Bile Ducts DFY27ZZ
Bladder DTY27ZZ
Bone, Other DPYC7ZZ
Brain D0Y07ZZ
Brain Stem D0Y17ZZ
Breast
Left DMY07ZZ
Right DMY17ZZ
Bronchus DBY17ZZ
Cervix DUY17ZZ
Chest DWY27ZZ
Chest Wall DBY77ZZ
Colon DDY57ZZ
Diaphragm DBY87ZZ
Duodenum DDY27ZZ
Ear D9Y07ZZ
Esophagus DDY07ZZ
Eye D8Y07ZZ
Femur DPY97ZZ
Fibula DPYB7ZZ
Gallbladder DFY17ZZ
Gland
Adrenal DGY27ZZ
Parathyroid DGY47ZZ
Pituitary DGY07ZZ
Thyroid DGY57ZZ
Glands, Salivary D9Y67ZZ
Head and Neck DWY17ZZ
Hemibody DWY47ZZ
Humerus DPY67ZZ
Hypopharynx D9Y37ZZ
Ileum DDY47ZZ
Jejunum DDY37ZZ
Kidney DTY07ZZ
Larynx D9YB7ZZ
Liver DFY07ZZ
Lung DBY27ZZ
Mandible DPY37ZZ
Maxilla DPY27ZZ
Mediastinum DBY67ZZ
Mouth D9Y47ZZ
Nasopharynx D9YD7ZZ

Contact Radiation—*continued*
Neck and Head DWY17ZZ
Nerve, Peripheral D0Y77ZZ
Nose D9Y17ZZ
Oropharynx D9YF7ZZ
Ovary DUY07ZZ
Palate
Hard D9Y87ZZ
Soft D9Y97ZZ
Pancreas DFY37ZZ
Parathyroid Gland DGY47ZZ
Pelvic Bones DPY87ZZ
Pelvic Region DWY67ZZ
Pineal Body DGY17ZZ
Pituitary Gland DGY07ZZ
Pleura DBY57ZZ
Prostate DVY07ZZ
Radius DPY77ZZ
Rectum DDY77ZZ
Rib DPY57ZZ
Sinuses D9Y77ZZ
Skin
Abdomen DHY87ZZ
Arm DHY47ZZ
Back DHY77ZZ
Buttock DHY97ZZ
Chest DHY67ZZ
Face DHY27ZZ
Leg DHYB7ZZ
Neck DHY37ZZ
Skull DPY07ZZ
Spinal Cord D0Y67ZZ
Sternum DPY47ZZ
Stomach DDY17ZZ
Testis DVY17ZZ
Thyroid Gland DGY57ZZ
Tibia DPYB7ZZ
Tongue D9Y57ZZ
Trachea DBY07ZZ
Ulna DPY77ZZ
Ureter DTY17ZZ
Urethra DTY37ZZ
Uterus DUY27ZZ
Whole Body DWY57ZZ
Continuous Negative Airway Pressure
24-96 Consecutive Hours, Ventilation 5A09459
Greater than 96 Consecutive Hours, Ventilation 5A09559
Less than 24 Consecutive Hours, Ventilation 5A09359
Continuous Positive Airway Pressure
24-96 Consecutive Hours, Ventilation 5A09457
Greater than 96 Consecutive Hours, Ventilation 5A09557
Less than 24 Consecutive Hours, Ventilation 5A09357
Contraceptive Device
Change device in, Uterus and Cervix 0U2DXHZ
Insertion of device in
Cervix 0UHC
Subcutaneous Tissue and Fascia
Abdomen 0JH8
Chest 0JH6
Lower Arm
Left 0JHH
Right 0JHG
Lower Leg
Left 0JHP
Right 0JHN
Upper Arm
Left 0JHF
Right 0JHD
Upper Leg
Left 0JHM
Sinus 0JHL
Uterus 0UH9
Removal of device from
Subcutaneous Tissue and Fascia
Lower Extremity 0JPW
Trunk 0JPT
Upper Extremity 0JPV
Uterus and Cervix 0UPD

Contraceptive Device—continued
Revision of device in
Subcutaneous Tissue and Fascia
Lower Extremity ØJWW
Trunk ØJWT
Upper Extremity ØJWV
Uterus and Cervix ØUWD
Control postprocedural bleeding in
Abdominal Wall ØW3F
Ankle Region
Left ØY3L
Right ØY3K
Arm
Lower
Left ØX3F
Right ØX3D
Upper
Left ØX39
Right ØX38
Axilla
Left ØX35
Right ØX34
Back
Lower ØW3L
Upper ØW3K
Buttock
Left ØY31
Right ØY30
Cavity, Cranial ØW31
Chest Wall ØW38
Elbow Region
Left ØX3C
Right ØX3B
Extremity
Lower
Left ØY3B
Right ØY39
Upper
Left ØX37
Right ØX36
Face ØW32
Femoral Region
Left ØY38
Right ØY37
Foot
Left ØY3N
Right ØY3M
Gastrointestinal Tract ØW3P
Genitourinary Tract ØW3R
Hand
Left ØX3K
Right ØX3J
Head ØW30
Inguinal Region
Left ØY36
Right ØY35
Jaw
Lower ØW35
Upper ØW34
Knee Region
Left ØY3G
Right ØY3F
Leg
Lower
Left ØY3J
Right ØY3H
Upper
Left ØY3D
Right ØY3C
Mediastinum ØW3C
Neck ØW36
Oral Cavity and Throat ØW33
Pelvic Cavity ØW3J
Pericardial Cavity ØW3D
Perineum
Female ØW3N
Male ØW3M
Peritoneal Cavity ØW3G
Pleural Cavity
Left ØW3B
Right ØW39
Respiratory Tract ØW3Q
Retroperitoneum ØW3H

Control postprocedural bleeding in—continued
Shoulder Region
Left ØX33
Right ØX32
Wrist Region
Left ØX3H
Right ØX3G
Conus arteriosus use Ventricle, Right
Conus medullaris use Spinal Cord, Lumbar
Conversion
Cardiac rhythm 5A2204Z
Gastrostomy to jejunostomy feeding device see
Insertion of device in, Jejunum ØDHA
Coracoacromial ligament
use Bursa and Ligament, Shoulder, Right
use Bursa and Ligament, Shoulder, Left
Coracobrachialis muscle
use Muscle, Upper Arm, Left
use Muscle, Upper Arm, Right
Coracoclavicular ligament
use Bursa and Ligament, Shoulder, Left
use Bursa and Ligament, Shoulder, Right
Coracohumeral ligament
use Bursa and Ligament, Shoulder, Left
use Bursa and Ligament, Shoulder, Right
Coracoid process
use Scapula, Right
use Scapula, Left
Cordotomy see Division, Central Nervous System ØØ8
Core needle biopsy see Excision, Diagnostic
Corniculate cartilage use Larynx
Coronary arteriography
see Plain Radiography, Heart B2Ø
see Fluoroscopy, Heart B21
Corpus callosum use Brain
Corpus cavernosum use Penis
Corpus spongiosum use Penis
Corpus striatum use Basal Ganglia
Corrugator supercilii muscle use Muscle, Facial
Costatectomy
see Excision, Upper Bones ØPB
see Resection, Upper Bones ØPT
Costectomy
see Excision, Upper Bones ØPB
see Resection, Upper Bones ØPT
Costocervical trunk
use Artery, Subclavian, Left
use Artery, Subclavian, Right
Costochondrectomy
see Excision, Upper Bones ØPB
see Resection, Upper Bones ØPT
Costoclavicular ligament
use Bursa and Ligament, Shoulder, Left
use Bursa and Ligament, Shoulder, Right
Costosternoplasty
see Repair, Upper Bones ØPQ
see Replacement, Upper Bones ØPR
see Supplement, Upper Bones ØPU
Costotomy
see Division, Upper Bones ØP8
see Drainage, Upper Bones ØP9
Costotransverse joint
use Joint, Thoracic Vertebral
use Joint, Thoracic Vertebral, 2 to 7
use Joint, Thoracic Vertebral, 8 or more
Costotransverse ligament
use Bursa and Ligament, Thorax, Right
use Bursa and Ligament, Thorax, Left
Costovertebral joint
use Joint, Thoracic Vertebral, 8 or more
use Joint, Thoracic Vertebral, 2 to 7
use Joint, Thoracic Vertebral
Costoxiphoid ligament
use Bursa and Ligament, Thorax, Right
use Bursa and Ligament, Thorax, Left
Counseling
Family, for substance abuse, Other Family
Counseling HZ63ZZZ
Group
12-Step HZ43ZZZ
Behavioral HZ41ZZZ
Cognitive HZ40ZZZ
Cognitive-Behavioral HZ42ZZZ

Counseling—continued
Group—continued
Confrontational HZ48ZZZ
Continuing Care HZ49ZZZ
Infectious disease
Post-Test HZ4CZZZ
Pre-Test HZ4CZZZ
Interpersonal HZ44ZZZ
Motivational Enhancement HZ47ZZZ
Psychoeducation HZ46ZZZ
Spiritual HZ4BZZZ
Vocational HZ45ZZZ
Individual
12-Step HZ33ZZZ
Behavioral HZ31ZZZ
Cognitive HZ30ZZZ
Cognitive-Behavioral HZ32ZZZ
Confrontational HZ38ZZZ
Continuing Care HZ39ZZZ
Infectious disease
Post-Test HZ3CZZZ
Pre-Test HZ3CZZZ
Interpersonal HZ34ZZZ
Motivational Enhancement HZ37ZZZ
Psychoeducation HZ36ZZZ
Spiritual HZ3BZZZ
Vocational HZ35ZZZ
Mental Health Services
Educational GZ60ZZZ
Other Counseling GZ63ZZZ
Vocational GZ61ZZZ
Countershock, cardiac 5A2204Z
Cowper's (bulbourethral) gland use Urethra
CPAP (continuous positive airway pressure) see
Assistance, Respiratory 5AØ9
Cranial dura mater use Dura Mater
Cranial epidural space use Epidural Space
Cranial subarachnoid space use Subarachnoid Space
Cranial subdural space use Subdural Space
Craniectomy
see Excision, Head and Facial Bones ØNB
see Resection, Head and Facial Bones ØNT
Cranioplasty
see Repair, Head and Facial Bones ØNQ
see Replacement, Head and Facial Bones ØNR
see Supplement, Head and Facial Bones ØNU
Craniotomy
see Drainage, Central Nervous System ØØ9
see Division, Head and Facial Bones ØN8
see Drainage, Head and Facial Bones ØN9
Creation
Female ØW4NØ
Male ØW4MØ
Cremaster muscle use Muscle, Perineum
Cribriform plate
use Bone, Ethmoid, Left
use Bone, Ethmoid, Right
Cricoid cartilage use Larynx
Cricoidectomy see Excision, Larynx ØCBS
Cricothyroid artery
use Artery, Thyroid, Left
use Artery, Thyroid, Right
Cricothyroid muscle
use Muscle, Neck, Right
use Muscle, Neck, Left
Crisis Intervention GZ2ZZZZ
Crural fascia
use Subcutaneous Tissue and Fascia, Upper Leg,
Right
use Subcutaneous Tissue and Fascia, Upper Leg, Left
Crushing, nerve
Cranial see Destruction, Central Nervous System ØØ5
Peripheral see Destruction, Peripheral Nervous
System Ø15
Cryoablation see Destruction
Cryotherapy see Destruction
Cryptorchidectomy
see Excision, Male Reproductive System ØVB
see Resection, Male Reproductive System ØVT
Cryptorchiectomy
see Excision, Male Reproductive System ØVB
see Resection, Male Reproductive System ØVT

Cryptotomy
see Division, Gastrointestinal System ØD8
see Drainage, Gastrointestinal System ØD9
CT scan use Computerized Tomography (CT Scan)
CT sialogram see Computerized Tomography (CT Scan), Ear, Nose, Mouth and Throat B92
Cubital lymph node
use Lymphatic, Upper Extremity, Left
use Lymphatic, Upper Extremity, Right
Cubital nerve use Nerve, Ulnar
Cuboid bone
use Tarsal, Left
use Tarsal, Right
Cuboideonavicular joint
use Joint, Tarsal, Right
use Joint, Tarsal, Left
Culdocentesis see Drainage, Cul-de-sac ØU9F
Culdoplasty
see Repair, Cul-de-sac ØUQF
see Supplement, Cul-de-sac ØUUF
Culdoscopy ØUJH8ZZ
Culdotomy see Drainage, Cul-de-sac ØU9F
Culmen use Cerebellum
Cuneiform cartilage use Larynx
Cuneonavicular joint
use Joint, Tarsal, Left
use Joint, Tarsal, Right
Cuneonavicular ligament
use Bursa and Ligament, Foot, Left
use Bursa and Ligament, Foot, Right
Curettage
see Excision
see Extraction
Cutaneous (transverse) cervical nerve use Nerve, Cervical Plexus
CVP (central venous pressure) see Measurement, Venous 4A04
Cyclodiathermy see Destruction, Eye Ø85
Cyclophotocoagulation see Destruction, Eye Ø85
Cystectomy
see Excision, Bladder ØTBB
see Resection, Bladder ØTTB
Cystocele repair see Repair, Subcutaneous Tissue and Fascia, Pelvic Region ØJQC
Cystography
see Plain Radiography, Urinary System BTØ
see Fluoroscopy, Urinary System BT1
Cystolithotomy see Extirpation, Bladder ØTCB
Cystopexy
see Repair, Bladder ØTQB
see Reposition, Bladder ØTSB
Cystoplasty
see Repair, Bladder ØTQB
see Replacement, Bladder ØTRB
see Supplement, Bladder ØTUB
Cystorrhaphy see Repair, Bladder ØTQB
Cystoscopy ØTJB8ZZ
Cystostomy see Bypass, Bladder ØT1B
Cystotomy see Drainage, Bladder ØT9B
Cystourethrography
see Plain Radiography, Urinary System BTØ
see Fluoroscopy, Urinary System BT1
Cystourethroplasty
see Repair, Urinary System ØTQ
see Replacement, Urinary System ØTR
see Supplement, Urinary System ØTU

D

Debridement
Excisiona see Excision
Non-excisional see Extraction
Decompression, Circulatory 6A15
Decortication, lung see Excision, Respiratory System ØBD
Deep cervical fascia use Subcutaneous Tissue and Fascia, Neck, Anterior
Deep cervical vein
use Vein, Vertebral, Left
use Vein, Vertebral, Right

Deep circumflex iliac artery
use Artery, External Iliac, Left
use Artery, External Iliac, Right
Deep facial vein
use Vein, Face, Left
use Vein, Face, Right
Deep femoral (profunda femoris) vein
use Vein, Femoral, Left
use Vein, Femoral, Right
Deep femoral artery
use Artery, Femoral, Right
use Artery, Femoral, Left
Deep Inferior Epigastric Artery Perforator Flap
Bilateral ØHRVØ77
Left ØHRUØ77
Right ØHRTØ77
Deep palmar arch
use Artery, Hand, Left
use Artery, Hand, Right
Deep transverse perineal muscle use Muscle, Perineum
Deferential artery
use Artery, Internal Iliac, Right
use Artery, Internal Iliac, Left
Defibrillator Lead
Atrium
Left Ø2H7
Right Ø2H6
Pericardium Ø2HN
Vein, Coronary Ø2H4
Ventricle
Left Ø2HL
Right Ø2HK
Delivery
Cesarean see Extraction, Products of Conception 1ØDØ
Forceps see Extraction, Products of Conception 1ØDØ
Manually assisted 1ØEØXZZ
Products of Conception 1ØEØXZZ
Vacuum assisted see Extraction, Products of Conception 1ØDØ
Deltoid fascia
use Subcutaneous Tissue and Fascia, Upper Arm, Right
use Subcutaneous Tissue and Fascia, Upper Arm, Left
Deltoid ligament
use Bursa and Ligament, Ankle, Left
use Bursa and Ligament, Ankle, Right
Deltoid muscle
use Muscle, Shoulder, Left
use Muscle, Shoulder, Right
Deltopectoral (infraclavicular) lymph node
use Lymphatic, Upper Extremity, Right
use Lymphatic, Upper Extremity, Left
Denervation
Cranial nerve see Destruction, Central Nervous System ØØ5
Peripheral nerve see Destruction, Peripheral Nervous System Ø15
Densitometry
Plain Radiography
Femur
Left BQ04ZZ1
Right BQ03ZZ1
Hip
Left BQ01ZZ1
Right BQ00ZZ1
Spine
Cervical BRØØZZ1
Lumbar BRØ9ZZ1
Thoracic BRØ7ZZ1
Whole BRØGZZ1
Ultrasonography
Elbow
Left BP4HZZ1
Right BP4GZZ1
Hand
Left BP4PZZ1
Right BP4NZZ1
Shoulder
Left BP49ZZ1
Right BP48ZZ1

Densitometry—continued
Ultrasonography—continued
Wrist
Left BP4MZZ1
Right BP4LZZ1
Dentate ligament use Dura Mater
Denticulate ligament use Spinal Cord
Depressor anguli oris muscle use Muscle, Facial
Depressor labii inferioris muscle use Muscle, Facial
Depressor septi nasi muscle use Muscle, Facial
Depressor supercilii muscle use Muscle, Facial
Dermabrasion see Extraction, Skin and Breast ØHD
Dermis use Skin
Descending genicular artery
use Artery, Femoral, Right
use Artery, Femoral, Left
Destruction
Acetabulum
Left ØQ55
Right ØQ54
Adenoids ØC5Q
Ampulla of Vater ØF5C
Anal Sphincter ØD5R
Anterior Chamber
Left Ø8533ZZ
Right Ø8523ZZ
Anus ØD5Q
Aorta
Abdominal Ø45Ø
Thoracic Ø25W
Aortic Body ØG5D
Appendix ØD5J
Artery
Anterior Tibial
Left Ø45Q
Right Ø45P
Axillary
Left Ø356
Right Ø355
Brachial
Left Ø358
Right Ø357
Celiac Ø451
Colic
Left Ø457
Middle Ø458
Right Ø456
Common Carotid
Left Ø35J
Right Ø35H
Common Iliac
Left Ø45D
Right Ø45C
External Carotid
Left Ø35N
Right Ø35M
External Iliac
Left Ø45J
Right Ø45H
Face Ø35R
Femoral
Left Ø45L
Right Ø45K
Foot
Left Ø45W
Right Ø45V
Gastric Ø452
Hand
Left Ø35F
Right Ø35D
Hepatic Ø453
Inferior Mesenteric Ø45B
Innominate Ø352
Internal Carotid
Left Ø35L
Right Ø35K
Internal Iliac
Left Ø45F
Right Ø45E
Internal Mammary
Left Ø351
Right Ø35Ø
Intracranial Ø35G

Destruction—*continued*
  Muscle—*continued*
    Upper Leg—*continued*
      Right ØK5Q
  Nasopharynx Ø95N
  Nerve
    Abdominal Sympathetic Ø15M
    Abducens ØØ5L
    Accessory ØØ5R
    Acoustic ØØ5N
    Brachial Plexus Ø153
    Cervical Ø151
    Cervical Plexus Ø150
    Facial ØØ5M
    Femoral Ø15D
    Glossopharyngeal ØØ5P
    Head and Neck Sympathetic Ø15K
    Hypoglossal ØØ5S
    Lumbar Ø15B
    Lumbar Plexus Ø159
    Lumbar Sympathetic Ø15N
    Lumbosacral Plexus Ø15A
    Median Ø155
    Oculomotor ØØ5H
    Olfactory ØØ5F
    Optic ØØ5G
    Peroneal Ø15H
    Phrenic Ø152
    Pudendal Ø15C
    Radial Ø156
    Sacral Ø15R
    Sacral Plexus Ø15Q
    Sacral Sympathetic Ø15P
    Sciatic Ø15F
    Thoracic Ø158
    Thoracic Sympathetic Ø15L
    Tibial Ø15G
    Trigeminal ØØ5K
    Trochlear ØØ5J
    Ulnar Ø154
    Vagus ØØ5Q
  Nipple
    Left ØH5X
    Right ØH5W
  Nose Ø95K
  Omentum
    Greater ØD5S
    Lesser ØD5T
  Orbit
    Left ØN5Q
    Right ØN5P
  Ovary
    Bilateral ØU52
    Left ØU51
    Right ØU50
  Palate
    Hard ØC52
    Soft ØC53
  Pancreas ØF5G
  Para-aortic Body ØG59
  Paraganglion Extremity ØG5F
  Parathyroid Gland ØG5R
    Inferior
      Left ØG5P
      Right ØG5N
    Multiple ØG5Q
    Superior
      Left ØG5M
      Right ØG5L
  Patella
    Left ØQ5F
    Right ØQ5D
  Penis ØV5S
  Pericardium Ø25N
  Peritoneum ØD5W
  Phalanx
    Finger
      Left ØP5V
      Right ØP5T
    Thumb
      Left ØP5S
      Right ØP5R

Destruction—*continued*
  Phalanx—*continued*
    Toe
      Left ØQ5R
      Right ØQ5Q
  Pharynx ØC5M
  Pineal Body ØG51
  Pleura
    Left ØB5P
    Right ØB5N
  Pons ØØ5B
  Prepuce ØV5T
  Prostate ØV50
  Radius
    Left ØP5J
    Right ØP5H
  Rectum ØD5P
  Retina
    Left Ø85F3ZZ
    Right Ø85E3ZZ
  Retinal Vessel
    Left Ø85H3ZZ
    Right Ø85G3ZZ
  Rib
    Left ØP52
    Right ØP51
  Sacrum ØQ51
  Scapula
    Left ØP56
    Right ØP55
  Sclera
    Left Ø857XZZ
    Right Ø856XZZ
  Scrotum ØV55
  Septum
    Atrial Ø255
    Nasal Ø95M
    Ventricular Ø25M
  Sinus
    Accessory Ø95P
    Ethmoid
      Left Ø95V
      Right Ø95U
    Frontal
      Left Ø95T
      Right Ø95S
    Mastoid
      Left Ø95C
      Right Ø95B
    Maxillary
      Left Ø95R
      Right Ø95Q
    Sphenoid
      Left Ø95X
      Right Ø95W
  Skin
    Abdomen ØH57XZ
    Back ØH56XZ
    Buttock ØH58XZ
    Chest ØH55XZ
    Ear
      Left ØH53XZ
      Right ØH52XZ
    Face ØH51XZ
    Foot
      Left ØH5NXZ
      Right ØH5MXZ
    Genitalia ØH5AXZ
    Hand
      Left ØH5GXZ
      Right ØH5FXZ
    Lower Arm
      Left ØH5EXZ
      Right ØH5DXZ
    Lower Leg
      Left ØH5LXZ
      Right ØH5KXZ
    Neck ØH54XZ
    Perineum ØH59XZ
    Scalp ØH50XZ
    Upper Arm
      Left ØH5CXZ
      Right ØH5BXZ

Destruction—*continued*
  Skin—*continued*
    Upper Leg
      Left ØH5JXZ
      Right ØH5HXZ
  Skull ØN50
  Spinal Cord
    Cervical ØØ5W
    Lumbar ØØ5Y
    Thoracic ØØ5X
  Spinal Meninges ØØ5T
  Spleen Ø75P
  Sternum ØP50
  Stomach ØD56
    Pylorus ØD57
  Subcutaneous Tissue and Fascia
    Abdomen ØJ58
    Back ØJ57
    Buttock ØJ59
    Chest ØJ56
    Face ØJ51
    Foot
      Left ØJ5R
      Right ØJ5Q
    Hand
      Left ØJ5K
      Right ØJ5J
    Lower Arm
      Left ØJ5H
      Right ØJ5G
    Lower Leg
      Left ØJ5P
      Right ØJ5N
    Neck
      Anterior ØJ54
      Posterior ØJ55
    Pelvic Region ØJ5C
    Perineum ØJ5B
    Scalp ØJ50
    Upper Arm
      Left ØJ5F
      Right ØJ5D
    Upper Leg
      Left ØJ5M
      Right ØJ5L
  Tarsal
    Left ØQ5M
    Right ØQ5L
  Tendon
    Abdomen
      Left ØL5G
      Right ØL5F
    Ankle
      Left ØL5T
      Right ØL5S
    Foot
      Left ØL5W
      Right ØL5V
    Hand
      Left ØL58
      Right ØL57
    Head and Neck ØL50
    Hip
      Left ØL5K
      Right ØL5J
    Knee
      Left ØL5R
      Right ØL5Q
    Lower Arm and Wrist
      Left ØL56
      Right ØL55
    Lower Leg
      Left ØL5P
      Right ØL5N
    Perineum ØL5H
    Shoulder
      Left ØL52
      Right ØL51
    Thorax
      Left ØL5D
      Right ØL5C

Dilation—*continued*
  Vein—*continued*
    Renal
      Left 067B
      Right 0679
    Splenic 0671
    Subclavian
      Left 0576
      Right 0575
    Superior Mesenteric 0675
    Upper 057Y
    Vertebral
      Left 057S
      Right 057R
  Vena Cava
    Inferior 0670
    Superior 027V
  Ventricle, Right 027K

Disarticulation *see* Detachment

Discectomy, diskectomy
  see Excision, Upper Joints 0RB
  see Resection, Upper Joints 0RT
  see Excision, Lower Joints 0SB
  see Resection, Lower Joints 0ST

Discography
  see Plain Radiography, Axial Skeleton, Except Skull and Facial Bones BR0
  see Fluoroscopy, Axial Skeleton, Except Skull and Facial Bones BR1

Distal radioulnar joint
  use Joint, Wrist, Right
  use Joint, Wrist, Left

Diversion *see* Bypass

Diverticulectomy *see* Excision, Gastrointestinal System 0DB

Division
  Acetabulum
    Left 0Q85
    Right 0Q84
  Anal Sphincter 0D8R
  Basal Ganglia 0088
  Bladder Neck 0T8C
  Bone
    Ethmoid
      Left 0N8G
      Right 0N8F
    Frontal
      Left 0N82
      Right 0N81
    Hyoid 0N8X
    Lacrimal
      Left 0N8J
      Right 0N8H
    Nasal 0N8B
    Occipital
      Left 0N88
      Right 0N87
    Palatine
      Left 0N8L
      Right 0N8K
    Parietal
      Left 0N84
      Right 0N83
    Pelvic
      Left 0Q83
      Right 0Q82
    Sphenoid
      Left 0N8D
      Right 0N8C
    Temporal
      Left 0N86
      Right 0N85
    Zygomatic
      Left 0N8N
      Right 0N8M
  Brain 0080
  Bursa and Ligament
    Abdomen
      Left 0M8J
      Right 0M8H
    Ankle
      Left 0M8R
      Right 0M8Q

Division
  Bursa and Ligament—*continued*
    Elbow
      Left 0M84
      Right 0M83
    Foot
      Left 0M8T
      Right 0M8S
    Hand
      Left 0M88
      Right 0M87
    Head and Neck 0M80
    Hip
      Left 0M8M
      Right 0M8L
    Knee
      Left 0M8P
      Right 0M8N
    Lower Extremity
      Left 0M8W
      Right 0M8V
    Perineum 0M8K
    Shoulder
      Left 0M82
      Right 0M81
    Thorax
      Left 0M8G
      Right 0M8F
    Trunk
      Left 0M8D
      Right 0M8C
    Upper Extremity
      Left 0M8B
      Right 0M89
    Wrist
      Left 0M86
      Right 0M85
  Carpal
    Left 0P8N
    Right 0P8M
  Cerebral Hemisphere 0087
  Chordae Tendineae 0289
  Clavicle
    Left 0P8B
    Right 0P89
  Coccyx 0Q8S
  Conduction Mechanism 0288
  Esophagogastric Junction 0D84
  Femoral Shaft
    Left 0Q89
    Right 0Q88
  Femur
    Lower
      Left 0Q8C
      Right 0Q8B
    Upper
      Left 0Q87
      Right 0Q86
  Fibula
    Left 0Q8K
    Right 0Q8J
  Gland, Pituitary 0G80
  Glenoid Cavity
    Left 0P88
    Right 0P87
  Humeral Head
    Left 0P8D
    Right 0P8C
  Humeral Shaft
    Left 0P8G
    Right 0P8F
  Hymen 0U8K
  Kidneys, Bilateral 0T82
  Mandible
    Left 0N8V
    Right 0N8T
  Maxilla
    Left 0N8S
    Right 0N8R
  Metacarpal
    Left 0P8Q
    Right 0P8P

Division—*continued*
  Metatarsal
    Left 0Q8P
    Right 0Q8N
  Muscle
    Abdomen
      Left 0K8L
      Right 0K8K
    Facial 0K81
    Foot
      Left 0K8W
      Right 0K8V
    Hand
      Left 0K8D
      Right 0K8C
    Head 0K80
    Hip
      Left 0K8P
      Right 0K8N
    Lower Arm and Wrist
      Left 0K8B
      Right 0K89
    Lower Leg
      Left 0K8T
      Right 0K8S
    Neck
      Left 0K83
      Right 0K82
    Papillary 028D
    Perineum 0K8M
    Shoulder
      Left 0K86
      Right 0K85
    Thorax
      Left 0K8J
      Right 0K8H
    Tongue, Palate, Pharynx 0K84
    Trunk
      Left 0K8G
      Right 0K8F
    Upper Arm
      Left 0K88
      Right 0K87
    Upper Leg
      Left 0K8R
      Right 0K8Q
  Nerve
    Abdominal Sympathetic 018M
    Abducens 008L
    Accessory 008R
    Acoustic 008N
    Brachial Plexus 0183
    Cervical 0181
    Cervical Plexus 0180
    Facial 008M
    Femoral 018D
    Glossopharyngeal 008P
    Head and Neck Sympathetic 018K
    Hypoglossal 008S
    Lumbar 018B
    Lumbar Plexus 0189
    Lumbar Sympathetic 018N
    Lumbosacral Plexus 018A
    Median 0185
    Oculomotor 008H
    Olfactory 008F
    Optic 008G
    Peroneal 018H
    Phrenic 0182
    Pudendal 018C
    Radial 0186
    Sacral 018R
    Sacral Plexus 018Q
    Sacral Sympathetic 018P
    Sciatic 018F
    Thoracic 0188
    Thoracic Sympathetic 018L
    Tibial 018G
    Trigeminal 008K
    Trochlear 008J
    Ulnar 0184
    Vagus 008Q

Division—*continued*
  Orbit
    Left ØN8Q
    Right ØN8P
  Ovary
    Bilateral ØU82
    Left ØU81
    Right ØU8Ø
  Pancreas ØF8G
  Patella
    Left ØQ8F
    Right ØQ8D
  Perineum, Female ØW8NXZZ
  Phalanx
    Finger
      Left ØP8V
      Right ØP8T
    Thumb
      Left ØP8S
      Right ØP8R
    Toe
      Left ØQ8R
      Right ØQ8Q
  Radius
    Left ØP8J
    Right ØP8H
  Rib
    Left ØP82
    Right ØP81
  Sacrum ØQ81
  Scapula
    Left ØP86
    Right ØP85
  Skin
    Abdomen ØH87XZZ
    Back ØH86XZZ
    Buttock ØH88XZZ
    Chest ØH85XZZ
    Ear
      Left ØH83XZZ
      Right ØH82XZZ
    Face ØH81XZZ
    Foot
      Left ØH8NXZZ
      Right ØH8MXZZ
    Genitalia ØH8AXZZ
    Hand
      Left ØH8GXZZ
      Right ØH8FXZZ
    Lower Arm
      Left ØH8EXZZ
      Right ØH8DXZZ
    Lower Leg
      Left ØH8LXZZ
      Right ØH8KXZZ
    Neck ØH84XZZ
    Perineum ØH89XZZ
    Scalp ØH8ØXZZ
    Upper Arm
      Left ØH8CXZZ
      Right ØH8BXZZ
    Upper Leg
      Left ØH8JXZZ
      Right ØH8HXZZ
  Skull ØN8Ø
  Spinal Cord
    Cervical ØØ8W
    Lumbar ØØ8Y
    Thoracic ØØ8X
  Sternum ØP8Ø
  Subcutaneous Tissue and Fascia
    Abdomen ØJ88
    Back ØJ87
    Buttock ØJ89
    Chest ØJ86
    Face ØJ81
    Foot
      Left ØJ8R
      Right ØJ8Q
    Hand
      Left ØJ8K
      Right ØJ8J
    Head and Neck ØJ8S

Division—*continued*
  Subcutaneous Tissue and Fascia—*continued*
    Lower Arm
      Left ØJ8H
      Right ØJ8G
    Lower Extremity ØJ8W
    Lower Leg
      Left ØJ8P
      Right ØJ8N
    Neck
      Anterior ØJ84
      Posterior ØJ85
    Pelvic Region ØJ8C
    Perineum ØJ8B
    Scalp ØJ8Ø
    Trunk ØJ8T
    Upper Arm
      Left ØJ8F
      Right ØJ8D
    Upper Extremity ØJ8V
    Upper Leg
      Left ØJ8M
      Right ØJ8L
  Tarsal
    Left ØQ8M
    Right ØQ8L
  Tendon
    Abdomen
      Left ØL8G
      Right ØL8F
    Ankle
      Left ØL8T
      Right ØL8S
    Foot
      Left ØL8W
      Right ØL8V
    Hand
      Left ØL88
      Right ØL87
    Head and Neck ØL8Ø
    Hip
      Left ØL8K
      Right ØL8J
    Knee
      Left ØL8R
      Right ØL8Q
    Lower Arm and Wrist
      Left ØL86
      Right ØL85
    Lower Leg
      Left ØL8P
      Right ØL8N
    Perineum ØL8H
    Shoulder
      Left ØL82
      Right ØL81
    Thorax
      Left ØL8D
      Right ØL8C
    Trunk
      Left ØL8B
      Right ØL89
    Upper Arm
      Left ØL84
      Right ØL83
    Upper Leg
      Left ØL8M
      Right ØL8L
  Thyroid Gland Isthmus ØG8J
  Tibia
    Left ØQ8H
    Right ØQ8G
  Turbinate, Nasal Ø98L
  Ulna
    Left ØP8L
    Right ØP8K
  Uterine Supporting Structure ØU84
  Vertebra
    Cervical ØP83
    Lumbar ØQ8Ø
    Thoracic ØP84
Doppler study *see* Ultrasonography
Dorsal digital nerve *use* Nerve, Radial

Dorsal metacarpal vein
  use Vein, Hand, Left
  use Vein, Hand, Right
Dorsal metatarsal artery
  use Artery, Foot, Left
  use Artery, Foot, Right
Dorsal metatarsal vein
  use Vein, Foot, Right
  use Vein, Foot, Left
Dorsal scapular artery
  use Artery, Subclavian, Right
  use Artery, Subclavian, Left
Dorsal scapular nerve *use* Nerve, Brachial Plexus
Dorsal venous arch
  use Vein, Foot, Right
  use Vein, Foot, Left
Dorsalis pedis artery
  use Artery, Anterior Tibial, Right
  use Artery, Anterior Tibial, Left
Drainage
  Abdominal Wall ØW9F
  Acetabulum
    Left ØQ95
    Right ØQ94
  Adenoids ØC9Q
  Ampulla of Vater ØF9C
  Anal Sphincter ØD9R
  Ankle Region
    Left ØY9L
    Right ØY9K
  Anterior Chamber
    Left Ø893
    Right Ø892
  Anus ØD9Q
  Aorta, Abdominal Ø49Ø
  Aortic Body ØG9D
  Appendix ØD9J
  Arm
    Lower
      Left ØX9F
      Right ØX9D
    Upper
      Left ØX99
      Right X98
  Artery
    Anterior Tibial
      Left Ø49Q
      Right Ø49P
    Axillary
      Left Ø396
      Right Ø395
    Brachial
      Left Ø398
      Right Ø397
    Celiac Ø491
    Colic
      Left Ø497
      Middle Ø498
      Right Ø496
    Common Carotid
      Left Ø39J
      Right Ø39H
    Common Iliac
      Left Ø49D
      Right Ø49C
    External Carotid
      Left Ø39N
      Right Ø39M
    External Iliac
      Left Ø49J
      Right Ø49H
    Face Ø39R
    Femoral
      Left Ø49L
      Right Ø49K
    Foot
      Left Ø49W
      Right Ø49V
    Gastric Ø492
    Hand
      Left Ø39F
      Right Ø39D
    Hepatic Ø493

Dressing—*continued*
  Leg
    Lower
      Left 2W2RX4Z
      Right 2W2QX4Z
    Upper
      Left 2W2PX4Z
      Right 2W2NX4Z
  Neck 2W22X4Z
  Thumb
    Left 2W2HX4Z
    Right 2W2GX4Z
  Toe
    Left 2W2VX4Z
    Right 2W2UX4Z
Drotrecogin alfa *see* Introduction, Recombinant Human-activated Protein C
Duct of Santorini *use* Duct, Pancreatic, Accessory
Duct of Wirsung *use* Duct, Pancreatic
Ductogram, mammary *see* Plain Radiography, Skin, Subcutaneous Tissue and Breast BHØ
Ductography, mammary *see* Plain Radiography, Skin, Subcutaneous Tissue and Breast BHØ
Ductus deferens
  use Vas Deferens, Left
  use Vas Deferens, Right
  use Vas Deferens
  use Vas Deferens, Bilateral
Duodenal ampulla *use* Ampulla of Vater
Duodenectomy
  see Excision, Duodenum ØDB9
  see Resection, Duodenum ØDT9
Duodenocholedochotomy *see* Drainage, Gallbladder ØF94
Duodenocystostomy
  see Bypass, Gallbladder ØF14
  see Drainage, Gallbladder ØF94
Duodenoenterostomy
  see Bypass, Gastrointestinal System ØD1
  see Drainage, Gastrointestinal System ØD9
Duodenojejunal flexure *use* Jejunum
Duodenolysis *see* Release, Duodenum ØDN9
Duodenorrhaphy *see* Repair, Duodenum ØDQ9
Duodenostomy
  see Bypass, Duodenum ØD19
  see Drainage, Duodenum ØD99
Duodenotomy *see* Drainage, Duodenum ØD99
Dural venous sinus *use* Vein, Intracranial

E

Earlobe
  use Ear, External, Bilateral
  use Ear, External, Left
  use Ear, External, Right
Echocardiogram *see* Ultrasonography, Heart B24
Echography *see* Ultrasonography
ECMO *see* Performance, Circulatory 5A15
EEG (electroencephalogram) *see* Measurement, Central Nervous 4A00
EGD (esophagogastroduodenoscopy) ØDJ08ZZ
Eighth cranial nerve *use* Nerve, Acoustic
Ejaculatory duct
  use Vas Deferens, Bilateral
  use Vas Deferens, Left
  use Vas Deferens, Right
  use Vas Deferens
EKG (electrocardiogram) *see* Measurement, Cardiac 4A02
Electrocautery
  Destruction *see* Destruction
  Repair *see* Repair
Electroconvulsive Therapy
  Bilateral-Multiple Seizure GZB3ZZZ
  Bilateral-Single Seizure GZB2ZZZ
  Electroconvulsive Therapy, Other GZB4ZZZ
  Unilateral-Multiple Seizure GZB1ZZZ
  Unilateral-Single Seizure GZB0ZZZ
Electroencephalogram (EEG) *see* Measurement, Central Nervous 4A00

Electromagnetic Therapy
  Central Nervous 6A22
  Urinary 6A21
Electrophysiologic stimulation (EPS) *see* Measurement, Cardiac 4A02
Electroshock therapy *see* Electroconvulsive Therapy
Elevation, bone fragments, skull *see* Reposition, Head and Facial Bones ØNS
Eleventh cranial nerve *use* Nerve, Accessory
Embolectomy *see* Extirpation
Embolization *see* Occlusion
EMG (electromyogram) *see* Measurement, Musculoskeletal 4A0F
Encephalon *use* Brain
Endarterectomy
  see Extirpation, Upper Arteries Ø3C
  see Extirpation, Lower Arteries Ø4C
Endobronchial Valve
  Insertion of device in
    Lingula ØBH9
    Lower Lobe
      Left ØBHB
      Right ØBH6
    Main
      Left ØBH7
      Right ØBH3
    Middle Lobe, Right ØBH5
    Upper Lobe
      Left ØBH8
      Right ØBH4
  Removal of device from, Tracheobronchial Tree ØBPØ
  Revision of device in, Tracheobronchial Tree ØBWØ
Endotracheal Airway
  Change device in, Trachea ØB21XEZ
  Insertion of device in, Trachea ØBH1
  Removal of device from, Trachea ØBP1
  Revision of device in, Trachea ØBW1
Enlargement
  see Dilation
  see Repair
Enterorrhaphy *see* Repair, Gastrointestinal System ØDQ
Enucleation
  Eyeball *see* Resection, Eye Ø8T
  Eyeball with prosthetic implant *see* Replacement, Eye Ø8R
Ependyma *use* Cerebral Ventricle
Epidermis *use* Skin
Epididymectomy
  see Excision, Male Reproductive System ØVB
  see Resection, Male Reproductive System ØVT
Epididymoplasty
  see Repair, Male Reproductive System ØVQ
  see Supplement, Male Reproductive System ØVU
Epididymorrhaphy *see* Repair, Male Reproductive System ØVQ
Epididymotomy *see* Drainage, Male Reproductive System ØV9
Epiphysiodesis
  see Fusion, Upper Joints ØRG
  see Fusion, Lower Joints ØSG
Epiploic foramen *use* Peritoneum
Episiorrhaphy *see* Repair, Perineum, Female ØWQN
Episiotomy *see* Division, Perineum, Female ØW8N
Epithalamus *use* Thalamus
Epitrochlear lymph node
  use Lymphatic, Upper Extremity, Left
  use Lymphatic, Upper Extremity, Right
EPS (electrophysiologic stimulation) *see* Measurement, Cardiac 4A02
Eptifibatide, infusion *see* Introduction, Platelet Inhibitor
ERCP (endoscopic retrograde cholangiopancreatography) *see* Fluoroscopy, Hepatobiliary System and Pancreas BF1
Erector spinae muscle
  use Muscle, Trunk, Left
  use Muscle, Trunk, Right
Esophageal artery *use* Aorta, Thoracic
Esophageal plexus *use* Nerve, Thoracic Sympathetic
Esophagectomy
  see Excision, Gastrointestinal System ØDB
  see Resection, Gastrointestinal System ØDT

Esophagocoloplasty
  see Repair, Gastrointestinal System ØDQ
  see Supplement, Gastrointestinal System ØDU
Esophagoenterostomy
  see Bypass, Gastrointestinal System ØD1
  see Drainage, Gastrointestinal System ØD9
Esophagoesophagostomy
  see Bypass, Gastrointestinal System ØD1
  see Drainage, Gastrointestinal System ØD9
Esophagogastrectomy
  see Excision, Gastrointestinal System ØDB
  see Resection, Gastrointestinal System ØDT
Esophagogastroplasty
  see Repair, Gastrointestinal System ØDQ
  see Supplement, Gastrointestinal System ØDU
Esophagogastroscopy ØDJ68ZZ
Esophagogastrostomy
  see Bypass, Gastrointestinal System ØD1
  see Drainage, Gastrointestinal System ØD9
Esophagojejunoplasty *see* Supplement, Gastrointestinal System ØDU
Esophagojejunostomy
  see Drainage, Gastrointestinal System ØD9
  see Bypass, Gastrointestinal System ØD1
Esophagomyotomy *see* Division, Esophagogastric Junction ØD84
Esophagoplasty
  see Repair, Gastrointestinal System ØDQ
  see Replacement, Esophagus ØDR5
  see Supplement, Gastrointestinal System ØDU
Esophagoplication *see* Restriction, Gastrointestinal System ØDV
Esophagorrhaphy *see* Repair, Gastrointestinal System ØDQ
Esophagoscopy ØDJ08ZZ
Esophagotomy *see* Drainage, Gastrointestinal System ØD9
ESWL (extracorporeal shock wave lithotripsy) *see* Fragmentation
Ethmoidal air cell
  use Sinus, Ethmoid, Left
  use Sinus, Ethmoid, Right
Ethmoidectomy
  see Excision, Ear, Nose, Sinus Ø9B
  see Resection, Ear, Nose, Sinus Ø9T
  see Excision, Head and Facial Bones ØNB
  see Resection, Head and Facial Bones ØNT
Ethmoidotomy *see* Drainage, Ear, Nose, Sinus Ø99
Evacuation
  Hematoma *see* Extirpation
  Other Fluid *see* Drainage
Evisceration
  Eyeball *see* Resection, Eye Ø8T
  Eyeball with prosthetic implant *see* Replacement, Eye Ø8R
Examination *see* Inspection
Exchange *see* Change device in
Excision
  Abdominal Wall ØWBF
  Acetabulum
    Left ØQB5
    Right ØQB4
  Adenoids ØCBQ
  Ampulla of Vater ØFBC
  Anal Sphincter ØDBR
  Ankle Region
    Left ØYBL
    Right ØYBK
  Anus ØDBQ
  Aorta
    Abdominal Ø4BØ
    Thoracic Ø2BW
  Aortic Body ØGBD
  Appendix ØDBJ
  Arm
    Lower
      Left ØXBF
      Right ØXBD
    Upper
      Left ØXB9
      Right ØXB8
  Artery
    Anterior Tibial

Excision—*continued*
  Diaphragm
    Left 0BBS
    Right 0BBR
  Disc
    Cervical Vertebral 0RB3
    Cervicothoracic Vertebral 0RB5
    Lumbar Vertebral 0SB2
    Lumbosacral 0SB4
    Thoracic Vertebral 0RB9
    Thoracolumbar Vertebral 0RBB
  Duct
    Common Bile 0FB9
    Cystic 0FB8
    Hepatic
      Left 0FB6
      Right 0FB5
    Lacrimal
      Left 08BY
      Right 08BX
    Pancreatic 0FBD
      Accessory 0FBF
    Parotid
      Left 0CBC
      Right 0CBB
  Duodenum 0DB9
  Dura Mater 00B2
  Ear
    External
      Left 09B1
      Right 09B0
    External Auditory Canal
      Left 09B4
      Right 09B3
    Inner
      Left 09BE0Z
      Right 09BD0Z
    Middle
      Left 09B60Z
      Right 09B50Z
  Elbow Region
    Left 0XBC
    Right 0XBB
  Epididymis
    Bilateral 0VBL
    Left 0VBK
    Right 0VBJ
  Epiglottis 0CBR
  Esophagogastric Junction 0DB4
  Esophagus 0DB5
    Lower 0DB3
    Middle 0DB2
    Upper 0DB1
  Eustachian Tube
    Left 09BG
    Right 09BF
  Extremity
    Lower
      Left 0YBB
      Right 0YB9
    Upper
      Left 0XB7
      Right 0XB6
  Eye
    Left 08B1
    Right 08B0
  Eyelid
    Lower
      Left 08BR
      Right 08BQ
    Upper
      Left 08BP
      Right 08BN
  Face 0WB2
  Fallopian Tube
    Left 0UB6
    Right 0UB5
  Fallopian Tubes, Bilateral 0UB7
  Femoral Region
    Left 0YB8
    Right 0YB7
  Femoral Shaft
    Left 0QB9

Excision—*continued*
  Femoral Shaft—*continued*
    Right 0QB8
  Femur
    Lower
      Left 0QBC
      Right 0QBB
    Upper
      Left 0QB7
      Right 0QB6
  Fibula
    Left 0QBK
    Right 0QBJ
  Finger Nail 0HBQXZ
  Foot
    Left 0YBN
    Right 0YBM
  Gallbladder 0FB4
  Gingiva
    Lower 0CB6
    Upper 0CB5
  Gland
    Adrenal
      Bilateral 0GB4
      Left 0GB2
      Right 0GB3
    Lacrimal
      Left 08BW
      Right 08BV
    Minor Salivary 0CBJ
    Parotid
      Left 0CB9
      Right 0CB8
    Pituitary 0GB0
    Sublingual
      Left 0CBF
      Right 0CBD
    Submaxillary
      Left 0CBH
      Right 0CBG
    Vestibular 0UBL
  Glenoid Cavity
    Left 0PB8
    Right 0PB7
  Glomus Jugulare 0GBC
  Hand
    Left 0XBK
    Right 0XBJ
  Head 0WB0
  Humeral Head
    Left 0PBD
    Right 0PBC
  Humeral Shaft
    Left 0PBG
    Right 0PBF
  Hymen 0UBK
  Hypothalamus 00BA
  Ileocecal Valve 0DBC
  Ileum 0DBB
  Inguinal Region
    Left 0YB6
    Right 0YB5
  Intestine
    Large 0DBE
    Left 0DBG
    Right 0DBF
    Small 0DB8
  Iris
    Left 08BD3Z
    Right 08BC3Z
  Jaw
    Lower 0WB5
    Upper 0WB4
  Jejunum 0DBA
  Joint
    Acromioclavicular
      Left 0RBH
      Right 0RBG
    Ankle
      Left 0SBG
      Right 0SBF
    Carpal
      Left 0RBR

Excision—*continued*
  Joint—*continued*
    Carpal—*continued*
      Right 0RBQ
    Cervical Vertebral 0RB1
    Cervicothoracic Vertebral 0RB4
    Coccygeal 0SB6
    Elbow
      Left 0RBM
      Right 0RBL
    Finger Phalangeal
      Left 0RBX
      Right 0RBW
    Hip
      Left 0SBB
      Right 0SB9
    Knee
      Left 0SBD
      Right 0SBC
    Lumbar Vertebral 0SB0
    Lumbosacral 0SB3
    Metacarpocarpal
      Left 0RBT
      Right 0RBS
    Metacarpophalangeal
      Left 0RBV
      Right 0RBU
    Metatarsal-Phalangeal
      Left 0SBN
      Right 0SBM
    Metatarsal-Tarsal
      Left 0SBL
      Right 0SBK
    Occipital-cervical 0RB0
    Sacrococcygeal 0SB5
    Sacroiliac
      Left 0SB8
      Right 0SB7
    Shoulder
      Left 0RBK
      Right 0RBJ
    Sternoclavicular
      Left 0RBF
      Right 0RBE
    Tarsal
      Left 0SBJ
      Right 0SBH
    Temporomandibular
      Left 0RBD
      Right 0RBC
    Thoracic Vertebral 0RB6
    Thoracolumbar Vertebral 0RBA
    Toe Phalangeal
      Left 0SBQ
      Right 0SBP
    Wrist
      Left 0RBP
      Right 0RBN
  Kidney
    Left 0TB1
    Right 0TB0
  Kidney Pelvis
    Left 0TB4
    Right 0TB3
  Knee Region
    Left 0YBG
    Right 0YBF
  Larynx 0CBS
  Leg
    Lower
      Left 0YBJ
      Right 0YBH
    Upper
      Left 0YBD
      Right 0YBC
  Lens
    Left 08BK3Z
    Right 08BJ3Z
  Lip
    Lower 0CB1
    Upper 0CB0

Excision—Excision

Excision—*continued*
  Skin—*continued*
    Face ØHB1XZ
    Foot
      Left ØHBNXZ
      Right ØHBMXZ
    Genitalia ØHBAXZ
    Hand
      Left ØHBGXZ
      Right ØHBFXZ
    Lower Arm
      Left ØHBEXZ
      Right ØHBDXZ
    Lower Leg
      Left ØHBLXZ
      Right ØHBKXZ
    Neck ØHB4XZ
    Perineum ØHB9XZ
    Scalp ØHBØXZ
    Upper Arm
      Left ØHBCXZ
      Right ØHBBXZ
    Upper Leg
      Left ØHBJXZ
      Right ØHBHXZ
  Skull ØNBØ
  Spinal Cord
    Cervical ØØBW
    Lumbar ØØBY
    Thoracic ØØBX
  Spinal Meninges ØØBT
  Spleen Ø7BP
  Sternum ØPBØ
  Stomach ØDB6
    Pylorus ØDB7
  Subcutaneous Tissue and Fascia
    Abdomen ØJB8
    Back ØJB7
    Buttock ØJB9
    Chest ØJB6
    Face ØJB1
    Foot
      Left ØJBR
      Right ØJBQ
    Hand
      Left ØJBK
      Right ØJBJ
    Lower Arm
      Left ØJBH
      Right ØJBG
    Lower Leg
      Left ØJBP
      Right ØJBN
    Neck
      Anterior ØJB4
      Posterior ØJB5
    Pelvic Region ØJBC
    Perineum ØJBB
    Scalp ØJBØ
    Upper Arm
      Left ØJBF
      Right ØJBD
    Upper Leg
      Left ØJBM
      Right ØJBL
  Tarsal
    Left ØQBM
    Right ØQBL
  Tendon
    Abdomen
      Left ØLBG
      Right ØLBF
    Ankle
      Left ØLBT
      Right ØLBS
    Foot
      Left ØLBW
      Right ØLBV
    Hand
      Left ØLB8
      Right ØLB7
    Head and Neck ØLBØ

Excision—*continued*
  Tendon—*continued*
    Hip
      Left ØLBK
      Right ØLBJ
    Knee
      Left ØLBR
      Right ØLBQ
    Lower Arm and Wrist
      Left ØLB6
      Right ØLB5
    Lower Leg
      Left ØLBP
      Right ØLBN
    Perineum ØLBH
    Shoulder
      Left ØLB2
      Right ØLB1
    Thorax
      Left ØLBD
      Right ØLBC
    Trunk
      Left ØLBB
      Right ØLB9
    Upper Arm
      Left ØLB4
      Right ØLB3
    Upper Leg
      Left ØLBM
      Right ØLBL
  Testis
    Bilateral ØVBC
    Left ØVBB
    Right ØVB9
  Thalamus ØØB9
  Thymus Ø7BM
  Thyroid Gland
    Left Lobe ØGBG
    Right Lobe ØGBH
  Tibia
    Left ØQBH
    Right ØQBG
  Toe Nail ØHBRXZ
  Tongue ØCB7
  Tonsils ØCBP
  Tooth
    Lower ØCBX
    Upper ØCBW
  Trachea ØBB1
  Tunica Vaginalis
    Left ØVB7
    Right ØVB6
  Turbinate, Nasal Ø9BL
  Tympanic Membrane
    Left Ø9B8
    Right Ø9B7
  Ulna
    Left ØPBL
    Right ØPBK
  Ureter
    Left ØTB7
    Right ØTB
  Urethra ØTBD
  Uterine Supporting Structure ØUB4
  Uterus ØUB9
  Uvula ØCBN
  Vagina ØUBG
  Valve
    Aortic Ø2BF
    Mitral Ø2BG
    Pulmonary Ø2BH
    Tricuspid Ø2BJ
  Vas Deferens
    Bilateral ØVBQ
    Left ØVBP
    Right ØVBN
  Vein
    Axillary
      Left Ø5B8
      Right Ø5B7
    Azygos Ø5BØ

Excision—*continued*
  Vein—*continued*
    Basilic
      Left Ø5BC
      Right Ø5BB
    Brachial
      Left Ø5BA
      Right Ø5B9
    Cephalic
      Left Ø5BF
      Right Ø5BD
    Colic Ø6B7
    Common Iliac
      Left Ø6BD
      Right Ø6BC
    Coronary Ø2B4
    Esophageal Ø6B3
    External Iliac
      Left Ø6BG
      Right Ø6BF
    External Jugular
      Left Ø5BQ
      Right Ø5BP
    Face
      Left Ø5BV
      Right Ø5BT
    Femoral
      Left Ø6BN
      Right Ø6BM
    Foot
      Left Ø6BV
      Right Ø6BT
    Gastric Ø6B2
    Greater Saphenous
      Left Ø6BQ
      Right Ø6BP
    Hand
      Left Ø5BH
      Right Ø5BG
    Hemiazygos Ø5B1
    Hepatic Ø6B4
    Hypogastric
      Left Ø6BJ
      Right Ø6BH
    Inferior Mesenteric Ø6B6
    Innominate
      Left Ø5B4
      Right Ø5B3
    Internal Jugular
      Left Ø5BN
      Right Ø5BM
    Intracranial Ø5BL
    Lesser Saphenous
      Left Ø6BS
      Right Ø6BR
    Lower Ø6BY
    Portal Ø6B8
    Pulmonary
      Left Ø2BT
      Right Ø2BS
    Renal
      Left Ø6BB
      Right Ø6B9
    Splenic Ø6B1
    Subclavian
      Left Ø5B6
      Right Ø5B5
    Superior Mesenteric Ø6B5
    Upper Ø5BY
    Vertebral
      Left Ø5BS
      Right Ø5BR
  Vena Cava
    Inferior Ø6BØ
    Superior Ø2BV
  Ventricle
    Left Ø2BL
    Right Ø2BK
  Vertebra
    Cervical ØPB3
    Lumbar ØQBØ
    Thoracic ØPB4

Excision—*continued*
- Vesicle
  - Bilateral ØVB3
  - Left ØVB2
  - Right ØVB1
- Vitreous
  - Left Ø8B53Z
  - Right Ø8B43Z
- Vocal Cord
  - Left ØCBV
  - Right ØCBT
- Vulva ØUBM
- Wrist Region
  - Left ØXBH
  - Right ØXBG

Exercise, rehabilitation *see* Motor Treatment, Rehabilitation FØ7

Exploration *see* Inspection

Extensor carpi radialis muscle
- *use* Muscle, Lower Arm and Wrist, Left
- *use* Muscle, Lower Arm and Wrist, Right

Extensor carpi ulnaris muscle
- *use* Muscle, Lower Arm and Wrist, Left
- *use* Muscle, Lower Arm and Wrist, Right

Extensor digitorum brevis muscle
- *use* Muscle, Foot, Right
- *use* Muscle, Foot, Left

Extensor digitorum longus muscle
- *use* Muscle, Lower Leg, Left
- *use* Muscle, Lower Leg, Right

Extensor hallucis brevis muscle
- *use* Muscle, Foot, Right
- *use* Muscle, Foot, Left

Extensor hallucis longus muscle
- *use* Muscle, Lower Leg, Right
- *use* Muscle, Lower Leg, Left

External anal sphincter *use* Anal Sphincter

External auditory meatus
- *use* Ear, External Auditory Canal, Left
- *use* Ear, External Auditory Canal, Right

External maxillary artery *use* Artery, Face

External naris *use* Nose

External oblique aponeurosis *use* Subcutaneous Tissue and Fascia, Trunk

External oblique muscle
- *use* Muscle, Abdomen, Left
- *use* Muscle, Abdomen, Right

External popliteal nerve *use* Nerve, Peroneal

External pudendal artery
- *use* Artery, Femoral, Right
- *use* Artery, Femoral, Left

External pudendal vein
- *use* Vein, Greater Saphenous, Right
- *use* Vein, Greater Saphenous, Left

External urethral sphincter *use* Urethra

Extirpation
- Acetabulum
  - Left ØQC5
  - Right ØQC4
- Adenoids ØCCQ
- Ampulla of Vater ØFCC
- Anal Sphincter ØDCR
- Anterior Chamber
  - Left Ø8C3
  - Right Ø8C2
- Anus ØDCQ
- Aorta
  - Abdominal Ø4CØ
  - Thoracic Ø2CW
- Aortic Body ØGCD
- Appendix ØDCJ
- Artery
  - Anterior Tibial
    - Left Ø4CQ
    - Right Ø4CP
  - Axillary
    - Left Ø3C6
    - Right Ø3C5
  - Brachial
    - Left Ø3C8
    - Right Ø3C7
  - Celiac Ø4C1

Extirpation—*continued*
- Artery—*continued*
  - Colic
    - Left Ø4C7
    - Middle Ø4C8
    - Right Ø4C6
  - Common Carotid
    - Left Ø3CJ
    - Right Ø3CH
  - Common Iliac
    - Left Ø4CD
    - Right Ø4CC
  - Coronary
    - Four or More Sites Ø2C3
    - One Site Ø2CØ
    - Three Sites Ø2C2
    - Two Sites Ø2C1
  - External Carotid
    - Left Ø3CN
    - Right Ø3CM
  - External Iliac
    - Left Ø4CJ
    - Right Ø4CH
  - Face Ø3CR
  - Femoral
    - Left Ø4CL
    - Right Ø4CK
  - Foot
    - Left Ø4CW
    - Right Ø4CV
  - Gastric Ø4C2
  - Hand
    - Left Ø3CF
    - Right Ø3CD
  - Hepatic Ø4C3
  - Inferior Mesenteric Ø4CB
  - Innominate Ø3C2
  - Internal Carotid
    - Left Ø3CL
    - Right Ø3CK
  - Internal Iliac
    - Left Ø4CF
    - Right Ø4CE
  - Internal Mammary
    - Left Ø3C1
    - Right Ø3CØ
  - Intracranial Ø3CG
  - Lower Ø4CY
  - Peroneal
    - Left Ø4CU
    - Right Ø4CT
  - Popliteal
    - Left Ø4CN
    - Right Ø4CM
  - Posterior Tibial
    - Left Ø4CS
    - Right Ø4CR
  - Pulmonary
    - Left Ø2CR
    - Right Ø2CQ
  - Pulmonary Trunk Ø2CP
  - Radial
    - Left Ø3CC
    - Right Ø3CB
  - Renal
    - Left Ø4CA
    - Right Ø4C9
  - Splenic Ø4C4
  - Subclavian
    - Left Ø3C4
    - Right Ø3C3
  - Superior Mesenteric Ø4C5
  - Temporal
    - Left Ø3CT
    - Right Ø3CS
  - Thyroid
    - Left Ø3CV
    - Right Ø3CU
  - Ulnar
    - Left Ø3CA
    - Right Ø3C9
  - Upper Ø3CY

Extirpation—*continued*
- Artery—*continued*
  - Vertebral
    - Left Ø3CQ
    - Right Ø3CP
- Atrium
  - Left Ø2C7
  - Right Ø2C6
- Auditory Ossicle
  - Left Ø9CAØZZ
  - Right Ø9C9ØZZ
- Basal Ganglia ØØC8
- Bladder ØTCB
- Bladder Neck ØTCC
- Bone
  - Ethmoid
    - Left ØNCG
    - Right ØNCF
  - Frontal
    - Left ØNC2
    - Right ØNC1
  - Hyoid ØNCX
  - Lacrimal
    - Left ØNCJ
    - Right ØNCH
  - Nasal ØNCB
  - Occipital
    - Left ØNC8
    - Right ØNC7
  - Palatine
    - Left ØNCL
    - Right ØNCK
  - Parietal
    - Left ØNC4
    - Right ØNC3
  - Pelvic
    - Left ØQC3
    - Right ØQC2
  - Sphenoid
    - Left ØNCD
    - Right ØNCC
  - Temporal
    - Left ØNC6
    - Right ØNC5
  - Zygomatic
    - Left ØNCN
    - Right ØNCM
- Brain ØØCØ
- Breast
  - Bilateral ØHCV
  - Left ØHCU
  - Right ØHCT
- Bronchus
  - Lingula ØBC9
  - Lower Lobe
    - Left ØBCB
    - Right ØBC6
  - Main
    - Left ØBC7
    - Right ØBC3
  - Middle Lobe, Right ØBC5
  - Upper Lobe
    - Left ØBC8
    - Right ØBC4
- Buccal Mucosa ØCC4
- Bursa and Ligament
  - Abdomen
    - Left ØMCJ
    - Right ØMCH
  - Ankle
    - Left ØMCR
    - Right ØMCQ
  - Elbow
    - Left ØMC4
    - Right ØMC3
  - Foot
    - Left ØMCT
    - Right ØMCS
  - Hand
    - Left ØMC8
    - Right ØMC7
  - Head and Neck ØMCØ

Extirpation—*continued*
  Bursa and Ligament—*continued*
    Hip
      Left ØMCM
      Right ØMCL
    Knee
      Left ØMCP
      Right ØMCN
    Lower Extremity
      Left ØMCW
      Right ØMCV
    Perineum ØMCK
    Shoulder
      Left ØMC2
      Right ØMC1
    Thorax
      Left ØMCG
      Right ØMCF
    Trunk
      Left ØMCD
      Right ØMCC
    Upper Extremity
      Left ØMCB
      Right ØMC9
    Wrist
      Left ØMC6
      Right ØMC5
  Carina ØBC2
  Carotid Bodies, Bilateral ØGC8
  Carotid Body
    Left ØGC6
    Right ØGC7
  Carpal
    Left ØPCN
    Right ØPCM
  Cavity, Cranial ØWC1
  Cecum ØDCH
  Cerebellum ØØCC
  Cerebral Hemisphere ØØC7
  Cerebral Meninges ØØC1
  Cerebral Ventricle ØØC6
  Cervix ØUCC
  Chordae Tendineae Ø2C9
  Choroid
    Left Ø8CB
    Right Ø8CA
  Cisterna Chyli Ø7CL
  Clavicle
    Left ØPCB
    Right ØPC9
  Clitoris ØUCJ
  Coccygeal Glomus ØGCB
  Coccyx ØQCS
  Colon
    Ascending ØDCK
    Descending ØDCM
    Sigmoid ØDCN
    Transverse ØDCL
  Conduction Mechanism Ø2C8
  Conjunctiva
    Left Ø8CTXZZ
    Right Ø8CSXZZ
  Cord
    Bilateral ØVCH
    Left ØVCG
    Right ØVCF
  Cornea
    Left Ø8C9XZZ
    Right Ø8C8XZZ
  Cul-de-sac ØUCF
  Diaphragm
    Left ØBCS
    Right ØBCR
  Disc
    Cervical Vertebral ØRC3
    Cervicothoracic Vertebral ØRC5
    Lumbar Vertebral ØSC2
    Lumbosacral ØSC4
    Thoracic Vertebral ØRC9
    Thoracolumbar Vertebral ØRCB
  Duct
    Common Bile ØFC9
    Cystic ØFC8

Extirpation—*continued*
  Duct—*continued*
    Hepatic
      Left ØFC6
      Right ØFC5
    Lacrimal
      Left Ø8CY
      Right Ø8CX
    Pancreatic ØFCD
      Accessory ØFCF
    Parotid
      Left ØCCC
      Right ØCCB
  Duodenum ØDC9
  Dura Mater ØØC2
  Ear
    External
      Left Ø9C1
      Right Ø9CØ
    External Auditory Canal
      Left Ø9C4
      Right Ø9C3
    Inner
      Left Ø9CEØZZ
      Right Ø9CDØZZ
    Middle
      Left Ø9C6ØZZ
      Right Ø9C5ØZZ
  Endometrium ØUCB
  Epididymis
    Bilateral ØVCL
    Left ØVCK
    Right ØVCJ
  Epidural Space ØØC3
  Epiglottis ØCCR
  Esophagogastric Junction ØDC4
  Esophagus ØDC5
    Lower ØDC3
    Middle ØDC2
    Upper ØDC1
  Eustachian Tube
    Left Ø9CG
    Right Ø9CF
  Eye
    Left Ø8C1XZZ
    Right Ø8CØXZZ
  Eyelid
    Lower
      Left Ø8CR
      Right Ø8CQ
    Upper
      Left Ø8CP
      Right Ø8CN
  Fallopian Tube
    Left ØUC6
    Right ØUC5
  Fallopian Tubes, Bilateral ØUC7
  Femoral Shaft
    Left ØQC9
    Right ØQC8
  Femur
    Lower
      Left ØQCC
      Right ØQCB
    Upper
      Left ØQC7
      Right ØQC6
  Fibula
    Left ØQCK
    Right ØQCJ
  Finger Nail ØHCQXZZ
  Gallbladder ØFC4
  Gastrointestinal Tract ØWCP
  Genitourinary Tract ØWCR
  Gingiva
    Lower ØCC6
    Upper ØCC5
  Gland
    Adrenal
      Bilateral ØGC4
      Left ØGC2
      Right ØGC3

Extirpation—*continued*
  Gland—*continued*
    Lacrimal
      Left Ø8CW
      Right Ø8CV
    Minor Salivary ØCCJ
    Parotid
      Left ØCC9
      Right ØCC8
    Pituitary ØGCØ
    Sublingual
      Left ØCCF
      Right ØCCD
    Submaxillary
      Left ØCCH
      Right ØCCG
    Vestibular ØUCL
  Glenoid Cavity
    Left ØPC8
    Right ØPC7
  Glomus Jugulare ØGCC
  Humeral Head
    Left ØPCD
    Right ØPCC
  Humeral Shaft
    Left ØPCG
    Right ØPCF
  Hymen ØUCK
  Hypothalamus ØØCA
  Ileocecal Valve ØDCC
  Ileum ØDCB
  Intestine
    Large ØDCE
      Left ØDCG
      Right ØDCF
    Small ØDC8
  Iris
    Left Ø8CD
    Right Ø8CC
  Jejunum ØDCA
  Joint
    Acromioclavicular
      Left ØRCH
      Right ØRCG
    Ankle
      Left ØSCG
      Right ØSCF
    Carpal
      Left ØRCR
      Right ØRCQ
    Cervical Vertebral ØRC1
    Cervicothoracic Vertebral ØRC4
    Coccygeal ØSC6
    Elbow
      Left ØRCM
      Right ØRCL
    Finger Phalangeal
      Left ØRCX
      Right ØRCW
    Hip
      Left ØSCB
      Right ØSC9
    Knee
      Left ØSCD
      Right ØSCC
    Lumbar Vertebral ØSCØ
    Lumbosacral ØSC3
    Metacarpocarpal
      Left ØRCT
      Right ØRCS
    Metacarpophalangeal
      Left ØRCV
      Right ØRCU
    Metatarsal-Phalangeal
      Left ØSCN
      Right ØSCM
    Metatarsal-Tarsal
      Left ØSCL
      Right ØSCK
    Occipital-cervical ØRCØ
    Sacrococcygeal ØSC5

Extirpation—*continued*
- Joint—*continued*
  - Sacroiliac
    - Left ØSC8
    - Right ØSC7
  - Shoulder
    - Left ØRCK
    - Right ØRCJ
  - Sternoclavicular
    - Left ØRCF
    - Right ØRCE
  - Tarsal
    - Left ØSCJ
    - Right ØSCH
  - Temporomandibular
    - Left ØRCD
    - Right ØRCC
  - Thoracic Vertebral ØRC6
  - Thoracolumbar Vertebral ØRCA
  - Toe Phalangeal
    - Left ØSCQ
    - Right ØSCP
  - Wrist
    - Left ØRCP
    - Right ØRCN
- Kidney
  - Left ØTC1
  - Right ØTCØ
- Kidney Pelvis
  - Left ØTC4
  - Right ØTC3
- Larynx ØCCS
- Lens
  - Left Ø8CK
  - Right Ø8CJ
- Lip
  - Lower ØCC1
  - Upper ØCCØ
- Liver ØFCØ
  - Left Lobe ØFC2
  - Right Lobe ØFC1
- Lung
  - Bilateral ØBCM
  - Left ØBCL
  - Lower Lobe
    - Left ØBCJ
    - Right ØBCF
  - Middle Lobe, Right ØBCD
  - Right ØBCK
  - Upper Lobe
    - Left ØBCG
    - Right ØBCC
- Lung Lingula ØBCH
- Lymphatic
  - Aortic Ø7CD
  - Axillary
    - Left Ø7C6
    - Right Ø7C5
  - Head Ø7CØ
  - Inguinal
    - Left Ø7CJ
    - Right Ø7CH
  - Internal Mammary
    - Left Ø7C9
    - Right Ø7C8
  - Lower Extremity
    - Left Ø7CG
    - Right Ø7CF
  - Mesenteric Ø7CB
  - Neck
    - Left Ø7C2
    - Right Ø7C1
  - Pelvis Ø7CC
  - Thoracic Duct Ø7CK
  - Thorax Ø7C7
  - Upper Extremity
    - Left Ø7C4
    - Right Ø7C3
- Mandible
  - Left ØNCV
  - Right ØNCT

Extirpation—*continued*
- Maxilla
  - Left ØNCS
  - Right ØNCR
- Mediastinum ØWCC
- Medulla Oblongata ØØCD
- Mesentery ØDCV
- Metacarpal
  - Left ØPCQ
  - Right ØPCP
- Metatarsal
  - Left ØQCP
  - Right ØQCN
- Muscle
  - Abdomen
    - Left ØKCL
    - Right ØKCK
  - Extraocular
    - Left Ø8CM
    - Right Ø8CL
  - Facial ØKC1
  - Foot
    - Left ØKCW
    - Right ØKCV
  - Hand
    - Left ØKCD
    - Right ØKCC
  - Head ØKCØ
  - Hip
    - Left ØKCP
    - Right ØKCN
  - Lower Arm and Wrist
    - Left ØKCB
    - Right ØKC9
  - Lower Leg
    - Left ØKCT
    - Right ØKCS
  - Neck
    - Left ØKC3
    - Right ØKC2
  - Papillary Ø2CD
  - Perineum ØKCM
  - Shoulder
    - Left ØKC6
    - Right ØKC5
  - Thorax
    - Left ØKCJ
    - Right ØKCH
  - Tongue, Palate, Pharynx ØKC4
  - Trunk
    - Left ØKCG
    - Right ØKCF
  - Upper Arm
    - Left ØKC8
    - Right ØKC7
  - Upper Leg
    - Left ØKCR
    - Right ØKCQ
- Nasopharynx Ø9CN
- Nerve
  - Abdominal Sympathetic Ø1CM
  - Abducens ØØCL
  - Accessory ØØCR
  - Acoustic ØØCN
  - Brachial Plexus Ø1C3
  - Cervical Ø1C1
  - Cervical Plexus Ø1CØ
  - Facial ØØCM
  - Femoral Ø1CD
  - Glossopharyngeal ØØCP
  - Head and Neck Sympathetic Ø1CK
  - Hypoglossal ØØCS
  - Lumbar Ø1CB
  - Lumbar Plexus Ø1C9
  - Lumbar Sympathetic Ø1CN
  - Lumbosacral Plexus Ø1CA
  - Median Ø1C5
  - Oculomotor ØØCH
  - Olfactory ØØCF
  - Optic ØØCG
  - Peroneal Ø1CH
  - Phrenic Ø1C2
  - Pudendal Ø1CC

Extirpation—*continued*
- Nerve—*continued*
  - Radial Ø1C6
  - Sacral Ø1CR
  - Sacral Plexus Ø1CQ
  - Sacral Sympathetic Ø1CP
  - Sciatic Ø1CF
  - Thoracic Ø1C8
  - Thoracic Sympathetic Ø1CL
  - Tibial Ø1CG
  - Trigeminal ØØCK
  - Trochlear ØØCJ
  - Ulnar Ø1C4
  - Vagus ØØCQ
- Nipple
  - Left ØHCX
  - Right ØHCW
- Nose Ø9CK
- Omentum
  - Greater ØDCS
  - Lesser ØDCT
- Oral Cavity and Throat ØWC3
- Orbit
  - Left ØNCQ
  - Right ØNCP
- Ovary
  - Bilateral ØUC2
  - Left ØUC1
  - Right ØUCØ
- Palate
  - Hard ØCC2
  - Soft ØCC3
- Pancreas ØFCG
- Para-aortic Body ØGC9
- Paraganglion Extremity ØGCF
- Parathyroid Gland ØGCR
  - Inferior
    - Left ØGCP
    - Right ØGCN
  - Multiple ØGCQ
  - Superior
    - Left ØGCM
    - Right ØGCL
- Patella
  - Left ØQCF
  - Right ØQCD
- Pelvic Cavity ØWCJ
- Penis ØVCS
- Pericardial Cavity ØWCD
- Pericardium Ø2CN
- Peritoneal Cavity ØWCG
- Peritoneum ØDCW
- Phalanx
  - Finger
    - Left ØPCV
    - Right ØPCT
  - Thumb
    - Left ØPCS
    - Right ØPCR
  - Toe
    - Left ØQCR
    - Right ØQCQ
- Pharynx ØCCM
- Pineal Body ØGC1
- Pleura
  - Left ØBCP
  - Right ØBCN
- Pleural Cavity
  - Left ØWCB
  - Right ØWC9
- Pons ØØCB
- Prepuce ØVCT
- Prostate ØVCØ
- Radius
  - Left ØPCJ
  - Right ØPCH
- Rectum ØDCP
- Respiratory Tract ØWCQ
- Retina
  - Left Ø8CF
  - Right Ø8CE

Extirpation—*continued*
- Retinal Vessel
  - Left 08CH
  - Right 08CG
- Rib
  - Left 0PC2
  - Right 0PC1
- Sacrum 0QC1
- Scapula
  - Left 0PC6
  - Right 0PC5
- Sclera
  - Left 08C7XZZ
  - Right 08C6XZZ
- Scrotum 0VC5
- Septum
  - Atrial 02C5
  - Nasal 09CM
  - Ventricular 02CM
- Sinus
  - Accessory 09CP
  - Ethmoid
    - Left 09CV
    - Right 09CU
  - Frontal
    - Left 09CT
    - Right 09CS
  - Mastoid
    - Left 09CC
    - Right 09CB
  - Maxillary
    - Left 09CR
    - Right 09CQ
  - Sphenoid
    - Left 09CX
    - Right 09CW
- Skin
  - Abdomen 0HC7XZZ
  - Back 0HC6XZZ
  - Buttock 0HC8XZZ
  - Chest 0HC5XZZ
  - Ear
    - Left 0HC3XZZ
    - Right 0HC2XZZ
  - Face 0HC1XZZ
  - Foot
    - Left 0HCNXZZ
    - Right 0HCMXZZ
  - Genitalia 0HCAXZZ
  - Hand
    - Left 0HCGXZZ
    - Right 0HCFXZZ
  - Lower Arm
    - Left 0HCEXZZ
    - Right 0HCDXZZ
  - Lower Leg
    - Left 0HCLXZZ
    - Right 0HCKXZZ
  - Neck 0HC4XZZ
  - Perineum 0HC9XZZ
  - Scalp 0HC0XZZ
  - Upper Arm
    - Left 0HCCXZZ
    - Right 0HCBXZZ
  - Upper Leg
    - Left 0HCJXZZ
    - Right 0HCHXZZ
- Spinal Cord
  - Cervical 00CW
  - Lumbar 00CY
  - Thoracic 00CX
- Spinal Meninges 00CT
- Spleen 07CP
- Sternum 0PC0
- Stomach 0DC6
  - Pylorus 0DC7
- Subarachnoid Space 00C5
- Subcutaneous Tissue and Fascia
  - Abdomen 0JC8
  - Back 0JC7
  - Buttock 0JC9
  - Chest 0JC6
  - Face 0JC1

Extirpation—*continued*
- Subcutaneous Tissue and Fascia—*continued*
  - Foot
    - Left 0JCR
    - Right 0JCQ
  - Hand
    - Left 0JCK
    - Right 0JCJ
  - Lower Arm
    - Left 0JCH
    - Right 0JCG
  - Lower Leg
    - Left 0JCP
    - Right 0JCN
  - Neck
    - Anterior 0JC4
    - Posterior 0JC5
  - Pelvic Region 0JCC
  - Perineum 0JCB
  - Scalp 0JC0
  - Upper Arm
    - Left 0JCF
    - Right 0JCD
  - Upper Leg
    - Left 0JCM
    - Right 0JCL
- Subdural Space 00C4
- Tarsal
  - Left 0QCM
  - Right 0QCL
- Tendon
  - Abdomen
    - Left 0LCG
    - Right 0LCF
  - Ankle
    - Left 0LCT
    - Right 0LCS
  - Foot
    - Left 0LCW
    - Right 0LCV
  - Hand
    - Left 0LC8
    - Right 0LC7
  - Head and Neck 0LC0
  - Hip
    - Left 0LCK
    - Right 0LCJ
  - Knee
    - Left 0LCR
    - Right 0LCQ
  - Lower Arm and Wrist
    - Left 0LC6
    - Right 0LC5
  - Lower Leg
    - Left 0LCP
    - Right 0LCN
  - Perineum 0LCH
  - Shoulder
    - Left 0LC2
    - Right 0LC1
  - Thorax
    - Left 0LCD
    - Right 0LCC
  - Trunk
    - Left 0LCB
    - Right 0LC9
  - Upper Arm
    - Left 0LC4
    - Right 0LC3
  - Upper Leg
    - Left 0LCM
    - Right 0LCL
- Testis
  - Bilateral 0VCC
  - Left 0VCB
  - Right 0VC9
- Thalamus 00C9
- Thymus 07CM
- Thyroid Gland 0GCK
  - Left Lobe 0GCG
  - Right Lobe 0GCH

Extirpation—*continued*
- Tibia
  - Left 0QCH
  - Right 0QCG
- Toe Nail 0HCRXZZ
- Tongue 0CC7
- Tonsils 0CCP
- Tooth
  - Lower 0CCX
  - Upper 0CCW
- Trachea 0BC1
- Tunica Vaginalis
  - Left 0VC7
  - Right 0VC6
- Turbinate, Nasal 09CL
- Tympanic Membrane
  - Left 09C8
  - Right 09C7
- Ulna
  - Left 0PCL
  - Right 0PCK
- Ureter
  - Left 0TC7
  - Right 0TC6
- Urethra 0TCD
- Uterine Supporting Structure 0UC4
- Uterus 0UC9
- Uvula 0CCN
- Vagina 0UCG
- Valve
  - Aortic 02CF
  - Mitral 02CG
  - Pulmonary 02CH
  - Tricuspid 02CJ
- Vas Deferens
  - Bilateral 0VCQ
  - Left 0VCP
  - Right 0VCN
- Vein
  - Axillary
    - Left 05C8
    - Right 05C7
  - Azygos 05C0
  - Basilic
    - Left 05CC
    - Right 05CB
  - Brachial
    - Left 05CA
    - Right 05C9
  - Cephalic
    - Left 05CF
    - Right 05CD
  - Colic 06C7
  - Common Iliac
    - Left 06CD
    - Right 06CC
  - Coronary 02C4
  - Esophageal 06C3
  - External Iliac
    - Left 06CG
    - Right 06CF
  - External Jugular
    - Left 05CQ
    - Right 05CP
  - Face
    - Left 05CV
    - Right 05CT
  - Femoral
    - Left 06CN
    - Right 06CM
  - Foot
    - Left 06CV
    - Right 06CT
  - Gastric 06C2
  - Greater Saphenous
    - Left 06CQ
    - Right 06CP
  - Hand
    - Left 05CH
    - Right 05CG
  - Hemiazygos 05C1
  - Hepatic 06C4

Extirpation—*continued*
  Vein—*continued*
    Hypogastric
      Left Ø6CJ
      Right Ø6CH
    Inferior Mesenteric Ø6C6
    Innominate
      Left Ø5C4
      Right Ø5C3
    Internal Jugular
      Left Ø5CN
      Right Ø5CM
    Intracranial Ø5CL
    Lesser Saphenous
      Left Ø6CS
      Right Ø6CR
    Lower Ø6CY
    Portal Ø6C8
    Pulmonary
      Left Ø2CT
      Right Ø2CS
    Renal
      Left Ø6CB
      Right Ø6C9
    Splenic Ø6C1
    Subclavian
      Left Ø5C6
      Right Ø5C5
    Superior Mesenteric Ø6C5
    Upper Ø5CY
    Vertebral
      Left Ø5CS
      Right Ø5CR
  Vena Cava
    Inferior Ø6CØ
    Superior Ø2CV
  Ventricle
    Left Ø2CL
    Right Ø2CK
  Vertebra
    Cervical ØPC3
    Lumbar ØQCØ
    Thoracic ØPC4
  Vesicle
    Bilateral ØVC3
    Left ØVC2
    Right ØVC1
  Vitreous
    Left Ø8C5
    Right Ø8C4
  Vocal Cord
    Left ØCCV
    Right ØCCT
  Vulva ØUCM
Extracorporeal shock wave lithotripsy *see*
    Fragmentation
Extracranial-intracranial bypass (EC-IC) *see* Bypass,
    Upper Arteries Ø31
Extraction
  Auditory Ossicle
    Left Ø9DAØZZ
    Right Ø9D9ØZZ
  Bone Marrow
    Iliac Ø7DR
    Sternum Ø7DQ
    Vertebral Ø7DS
  Bursa and Ligament
    Abdomen
      Left ØMDJ
      Right ØMDH
    Ankle
      Left ØMDR
      Right ØMDQ
    Elbow
      Left ØMD4
      Right ØMD3
    Foot
      Left ØMDT
      Right ØMDS
    Hand
      Left ØMD8
      Right ØMD7
    Head and Neck ØMDØ

Extraction—*continued*
  Bursa and Ligament—*continued*
    Hip
      Left ØMDM
      Right ØMDL
    Knee
      Left ØMDP
      Right ØMDN
    Lower Extremity
      Left ØMDW
      Right ØMDV
    Perineum ØMDK
    Shoulder
      Left ØMD2
      Right ØMD1
    Thorax
      Left ØMDG
      Right ØMDF
    Trunk
      Left ØMDD
      Right ØMDC
    Upper Extremity
      Left ØMDB
      Right ØMD9
    Wrist
      Left ØMD6
      Right ØMD5
  Cerebral Meninges ØØD1
  Cornea
    Left Ø8D9XZ
    Right Ø8D8XZ
  Dura Mater ØØD2
  Endometrium ØUDB
  Finger Nail ØHDQXZZ
  Hair ØHDSXZZ
  Kidney
    Left ØTD1
    Right ØTDØ
  Lens
    Left Ø8DK3ZZ
    Right Ø8DJ3ZZ
  Nerve
    Abdominal Sympathetic Ø1DM
    Abducens ØØDL
    Accessory ØØDR
    Acoustic ØØDN
    Brachial Plexus Ø1D3
    Cervical Ø1D1
    Cervical Plexus Ø1DØ
    Facial ØØDM
    Femoral Ø1DD
    Glossopharyngeal ØØDP
    Head and Neck Sympathetic Ø1DK
    Hypoglossal ØØDS
    Lumbar Ø1DB
    Lumbar Plexus Ø1D9
    Lumbar Sympathetic Ø1DN
    Lumbosacral Plexus Ø1DA
    Median Ø1D5
    Oculomotor ØØDH
    Olfactory ØØDF
    Optic ØØDG
    Peroneal Ø1DH
    Phrenic Ø1D2
    Pudendal Ø1DC
    Radial Ø1D6
    Sacral Ø1DR
    Sacral Plexus Ø1DQ
    Sacral Sympathetic Ø1DP
    Sciatic Ø1DF
    Thoracic Ø1D8
    Thoracic Sympathetic Ø1DL
    Tibial Ø1DG
    Trigeminal ØØDK
    Trochlear ØØDJ
    Ulnar Ø1D4
    Vagus ØØDQ
  Ova ØUDN
  Pleura
    Left ØBDP
    Right ØBDN
  Products of Conception
    Classical 1ØDØØZØ

Extraction—*continued*
  Products of Conception—*continued*
    Ectopic 1ØD2
    Extraperitoneal 1ØDØØZ2
    High Forceps 1ØDØ7Z5
    Internal Version 1ØDØ7Z7
    Low Cervical 1ØDØØZ1
    Low Forceps 1ØDØ7Z3
    Mid Forceps 1ØDØ7Z4
    Other 1ØDØ7Z8
    Retained 1ØD1
    Vacuum 1ØDØ7Z6
  Septum, Nasal Ø9DM
  Sinus
    Accessory Ø9DP
    Ethmoid
      Left Ø9DV
      Right Ø9DU
    Frontal
      Left Ø9DT
      Right Ø9DS
    Mastoid
      Left Ø9DC
      Right Ø9DB
    Maxillary
      Left Ø9DR
      Right Ø9DQ
    Sphenoid
      Left Ø9DX
      Right Ø9DW
  Skin
    Abdomen ØHD7XZZ
    Back ØHD6XZZ
    Buttock ØHD8XZZ
    Chest ØHD5XZZ
    Ear
      Left ØHD3XZZ
      Right ØHD2XZZ
    Face ØHD1XZZ
    Foot
      Left ØHDNXZZ
      Right ØHDMXZZ
    Genitalia ØHDAXZZ
    Hand
      Left ØHDGXZZ
      Right ØHDFXZZ
    Lower Arm
      Left ØHDEXZZ
      Right ØHDDXZZ
    Lower Leg
      Left ØHDLXZZ
      Right ØHDKXZZ
    Neck ØHD4XZZ
    Perineum ØHD9XZZ
    Scalp ØHDØXZZ
    Upper Arm
      Left ØHDCXZZ
      Right ØHDBXZZ
    Upper Leg
      Left ØHDJXZZ
      Right ØHDHXZZ
  Spinal Meninges ØØDT
  Subcutaneous Tissue and Fascia
    Abdomen ØJD8
    Back ØJD7
    Buttock ØJD9
    Chest ØJD6
    Face ØJD1
    Foot
      Left ØJDR
      Right ØJDQ
    Hand
      Left ØJDK
      Right ØJDJ
    Lower Arm
      Left ØJDH
      Right ØJDG
    Lower Leg
      Left ØJDP
      Right ØJDN
    Neck
      Anterior ØJD4
      Posterior ØJD5

Extraction—*continued*
  Subcutaneous Tissue and Fascia—*continued*
    Pelvic Region ØJDC
    Perineum ØJDB
    Scalp ØJDØ
    Upper Arm
      Left ØJDF
      Right ØJDD
    Upper Leg
      Left ØJDM
      Right ØJDL
  Toe Nail ØHDRXZZ
  Tooth
    Lower ØCDXXZ
    Upper ØCDWXZ
  Turbinate, Nasal Ø9DL
  Tympanic Membrane
    Left Ø9D8
    Right Ø9D7
  Vein
    Basilic
      Left Ø5DC
      Right Ø5DB
    Brachial
      Left Ø5DA
      Right Ø5D9
    Cephalic
      Left Ø5DF
      Right Ø5DD
    Femoral
      Left Ø6DN
      Right Ø6DM
    Foot
      Left Ø6DV
      Right Ø6DT
    Greater Saphenous
      Left Ø6DQ
      Right Ø6DP
    Hand
      Left Ø5DH
      Right Ø5DG
    Lesser Saphenous
      Left Ø6DS
      Right Ø6DR
    Lower Ø6DY
    Upper Ø5DY
  Vocal Cord
    Left ØCDV
    Right ØCDT
Extradural space *use* Epidural Space

F

Face lift *see* Alteration, Face ØWØ2
Facial artery *use* Artery, Face
False vocal cord *use* Larynx
Falx cerebri *use* Dura Mater
Fascia lata
  use Subcutaneous Tissue and Fascia, Upper Leg, Left
  use Subcutaneous Tissue and Fascia, Upper Leg, Right
Fasciaplasty, fascioplasty
  see Repair, Subcutaneous Tissue and Fascia ØJQ
  see Replacement, Subcutaneous Tissue and Fascia ØJR
Fasciectomy *see* Excision, Subcutaneous Tissue and Fascia ØJB
Fasciorrhaphy *see* Repair, Subcutaneous Tissue and Fascia ØJQ
Fasciotomy
  see Division, Subcutaneous Tissue and Fascia ØJ8
  see Drainage, Subcutaneous Tissue and Fascia ØJ9
Feeding Device
  Change device in
    Lower ØD2DXUZ
    Upper ØD2ØXUZ
  Insertion of device in
    Duodenum ØDH9
    Esophagus ØDH5
    Ileum ØDHB
    Intestine, Small ØDH8

Feeding Device—*continued*
  Insertion of device in—*continued*
    Jejunum ØDHA
    Stomach ØDH6
  Removal of device from
    Esophagus ØDP5
    Intestinal Tract
      Lower ØDPD
      Upper ØDPØ
    Stomach ØDP6
  Revision of device in
    Intestinal Tract
      Lower ØDWD
      Upper ØDWØ
    Stomach ØDW6
Femoral head
  use Femur, Upper, Right
  use Femur, Upper, Left
Femoral lymph node
  use Lymphatic, Lower Extremity, Left
  use Lymphatic, Lower Extremity, Right
Femoropatellar joint
  use Joint, Knee, Right
  use Joint, Knee, Left
Femorotibial joint
  use Joint, Knee, Right
  use Joint, Knee, Left
Fibular artery
  use Artery, Peroneal, Right
  use Artery, Peroneal, Left
Fibularis brevis muscle
  use Muscle, Lower Leg, Left
  use Muscle, Lower Leg, Right
Fibularis longus muscle
  use Muscle, Lower Leg, Left
  use Muscle, Lower Leg, Right
Fifth cranial nerve *use* Nerve, Trigeminal
Fimbriectomy
  see Excision, Female Reproductive System ØUB
  see Resection, Female Reproductive System ØUT
First cranial nerve *use* Nerve, Olfactory
First intercostal nerve *use* Nerve, Brachial Plexus
Fistulization
  see Bypass
  see Drainage
  see Repair
Fitting
  Arch bars, for fracture reduction *see* Reposition, Mouth and Throat ØCS
  Arch bars, for immobilization *see* Immobilization, Face 2W31
  Artificial limb *see* Device Fitting, Rehabilitation FØD
  Hearing aid *see* Device Fitting, Rehabilitation FØD
  Ocular prosthesis FØDZ8UZ
  Prosthesis, limb *see* Device Fitting, Rehabilitation FØD
  Prosthesis, ocular FØDZ8UZ
Fixation, bone
  External, with fracture reduction *see* Reposition
  External, without fracture reduction *see* Insertion
  Internal, with fracture reduction *see* Reposition
  Internal, without fracture reduction *see* Insertion
Flexor carpi radialis muscle
  use Muscle, Lower Arm and Wrist, Right
  use Muscle, Lower Arm and Wrist, Left
Flexor carpi ulnaris muscle
  use Muscle, Lower Arm and Wrist, Right
  use Muscle, Lower Arm and Wrist, Left
Flexor digitorum brevis muscle
  use Muscle, Foot, Left
  use Muscle, Foot, Right
Flexor digitorum longus muscle
  use Muscle, Lower Leg, Left
  use Muscle, Lower Leg, Right
Flexor hallucis brevis muscle
  use Muscle, Foot, Left
  use Muscle, Foot, Right
Flexor hallucis longus muscle
  use Muscle, Lower Leg, Right
  use Muscle, Lower Leg, Left
Flexor pollicis longus muscle
  use Muscle, Lower Arm and Wrist, Left
  use Muscle, Lower Arm and Wrist, Right

Fluoroscopy
  Abdomen and Pelvis BW11
  Airway, Upper BB1DZZZ
  Ankle
    Left BQ1H
    Right BQ1G
  Aorta
    Abdominal B41Ø
      Laser, Intraoperative B41Ø
    Thoracic B31Ø
      Laser, Intraoperative B31Ø
    Thoraco-Abdominal B31P
      Laser, Intraoperative B31P
  Aorta and Bilateral Lower Extremity Arteries B41D
    Laser, Intraoperative B41D
  Arm
    Left BP1FZZZ
    Right BP1EZZZ
  Artery
    Brachiocephalic-Subclavian
      Right B311
        Laser, Intraoperative B311
    Bronchial B31L
      Laser, Intraoperative B31L
    Bypass Graft, Other B21F
    Cervico-Cerebral Arch B31Q
      Laser, Intraoperative B31Q
    Common Carotid
      Bilateral B315
        Laser, Intraoperative B315
      Left B314
        Laser, Intraoperative B314
      Right B313
        Laser, Intraoperative B313
    Coronary
      Bypass Graft
        Multiple B213
          Laser, Intraoperative B213
        Single B212
          Laser, Intraoperative B212
      Multiple B211
        Laser, Intraoperative B211
      Single B21Ø
        Laser, Intraoperative B21Ø
    External Carotid
      Bilateral B31C
        Laser, Intraoperative B31C
      Left B31B
        Laser, Intraoperative B31B
      Right B319
        Laser, Intraoperative B319
    Hepatic B412
      Laser, Intraoperative B412
    Inferior Mesenteric B415
      Laser, Intraoperative B415
    Intercostal B31L
      Laser, Intraoperative B31L
    Internal Carotid
      Bilateral B318
        Laser, Intraoperative B318
      Left B317
        Laser, Intraoperative B317
      Right B316
        Laser, Intraoperative B316
    Internal Mammary Bypass Graft
      Left B218
      Right B217
    Intra-Abdominal
      Other B41B
      Laser, Intraoperative B41B
    Intracranial B31R
      Laser, Intraoperative B31R
    Lower
      Other B41J
      Laser, Intraoperative B41J
    Lower Extremity
      Bilateral and Aorta B41D
        Laser, Intraoperative B41D
      Left B41G
        Laser, Intraoperative B41G
      Right B41F
        Laser, Intraoperative B41F

Fluoroscopy—*continued*
  Vein—*continued*
    Upper Extremity
      Bilateral B51P
      Left B51N
      Right B51M
    Vena Cava
      Inferior B519
      Superior B518
    Wrist
      Left BP1M
      Right BP1L
Flushing *see* Irrigation
Foramen magnum
  use Bone, Occipital, Right
  use Bone, Occipital, Left
Foramen of Monro (intraventricular) *use* Cerebral
  Ventricle
Foreskin *use* Prepuce
Fossa of Rosenmuller *use* Nasopharynx
Fourth cranial nerve *use* Nerve, Trochlear
Fourth ventricle *use* Cerebral Ventricle
Fovea
  use Retina, Right
  use Retina, Left
Fragmentation
  Ampulla of Vater ØFFC
  Anus ØDFQ
  Appendix ØDFJ
  Bladder ØTFB
  Bladder Neck ØTFC
  Bronchus
    Lingula ØBF9
    Lower Lobe
      Left ØBFB
      Right ØBF6
    Main
      Left ØBF7
      Right ØBF3
    Middle Lobe, Right ØBF5
    Upper Lobe
      Left ØBF8
      Right ØBF4
  Carina ØBF2
  Cavity, Cranial ØWF1
  Cecum ØDFH
  Cerebral Ventricle ØØF6
  Colon
    Ascending ØDFK
    Descending ØDFM
    Sigmoid ØDFN
    Transverse ØDFL
  Duct
    Common Bile ØFF9
    Cystic ØFF8
    Hepatic
      Left ØFF6
      Right ØFF5
    Pancreatic ØFFD
      Accessory ØFFF
    Parotid
      Left ØCFC
      Right ØCFB
  Duodenum ØDF9
  Epidural Space ØØF3
  Esophagus ØDF5
  Fallopian Tube
    Left ØUF6
    Right ØUF5
  Fallopian Tubes, Bilateral ØUF7
  Gallbladder ØFF4
  Gastrointestinal Tract ØWFP
  Genitourinary Tract ØWFR
  Ileum ØDFB
  Intestine
    Large ØDFE
      Left ØDFG
      Right ØDFF
    Small ØDF8
  Jejunum ØDFA
  Kidney Pelvis
    Left ØTF4
    Right ØTF3

Fragmentation—*continued*
  Mediastinum ØWFC
  Oral Cavity and Throat ØWF3
  Pelvic Cavity ØWFJ
  Pericardial Cavity ØWFD
  Pericardium Ø2FN
  Peritoneal Cavity ØWFG
  Pleural Cavity
    Left ØWFB
    Right ØWF9
  Rectum ØDFP
  Respiratory Tract ØWFQ
  Spinal Canal ØØFU
  Stomach ØDF6
  Subarachnoid Space ØØF5
  Subdural Space ØØF4
  Trachea ØBF1
  Ureter
    Left ØTF7
    Right ØTF6
  Urethra ØTFD
  Uterus ØUF9
  Vitreous
    Left Ø8F5
    Right Ø8F4
Frenectomy
  see Excision, Mouth and Throat ØCB
  see Resection, Mouth and Throat ØCT
Frenoplasty, frenuloplasty
  see Repair, Mouth and Throat ØCQ
  see Replacement, Mouth and Throat ØCR
  see Supplement, Mouth and Throat ØCU
Frenotomy
  see Drainage, Mouth and Throat ØC9
  see Release, Mouth and Throat ØCN
Frenulotomy
  see Drainage, Mouth and Throat ØC9
  see Release, Mouth and Throat ØCN
Frenulum labii inferioris *use* Lip, Lower
Frenulum labii superioris *use* Lip, Upper
Frenulum linguae *use* Tongue
Frenulumectomy
  see Excision, Mouth and Throat ØCB
  see Resection, Mouth and Throat ØCT
Frontal lobe *use* Cerebral Hemisphere
Frontal vein
  use Vein, Face, Right
  use Vein, Face, Left
Fulguration *see* Destruction
Fundoplication, gastroesophageal *see* Restriction,
  Esophagogastric Junction ØDV4
Fundus uteri *use* Uterus
Fusion
  Acromioclavicular
    Left ØRGH
    Right ØRGG
  Ankle
    Left ØSGG
    Right ØSGF
  Carpal
    Left ØRGR
    Right ØRGQ
  Cervical Vertebral ØRG1
    2 or more ØRG2
  Cervicothoracic Vertebral ØRG4
  Coccygeal ØSG6
  Elbow
    Left ØRGM
    Right ØRGL
  Finger Phalangeal
    Left ØRGX
    Right ØRGW
  Hip
    Left ØSGB
    Right ØSG9
  Knee
    Left ØSGD
    Right ØSGC
  Lumbar Vertebral ØSGØ
    2 or more ØSG1
  Lumbosacral ØSG3

Fusion—*continued*
  Metacarpocarpal
    Left ØRGT
    Right ØRGS
  Metacarpophalangeal
    Left ØRGV
    Right ØRGU
  Metatarsal-Phalangeal
    Left ØSGN
    Right ØSGM
  Metatarsal-Tarsal
    Left ØSGL
    Right ØSGK
  Occipital-cervical ØRGØ
  Sacrococcygeal ØSG5
  Sacroiliac
    Left ØSG8
    Right ØSG7
  Shoulder
    Left ØRGK
    Right ØRGJ
  Sternoclavicular
    Left ØRGF
    Right ØRGE
  Tarsal
    Left ØSGJ
    Right ØSGH
  Temporomandibular
    Left ØRGD
    Right ØRGC
  Thoracic Vertebral ØRG6
    2 to 7 ØRG7
    8 or more ØRG8
  Thoracolumbar Vertebral ØRGA
  Toe Phalangeal
    Left ØSGQ
    Right ØSGP
  Wrist
    Left ØRGP
    Right ØRGN

G

Gait training *see* Motor Treatment, Rehabilitation FØ7
Galea aponeurotica *use* Subcutaneous Tissue and
  Fascia, Scalp
Ganglion impar (ganglion of Walther) *use* Nerve,
  Sacral Sympathetic
Ganglionectomy
  Destruction of lesion *see* Destruction
  Excision of lesion *see* Excision
Gasserian ganglion *use* Nerve, Trigeminal
Gastrectomy
  see Excision, Stomach ØDB6
  see Resection, Stomach ØDT6
Gastric lymph node *use* Lymphatic, Aortic
Gastric plexus *use* Nerve, Abdominal Sympathetic
Gastrocnemius muscle
  use Muscle, Lower Leg, Left
  use Muscle, Lower Leg, Right
Gastrocolic ligament *use* Omentum, Greater
Gastrocolic omentum *use* Omentum, Greater
Gastrocolostomy
  see Bypass, Gastrointestinal System ØD1
  see Drainage, Gastrointestinal System ØD9
Gastroduodenal artery *use* Artery, Hepatic
Gastroduodenectomy
  see Excision, Gastrointestinal System ØDB
  see Resection, Gastrointestinal System ØDT
Gastroduodenoscopy ØDJØ8ZZ
Gastroenteroplasty
  see Repair, Gastrointestinal System ØDQ
  see Supplement, Gastrointestinal System ØDU
Gastroenterostomy
  see Bypass, Gastrointestinal System ØD1
  see Drainage, Gastrointestinal System ØD9
Gastroesophageal (GE) junction *use* Esophagogastric
  Junction
Gastrogastrostomy
  see Bypass, Stomach ØD16
  see Drainage, Stomach ØD96

Gastrohepatic omentum—Hymenectomy

Index

Gastrohepatic omentum *use* Omentum, Lesser
Gastrojejunostomy
   see Bypass, Stomach ØD16
   see Drainage, Stomach ØD96
Gastrolysis *see* Release, Stomach ØDN6
Gastropexy
   see Repair, Stomach ØDQ6
   see Reposition, Stomach ØDS6
Gastrophrenic ligament *use* Omentum, Greater
Gastroplasty
   see Repair, Stomach ØDQ6
   see Supplement, Stomach ØDU6
Gastroplication *see* Restriction, Stomach ØDV6
Gastropylorectomy *see* Excision, Gastrointestinal
   System ØDB
Gastrorrhaphy *see* Repair, Stomach ØDQ6
Gastroscopy ØDJ68ZZ
Gastrosplenic ligament *use* Omentum, Greater
Gastrostomy
   see Bypass, Stomach ØD16
   see Drainage, Stomach ØD96
Gastrotomy *see* Drainage, Stomach ØD96
Gemellus muscle
   use Muscle, Hip, Left
   use Muscle, Hip, Right
Geniculate ganglion *use* Nerve, Facial
Geniculate nucleus *use* Thalamus
Genioglossus muscle *use* Muscle, Tongue, Palate,
   Pharynx
Genioplasty *see* Alteration, Jaw, Lower ØW05
Genitofemoral nerve *use* Nerve, Lumbar Plexus
Gingivectomy *see* Excision, Mouth and Throat ØCB
Gingivoplasty
   see Repair, Mouth and Throat ØCQ
   see Replacement, Mouth and Throat ØCR
   see Supplement, Mouth and Throat ØCU
Glans penis *use* Prepuce
Glenohumeral joint
   use Joint, Shoulder, Left
   use Joint, Shoulder, Right
Glenohumeral ligament
   use Bursa and Ligament, Shoulder, Right
   use Bursa and Ligament, Shoulder, Left
Glenoid fossa (of scapula)
   use Glenoid Cavity, Left
   use Glenoid Cavity, Right
Glenoid ligament (labrum)
   use Bursa and Ligament, Shoulder, Right
   use Bursa and Ligament, Shoulder, Left
Globus pallidus *use* Basal Ganglia
Glomectomy
   see Excision, Endocrine System ØGB
   see Resection, Endocrine System ØGT
Glossectomy
   see Excision, Tongue ØCB7
   see Resection, Tongue ØCT7
Glossoepiglottic fold *use* Epiglottis
Glossopexy
   see Repair, Tongue ØCQ7
   see Reposition, Tongue ØCS7
Glossoplasty
   see Repair, Tongue ØCQ7
   see Replacement, Tongue ØCR7
   see Supplement, Tongue ØCU7
Glossorrhaphy *see* Repair, Tongue ØCQ7
Glossotomy *see* Drainage, Tongue ØC97
Glottis *use* Larynx
Gluteal Artery Perforator Flap
   Bilateral ØHRVØ79
   Left ØHRUØ79
   Right ØHRTØ79
Gluteal lymph node *use* Lymphatic, Pelvis
Gluteal vein
   use Vein, Hypogastric, Right
   use Vein, Hypogastric, Left
Gluteus maximus muscle
   use Muscle, Hip, Right
   use Muscle, Hip, Left
Gluteus medius muscle
   use Muscle, Hip, Right
   use Muscle, Hip, Left

Gluteus minimus muscle
   use Muscle, Hip, Left
   use Muscle, Hip, Right
Gracilis muscle
   use Muscle, Upper Leg, Left
   use Muscle, Upper Leg, Right
Graft
   see Replacement
   see Supplement
Great auricular nerve *use* Nerve, Cervical Plexus
Great cerebral vein *use* Vein, Intracranial
Great saphenous vein
   use Vein, Greater Saphenous, Left
   use Vein, Greater Saphenous, Right
Greater alar cartilage *use* Nose
Greater occipital nerve *use* Nerve, Cervical
Greater splanchnic nerve *use* Nerve, Thoracic
   Sympathetic
Greater superficial petrosal nerve *use* Nerve, Facial
Greater trochanter
   use Femur, Upper, Left
   use Femur, Upper, Right
Greater tuberosity
   use Humeral Head, Right
   use Humeral Head, Left
Greater vestibular (Bartholin's) gland *use* Gland,
   Vestibular
Greater wing
   use Bone, Sphenoid, Left
   use Bone, Sphenoid, Right
Guidance
   Catheter placement
      EKG *see* Measurement, Physiological Systems 4AØ
      Fluoroscopy *see* Fluoroscopy, Veins B51
      Ultrasound *see* Ultrasonography, Veins B54

H

Hallux
   use Toe, 1st, Right
   use Toe, 1st, Left
Hamate bone
   use Carpal, Right
   use Carpal, Left
Harvesting, stem cells *see* Pheresis, Circulatory 6A55
Head of fibula
   use Fibula, Right
   use Fibula, Left
Hearing Aid Assessment F14Z
Hearing Assessment F13Z
Hearing Device
   Insertion of device in
      Bone
         Left ØNH6
         Right ØNH5
      Ear
         Left Ø9HE
            Other Hearing Device Ø9HEØSY
         Right Ø9HD
            Other Hearing Device Ø9HDØSY
   Removal of device from
      Ear
         Left Ø9PE
         Right Ø9PD
      Skull ØNPØ
   Revision of device in
      Ear
         Left Ø9WE
         Right Ø9WD
      Skull ØNWØ
Hearing Treatment F09Z
Heart Assist System
   External
      Insertion of device in, Heart Ø2HA
      Removal of device from, Heart Ø2PA
      Revision of device in, Heart Ø2WA
   Implantable
      Insertion of device in, Heart Ø2HA
      Removal of device from, Heart Ø2PA
      Revision of device in, Heart Ø2WA

HeartMate® implantable heart assist system *see*
   Insertion of device in, Heart Ø2HA
Helix
   use Ear, External, Bilateral
   use Ear, External, Right
   use Ear, External, Left
Hemicolectomy *see* Resection, Gastrointestinal
   System ØDT
Hemicystectomy *see* Excision, Urinary System ØTB
Hemigastrectomy *see* Excision, Gastrointestinal
   System ØDB
Hemiglossectomy *see* Excision, Mouth and Throat ØCB
Hemilaminectomy
   see Excision, Upper Joints ØRB
   see Excision, Lower Joints ØSB
Hemilaryngectomy *see* Excision, Larynx ØCBS
Hemimandibulectomy *see* Excision, Head and Facial
   Bones ØNB
Hemimaxillectomy *see* Excision, Head and Facial
   Bones ØNB
Hemipylorectomy *see* Excision, Gastrointestinal
   System ØDB
Hemispherectomy
   see Excision, Central Nervous System ØØB
   see Resection, Central Nervous System ØØT
Hemithyroidectomy
   see Resection, Endocrine System ØGT
   see Excision, Endocrine System ØGB
Hemodialysis 5A1DØØZ
Hepatectomy
   see Excision, Hepatobiliary System and Pancreas ØFB
   see Resection, Hepatobiliary System and Pancreas
      ØFT
Hepatic artery proper *use* Artery, Hepatic
Hepatic flexure *use* Colon, Ascending
Hepatic lymph node *use* Lymphatic, Aortic
Hepatic plexus *use* Nerve, Abdominal Sympathetic
Hepatic portal vein *use* Vein, Portal
Hepaticoduodenostomy
   see Bypass, Hepatobiliary System and Pancreas ØF1
   see Drainage, Hepatobiliary System and Pancreas
      ØF9
Hepaticotomy *see* Drainage, Hepatobiliary System and
   Pancreas ØF9
Hepatocholedochostomy *see* Drainage, Duct,
   Common Bile ØF99
Hepatogastric ligament *use* Omentum, Lesser
Hepatopancreatic ampulla *use* Ampulla of Vater
Hepatopexy
   see Repair, Hepatobiliary System and Pancreas ØFQ
   see Reposition, Hepatobiliary System and Pancreas
      ØFS
Hepatorrhaphy *see* Repair, Hepatobiliary System and
   Pancreas ØFQ
Hepatotomy *see* Drainage, Hepatobiliary System and
   Pancreas ØF9
Herniorrhaphy
   see Repair, Anatomical Regions, General ØWQ
   see Repair, Anatomical Regions, Lower Extremities
      ØYQ
   with synthetic substitute
      see Supplement, Anatomical Regions, General
         ØWU
      see Supplement, Anatomical Regions, Lower
         Extremities ØYU
Holter Monitoring 4A12X45
Humeroradial joint
   use Joint, Elbow, Right
   use Joint, Elbow, Left
Humeroulnar joint
   use Joint, Elbow, Left
   use Joint, Elbow, Right
Hydrocelectomy *see* Excision, Male Reproductive
   System ØVB
Hydrotherapy
   Assisted exercise in pool *see* Motor Treatment,
      Rehabilitation F07
   Whirlpool *see* Activities of Daily Living Treatment,
      Rehabilitation F08
Hymenectomy
   see Excision, Hymen ØUBK
   see Resection, Hymen ØUTK

Hymenoplasty
see Repair, Hymen ØUQK
see Supplement, Hymen ØUUK
Hymenorrhaphy see Repair, Hymen ØUQK
Hymenotomy
see Division, Hymen ØU8K
see Drainage, Hymen ØU9K
Hyoglossus muscle use Muscle, Tongue, Palate, Pharynx
Hyoid artery
use Artery, Thyroid, Right
use Artery, Thyroid, Left
Hyperalimentation see Introduction
Hyperbaric oxygenation
Decompression sickness treatment see Decompression, Circulatory 6A15
Wound treatment see Assistance, Circulatory 5AØ5
Hyperthermia
Radiation Oncology
Abdomen DWY38ZZ
Adrenal Gland DGY28ZZ
Bile Ducts DFY28ZZ
Bladder DTY28ZZ
Bone, Other DPYC8ZZ
Bone Marrow D7YØ8ZZ
Brain DØYØ8ZZ
Brain Stem DØY18ZZ
Breast
Left DMYØ8ZZ
Right DMY18ZZ
Bronchus DBY18ZZ
Cervix DUY18ZZ
Chest DWY28ZZ
Chest Wall DBY78ZZ
Colon DDY58ZZ
Diaphragm DBY88ZZ
Duodenum DDY28ZZ
Ear D9YØ8ZZ
Esophagus DDYØ8ZZ
Eye D8YØ8ZZ
Femur DPY98ZZ
Fibula DPYB8ZZ
Gallbladder DFY18ZZ
Gland
Adrenal DGY28ZZ
Parathyroid DGY48ZZ
Pituitary DGYØ8ZZ
Thyroid DGY58ZZ
Glands, Salivary D9Y68ZZ
Head and Neck DWY18ZZ
Hemibody DWY48ZZ
Humerus DPY68ZZ
Hypopharynx D9Y38ZZ
Ileum DDY48ZZ
Jejunum DDY38ZZ
Kidney DTYØ8ZZ
Larynx D9YB8ZZ
Liver DFYØ8ZZ
Lung DBY28ZZ
Lymphatics
Abdomen D7Y68ZZ
Axillary D7Y48ZZ
Inguinal D7Y88ZZ
Neck D7Y38ZZ
Pelvis D7Y78ZZ
Thorax D7Y58ZZ
Mandible DPY38ZZ
Maxilla DPY28ZZ
Mediastinum DBY68ZZ
Mouth D9Y48ZZ
Nasopharynx D9YD8ZZ
Neck and Head DWY18ZZ
Nerve, Peripheral DØY78ZZ
Nose D9Y18ZZ
Oropharynx D9YF8ZZ
Ovary DUYØ8ZZ
Palate
Hard D9Y88ZZ
Soft D9Y98ZZ
Pancreas DFY38ZZ
Parathyroid Gland DGY48ZZ
Pelvic Bones DPY88ZZ
Pelvic Region DWY68ZZ

Hyperthermia—continued
Radiation Oncology—continued
Pineal Body DGY18ZZ
Pituitary Gland DGYØ8ZZ
Pleura DBY58ZZ
Prostate DVYØ8ZZ
Radius DPY78ZZ
Rectum DDY78ZZ
Rib DPY58ZZ
Sinuses D9Y78ZZ
Skin
Abdomen DHY88ZZ
Arm DHY48ZZ
Back DHY78ZZ
Buttock DHY98ZZ
Chest DHY68ZZ
Face DHY28ZZ
Leg DHYB8ZZ
Neck DHY38ZZ
Skull DPYØ8ZZ
Spinal Cord DØY68ZZ
Spleen D7Y28ZZ
Sternum DPY48ZZ
Stomach DDY18ZZ
Testis DVY18ZZ
Thymus D7Y18ZZ
Thyroid Gland DGY58ZZ
Tibia DPYB8ZZ
Tongue D9Y58ZZ
Trachea DBYØ8ZZ
Ulna DPY78ZZ
Ureter DTY18ZZ
Urethra DTY38ZZ
Uterus DUY28ZZ
Whole Body DWY58ZZ
Whole Body 6A3Z
Hypnosis GZFZZZZ
Hypogastric artery
use Artery, Internal Iliac, Right
use Artery, Internal Iliac, Left
Hypopharynx use Pharynx
Hypophysectomy
see Excision, Gland, Pituitary ØGBØ
see Resection, Gland, Pituitary ØGTØ
Hypophysis use Gland, Pituitary
Hypothalamotomy see Destruction, Thalamus ØØ59
Hypothenar muscle
use Muscle, Hand, Right
use Muscle, Hand, Left
Hypothermia, Whole Body 6A4Z
Hysterectomy
see Excision, Uterus ØUB9
see Resection, Uterus ØUT9
Hysterolysis see Release, Uterus ØUN9
Hysteropexy
see Repair, Uterus ØUQ9
see Reposition, Uterus ØUS9
Hysteroplasty see Repair, Uterus ØUQ9
Hysterorrhaphy see Repair, Uterus ØUQ9
Hysteroscopy ØUJD8ZZ
Hysterotomy see Drainage, Uterus ØU99
Hysterotrachelectomy see Resection, Uterus ØUT9
Hysterotracheloplasty see Repair, Uterus ØUQ9
Hysterotrachelorrhaphy see Repair, Uterus ØUQ9

I

IABP (intra-aortic balloon pump) see Assistance, Cardiac 5AØ2
IAEMT (intraoperative anesthetic effect monitoring and titration) see Monitoring, Central Nervous 4A1Ø
Ileal artery use Artery, Superior Mesenteric
Ileectomy
see Excision, Ileum ØDBB
see Resection, Ileum ØDTB
Ileocolic artery use Artery, Superior Mesenteric
Ileocolic vein use Vein, Colic
Ileopexy
see Repair, Ileum ØDQB
see Reposition, Ileum ØDSB

Ileorrhaphy see Repair, Ileum ØDQB
Ileoscopy ØDJD8ZZ
Ileostomy
see Bypass, Ileum ØD1B
see Drainage, Ileum ØD9B
Ileotomy see Drainage, Ileum ØD9B
Ileoureterostomy see Bypass, Urinary System ØT1
Iliac crest
use Bone, Pelvic, Left
use Bone, Pelvic, Right
Iliac fascia
use Subcutaneous Tissue and Fascia, Upper Leg, Left
use Subcutaneous Tissue and Fascia, Upper Leg, Right
Iliac lymph node use Lymphatic, Pelvis
Iliacus muscle
use Muscle, Hip, Right
use Muscle, Hip, Left
Iliofemoral ligament
use Bursa and Ligament, Hip, Left
use Bursa and Ligament, Hip, Right
Iliohypogastric nerve use Nerve, Lumbar Plexus
Ilioinguinal nerve use Nerve, Lumbar Plexus
Iliolumbar artery
use Artery, Internal Iliac, Left
use Artery, Internal Iliac, Right
Iliolumbar ligament
use Bursa and Ligament, Trunk, Left
use Bursa and Ligament, Trunk, Right
Iliotibial tract (band)
use Subcutaneous Tissue and Fascia, Upper Leg, Right
use Subcutaneous Tissue and Fascia, Upper Leg, Left
Ilium
use Bone, Pelvic, Left
use Bone, Pelvic, Right
Imaging, diagnostic
see Computerized Tomography (CT Scan)
see Fluoroscopy
see Magnetic Resonance Imaging (MRI)
see Plain Radiography
see Ultrasonography
Immobilization
Abdominal Wall 2W33X
Arm
Lower
Left 2W3DX
Right 2W3CX
Upper
Left 2W3BX
Right 2W3AX
Back 2W35X
Chest Wall 2W34X
Extremity
Lower
Left 2W3MX
Right 2W3LX
Upper
Left 2W39X
Right 2W38X
Face 2W31X
Finger
Left 2W3KX
Right 2W3JX
Foot
Left 2W3TX
Right 2W3SX
Hand
Left 2W3FX
Right 2W3EX
Head 2W3ØX
Inguinal Region
Left 2W37X
Right 2W36X
Leg
Lower
Left 2W3RX
Right 2W3QX
Upper
Left 2W3PX
Right 2W3NX
Neck 2W32X

Immobilization—continued
Thumb
Left 2W3HX
Right 2W3GX
Toe
Left 2W3VX
Right 2W3UX
Immunization see Introduction, Serum, Toxoid, and Vaccine
Immunotherapy see Introduction, Immunotherapeutic Substance
Immunotherapy, antineoplastic
Interferon see Introduction, Low-dose Interleukin-2
Interleukin-2, high-dose see Introduction, High-dose Interleukin-2
Interleukin-2, low-dose see Introduction, Low-dose Interleukin-2
Monoclonal antibody see Introduction, Monoclonal Antibody
Proleukin, high-dose see Introduction, High-dose Interleukin-2
Proleukin, low-dose see Introduction, Low-dose Interleukin-2
Impeller Pump
Continuous, Output 5A0221D
Intermittent, Output 5A0211D
Implantation
see Insertion
see Replacement
IMV (intermittent mandatory ventilation) see Assistance, Respiratory 5A09
In Vitro Fertilization 8E0ZXY1
Incision, abscess see Drainage
Incudectomy
see Excision, Ear, Nose, Sinus 09B
see Resection, Ear, Nose, Sinus 09T
Incudopexy
see Reposition, Ear, Nose, Sinus 09S
see Repair, Ear, Nose, Sinus 09Q
Incus
use Auditory Ossicle, Left
use Auditory Ossicle, Right
Induction of labor
Artificial rupture of membranes see Drainage, Pregnancy 109
Oxytocin see Introduction, Hormone
Inferior cardiac nerve use Nerve, Thoracic Sympathetic
Inferior cerebellar vein use Vein, Intracranial
Inferior cerebral vein use Vein, Intracranial
Inferior epigastric artery
use Artery, External Iliac, Right
use Artery, External Iliac, Left
Inferior epigastric lymph node use Lymphatic, Pelvis
Inferior genicular artery
use Artery, Popliteal, Left
use Artery, Popliteal, Right
Inferior gluteal artery
use Artery, Internal Iliac, Right
use Artery, Internal Iliac, Left
Inferior gluteal nerve use Nerve, Sacral Plexus
Inferior hypogastric plexus use Nerve, Abdominal Sympathetic
Inferior labial artery use Artery, Face
Inferior longitudinal muscle use Muscle, Tongue, Palate, Pharynx
Inferior mesenteric ganglion use Nerve, Abdominal Sympathetic
Inferior mesenteric lymph node use Lymphatic, Mesenteric
Inferior mesenteric plexus use Nerve, Abdominal Sympathetic
Inferior oblique muscle
use Muscle, Extraocular, Right
use Muscle, Extraocular, Left
Inferior pancreaticoduodenal artery use Artery, Superior Mesenteric
Inferior phrenic artery use Aorta, Abdominal
Inferior rectus muscle
use Muscle, Extraocular, Right
use Muscle, Extraocular, Left

Inferior suprarenal artery
use Artery, Renal, Left
use Artery, Renal, Right
Inferior tarsal plate
use Eyelid, Lower, Right
use Eyelid, Lower, Left
Inferior thyroid vein
use Vein, Innominate, Left
use Vein, Innominate, Right
Inferior tibiofibular joint
use Joint, Ankle, Right
use Joint, Ankle, Left
Inferior turbinate use Turbinate, Nasal
Inferior ulnar collateral artery
use Artery, Brachial, Right
use Artery, Brachial, Left
Inferior vesical artery
use Artery, Internal Iliac, Right
use Artery, Internal Iliac, Left
Infraauricular lymph node use Lymphatic, Head
Infraclavicular (deltopectoral) lymph node
use Lymphatic, Upper Extremity, Left
use Lymphatic, Upper Extremity, Right
Infrahyoid muscle
use Muscle, Neck, Left
use Muscle, Neck, Right
Infraparotid lymph node use Lymphatic, Head
Infraspinatus fascia
use Subcutaneous Tissue and Fascia, Upper Arm, Right
use Subcutaneous Tissue and Fascia, Upper Arm, Left
Infraspinatus muscle
use Muscle, Shoulder, Right
use Muscle, Shoulder, Left
Infundibulopelvic ligament use Uterine Supporting Structure
Infusion see Introduction
Infusion Pump
Insertion of device in
Abdomen 0JH8
Back 0JH7
Chest 0JH6
Lower Arm
Left 0JHH
Right 0JHG
Lower Leg
Left 0JHP
Right 0JHN
Trunk 0JHT
Upper Arm
Left 0JHF
Right 0JHD
Upper Leg
Left 0JHM
Right 0JHL
Removal of device from
Lower Extremity 0JPW
Trunk 0JPT
Upper Extremity 0JPV
Revision of device in
Lower Extremity 0JWW
Trunk 0JWT
Upper Extremity 0JWV
Inguinal canal
use Inguinal Region, Right
use Inguinal Region, Left
use Inguinal Region, Bilateral
Inguinal triangle
use Inguinal Region, Right
use Inguinal Region, Bilateral
use Inguinal Region, Left
Injection see Introduction
Insemination, artificial 3E0P7LZ
Insertion, Products of Conception 10H0
Insertion of device in
Abdominal Wall 0WHF
Acetabulum
Left 0QH5
Right 0QH4
Anal Sphincter 0DHR

Insertion of device in—continued
Ankle Region
Left 0YHL
Right 0YHK
Anus 0DHQ
Aorta
Abdominal 04H0
Thoracic 02HW
Arm
Lower
Left 0XHF
Right 0XHD
Upper
Left 0XH9
Right 0XH8
Artery
Anterior Tibial
Left 04HQ
Right 04HP
Axillary
Left 03H6
Right 03H5
Brachial
Left 03H8
Right 03H7
Celiac 04H1
Colic
Left 04H7
Middle 04H8
Right 04H6
Common Carotid
Left 03HJ
Right 03HH
Common Iliac
Left 04HD
Right 04HC
External Carotid
Left 03HN
Right 03HM
External Iliac
Left 04HJ
Right 04HH
Face 03HR
Femoral
Left 04HL
Right 04HK
Foot
Left 04HW
Right 04HV
Gastric 04H2
Hand
Left 03HF
Right 03HD
Hepatic 04H3
Inferior Mesenteric 04HB
Innominate 03H2
Internal Carotid
Left 03HL
Right 03HK
Internal Iliac
Left 04HF
Right 04HE
Internal Mammary
Left 03H1
Right 03H0
Intracranial 03HG
Lower 04HY
Peroneal
Left 04HU
Right 04HT
Popliteal
Left 04HN
Right 04HM
Posterior Tibial
Left 04HS
Right 04HR
Pulmonary
Left 02HR
Right 02HQ
Pulmonary Trunk 02HP
Radial
Left 03HC
Right 03HB

Insertion of device in—*continued*

Anterior Tibial—*continued*

Renal
Left Ø4HA
Right Ø4H9

Splenic Ø4H4

Subclavian
Left Ø3H4
Right Ø3H3

Superior Mesenteric Ø4H5

Temporal
Left Ø3HT
Right Ø3HS

Thyroid
Left Ø3HV
Right Ø3HU

Ulnar
Left Ø3HA
Right Ø3H9

Upper Ø3HY

Vertebral
Left Ø3HQ
Right Ø3HP

Atrium
Left Ø2H7
Right Ø2H6

Axilla
Left ØXH5
Right ØXH4

Back
Lower ØWHL
Upper ØWHK

Bladder ØTHB

Bladder Neck ØTHC

Bone

Ethmoid
Left ØNHG
Right ØNHF

Facial ØNHW

Frontal
Left ØNH2
Right ØNH1

Hyoid ØNHX

Lacrimal
Left ØNHJ
Right ØNHH

Lower ØQHY

Nasal ØNHB

Occipital
Left ØNH8
Right ØNH7

Palatine
Left ØNHL
Right ØNHK

Parietal
Left ØNH4
Right ØNH3

Pelvic
Left ØQH3
Right ØQH2

Sphenoid
Left ØNHD
Right ØNHC

Temporal
Left ØNH6
Right ØNH5

Upper ØPHY

Zygomatic
Left ØNHN
Right ØNHM

Brain ØØHØ

Breast
Bilateral ØHHV
Left ØHHU
Right ØHHT

Bronchus
Lingula ØBH9

Lower Lobe
Left ØBHB
Right ØBH6

Main
Left ØBH7
Right ØBH3

Insertion of device in—*continued*

Bronchus—*continued*
Middle Lobe, Right ØBH5

Upper Lobe
Left ØBH8
Right ØBH4

Buttock
Left ØYH1
Right ØYHØ

Carpal
Left ØPHN
Right ØPHM

Cavity, Cranial ØWH1

Cerebral Ventricle ØØH6

Cervix ØUHC

Chest Wall ØWH8

Cisterna Chyli Ø7HL

Clavicle
Left ØPHB
Right ØPH9

Coccyx ØQHS

Cul-de-sac ØUHF

Diaphragm
Left ØBHS
Right ØBHR

Disc
Cervical Vertebral ØRH3
Cervicothoracic Vertebral ØRH5
Lumbar Vertebral ØSH2
Lumbosacral ØSH4
Thoracic Vertebral ØRH9
Thoracolumbar Vertebral ØRHB

Duct
Hepatobiliary ØFHB
Pancreatic ØFHD

Duodenum ØDH9

Ear
Left Ø9HE
Other Hearing Device Ø9HEØSY
Right Ø9HD
Other Hearing Device Ø9HDØSY

Elbow Region
Left ØXHC
Right ØXHB

Epididymis and Spermatic Cord ØVHM

Esophagus ØDH5

Extremity
Lower
Left ØYHB
Right ØYH9
Upper
Left ØXH7
Right ØXH6

Eye
Left Ø8H1
Right Ø8HØ

Face ØWH2

Fallopian Tube ØUH8

Femoral Region
Left ØYH8
Right ØYH7

Femoral Shaft
Left ØQH9
Right ØQH8

Femur
Lower
Left ØQHC
Right ØQHB
Upper
Left ØQH7
Right ØQH6

Fibula
Left ØQHK
Right ØQHJ

Foot
Left ØYHN
Right ØYHM

Gallbladder ØFH4

Gastrointestinal Tract ØWHP

Genitourinary Tract ØWHR

Gland, Endocrine ØGHS

Insertion of device in—*continued*

Glenoid Cavity
Left ØPH8
Right ØPH7

Hand
Left ØXHK
Right ØXHJ

Head ØWHØ

Heart Ø2HA

Humeral Head
Left ØPHD
Right ØPHC

Humeral Shaft
Left ØPHG
Right ØPHF

Ileum ØDHB

Inguinal Region
Left ØYH6
Right ØYH5

Intestine, Small ØDH8

Jaw
Lower ØWH5
Upper ØWH4

Jejunum ØDHA

Joint

Acromioclavicular
Left ØRHH
Right ØRHG

Ankle
Left ØSHG
Right ØSHF

Carpal
Left ØRHR
Right ØRHQ

Cervical Vertebral ØRH1

Cervicothoracic Vertebral ØRH4

Coccygeal ØSH6

Elbow
Left ØRHM
Right ØRHL

Finger Phalangeal
Left ØRHX
Right ØRHW

Hip
Left ØSHB
Right ØSH9

Knee
Left ØSHD
Right ØSHC

Lumbar Vertebral ØSHØ

Lumbosacral ØSH3

Metacarpocarpal
Left ØRHT
Right ØRHS

Metacarpophalangeal
Left ØRHV
Right ØRHU

Metatarsal-Phalangeal
Left ØSHN
Right ØSHM

Metatarsal-Tarsal
Left ØSHL
Right ØSHK

Occipital-cervical ØRHØ

Sacrococcygeal ØSH5

Sacroiliac
Left ØSH8
Right ØSH7

Shoulder
Left ØRHK
Right ØRHJ

Sternoclavicular
Left ØRHF
Right ØRHE

Tarsal
Left ØSHJ
Right ØSHH

Temporomandibular
Left ØRHD
Right ØRHC

Thoracic Vertebral ØRH6

Thoracolumbar Vertebral ØRHA

Insertion of device in—*continued*
- Vein—*continued*
  - Pulmonary
    - Left 02HT
    - Right 02HS
  - Renal
    - Left 06HB
    - Right 06H9
  - Splenic 06H1
  - Subclavian
    - Left 05H6
    - Right 05H5
  - Superior Mesenteric 06H5
  - Upper 05HY
  - Vertebral
    - Left 05HS
    - Right 05HR
- Vena Cava
  - Inferior 06H0
  - Superior 02HV
- Ventricle
  - Left 02HL
  - Right 02HK
- Vertebra
  - Cervical 0PH3
  - Lumbar 0QH0
  - Thoracic 0PH4
- Wrist Region
  - Left 0XHH
  - Right 0XHG

Inspection
- Abdominal Wall 0WJF
- Ankle Region
  - Left 0YJL
  - Right 0YJK
- Arm
  - Lower
    - Left 0XJF
    - Right 0XJD
  - Upper
    - Left 0XJ9
    - Right 0XJ8
- Artery
  - Lower 04JY
  - Upper 03JY
- Axilla
  - Left 0XJ5
  - Right 0XJ4
- Back
  - Lower 0WJL
  - Upper 0WJK
- Bladder 0TJB
- Bone
  - Facial 0NJW
  - Lower 0QJY
  - Nasal 0NJB
  - Upper 0PJY
- Bone Marrow 07JT
- Brain 00J0
- Breast
  - Left 0HJU
  - Right 0HJT
- Bursa and Ligament
  - Lower 0MJY
  - Upper 0MJX
- Buttock
  - Left 0YJ1
  - Right 0YJ0
- Cavity, Cranial 0WJ1
- Chest Wall 0WJ8
- Cisterna Chyli 07JL
- Diaphragm 0BJT
- Disc
  - Cervical Vertebral 0RJ3
  - Cervicothoracic Vertebral 0RJ5
  - Lumbar Vertebral 0SJ2
  - Lumbosacral 0SJ4
  - Thoracic Vertebral 0RJ9
  - Thoracolumbar Vertebral 0RJB
- Duct
  - Hepatobiliary 0FJB
  - Pancreatic 0FJD

Inspection—*continued*
- Ear
  - Inner
    - Left 09JE
    - Right 09JD
  - Left 09JJ
  - Right 09JH
- Elbow Region
  - Left 0XJC
  - Right 0XJB
- Epididymis and Spermatic Cord 0VJM
- Extremity
  - Lower
    - Left 0YJB
    - Right 0YJ9
  - Upper
    - Left 0XJ7
    - Right 0XJ6
- Eye
  - Left 08J1XZZ
  - Right 08J0XZZ
- Face 0WJ2
- Fallopian Tube 0UJ8
- Femoral Region
  - Bilateral 0YJE
  - Left 0YJ8
  - Right 0YJ7
- Finger Nail 0HJQXZZ
- Foot
  - Left 0YJN
  - Right 0YJM
- Gallbladder 0FJ4
- Gastrointestinal Tract 0WJP
- Genitourinary Tract 0WJR
- Gland
  - Adrenal 0GJ5
  - Endocrine 0GJS
  - Pituitary 0GJ0
  - Salivary 0CJA
- Great Vessel 02JY
- Hand
  - Left 0XJK
  - Right 0XJJ
- Head 0WJ0
- Heart 02JA
- Inguinal Region
  - Bilateral 0YJA
  - Left 0YJ6
  - Right 0YJ5
- Intestinal Tract
  - Lower 0DJD
  - Upper 0DJ0
- Jaw
  - Lower 0WJ5
  - Upper 0WJ4
- Joint
  - Acromioclavicular
    - Left 0RJH
    - Right 0RJG
  - Ankle
    - Left 0SJG
    - Right 0SJF
  - Carpal
    - Left 0RJR
    - Right 0RJQ
  - Cervical Vertebral 0RJ1
  - Cervicothoracic Vertebral 0RJ4
  - Coccygeal 0SJ6
  - Elbow
    - Left 0RJM
    - Right 0RJL
  - Finger Phalangeal
    - Left 0RJX
    - Right 0RJW
  - Hip
    - Left 0SJB
    - Right 0SJ9
  - Knee
    - Left 0SJD
    - Right 0SJC
  - Lumbar Vertebral 0SJ0
  - Lumbosacral 0SJ3

Inspection—*continued*
- Joint—*continued*
  - Metacarpocarpal
    - Left 0RJT
    - Right 0RJS
  - Metacarpophalangeal
    - Left 0RJV
    - Right 0RJU
  - Metatarsal-Phalangeal
    - Left 0SJN
    - Right 0SJM
  - Metatarsal-Tarsal
    - Left 0SJL
    - Right 0SJK
  - Occipital-cervical 0RJ0
  - Sacrococcygeal 0SJ5
  - Sacroiliac
    - Left 0SJ8
    - Right 0SJ7
  - Shoulder
    - Left 0RJK
    - Right 0RJJ
  - Sternoclavicular
    - Left 0RJF
    - Right 0RJE
  - Tarsal
    - Left 0SJJ
    - Right 0SJH
  - Temporomandibular
    - Left 0RJD
    - Right 0RJC
  - Thoracic Vertebral 0RJ6
  - Thoracolumbar Vertebral 0RJA
  - Toe Phalangeal
    - Left 0SJQ
    - Right 0SJP
  - Wrist
    - Left 0RJP
    - Right 0RJN
- Kidney 0TJ5
- Knee Region
  - Left 0YJG
  - Right 0YJF
- Larynx 0CJS
- Leg
  - Lower
    - Left 0YJJ
    - Right 0YJH
  - Upper
    - Left 0YJD
    - Right 0YJC
- Lens
  - Left 08JKXZZ
  - Right 08JJXZZ
- Liver 0FJ0
- Lung
  - Left 0BJL
  - Right 0BJK
- Lymphatic 07JN
  - Thoracic Duct 07JK
- Mediastinum 0WJC
- Mesentery 0DJV
- Mouth and Throat 0CJY
- Muscle
  - Extraocular
    - Left 08JM
    - Right 08JL
  - Lower 0KJY
  - Upper 0KJX
- Neck 0WJ6
- Nerve
  - Cranial 00JE
  - Peripheral 01JY
- Nose 09JK
- Omentum 0DJU
- Oral Cavity and Throat 0WJ3
- Ovary 0UJ3
- Pancreas 0FJG
- Parathyroid Gland 0GJR
- Pelvic Cavity 0WJJ
- Penis 0VJS
- Pericardial Cavity 0WJD

Inspection—*continued*
  Perineum
    Female ØWJN
    Male ØWJM
  Peritoneal Cavity ØWJG
  Peritoneum ØDJW
  Pineal Body ØGJ1
  Pleura ØBJQ
  Pleural Cavity
    Left ØWJB
    Right ØWJ9
  Products of Conception 1ØJØ
    Ectopic 1ØJ2
    Retained 1ØJ1
  Prostate and Seminal Vesicles ØVJ4
  Respiratory Tract ØWJQ
  Retroperitoneum ØWJH
  Scrotum and Tunica Vaginalis ØVJ8
  Shoulder Region
    Left ØXJ3
    Right ØXJ2
  Sinus Ø9JY
  Skin ØHJPXZZ
  Skull ØNJØ
  Spinal Canal ØØJU
  Spinal Cord ØØJV
  Spleen Ø7JP
  Stomach ØDJ6
  Subcutaneous Tissue and Fascia
    Head and Neck ØJJS
    Lower Extremity ØJJW
    Trunk ØJJT
    Upper Extremity ØJJV
  Tendon
    Lower ØLJY
    Upper ØLJX
  Testis ØVJD
  Thymus Ø7JM
  Thyroid Gland ØGJK
  Toe Nail ØHJRXZZ
  Trachea ØBJ1
  Tracheobronchial Tree ØBJØ
  Tympanic Membrane
    Left Ø9J8
    Right Ø9J7
  Ureter ØTJ9
  Urethra ØTJD
  Uterus and Cervix ØUJD
  Vagina and Cul-de-sac ØUJH
  Vas Deferens ØVJR
  Vein
    Lower Ø6JY
    Upper Ø5JY
  Vulva ØUJM
  Wrist Region
    Left ØXJH
    Right ØXJG
Instillation *see* Introduction
Insufflation *see* Introduction
Interatrial septum *use* Septum, Atrial
Intercarpal joint
  use Joint, Carpal, Right
  use Joint, Carpal, Left
Intercarpal ligament
  use Bursa and Ligament, Hand, Right
  use Bursa and Ligament, Hand, Left
Interclavicular ligament
  use Bursa and Ligament, Shoulder, Right
  use Bursa and Ligament, Shoulder, Left
Intercostal lymph node *use* Lymphatic, Thorax
Intercostal muscle
  use Muscle, Thorax, Right
  use Muscle, Thorax, Left
Intercostal nerve *use* Nerve, Thoracic
Intercostobrachial nerve *use* Nerve, Thoracic
Intercuneiform joint
  use Joint, Tarsal, Right
  use Joint, Tarsal, Left
Intercuneiform ligament
  use Bursa and Ligament, Foot, Left
  use Bursa and Ligament, Foot, Right

Intermediate cuneiform bone
  use Tarsal, Right
  use Tarsal, Left
Intermittent mandatory ventilation *see* Assistance, Respiratory 5AØ9
Intermittent Negative Airway Pressure
  24-96 Consecutive Hours, Ventilation 5AØ945B
  Greater than 96 Consecutive Hours, Ventilation 5AØ955B
  Less than 24 Consecutive Hours, Ventilation 5AØ935B
Intermittent Positive Airway Pressure
  24-96 Consecutive Hours, Ventilation 5AØ9458
  Greater than 96 Consecutive Hours, Ventilation 5AØ9558
  Less than 24 Consecutive Hours, Ventilation 5AØ9358
Intermittent positive pressure breathing *see* Assistance, Respiratory 5AØ9
Internal (basal) cerebral vein *use* Vein, Intracranial
Internal anal sphincter *use* Anal Sphincter
Internal carotid plexus *use* Nerve, Head and Neck Sympathetic
Internal iliac vein
  use Vein, Hypogastric, Right
  use Vein, Hypogastric, Left
Internal maxillary artery
  use Artery, External Carotid, Left
  use Artery, External Carotid, Right
Internal naris *use* Nose
Internal oblique muscle
  use Muscle, Abdomen, Right
  use Muscle, Abdomen, Left
Internal pudendal artery
  use Artery, Internal Iliac, Right
  use Artery, Internal Iliac, Left
Internal pudendal vein
  use Vein, Hypogastric, Right
  use Vein, Hypogastric, Left
Internal thoracic artery
  use Artery, Subclavian, Right
  use Artery, Subclavian, Left
  use Artery, Internal Mammary, Left
  use Artery, Internal Mammary, Right
Internal urethral sphincter *use* Urethra
Interphalangeal (IP) joint
  use Joint, Finger Phalangeal, Left
  use Joint, Toe Phalangeal, Right
  use Joint, Toe Phalangeal, Left
  use Joint, Finger Phalangeal, Right
Interphalangeal ligament
  use Bursa and Ligament, Hand, Left
  use Bursa and Ligament, Hand, Right
  use Bursa and Ligament, Foot, Right
  use Bursa and Ligament, Foot, Left
Interrogation, cardiac rhythm related device
  Interrogation only *see* Measurement, Cardiac 4BØ2
  With cardiac function testing *see* Measurement, Cardiac 4AØ2
Interruption *see* Occlusion
Interspinalis muscle
  use Muscle, Trunk, Right
  use Muscle, Trunk, Left
Interspinous ligament
  use Bursa and Ligament, Trunk, Right
  use Bursa and Ligament, Trunk, Left
Intertransversarius muscle
  use Muscle, Trunk, Left
  use Muscle, Trunk, Right
Intertransverse ligament
  use Bursa and Ligament, Trunk, Right
  use Bursa and Ligament, Trunk, Left
Interventricular foramen (Monro) *use* Cerebral Ventricle
Interventricular septum *use* Septum, Ventricular
Intestinal lymphatic trunk *use* Cisterna Chyli
Intraocular Telescope
  Left Ø8RK3J5
  Right Ø8RJ3J5
Intraoperative Radiation Therapy (IORT)
  Anus DDY8CZZ
  Bile Ducts DFY2CZZ
  Bladder DTY2CZZ

Intraoperative Radiation Therapy (IORT)—
    continued
  Cervix DUY1CZZ
  Colon DDY5CZZ
  Duodenum DDY2CZZ
  Gallbladder DFY1CZZ
  Ileum DDY4CZZ
  Jejunum DDY3CZZ
  Kidney DTYØCZZ
  Larynx D9YBCZZ
  Liver DFYØCZZ
  Mouth D9Y4CZZ
  Nasopharynx D9YDCZZ
  Ovary DUYØCZZ
  Pancreas DFY3CZZ
  Pharynx D9YCCZZ
  Prostate DVYØCZZ
  Rectum DDY7CZZ
  Stomach DDY1CZZ
  Ureter DTY1CZZ
  Urethra DTY3CZZ
  Uterus DUY2CZZ
Introduction
  Artery
    Central 3EØ6
      Analgesics 3EØ6
      Anesthetic, Intracirculatory 3EØ6
      Anti-infective 3EØ6
      Anti-inflammatory 3EØ6
      Antiarrhythmic 3EØ6
      Antineoplastic 3EØ6
      Contrast Agent 3EØ6
      Destructive Agent 3EØ6
      Diagnostic Substance, Other 3EØ6
      Electrolytic Substance 3EØ6
      Hormone 3EØ6
      Hypnotics 3EØ6
      Immunotherapeutic 3EØ6
      Nutritional Substance 3EØ6
      Platelet Inhibitor 3EØ6
      Radioactive Substance 3EØ6
      Sedatives 3EØ6
      Serum 3EØ6
      Thrombolytic 3EØ6
      Toxoid 3EØ6
      Vaccine 3EØ6
      Vasopressor 3EØ6
      Water Balance Substance 3EØ6
    Coronary 3EØ7
      Contrast Agent 3EØ7
      Diagnostic Substance, Other 3EØ7
      Platelet Inhibitor 3EØ7
      Thrombolytic 3EØ7
    Peripheral 3EØ5
      Analgesics 3EØ5
      Anesthetic, Intracirculatory 3EØ5
      Anti-infective 3EØ5
      Anti-inflammatory 3EØ5
      Antiarrhythmic 3EØ5
      Antineoplastic 3EØ5
      Contrast Agent 3EØ5
      Destructive Agent 3EØ5
      Diagnostic Substance, Other 3EØ5
      Electrolytic Substance 3EØ5
      Hormone 3EØ5
      Hypnotics 3EØ5
      Immunotherapeutic 3EØ5
      Nutritional Substance 3EØ5
      Platelet Inhibitor 3EØ5
      Radioactive Substance 3EØ5
      Sedatives 3EØ5
      Serum 3EØ5
      Thrombolytic 3EØ5
      Toxoid 3EØ5
      Vaccine 3EØ5
      Vasopressor 3EØ5
      Water Balance Substance 3EØ5
  Biliary Tract 3EØJ
    Analgesics 3EØJ
    Anesthetic, Local 3EØJ
    Anti-infective 3EØJ
    Anti-inflammatory 3EØJ
    Antineoplastic 3EØJ

Introduction—*continued*
Vein
Central 3E04
Analgesics 3E04
Anesthetic, Intracirculatory 3E04
Anti-infective 3E04
Anti-inflammatory 3E04
Antiarrhythmic 3E04
Antineoplastic 3E04
Contrast Agent 3E04
Destructive Agent 3E04
Diagnostic Substance, Other 3E04
Electrolytic Substance 3E04
Hormone 3E04
Hypnotics 3E04
Immunotherapeutic 3E04
Nutritional Substance 3E04
Platelet Inhibitor 3E04
Radioactive Substance 3E04
Sedatives 3E04
Serum 3E04
Thrombolytic 3E04
Toxoid 3E04
Vaccine 3E04
Vasopressor 3E04
Water Balance Substance 3E04
Peripheral 3E03
Analgesics 3E03
Anesthetic, Intracirculatory 3E03
Anti-infective 3E03
Anti-inflammatory 3E03
Antiarrhythmic 3E03
Antineoplastic 3E03
Contrast Agent 3E03
Destructive Agent 3E03
Diagnostic Substance, Other 3E03
Electrolytic Substance 3E03
Hormone 3E03
Hypnotics 3E03
Immunotherapeutic 3E03
Islet Cells, Pancreatic 3E03
Nutritional Substance 3E03
Platelet Inhibitor 3E03
Radioactive Substance 3E03
Sedatives 3E03
Serum 3E03
Thrombolytic 3E03
Toxoid 3E03
Vaccine 3E03
Vasopressor 3E03
Water Balance Substance 3E03
Intubation
Airway
see Insertion of device in, Trachea 0BH1
see Insertion of device in, Mouth and Throat 0CHY
see Insertion of device in, Esophagus 0DH5
Drainage device *see* Drainage
Feeding Device *see* Insertion of device in, Gastrointestinal System 0DH
IPPB (intermittent positive pressure breathing) *see* Assistance, Respiratory 5A09
Iridectomy
see Excision, Eye 08B
see Resection, Eye 08T
Iridoplasty
see Repair, Eye 08Q
see Replacement, Eye 08R
see Supplement, Eye 08U
Iridotomy *see* Drainage, Eye 089
Irrigation
Biliary Tract, Irrigating Substance 3E1J
Brain, Irrigating Substance 3E1Q38Z
Cranial Cavity, Irrigating Substance 3E1Q38Z
Ear, Irrigating Substance 3E1B
Epidural Space, Irrigating Substance 3E1S38Z
Eye, Irrigating Substance 3E1C
Gastrointestinal Tract
Lower, Irrigating Substance 3E1H
Upper, Irrigating Substance 3E1G
Genitourinary Tract, Irrigating Substance 3E1K
Irrigating Substance 3C1ZX8Z
Joint, Irrigating Substance 3E1U38Z

Irrigation—*continued*
Mucous Membrane, Irrigating Substance 3E10
Nose, Irrigating Substance 3E19
Pancreatic Tract, Irrigating Substance 3E1J
Pericardial Cavity, Irrigating Substance 3E1Y38Z
Peritoneal Cavity
Dialysate 3E1M39Z
Irrigating Substance 3E1M38Z
Pleural Cavity, Irrigating Substance 3E1L38Z
Reproductive
Female, Irrigating Substance 3E1P
Male, Irrigating Substance 3E1N
Respiratory Tract, Irrigating Substance 3E1F
Skin, Irrigating Substance 3E10
Spinal Canal, Irrigating Substance 3E1R38Z
Ischiatic nerve *use* Nerve, Sciatic
Ischiocavernosus muscle *use* Muscle, Perineum
Ischiofemoral ligament
use Bursa and Ligament, Hip, Left
use Bursa and Ligament, Hip, Right
Ischium
use Bone, Pelvic, Right
use Bone, Pelvic, Left
Isolation 8E0ZXY6
Isotope Administration, Whole Body DWY5G

J

Jejunal artery *use* Artery, Superior Mesenteric
Jejunectomy
see Excision, Jejunum 0DBA
see Resection, Jejunum 0DTA
Jejunocolostomy
see Bypass, Gastrointestinal System 0D1
see Drainage, Gastrointestinal System 0D9
Jejunopexy
see Repair, Jejunum 0DQA
see Reposition, Jejunum 0DSA
Jejunostomy
see Bypass, Jejunum 0D1A
see Drainage, Jejunum 0D9A
Jejunotomy *see* Drainage, Jejunum 0D9A
Jugular body *use* Glomus Jugulare
Jugular lymph node
use Lymphatic, Neck, Left
use Lymphatic, Neck, Right

K

Keratectomy, kerectomy
see Excision, Eye 08B
see Resection, Eye 08T
Keratocentesis *see* Drainage, Eye 089
Keratoplasty
see Repair, Eye 08Q
see Replacement, Eye 08R
see Supplement, Eye 08U
Keratotomy
see Drainage, Eye 089
see Repair, Eye 08Q
KUB x-ray *see* Plain Radiography, Kidney, Ureter and Bladder BT04

L

Labia majora *use* Vulva
Labia minora *use* Vulva
Labial gland *use* Buccal Mucosa
Labiectomy
see Excision, Female Reproductive System 0UB
see Resection, Female Reproductive System 0UT
Lacrimal canaliculus
use Duct, Lacrimal, Left
use Duct, Lacrimal, Right
Lacrimal punctum
use Duct, Lacrimal, Right
use Duct, Lacrimal, Left

Lacrimal sac
use Duct, Lacrimal, Right
use Duct, Lacrimal, Left
Laminectomy
see Excision, Upper Joints 0RB
see Excision, Lower Joints 0SB
Laminotomy
see Drainage, Upper Joints 0R9
see Drainage, Lower Joints 0S9
Laparoscopy *see* Inspection
Laparotomy
Drainage *see* Drainage, Peritoneal Cavity 0W9G
Exploratory *see* Inspection, Peritoneal Cavity 0WJG
Laryngectomy
see Excision, Larynx 0CBS
see Resection, Larynx 0CTS
Laryngocentesis *see* Drainage, Larynx 0C9S
Laryngogram *see* Fluoroscopy, Larynx B91J
Laryngopexy *see* Repair, Larynx 0CQS
Laryngopharynx *use* Pharynx
Laryngoplasty
see Repair, Larynx 0CQS
see Replacement, Larynx 0CRS
see Supplement, Larynx 0CUS
Laryngorrhaphy *see* Repair, Larynx 0CQS
Laryngoscopy 0CJS8ZZ
Laryngotomy *see* Drainage, Larynx 0C9S
Laser Interstitial Thermal Therapy
Adrenal Gland DGY2KZZ
Anus DDY8KZZ
Bile Ducts DFY2KZZ
Brain D0Y0KZZ
Brain Stem D0Y1KZZ
Colon DDY5KZZ
Duodenum DDY2KZZ
Esophagus DDY0KZZ
Gallbladder DFY1KZZ
Gland
Adrenal DGY2KZ
Parathyroid DGY4KZZ
Pituitary DGY0KZZ
Thyroid DGY5KZZ
Ileum DDY4KZZ
Jejunum DDY3KZZ
Liver DFY0KZZ
Nerve, Peripheral D0Y7KZZ
Pancreas DFY3KZZ
Parathyroid Gland DGY4KZZ
Pineal Body DGY1KZZ
Pituitary Gland DGY0KZZ
Rectum DDY7KZZ
Spinal Cord D0Y6KZZ
Stomach DDY1KZZ
Thyroid Gland DGY5KZZ
Lateral (brachial) lymph node
use Lymphatic, Axillary, Left
use Lymphatic, Axillary, Right
Lateral canthus
use Eyelid, Upper, Right
use Eyelid, Upper, Left
Lateral collateral ligament (LCL)
use Bursa and Ligament, Knee, Right
use Bursa and Ligament, Knee, Left
Lateral condyle of femur
use Femur, Lower, Right
use Femur, Lower, Left
Lateral condyle of tibia
use Tibia, Left
use Tibia, Right
Lateral cuneiform bone
use Tarsal, Right
use Tarsal, Left
Lateral epicondyle of femur
use Femur, Lower, Left
use Femur, Lower, Right
Lateral epicondyle of humerus
use Humeral Shaft, Right
use Humeral Shaft, Left
Lateral femoral cutaneous nerve *use* Nerve, Lumbar Plexus
Lateral malleolus
use Fibula, Right
use Fibula, Left

Magnetic Resonance Imaging (MRI)
Abdomen BW3Ø
Ankle
   Left BQ3H
   Right BQ3G
Aorta
   Abdominal B43Ø
   Thoracic B33Ø
Arm
   Left BP3F
   Right BP3E
Artery
   Celiac B431
   Cervico-Cerebral Arch B33Q
   Common Carotid, Bilateral B335
   Coronary
      Bypass Graft, Multiple B233
      Multiple B231
   Internal Carotid, Bilateral B338
   Intracranial B33R
   Lower Extremity
      Bilateral B43H
      Left B43G
      Right B43F
   Pelvic B43C
   Renal, Bilateral B438
   Spinal B33M
   Superior Mesenteric B434
   Upper Extremity
      Bilateral B33K
      Left B33J
      Right B33H
   Vertebral, Bilateral B33G
Bladder BT3Ø
Brachial Plexus BW3P
Brain BØ3Ø
Breast
   Bilateral BH32
   Left BH31
   Right BH3Ø
Calcaneus
   Left BQ3K
   Right BQ3J
Chest BW33Y
Coccyx BR3F
Connective Tissue
   Lower Extremity BL31
   Upper Extremity BL3Ø
Corpora Cavernosa BV3Ø
Disc
   Cervical BR31
   Lumbar BR33
   Thoracic BR32
Ear B93Ø
Elbow
   Left BP3H
   Right BP3G
Eye
   Bilateral B837
   Left B836
   Right B835
Femur
   Left BQ34
   Right BQ33
Fetal Abdomen BY33
Fetal Extremity BY35
Fetal Head BY3Ø
Fetal Heart BY31
Fetal Spine BY34
Fetal Thorax BY32
Fetus, Whole BY36
Foot
   Left BQ3M
   Right BQ3L
Forearm
   Left BP3K
   Right BP3J
Gland
   Adrenal, Bilateral BG32
   Parathyroid BG33
   Parotid, Bilateral B936
   Salivary, Bilateral B93D
   Submandibular, Bilateral B939

Magnetic Resonance Imaging (MRI)—*continued*
Gland—*continued*
   Thyroid BG34
Head BW38
Heart, Right and Left B236
Hip
   Left BQ31
   Right BQ3Ø
Intracranial Sinus B532
Joint
   Finger
      Left BP3D
      Right BP3C
   Hand
      Left BP3D
      Right BP3C
   Temporomandibular, Bilateral BN39
Kidney
   Bilateral BT33
   Left BT32
   Right BT31
   Transplant BT39
Knee
   Left BQ38
   Right BQ37
Larynx B93J
Leg
   Left BQ3F
   Right BQ3D
Liver BF35
Liver and Spleen BF36
Lung Apices BB3G
Nasopharynx B93F
Neck BW3F
Nerve
   Acoustic BØ3C
   Brachial Plexus BW3P
Oropharynx B93F
Ovary
   Bilateral BU35
   Left BU34
   Right BU33
Ovary and Uterus BU3C
Pancreas BF37
Patella
   Left BQ3W
   Right BQ3V
Pelvic Region BW3G
Pelvis BR3C
Pituitary Gland BØ39
Plexus, Brachial BW3P
Prostate BV33
Retroperitoneum BW3H
Sacrum BR3F
Scrotum BV34
Sella Turcica BØ39
Shoulder
   Left BP39
   Right BP38
Sinus
   Intracranial B532
   Paranasal B932
Spinal Cord BØ3B
Spine
   Cervical BR3Ø
   Lumbar BR39
   Thoracic BR37
Spleen and Liver BF36
Subcutaneous Tissue
   Abdomen BH3H
   Extremity
      Lower BH3J
      Upper BH3F
   Head BH3D
   Neck BH3D
   Pelvis BH3H
   Thorax BH3G
Tendon
   Lower Extremity BL33
   Upper Extremity BL32
Testicle
   Bilateral BV37
   Left BV36

Magnetic Resonance Imaging (MRI)—*continued*
Testicle—*continued*
   Right BV35
Toe
   Left BQ3Q
   Right BQ3P
Uterus BU36
   Pregnant BU3B
Uterus and Ovary BU3C
Vagina BU39
Vein
   Cerebellar B531
   Cerebral B531
   Jugular, Bilateral B535
   Lower Extremity
      Bilateral B53D
      Left B53C
      Right B53B
   Other B53V
   Pelvic (Iliac) Bilateral B53H
   Portal B53T
   Pulmonary, Bilateral B53S
   Renal, Bilateral B53L
   Spanchnic B53T
   Upper Extremity
      Bilateral B53P
      Left B53N
      Right B53M
Vena Cava
   Inferior B539
   Superior B538
Wrist
   Left BP3M
   Right BP3L
Malleotomy *see* Drainage, Ear, Nose, Sinus Ø99
Malleus
   use Auditory Ossicle, Right
   use Auditory Ossicle, Left
Mammaplasty, mammoplasty
   see Alteration, Skin and Breast ØHØ
   see Repair, Skin and Breast ØHQ
   see Replacement, Skin and Breast ØHR
   see Supplement, Skin and Breast ØHU
Mammary duct
   use Breast, Bilateral
   use Breast, Right
   use Breast, Left
Mammary gland
   use Breast, Bilateral
   use Breast, Right
   use Breast, Left
Mammectomy
   see Excision, Skin and Breast ØHB
   see Resection, Skin and Breast ØHT
Mammillary body *use* Hypothalamus
Mammography *see* Plain Radiography, Skin,
      Subcutaneous Tissue and Breast BHØ
Mammotomy *see* Drainage, Skin and Breast ØH9
Mandibular nerve *use* Nerve, Trigeminal
Mandibular notch
   use Mandible, Right
   use Mandible, Left
Mandibulectomy
   see Excision, Head and Facial Bones ØNB
   see Resection, Head and Facial Bones ØNT
Manipulation
   Adhesions *see* Release
   Chiropractic *see* Chiropractic Manipulation
Manubrium *use* Sternum
Map
   Basal Ganglia ØØK8
   Brain ØØKØ
   Cerebellum ØØKC
   Cerebral Hemisphere ØØK7
   Conduction Mechanism Ø2K8
   Hypothalamus ØØKA
   Medulla Oblongata ØØKD
   Pons ØØKB
   Thalamus ØØK9
Mapping
   Doppler ultrasound *see* Ultrasonography
   Electrocardiogram only *see* Measurement, Cardiac
      4AØ2

Marsupialization
  see Drainage
  see Excision
Massage, cardiac
  External 5A12012
  Open 02QA0ZZ
Masseter muscle *use* Muscle, Head
Masseteric fascia *use* Subcutaneous Tissue and Fascia, Face
Mastectomy
  see Excision, Skin and Breast 0HB
  see Resection, Skin and Breast 0HT
Mastoid (postauricular) lymph node
  use Lymphatic, Neck, Left
  use Lymphatic, Neck, Right
Mastoid air cells
  use Sinus, Mastoid, Left
  use Sinus, Mastoid, Right
Mastoid process
  use Bone, Temporal, Right
  use Bone, Temporal, Left
Mastoidectomy
  see Excision, Ear, Nose, Sinus 09B
  see Resection, Ear, Nose, Sinus 09T
Mastoidotomy *see* Drainage, Ear, Nose, Sinus 099
Mastopexy
  see Reposition, Skin and Breast 0HS
  see Repair, Skin and Breast 0HQ
Mastorrhaphy *see* Repair, Skin and Breast 0HQ
Mastotomy *see* Drainage, Skin and Breast 0H9
Maxillary artery
  use Artery, External Carotid, Right
  use Artery, External Carotid, Left
Maxillary nerve *use* Nerve, Trigeminal
Measurement
  Arterial
    Flow
      Coronary 4A03
      Peripheral 4A03
      Pulmonary 4A03
    Pressure
      Coronary 4A03
      Peripheral 4A03
      Pulmonary 4A03
      Thoracic, Other 4A03
    Pulse
      Coronary 4A03
      Peripheral 4A03
      Pulmonary 4A03
    Saturation, Peripheral 4A03
    Sound, Peripheral 4A03
  Biliary
    Flow 4A0C
    Pressure 4A0C
  Cardiac
    Action Currents 4A02
    Defibrillator 4B02XTZ
    Electrical Activity 4A02
      Guidance 4A02X4A
      No Qualifier 4A02X4Z
    Output 4A02
    Pacemaker 4B02XSZ
    Rate 4A02
    Rhythm 4A02
    Sampling and Pressure
      Bilateral 4A02
      Left Heart 4A02
      Right Heart 4A02
    Sound 4A02
    Total Activity, Stress 4A02XM4
  Central Nervous
    Conductivity 4A00
    Electrical Activity 4A00
    Pressure 4A000BZ
      Intracranial 4A00
    Saturation, Intracranial 4A00
    Stimulator 4B00XVZ
    Temperature, Intracranial 4A00
  Circulatory, Volume 4A05XLZ
  Gastrointestinal
    Motility 4A0B
    Pressure 4A0B
    Secretion 4A0B

Measurement—*continued*
  Lymphatic
    Flow 4A06
    Pressure 4A06
  Metabolism 4A0Z
  Musculoskeletal
    Contractility 4A0F
    Stimulator 4B0FXVZ
  Olfactory, Acuity 4A08X0Z
  Peripheral Nervous
    Conductivity
      Motor 4A01
      Sensory 4A01
    Stimulator 4B01XVZ
  Products of Conception
    Cardiac
      Electrical Activity 4A0H
      Rate 4A0H
      Rhythm 4A0H
      Sound 4A0H
    Nervous
      Conductivity 4A0J
      Electrical Activity 4A0J
      Pressure 4A0J
  Respiratory
    Capacity 4A09
    Flow 4A09
    Pacemaker 4B09XSZ
    Rate 4A09
    Resistance 4A09
    Total Activity 4A09
    Volume 4A09
  Sleep 4A0ZXQZ
  Temperature 4A0Z
  Urinary
    Contractility 4A0D73Z
    Flow 4A0D75Z
    Pressure 4A0D7BZ
    Resistance 4A0D7DZ
    Volume 4A0D7LZ
  Venous
    Flow
      Central 4A04
      Peripheral 4A04
      Portal 4A04
      Pulmonary 4A04
    Pressure
      Central 4A04
      Peripheral 4A04
      Portal 4A04
      Pulmonary 4A04
    Pulse
      Central 4A04
      Peripheral 4A04
      Portal 4A04
      Pulmonary 4A04
    Saturation, Peripheral 4A04
  Visual
    Acuity 4A07X0Z
    Mobility 4A07X7Z
    Pressure 4A07XBZ
Meatoplasty, urethra *see* Repair, Urethra 0TQD
Meatotomy *see* Drainage, Urinary System 0T9
Mechanical ventilation *see* Performance, Respiratory 5A19
Medial canthus
  use Eyelid, Lower, Left
  use Eyelid, Lower, Right
Medial collateral ligament (MCL)
  use Bursa and Ligament, Knee, Left
  use Bursa and Ligament, Knee, Right
Medial condyle of femur
  use Femur, Lower, Right
  use Femur, Lower, Left
Medial condyle of tibia
  use Tibia, Left
  use Tibia, Right
Medial cuneiform bone
  use Tarsal, Right
  use Tarsal, Left
Medial epicondyle of femur
  use Femur, Lower, Right
  use Femur, Lower, Left

Medial epicondyle of humerus
  use Humeral Shaft, Left
  use Humeral Shaft, Right
Medial malleolus
  use Tibia, Right
  use Tibia, Left
Medial meniscus
  use Joint, Knee, Right
  use Joint, Knee, Left
Medial plantar artery
  use Artery, Foot, Right
  use Artery, Foot, Left
Medial plantar nerve *use* Nerve, Tibial
Medial popliteal nerve *use* Nerve, Tibial
Medial rectus muscle
  use Muscle, Extraocular, Right
  use Muscle, Extraocular, Left
Medial sural cutaneous nerve *use* Nerve, Tibial
Median antebrachial vein
  use Vein, Basilic, Left
  use Vein, Basilic, Right
Median cubital vein
  use Vein, Basilic, Left
  use Vein, Basilic, Right
Median sacral artery *use* Aorta, Abdominal
Mediastinal lymph node *use* Lymphatic, Thorax
Mediastinoscopy 0WJC4ZZ
Medication Management GZ3ZZZZ
  for substance abuse
    Antabuse HZ83ZZZ
    Bupropion HZ87ZZZ
    Clonidine HZ86ZZZ
    Levo-alpha-acetyl-methadol (LAAM) HZ82ZZZ
    Methadone Maintenance HZ81ZZZ
    Naloxone HZ85ZZZ
    Naltrexone HZ84ZZZ
    Nicotine Replacement HZ80ZZZ
    Other Replacement Medication HZ89ZZZ
    Psychiatric Medication HZ88ZZZ
Meditation 8E0ZXY5
Meissner's (submucous) plexus *use* Nerve, Abdominal Sympathetic
Membranous urethra *use* Urethra
Meningeorrhaphy
  see Repair, Cerebral Meninges 00Q1
  see Repair, Spinal Meninges 00QT
Meniscectomy
  see Excision, Lower Joints 0SB
  see Resection, Lower Joints 0ST
Mental foramen
  use Mandible, Left
  use Mandible, Right
Mentalis muscle *use* Muscle, Facial
Mentoplasty *see* Alteration, Jaw, Lower 0W05
Mesenterectomy *see* Excision, Mesentery 0DBV
Mesenteriorrhaphy, mesenterorrhaphy *see* Repair, Mesentery 0DQV
Mesenteriplication *see* Repair, Mesentery 0DQV
Mesoappendix *use* Mesentery
Mesocolon *use* Mesentery
Metacarpal ligament
  use Bursa and Ligament, Hand, Left
  use Bursa and Ligament, Hand, Right
Metacarpophalangeal ligament
  use Bursa and Ligament, Hand, Right
  use Bursa and Ligament, Hand, Left
Metatarsal ligament
  use Bursa and Ligament, Foot, Right
  use Bursa and Ligament, Foot, Left
Metatarsectomy
  see Excision, Lower Bones 0QB
  see Resection, Lower Bones 0QT
Metatarsophalangeal (MTP) joint
  use Joint, Metatarsal-Phalangeal, Left
  use Joint, Metatarsal-Phalangeal, Right
Metatarsophalangeal ligament
  use Bursa and Ligament, Foot, Right
  use Bursa and Ligament, Foot, Left
Metathalamus *use* Thalamus
Midcarpal joint
  use Joint, Carpal, Right
  use Joint, Carpal, Left

Middle cardiac nerve *use* Nerve, Thoracic
    Sympathetic
Middle cerebral artery *use* Artery, Intracranial
Middle cerebral vein *use* Vein, Intracranial
Middle colic vein *use* Vein, Colic
Middle genicular artery
    use Artery, Popliteal, Left
    use Artery, Popliteal, Right
Middle hemorrhoidal vein
    use Vein, Hypogastric, Left
    use Vein, Hypogastric, Right
Middle rectal artery
    use Artery, Internal Iliac, Right
    use Artery, Internal Iliac, Left
Middle suprarenal artery *use* Aorta, Abdominal
Middle temporal artery
    use Artery, Temporal, Left
    use Artery, Temporal, Right
Middle turbinate *use* Turbinate, Nasal
Mitral annulus *use* Valve, Mitral
Mobilization, adhesions *see* Release
Molar gland *use* Buccal Mucosa
Monitoring
  Arterial
    Flow
      Coronary 4A13
      Peripheral 4A13
      Pulmonary 4A13
    Pressure
      Coronary 4A13
      Peripheral 4A13
      Pulmonary 4A13
    Pulse
      Coronary 4A13
      Peripheral 4A13
      Pulmonary 4A13
    Saturation, Peripheral 4A13
    Sound, Peripheral 4A13
  Cardiac
    Electrical Activity 4A12
      Ambulatory 4A12X45
      No Qualifier 4A12X4Z
    Output 4A12
    Rate 4A12
    Rhythm 4A12
    Sound 4A12
    Total Activity, Stress 4A12XM4
  Central Nervous
    Conductivity 4A10
    Electrical Activity
      Intraoperative 4A10
      No Qualifier 4A10
    Pressure 4A100BZ
      Intracranial 4A10
    Saturation, Intracranial 4A10
    Temperature, Intracranial 4A10
  Gastrointestinal
    Motility 4A1B
    Pressure 4A1B
    Secretion 4A1B
  Lymphatic
    Flow 4A16
    Pressure 4A16
  Peripheral Nervous
    Motor 4A11
    Sensory 4A11
  Products of Conception
    Cardiac
      Electrical Activity 4A1H
      Rate 4A1H
      Rhythm 4A1H
      Sound 4A1H
    Nervous
      Conductivity 4A1J
      Electrical Activity 4A1J
      Pressure 4A1J
  Respiratory
    Capacity 4A19
    Flow 4A19
    Rate 4A19
    Resistance 4A19
    Volume 4A19

Monitoring—*continued*
  Sleep 4A1ZXQZ
  Temperature 4A1Z
  Urinary
    Contractility 4A1D73Z
    Flow 4A1D75Z
    Pressure 4A1D7BZ
    Resistance 4A1D7DZ
    Volume 4A1D7LZ
  Venous
    Flow
      Central 4A14
      Peripheral 4A14
      Portal 4A14
      Pulmonary 4A14
    Pressure
      Central 4A14
      Peripheral 4A14
      Portal 4A14
      Pulmonary 4A14
    Pulse
      Central 4A14
      Peripheral 4A14
      Portal 4A14
      Pulmonary 4A14
    Saturation
      Central 4A14
      Portal 4A14
      Pulmonary 4A14
Motor Function Assessment F01
Motor Treatment F07
MR angiography
    see Magnetic Resonance Imaging (MRI), Heart B23
    see Magnetic Resonance Imaging (MRI), Upper
      Arteries B33
    see Magnetic Resonance Imaging (MRI), Lower
      Arteries B43
Multiple sleep latency test 4A0ZXQZ
Musculocutaneous nerve *use* Nerve, Brachial Plexus
Musculopexy
    see Repair, Muscles 0KQ
    see Reposition, Muscles 0KS
Musculophrenic artery
    use Artery, Internal Mammary, Left
    use Artery, Internal Mammary, Right
Musculoplasty
    see Repair, Muscles 0KQ
    see Supplement, Muscles 0KU
Musculorrhaphy *see* Repair, Muscles 0KQ
Musculospiral nerve *use* Nerve, Radial
Myectomy
    see Excision, Muscles 0KB
    see Resection, Muscles 0KT
Myelencephalon *use* Medulla Oblongata
Myelogram
    CT *see* Computerized Tomography (CT Scan), Central
      Nervous System B02
    MRI *see* Magnetic Resonance Imaging (MRI), Central
      Nervous System B03
Myenteric (Auerbach's) plexus *use* Nerve, Abdominal
    Sympathetic
Myomectomy *see* Excision, Female Reproductive
    System 0UB
Myometrium *use* Uterus
Myopexy
    see Repair, Muscles 0KQ
    see Reposition, Muscles 0KS
Myoplasty
    see Repair, Muscles 0KQ
    see Supplement, Muscles 0KU
Myorrhaphy *see* Repair, Muscles 0KQ
Myoscopy *see* Inspection, Muscles 0KJ
Myotomy
    see Division, Muscles 0K8
    see Drainage, Muscles 0K9
Myringectomy
    see Excision, Ear, Nose, Sinus 09B
    see Resection, Ear, Nose, Sinus 09T
Myringoplasty
    see Repair, Ear, Nose, Sinus 09Q
    see Replacement, Ear, Nose, Sinus 09R
    see Supplement, Ear, Nose, Sinus 09U
Myringostomy *see* Drainage, Ear, Nose, Sinus 099

Myringotomy *see* Drainage, Ear, Nose, Sinus 099

N

Nail bed
    use Finger Nail
    use Toe Nail
Nail plate
    use Finger Nail
    use Toe Nail
Narcosynthesis GZGZZZZ
Nasal cavity *use* Nose
Nasal concha *use* Turbinate, Nasal
Nasalis muscle *use* Muscle, Facial
Nasolacrimal duct
    use Duct, Lacrimal, Right
    use Duct, Lacrimal, Left
Navicular bone
    use Tarsal, Left
    use Tarsal, Right
Near Infrared Spectroscopy, Circulatory System
    8E023DZ
Neck of femur
    use Femur, Upper, Right
    use Femur, Upper, Left
Neck of humerus (anatomical)(surgical)
    use Humeral Head, Right
    use Humeral Head, Left
Nephrectomy
    see Excision, Urinary System 0TB
    see Resection, Urinary System 0TT
Nephrolithotomy *see* Extirpation, Urinary System 0TC
Nephrolysis *see* Release, Urinary System 0TN
Nephropexy
    see Repair, Urinary System 0TQ
    see Reposition, Urinary System 0TS
Nephroplasty
    see Repair, Urinary System 0TQ
    see Supplement, Urinary System 0TU
Nephropyeloureterostomy
    see Bypass, Urinary System 0T1
    see Drainage, Urinary System 0T9
Nephrorrhaphy *see* Repair, Urinary System 0TQ
Nephroscopy, transurethral 0TJ58ZZ
Nephrostomy
    see Bypass, Urinary System 0T1
    see Drainage, Urinary System 0T9
Nephrotomography
    see Plain Radiography, Urinary System BT0
    see Fluoroscopy, Urinary System BT1
Nephrotomy
    see Drainage, Urinary System 0T9
    see Division, Urinary System 0T8
Nerve conduction study
    see Measurement, Central Nervous 4A00
    see Measurement, Peripheral Nervous 4A01
Nerve Function Assessment F01
Nerve to the stapedius *use* Nerve, Facial
Neurectomy
    see Excision, Central Nervous System 00B
    see Excision, Peripheral Nervous System 01B
Neurexeresis
    see Extraction, Central Nervous System 00D
    see Extraction, Peripheral Nervous System 01D
Neurohypophysis *use* Gland, Pituitary
Neurolysis
    see Release, Central Nervous System 00N
    see Release, Peripheral Nervous System 01N
Neurophysiologic monitoring *see* Monitoring,
    Central Nervous 4A10
Neuroplasty
    see Repair, Central Nervous System 00Q
    see Repair, Peripheral Nervous System 01Q
    see Supplement, Central Nervous System 00U
    see Supplement, Peripheral Nervous System 01U
Neurorrhaphy
    see Repair, Central Nervous System 00Q
    see Repair, Peripheral Nervous System 01Q
Neurostimulator Generator
    Insertion of device in, Skull 0NH00NZ
    Removal of device from, Skull 0NP00NZ

Neurostimulator Generator—*continued*
Revision of device in, Skull 0NW00NZ
Neurostimulator Lead
Insertion of device in
Brain 00H0
Cerebral Ventricle 00H6
Nerve
Cranial 00HE
Peripheral 01HY
Spinal Canal 00HU
Spinal Cord 00HV
Removal of device from
Brain 00P0
Cerebral Ventricle 00P6
Nerve
Cranial 00PE
Peripheral 01PY
Spinal Canal 00PU
Spinal Cord 00PV
Revision of device in
Brain 00W0
Cerebral Ventricle 00W6
Nerve
Cranial 00WE
Peripheral 01WY
Spinal Canal 00WU
Spinal Cord 00WV
Neurotomy
see Division, Central Nervous System 008
see Division, Peripheral Nervous System 018
Neurotripsy
see Destruction, Central Nervous System 005
see Destruction, Peripheral Nervous System 015
Ninth cranial nerve *use* Nerve, Glossopharyngeal
Nonimaging Nuclear Medicine Assay
Bladder, Kidneys and Ureters CT63
Blood C763
Kidneys, Ureters and Bladder CT63
Lymphatics and Hematologic System C76YYZZ
Ureters, Kidneys and Bladder CT63
Urinary System CT6YYZZ
Nonimaging Nuclear Medicine Probe CP5YYZZ
Abdomen CW50
Abdomen and Chest CW54
Abdomen and Pelvis CW51
Brain C050
Central Nervous System C05YYZZ
Chest CW53
Chest and Abdomen CW54
Chest and Neck CW56
Extremity
Lower CP5
Upper CP5
Head and Neck CW5B
Heart C25YYZZ
Right and Left C256
Lymphatics
Head C75J
Head and Neck C755
Lower Extremity C75P
Neck C75K
Pelvic C75D
Trunk C75M
Upper Chest C75L
Upper Extremity C75N
Lymphatics and Hematologic System C75YYZZ
Neck and Chest CW56
Neck and Head CW5B
Pelvic Region CW5J
Pelvis and Abdomen CW51
Spine CP55ZZZ
Nonimaging Nuclear Medicine Uptake
Endocrine System CG4YYZZ
Gland, Thyroid CG42
Nostril *use* Nose
Nuclear medicine
use Planar Nuclear Medicine Imaging
use Tomographic (Tomo) Nuclear Medicine Imaging
use Positron Emission Tomographic (PET) Imaging
use Nonimaging Nuclear Medicine Uptake
use Nonimaging Nuclear Medicine Probe
use Nonimaging Nuclear Medicine Assay
use Systemic Nuclear Medicine Therapy

Nuclear scintigraphy *use* Nuclear Medicine
Nutrition, concentrated substances
Enteral infusion 3E0G36Z
Parenteral (peripheral) infusion *see* Introduction, Nutritional Substance

O

Obliteration *see* Destruction
Obturator artery
use Artery, Internal Iliac, Left
use Artery, Internal Iliac, Right
Obturator lymph node *use* Lymphatic, Pelvis
Obturator muscle
use Muscle, Hip, Left
use Muscle, Hip, Right
Obturator nerve *use* Nerve, Lumbar Plexus
Obturator vein
use Vein, Hypogastric, Right
use Vein, Hypogastric, Left
Obtuse margin *use* Heart, Left
Occipital artery
use Artery, External Carotid, Right
use Artery, External Carotid, Left
Occipital lobe *use* Cerebral Hemisphere
Occipital lymph node
use Lymphatic, Neck, Left
use Lymphatic, Neck, Right
Occipitofrontalis muscle *use* Muscle, Facial
Occlusion
Ampulla of Vater 0FLC
Anus 0DLQ
Aorta, Abdominal 04L0
Artery
Anterior Tibial
Left 04LQ
Right 04LP
Axillary
Left 03L6
Right 03L5
Brachial
Left 03L8
Right 03L7
Celiac 04L1
Colic
Left 04L7
Middle 04L8
Right 04L6
Common Carotid
Left 03LJ
Right 03LH
Common Iliac
Left 04LD
Right 04LC
External Carotid
Left 03LN
Right 03LM
External Iliac
Left 04LJ
Right 04LH
Face 03LR
Femoral
Left 04LL
Right 04LK
Foot
Left 04LW
Right 04LV
Gastric 04L2
Hand
Left 03LF
Right 03LD
Hepatic 04L3
Inferior Mesenteric 04LB
Innominate 03L2
Internal Carotid
Left 03LL
Right 03LK
Internal Iliac
Left 04LF
Right 04LE

Occlusion—*continued*
Artery—*continued*
Internal Mammary
Left 03L1
Right 03L0
Intracranial 03LG
Lower 04LY
Peroneal
Left 04LU
Right 04LT
Popliteal
Left 04LN
Right 04LM
Posterior Tibial
Left 04LS
Right 04LR
Pulmonary, Left 02LR
Radial
Left 03LC
Right 03LB
Renal
Left 04LA
Right 04L9
Splenic 04L4
Subclavian
Left 03L4
Right 03L3
Superior Mesenteric 04L5
Temporal
Left 03LT
Right 03LS
Thyroid
Left 03LV
Right 03LU
Ulnar
Left 03LA
Right 03L9
Upper 03LY
Vertebral
Left 03LQ
Right 03LP
Bladder 0TLB
Bladder Neck 0TLC
Bronchus
Lingula 0BL9
Lower Lobe
Left 0BLB
Right 0BL6
Main
Left 0BL7
Right 0BL3
Middle Lobe, Right 0BL5
Upper Lobe
Left 0BL8
Right 0BL4
Carina 0BL2
Cecum 0DLH
Cisterna Chyli 07LL
Colon
Ascending 0DLK
Descending 0DLM
Sigmoid 0DLN
Transverse 0DLL
Cord
Bilateral 0VLH
Left 0VLG
Right 0VLF
Cul-de-sac 0ULF
Duct
Common Bile 0FL9
Cystic 0FL8
Hepatic
Left 0FL6
Right 0FL5
Lacrimal
Left 08LY
Right 08LX
Pancreatic 0FLD
Accessory 0FLF
Parotid
Left 0CLC
Right 0CLB

Occlusion—*continued*
Duodenum ØDL9
Esophagogastric Junction ØDL4
Esophagus ØDL5
Lower ØDL3
Middle ØDL2
Upper ØDL1
Fallopian Tube
Left ØUL6
Right ØUL5
Fallopian Tubes, Bilateral ØUL7
Ileocecal Valve ØDLC
Ileum ØDLB
Intestine
Large ØDLE
Left ØDLG
Right ØDLF
Small ØDL8
Jejunum ØDLA
Kidney Pelvis
Left ØTL4
Right ØTL3
Lymphatic
Aortic 07LD
Axillary
Left 07L6
Right 07L5
Head 07LØ
Inguinal
Left 07LJ
Right 07LH
Internal Mammary
Left 07L9
Right 07L8
Lower Extremity
Left 07LG
Right 07LF
Mesenteric 07LB
Neck
Left 07L2
Right 07L1
Pelvis 07LC
Thoracic Duct 07LK
Thorax 07L7
Upper Extremity
Left 07L4
Right 07L3
Rectum ØDLP
Stomach ØDL6
Pylorus ØDL7
Trachea ØBL1
Ureter
Left ØTL7
Right ØTL6
Urethra ØTLD
Vagina ØULG
Vas Deferens
Bilateral ØVLQ
Left ØVLP
Right ØVLN
Vein
Axillary
Left 05L8
Right 05L7
Azygos 05LØ
Basilic
Left 05LC
Right 05LB
Brachial
Left 05LA
Right 05L9
Cephalic
Left 05LF
Right 05LD
Colic 06L7
Common Iliac
Left 06LD
Right 06LC
Esophageal 06L3
External Iliac
Left 06LG
Right 06LF

Occlusion—*continued*
Vein—*continued*
External Jugular
Left 05LQ
Right 05LP
Face
Left 05LV
Right 05LT
Femoral
Left 06LN
Right 06LM
Foot
Left 06LV
Right 06LT
Gastric 06L2
Greater Saphenous
Left 06LQ
Right 06LP
Hand
Left 05LH
Right 05LG
Hemiazygos 05L1
Hepatic 06L4
Hypogastric
Left 06LJ
Right 06LH
Inferior Mesenteric 06L6
Innominate
Left 05L4
Right 05L3
Internal Jugular
Left 05LN
Right 05LM
Intracranial 05LL
Lesser Saphenous
Left 06LS
Right 06LR
Lower 06LY
Portal 06L8
Pulmonary
Left 02LT
Right 02LS
Renal
Left 06LB
Right 06L9
Splenic 06L1
Subclavian
Left 05L6
Right 05L5
Superior Mesenteric 06L5
Upper 05LY
Vertebral
Left 05LS
Right 05LR
Vena Cava
Inferior 06LØ
Superior 02LV
Occupational therapy *see* Activities of Daily Living Treatment, Rehabilitation FØ8
Odentectomy
see Excision, Mouth and Throat ØCB
see Resection, Mouth and Throat ØCT
Olecranon bursa
use Bursa and Ligament, Elbow, Left
use Bursa and Ligament, Elbow, Right
Olecranon process
use Ulna, Left
use Ulna, Right
Olfactory bulb *use* Nerve, Olfactory
Omentectomy, omentumectomy
see Excision, Gastrointestinal System ØDB
see Resection, Gastrointestinal System ØDT
Omentofixation *see* Repair, Gastrointestinal System ØDQ
Omentoplasty
see Repair, Gastrointestinal System ØDQ
see Replacement, Gastrointestinal System ØDR
see Supplement, Gastrointestinal System ØDU
Omentorrhaphy *see* Repair, Gastrointestinal System ØDQ
Omentotomy *see* Drainage, Gastrointestinal System ØD9

Onychectomy
see Excision, Skin and Breast ØHB
see Resection, Skin and Breast ØHT
Onychoplasty
see Repair, Skin and Breast ØHQ
see Replacement, Skin and Breast ØHR
Onychotomy *see* Drainage, Skin and Breast ØH9
Oophorectomy
see Excision, Female Reproductive System ØUB
see Resection, Female Reproductive System ØUT
Oophoropexy
see Repair, Female Reproductive System ØUQ
see Reposition, Female Reproductive System ØUS
Oophoroplasty
see Repair, Female Reproductive System ØUQ
see Supplement, Female Reproductive System ØUU
Oophororrhaphy *see* Repair, Female Reproductive System ØUQ
Oophorostomy *see* Drainage, Female Reproductive System ØU9
Oophorotomy
see Drainage, Female Reproductive System ØU9
see Division, Female Reproductive System ØU8
Oophorrhaphy *see* Repair, Female Reproductive System ØUQ
Ophthalmic artery
use Artery, Internal Carotid, Right
use Artery, Internal Carotid, Left
Ophthalmic nerve *use* Nerve, Trigeminal
Ophthalmic vein *use* Vein, Intracranial
Opponensplasty
Tendon replacement *see* Replacement, Tendons ØLR
Tendon transfer *see* Transfer, Tendons ØLX
Optic chiasma *use* Nerve, Optic
Optic disc
use Retina, Left
use Retina, Right
Optic foramen
use Bone, Sphenoid, Right
use Bone, Sphenoid, Left
Optical coherence tomography, intravascular *use* Computerized Tomography (CT Scan)
Orbicularis oculi muscle
use Eyelid, Upper, Left
use Eyelid, Upper, Right
Orbicularis oris muscle *use* Muscle, Facial
Orbital fascia *use* Subcutaneous Tissue and Fascia, Face
Orbital portion of ethmoid bone
use Orbit, Left
use Orbit, Right
Orbital portion of frontal bone
use Orbit, Right
use Orbit, Left
Orbital portion of lacrimal bone
use Orbit, Left
use Orbit, Right
Orbital portion of maxilla
use Orbit, Left
use Orbit, Right
Orbital portion of palatine bone
use Orbit, Right
use Orbit, Left
Orbital portion of sphenoid bone
use Orbit, Right
use Orbit, Left
Orbital portion of zygomatic bone
use Orbit, Left
use Orbit, Right
Orchectomy, orchidectomy, orchiectomy
see Excision, Male Reproductive System ØVB
see Resection, Male Reproductive System ØVT
Orchidoplasty, orchioplasty
see Repair, Male Reproductive System ØVQ
see Replacement, Male Reproductive System ØVR
see Supplement, Male Reproductive System ØVU
Orchidorrhaphy, orchiorrhaphy *see* Repair, Male Reproductive System ØVQ
Orchidotomy, orchiotomy, orchotomy *see* Drainage, Male Reproductive System ØV9
Orchiopexy
see Repair, Male Reproductive System ØVQ
see Reposition, Male Reproductive System ØVS

Oropharynx *use* Pharynx
Ossicular chain
    use Auditory Ossicle, Left
    use Auditory Ossicle, Right
Ossiculectomy
    see Excision, Ear, Nose, Sinus 09B
    see Resection, Ear, Nose, Sinus 09T
Ossiculotomy *see* Drainage, Ear, Nose, Sinus 099
Ostectomy
    see Excision, Head and Facial Bones 0NB
    see Resection, Head and Facial Bones 0NT
    see Excision, Upper Bones 0PB
    see Resection, Upper Bones 0PT
    see Excision, Lower Bones 0QB
    see Resection, Lower Bones 0QT
Osteoclasis
    see Division, Head and Facial Bones 0N8
    see Division, Upper Bones 0P8
    see Division, Lower Bones 0Q8
Osteolysis
    see Release, Head and Facial Bones 0NN
    see Release, Upper Bones 0PN
    see Release, Lower Bones 0QN
Osteopathic Treatment
    Abdomen 7W09X
    Cervical 7W01X
    Extremity
        Lower 7W06X
        Upper 7W07X
    Head 7W00X
    Lumbar 7W03X
    Pelvis 7W05X
    Rib Cage 7W08X
    Sacrum 7W04X
    Thoracic 7W02X
Osteopexy
    see Repair, Head and Facial Bones 0NQ
    see Reposition, Head and Facial Bones 0NS
    see Repair, Upper Bones 0PQ
    see Reposition, Upper Bones 0PS
    see Repair, Lower Bones 0QQ
    see Reposition, Lower Bones 0QS
Osteoplasty
    see Repair, Head and Facial Bones 0NQ
    see Replacement, Head and Facial Bones 0NR
    see Repair, Upper Bones 0PQ
    see Replacement, Upper Bones 0PR
    see Repair, Lower Bones 0QQ
    see Replacement, Lower Bones 0QR
    see Supplement, Lower Bones 0QU
    see Supplement, Head and Facial Bones 0NU
    see Supplement, Upper Bones 0PU
Osteorrhaphy
    see Repair, Head and Facial Bones 0NQ
    see Repair, Upper Bones 0PQ
    see Repair, Lower Bones 0QQ
Osteotomy, ostotomy
    see Division, Head and Facial Bones 0N8
    see Drainage, Head and Facial Bones 0N9
    see Division, Upper Bones 0P8
    see Drainage, Upper Bones 0P9
    see Division, Lower Bones 0Q8
    see Drainage, Lower Bones 0Q9
Otic ganglion *use* Nerve, Head and Neck Sympathetic
Otoplasty
    see Repair, Ear, Nose, Sinus 09Q
    see Replacement, Ear, Nose, Sinus 09R
    see Supplement, Ear, Nose, Sinus 09U
Otoscopy *see* Inspection, Ear, Nose, Sinus 09J
Oval window
    use Ear, Inner, Left
    use Ear, Inner, Right
Ovarian artery *use* Aorta, Abdominal
Ovarian ligament *use* Uterine Supporting Structure
Ovariectomy
    see Excision, Female Reproductive System 0UB
    see Resection, Female Reproductive System 0UT
Ovariocentesis *see* Drainage, Female Reproductive System 0U9
Ovariopexy
    see Repair, Female Reproductive System 0UQ
    see Reposition, Female Reproductive System 0US

Ovariotomy
    see Drainage, Female Reproductive System 0U9
    see Division, Female Reproductive System 0U8
Oversewing
    Gastrointestinal ulcer *see* Repair, Gastrointestinal System 0DQ
    Pleural bleb *see* Repair, Respiratory System 0BQ
Oviduct
    use Fallopian Tube, Right
    use Fallopian Tube, Left
Oximetry, Fetal pulse 10H073Z
Oxygenation
    Extracorporeal membrane (ECMO) *see* Assistance, Circulatory 5A05
    Hyperbaric *see* Assistance, Circulatory 5A05
    Supersaturated *see* Assistance, Circulatory 5A05

P

Pacemaker Lead
    Atrium
        Left 02H7
        Right 02H6
    Pericardium 02HN
    Vein, Coronary 02H4
    Ventricle
        Left 02HL
        Right 02HK
Packing
    Abdominal Wall 2W43X5Z
    Anorectal 2Y43X5Z
    Arm
        Lower
            Left 2W4DX5Z
            Right 2W4CX5Z
        Upper
            Left 2W4BX5Z
            Right 2W4AX5Z
    Back 2W45X5Z
    Chest Wall 2W44X5Z
    Ear 2Y42X5Z
    Extremity
        Lower
            Left 2W4MX5Z
            Right 2W4LX5Z
        Upper
            Left 2W49X5Z
            Right 2W48X5Z
    Face 2W41X5Z
    Finger
        Left 2W4KX5Z
        Right 2W4JX5Z
    Foot
        Left 2W4TX5Z
        Right 2W4SX5Z
    Genital Tract, Female 2Y44X5Z
    Hand
        Left 2W4FX5Z
        Right 2W4EX5Z
    Head 2W40X5Z
    Inguinal Region
        Left 2W47X5Z
        Right 2W46X5Z
    Leg
        Lower
            Left 2W4RX5Z
            Right 2W4QX5Z
        Upper
            Left 2W4PX5Z
            Right 2W4NX5Z
    Mouth and Pharynx 2Y40X5Z
    Nasal 2Y41X5Z
    Neck 2W42X5Z
    Thumb
        Left 2W4HX5Z
        Right 2W4GX5Z
    Toe
        Left 2W4VX5Z
        Right 2W4UX5Z
    Urethra 2Y45X5Z
Palatine gland *use* Buccal Mucosa

Palatine tonsil *use* Tonsils
Palatine uvula *use* Uvula
Palatoglossal muscle *use* Muscle, Tongue, Palate, Pharynx
Palatopharyngeal muscle *use* Muscle, Tongue, Palate, Pharynx
Palatoplasty
    see Repair, Mouth and Throat 0CQ
    see Replacement, Mouth and Throat 0CR
    see Supplement, Mouth and Throat 0CU
Palatorrhaphy *see* Repair, Mouth and Throat 0CQ
Palmar (volar) digital vein
    use Vein, Hand, Right
    use Vein, Hand, Left
Palmar (volar) metacarpal vein
    use Vein, Hand, Left
    use Vein, Hand, Right
Palmar cutaneous nerve
    use Nerve, Radial
    use Nerve, Median
Palmar fascia (aponeurosis)
    use Subcutaneous Tissue and Fascia, Hand, Left
    use Subcutaneous Tissue and Fascia, Hand, Right
Palmar interosseous muscle
    use Muscle, Hand, Left
    use Muscle, Hand, Right
Palmar ulnocarpal ligament
    use Bursa and Ligament, Wrist, Right
    use Bursa and Ligament, Wrist, Left
Palmaris longus muscle
    use Muscle, Lower Arm and Wrist, Left
    use Muscle, Lower Arm and Wrist, Right
Pancreatectomy
    see Excision, Pancreas 0FBG
    see Resection, Pancreas 0FTG
Pancreatic artery *use* Artery, Splenic
Pancreatic plexus *use* Nerve, Abdominal Sympathetic
Pancreatic vein *use* Vein, Splenic
Pancreaticoduodenostomy *see* Bypass, Hepatobiliary System and Pancreas 0F1
Pancreaticosplenic lymph node *use* Lymphatic, Aortic
Pancreatogram, endoscopic retrograde *see* Fluoroscopy, Pancreatic Duct BF18
Pancreatolithotomy *see* Extirpation, Pancreas 0FCG
Pancreatotomy
    see Drainage, Pancreas 0F9G
    see Division, Pancreas 0F8G
Panniculectomy
    see Excision, Skin, Abdomen 0HB7
    see Excision, Abdominal Wall 0WBF
Paraaortic lymph node *use* Lymphatic, Aortic
Paracentesis
    Eye *see* Drainage, Eye 089
    Peritoneal Cavity *see* Drainage, Peritoneal Cavity 0W9G
    Tympanum *see* Drainage, Ear, Nose, Sinus 099
Pararectal lymph node *use* Lymphatic, Mesenteric
Parasternal lymph node *use* Lymphatic, Thorax
Parathyroidectomy
    see Excision, Endocrine System 0GB
    see Resection, Endocrine System 0GT
Paratracheal lymph node *use* Lymphatic, Thorax
Paraurethral (Skene's) gland *use* Gland, Vestibular
Parenteral nutrition, total *see* Introduction, Nutritional Substance
Parietal lobe *use* Cerebral Hemisphere
Parotid lymph node *use* Lymphatic, Head
Parotid plexus *use* Nerve, Facial
Parotidectomy
    see Excision, Mouth and Throat 0CB
    see Resection, Mouth and Throat 0CT
Pars flaccida
    use Tympanic Membrane, Right
    use Tympanic Membrane, Left
Patch, blood, spinal 3E0S3GC
Patellapexy
    see Repair, Lower Bones 0QQ
    see Reposition, Lower Bones 0QS
Patellaplasty
    see Repair, Lower Bones 0QQ
    see Replacement, Lower Bones 0QR
    see Supplement, Lower Bones 0QU

Patellar ligament
use Bursa and Ligament, Knee, Right
use Bursa and Ligament, Knee, Left
Patellar tendon
use Tendon, Knee, Left
use Tendon, Knee, Right
Patellectomy
see Excision, Lower Bones 0QB
see Resection, Lower Bones 0QT
Pectineus muscle
use Muscle, Upper Leg, Left
use Muscle, Upper Leg, Right
Pectoral (anterior) lymph node
use Lymphatic, Axillary, Right
use Lymphatic, Axillary, Left
Pectoral fascia use Subcutaneous Tissue and Fascia,
Chest
Pectoralis major muscle
use Muscle, Thorax, Left
use Muscle, Thorax, Right
Pectoralis minor muscle
use Muscle, Thorax, Right
use Muscle, Thorax, Left
PEEP (positive end expiratory pressure) see Assistance,
Respiratory 5A09
PEG (percutaneous endoscopic gastrostomy)
0DH64UZ
PEJ (percutaneous endoscopic jejunostomy)
0DHA4UZ
Pelvic splanchnic nerve
use Nerve, Abdominal Sympathetic
use Nerve, Sacral Sympathetic
Penectomy
see Excision, Male Reproductive System 0VB
see Resection, Male Reproductive System 0VT
Penile urethra use Urethra
**Percutaneous transluminal coronary angioplasty
(PTCA)** see Dilation, Heart and Great Vessels 027
Performance
Biliary
Multiple, Filtration 5A1C60Z
Single, Filtration 5A1C00Z
Cardiac
Continuous
Output 5A1221Z
Pacing 5A1223Z
Intermittent, Pacing 5A1213Z
Single, Output, Manual 5A12012
Circulatory, Continuous, Oxygenation, Membrane
5A15223
Respiratory
24-96 Consecutive Hours, Ventilation 5A1945Z
Greater than 96 Consecutive Hours, Ventilation
5A1955Z
Less than 24 Consecutive Hours, Ventilation
5A1935Z
Single, Ventilation, Nonmechanical 5A19054
Urinary
Multiple, Filtration 5A1D60Z
Single, Filtration 5A1D00Z
Perfusion see Introduction
Pericardiectomy
see Excision, Pericardium 02BN
see Resection, Pericardium 02TN
Pericardiocentesis see Drainage, Pericardial Cavity
0W9D
Pericardiolysis see Release, Pericardium 02NN
Pericardiophrenic artery
use Artery, Internal Mammary, Left
use Artery, Internal Mammary, Right
Pericardioplasty
see Repair, Pericardium 02QN
see Replacement, Pericardium 02RN
see Supplement, Pericardium 02UN
Pericardiorrhaphy see Repair, Pericardium 02QN
Pericardiostomy see Drainage, Pericardial Cavity
0W9D
Pericardiotomy see Drainage, Pericardial Cavity 0W9D
Perimetrium use Uterus
Peripheral parenteral nutrition see Introduction,
Nutritional Substance
Peritoneal dialysis 3E1M39Z

Peritoneocentesis
see Drainage, Peritoneum 0D9W
see Drainage, Peritoneal Cavity 0W9G
Peritoneoplasty
see Repair, Peritoneum 0DQW
see Replacement, Peritoneum 0DRW
see Supplement, Peritoneum 0DUW
Peritoneoscopy 0DJW4ZZ
Peritoneotomy see Drainage, Peritoneum 0D9W
Peritoneumectomy see Excision, Peritoneum 0DBW
Peroneus brevis muscle
use Muscle, Lower Leg, Left
use Muscle, Lower Leg, Right
Peroneus longus muscle
use Muscle, Lower Leg, Right
use Muscle, Lower Leg, Left
Pessary
Change device in, Vagina and Cul-de-sac 0U2HXGZ
Insertion of device in
Cul-de-sac 0UHF
Vagina 0UHG
Removal of device from, Vagina and Cul-de-sac
0UPH
Revision of device in, Vagina and Cul-de-sac 0UWH
PET scan use Positron Emission Tomographic (PET)
Imaging
Petrous part of temoporal bone
use Bone, Temporal, Right
use Bone, Temporal, Left
Phacoemulsification, lens
With IOL implant see Replacement, Eye 08R
Without IOL implant see Extraction, Eye 08D
Phalangectomy
see Excision, Upper Bones 0PB
see Resection, Upper Bones 0PT
see Excision, Lower Bones 0QB
see Resection, Lower Bones 0QT
Phallectomy
see Excision, Penis 0VBS
see Resection, Penis 0VTS
Phalloplasty
see Repair, Penis 0VQS
see Supplement, Penis 0VUS
Phallotomy see Drainage, Penis 0V9S
Pharmacotherapy
Antabuse HZ93ZZZ
Bupropion HZ97ZZZ
Clonidine HZ96ZZZ
Levo-alpha-acetyl-methadol (LAAM) HZ92ZZZ
Methadone Maintenance HZ91ZZZ
Naloxone HZ95ZZZ
Naltrexone HZ94ZZZ
Nicotine Replacement HZ90ZZZ
Psychiatric Medication HZ98ZZZ
Replacement Medication, Other HZ99ZZZ
Pharyngeal constrictor muscle use Muscle, Tongue,
Palate, Pharynx
Pharyngeal plexus use Nerve, Vagus
Pharyngeal recess use Nasopharynx
Pharyngeal tonsil use Adenoids
Pharyngogram see Fluoroscopy, Pharynix B91G
Pharyngoplasty
see Repair, Mouth and Throat 0CQ
see Replacement, Mouth and Throat 0CR
see Supplement, Mouth and Throat 0CU
Pharyngorrhaphy see Repair, Mouth and Throat 0CQ
Pharyngotomy see Drainage, Mouth and Throat 0C9
Pharyngotympanic tube
use Eustachian Tube, Right
use Eustachian Tube, Left
Pheresis
Erythrocytes 6A55
Leukocytes 6A55
Plasma 6A55
Platelets 6A55
Stem Cells
Cord Blood 6A55
Hematopoietic 6A55
Phlebectomy
see Excision, Upper Veins 05B
see Extraction, Upper Veins 05D
see Excision, Lower Veins 06B
see Extraction, Lower Veins 06D

Phlebography
see Plain Radiography, Veins B50
Impedance 4A04X51
Phleborrhaphy
see Repair, Upper Veins 05Q
see Repair, Lower Veins 06Q
Phlebotomy
see Drainage, Upper Veins 059
see Drainage, Lower Veins 069
Photocoagulation
for Destruction see Destruction
for Repair see Repair
Photopheresis, therapeutic see Phototherapy,
Circulatory 6A65
Phototherapy
Circulatory 6A65
Skin 6A60
Phrenectomy, phrenoneurectomy see Excision,
Nerve, Phrenic 01B2
Phrenemphraxis see Destruction, Nerve, Phrenic 0152
Phreniclasis see Destruction, Nerve, Phrenic 0152
Phrenicoexeresis see Extraction, Nerve, Phrenic 01D2
Phrenicotomy see Division, Nerve, Phrenic 0182
Phrenicotripsy see Destruction, Nerve, Phrenic 0152
Phrenoplasty
see Repair, Respiratory System 0BQ
see Supplement, Respiratory System 0BU
Phrenotomy see Drainage, Respiratory System 0B9
Physiatry see Motor Treatment, Rehabilitation F07
Physical medicine see Motor Treatment,
Rehabilitation F07
Physical therapy see Motor Treatment, Rehabilitation
F07
Pia mater
use Spinal Meninges
use Cerebral Meninges
Pinealectomy
see Excision, Pineal Body 0GB1
see Resection, Pineal Body 0GT1
Pinealoscopy 0GJ14ZZ
Pinealotomy see Drainage, Pineal Body 0G91
Pinna
use Ear, External, Left
use Ear, External, Bilateral
use Ear, External, Right
Piriform recess (sinus) use Pharynx
Piriformis muscle
use Muscle, Hip, Left
use Muscle, Hip, Right
Pisiform bone
use Carpal, Left
use Carpal, Right
Pisohamate ligament
use Bursa and Ligament, Hand, Right
use Bursa and Ligament, Hand, Left
Pisometacarpal ligament
use Bursa and Ligament, Hand, Left
use Bursa and Ligament, Hand, Right
Pituitectomy
see Excision, Gland, Pituitary 0GB0
see Resection, Gland, Pituitary 0GT0
Plain film radiology see Plain Radiography
Plain Radiography
Abdomen BW00ZZZ
Abdomen and Pelvis BW01ZZZ
Abdominal Lymphatic
Bilateral B701
Unilateral B700
Airway, Upper BB0DZZZ
Ankle
Left BQ0H
Right BQ0G
Aorta
Abdominal B400
Thoracic B300
Thoraco-Abdominal B30P
Aorta and Bilateral Lower Extremity Arteries B40D
Arch
Bilateral BN0DZZZ
Left BN0CZZZ
Right BN0BZZZ
Arm
Left BP0FZZZ

Plain Radiography—*continued*
  Arm—*continued*
    Right BP0EZZZ
  Artery
    Brachiocephalic-Subclavian, Right B301
    Bronchial B30L
    Bypass Graft, Other B20F
    Cervico-Cerebral Arch B30Q
    Common Carotid
      Bilateral B305
      Left B304
      Right B303
    Coronary
      Bypass Graft
        Multiple B203
        Single B202
      Multiple B201
      Single B200
    External Carotid
      Bilateral B30C
      Left B30B
      Right B309
    Hepatic B402
    Inferior Mesenteric B405
    Intercostal B30L
    Internal Carotid
      Bilateral B308
      Left B307
      Right B306
    Internal Mammary Bypass Graft
      Left B208
      Right B207
    Intra-Abdominal, Other B40B
    Intracranial B30R
    Lower, Other B40J
    Lower Extremity
      Bilateral and Aorta B40D
      Left B40G
      Right B40F
    Lumbar B409
    Pelvic B40C
    Pulmonary
      Left B30T
      Right B30S
    Renal
      Bilateral B408
      Left B407
      Right B406
      Transplant B40M
    Spinal B30M
    Splenic B403
    Subclavian, Left B302
    Superior Mesenteric B404
    Upper, Other B30N
    Upper Extremity
      Bilateral B30K
      Left B30J
      Right B30H
    Vertebral
      Bilateral B30G
      Left B30F
      Right B30D
  Bile Duct BF00
  Bile Duct and Gallbladder BF03
  Bladder BT00
    Kidney and Ureter BT04
  Bladder and Urethra BT0B
  Bone
    Facial BN05ZZZ
    Nasal BN04ZZZ
  Bones, Long, All BW0BZZZ
  Breast
    Bilateral BH02ZZZ
    Left BH01ZZZ
    Right BH00ZZZ
  Calcaneus
    Left BQ0KZZZ
    Right BQ0JZZZ
  Chest BW03ZZZ
  Clavicle
    Left BP05ZZZ
    Right BP04ZZZ
  Coccyx BR0FZZZ

Plain Radiography—*continued*
  Corpora Cavernosa BV00
  Dialysis Fistula B50W
  Dialysis Shunt B50W
  Disc
    Cervical BR01
    Lumbar BR03
    Thoracic BR02
  Duct
    Lacrimal
      Bilateral B802
      Left B801
      Right B800
    Mammary
      Multiple
        Left BH06
        Right BH05
      Single
        Left BH04
        Right BH03
  Elbow
    Left BP0H
    Right BP0G
  Epididymis
    Left BV02
    Right BV01
  Extremity
    Lower BW0CZZZ
    Upper BW0JZZZ
  Eye
    Bilateral B807ZZZ
    Left B806ZZZ
    Right B805ZZZ
  Facet Joint
    Cervical BR04
    Lumbar BR06
    Thoracic BR05
  Fallopian Tube
    Bilateral BU02
    Left BU01
    Right BU00
  Fallopian Tube and Uterus BU08
  Femur
    Left, Densitometry BQ04ZZ1
    Right, Densitometry BQ03ZZ1
  Finger
    Left BP0SZZZ
    Right BP0RZZZ
  Foot
    Left BQ0MZZZ
    Right BQ0LZZZ
  Forearm
    Left BP0KZZZ
    Right BP0JZZZ
  Gallbladder and Bile Duct BF03
  Gland
    Parotid
      Bilateral B906
      Left B905
      Right B904
    Salivary
      Bilateral B90D
      Left B90C
      Right B90B
    Submandibular
      Bilateral B909
      Left B908
      Right B907
  Hand
    Left BP0PZZZ
    Right BP0NZZZ
  Heart
    Left B205
    Right B204
    Right and Left B206
  Hepatobiliary System, All BF0C
  Hip
    Left BQ01
      Densitometry BQ01ZZ1
    Right BQ00
      Densitometry BQ00ZZ1

Plain Radiography—*continued*
  Humerus
    Left BP0BZZZ
    Right BP0AZZZ
  Ileal Diversion Loop BT0C
  Intracranial Sinus B502
  Joint
    Acromioclavicular, Bilateral BP03ZZZ
    Finger
      Left BP0D
      Right BP0C
    Foot
      Left BQ0Y
      Right BQ0X
    Hand
      Left BP0D
      Right BP0C
    Lumbosacral BR0BZZZ
    Sacroiliac BR0D
    Sternoclavicular
      Bilateral BP02ZZZ
      Left BP01ZZZ
      Right BP00ZZZ
    Temporomandibular
      Bilateral BN09
      Left BN08
      Right BN07
    Thoracolumbar BR08ZZZ
    Toe
      Left BQ0Y
      Right BQ0X
  Kidney
    Bilateral BT03
    Left BT02
    Right BT01
    Ureter and Bladder BT04
  Knee
    Left BQ08
    Right BQ07
  Leg
    Left BQ0FZZZ
    Right BQ0DZZZ
  Lymphatic
    Head B704
    Lower Extremity
      Bilateral B70B
      Left B709
      Right B708
    Neck B704
    Pelvic B70C
    Upper Extremity
      Bilateral B707
      Left B706
      Right B705
  Mandible BN06ZZZ
  Mastoid B90HZZZ
  Nasopharynx B90FZZZ
  Optic Foramina
    Left B804ZZZ
    Right B803ZZZ
  Orbit
    Bilateral BN03ZZZ
    Left BN02ZZZ
    Right BN01ZZZ
  Oropharynx B90FZZZ
  Patella
    Left BQ0WZZZ
    Right BQ0VZZZ
  Pelvis BR0CZZZ
  Pelvis and Abdomen BW01ZZZ
  Prostate BV03
  Retroperitoneal Lymphatic
    Bilateral B701
    Unilateral B700
  Ribs
    Left BP0YZZZ
    Right BP0XZZZ
  Sacrum BR0FZZZ
  Scapula
    Left BP07ZZZ
    Right BP06ZZZ

Plain Radiography—*continued*

Shoulder
Left BP09
Right BP08
Sinus
Intracranial B502
Paranasal B902ZZZ
Skull BN00ZZZ
Spinal Cord B00B
Spine
Cervical, Densitometry BR00ZZ1
Lumbar, Densitometry BR09ZZ1
Thoracic, Densitometry BR07ZZ1
Whole, Densitometry BR0GZZ1
Sternum BR0HZZZ
Teeth
All BN0JZZZ
Multiple BN0HZZZ
Testicle
Left BV06
Right BV05
Toe
Left BQ0QZZZ
Right BQ0PZZZ
Tooth, Single BN0GZZZ
Tracheobronchial Tree
Bilateral BB09YZZ
Left BB08YZZ
Right BB07YZZ
Ureter
Bilateral BT08
Kidney and Bladder BT04
Left BT07
Right BT06
Urethra BT05
Urethra and Bladder BT0B
Uterus BU06
Uterus and Fallopian Tube BU08
Vagina BU09
Vasa Vasorum BV08
Vein
Cerebellar B501
Cerebral B501
Epidural B500
Jugular
Bilateral B505
Left B504
Right B503
Lower Extremity
Bilateral B50D
Left B50C
Right B50B
Other B50V
Pelvic (Iliac)
Left B50G
Right B50F
Pelvic (Iliac) Bilateral B50H
Portal B50T
Pulmonary
Bilateral B50S
Left B50R
Right B50Q
Renal
Bilateral B50L
Left B50K
Right B50J
Spanchnic B50T
Subclavian
Left B507
Right B506
Upper Extremity
Bilateral B50P
Left B50N
Right B50M
Vena Cava
Inferior B509
Superior B508
Whole Body BW0KZZZ
Infant BW0MZZZ
Whole Skeleton BW0LZZZ
Wrist
Left BP0M
Right BP0L

Planar Nuclear Medicine Imaging CP1

Abdomen CW10
Abdomen and Chest CW14
Abdomen and Pelvis CW11
Anatomical Regions, Multiple CW1YYZZ
Bladder, Kidneys and Ureters CT13
Bladder and Ureters CT1H
Blood C713
Bone Marrow C710
Brain C010
Breast CH1YYZZ
Bilateral CH12
Left CH11
Right CH10
Bronchi and Lungs CB12
Central Nervous System C01YYZZ
Cerebrospinal Fluid C015
Chest CW13
Chest and Abdomen CW14
Chest and Neck CW16
Digestive System CD1YYZZ
Ducts, Lacrimal, Bilateral C819
Ear, Nose, Mouth and Throat C91YYZZ
Endocrine System CG1YYZZ
Extremity
Lower CW1D
Bilateral CP1F
Left CP1D
Right CP1C
Upper CW1M
Bilateral CP1B
Left CP19
Right CP18
Eye C81YYZZ
Gallbladder CF14
Gastrointestinal Tract CD17
Upper CD15
Gland
Adrenal, Bilateral CG14
Parathyroid CG11
Thyroid CG12
Glands, Salivary, Bilateral C91B
Head and Neck CW1B
Heart C21YYZZ
Right and Left C216
Hepatobiliary System, All CF1C
Hepatobiliary System and Pancreas CF1YYZZ
Kidneys, Ureters and Bladder CT13
Liver CF15
Liver and Spleen CF16
Lungs and Bronchi CB12
Lymphatics
Head C71J
Head and Neck C715
Lower Extremity C71P
Neck C71K
Pelvic C71D
Trunk C71M
Upper Chest C71L
Upper Extremity C71N
Lymphatics and Hematologic System C71YYZZ
Musculoskeletal System, All CP1Z
Myocardium C21G
Neck and Chest CW16
Neck and Head CW1B
Pancreas and Hepatobiliary System CF1YYZZ
Pelvic Region CW1J
Pelvis CP16
Pelvis and Abdomen CW11
Pelvis and Spine CP17
Reproductive System, Male CV1YYZZ
Respiratory System CB1YYZZ
Skin CH1YYZZ
Skull CP11
Spine CP15
Spine and Pelvis CP17
Spleen C712
Spleen and Liver CF16
Subcutaneous Tissue CH1YYZZ
Testicles, Bilateral CV19
Thorax CP14
Ureters, Kidneys and Bladder CT13
Ureters and Bladder CT1H

Planar Nuclear Medicine Imaging —*continued*

Urinary System CT1YYZZ
Veins C51YYZZ
Central C51R
Lower Extremity
Bilateral C51D
Left C51C
Right C51B
Upper Extremity
Bilateral C51Q
Left C51P
Right C51N
Whole Body CW1N

Plantar digital vein

use Vein, Foot, Right
use Vein, Foot, Left

Plantar fascia (aponeurosis)

use Subcutaneous Tissue and Fascia, Foot, Right
use Subcutaneous Tissue and Fascia, Foot, Left

Plantar metatarsal vein

use Vein, Foot, Right
use Vein, Foot, Left

Plantar venous arch

use Vein, Foot, Right
use Vein, Foot, Left

Plaque Radiation

Abdomen DWY3FZZ
Adrenal Gland DGY2FZZ
Anus DDY8FZZ
Bile Ducts DFY2FZZ
Bladder DTY2FZZ
Bone, Other DPYCFZZ
Bone Marrow D7Y0FZZ
Brain D0Y0FZZ
Brain Stem D0Y1FZZ
Breast
Left DMY0FZZ
Right DMY1FZZ
Bronchus DBY1FZZ
Cervix DUY1FZZ
Chest DWY2FZZ
Chest Wall DBY7FZZ
Colon DDY5FZZ
Diaphragm DBY8FZZ
Duodenum DDY2FZZ
Ear D9Y0FZZ
Esophagus DDY0FZZ
Eye D8Y0FZZ
Femur DPY9FZZ
Fibula DPYBFZZ
Gallbladder DFY1FZZ
Gland
Adrenal DGY2FZZ
Parathyroid DGY4FZZ
Pituitary DGY0FZZ
Thyroid DGY5FZZ
Glands, Salivary D9Y6FZZ
Head and Neck DWY1FZZ
Hemibody DWY4FZZ
Humerus DPY6FZZ
Ileum DDY4FZZ
Jejunum DDY3FZZ
Kidney DTY0FZZ
Larynx D9YBFZZ
Liver DFY0FZZ
Lung DBY2FZZ
Lymphatics
Abdomen D7Y6FZZ
Axillary D7Y4FZZ
Inguinal D7Y8FZZ
Neck D7Y3FZZ
Pelvis D7Y7FZZ
Thorax D7Y5FZZ
Mandible DPY3FZZ
Maxilla DPY2FZZ
Mediastinum DBY6FZZ
Mouth D9Y4FZZ
Nasopharynx D9YDFZZ
Neck and Head DWY1FZZ
Nerve, Peripheral D0Y7FZZ
Nose D9Y1FZZ
Ovary DUY0FZZ

Plaque Radiation—*continued*
Palate
  Hard D9Y8FZZ
  Soft D9Y9FZZ
Pancreas DFY3FZZ
Parathyroid Gland DGY4FZZ
Pelvic Bones DPY8FZZ
Pelvic Region DWY6FZZ
Pharynx D9YCFZZ
Pineal Body DGY1FZZ
Pituitary Gland DGY0FZZ
Pleura DBY5FZZ
Prostate DVY0FZZ
Radius DPY7FZZ
Rectum DDY7FZZ
Rib DPY5FZZ
Sinuses D9Y7FZZ
Skin
  Abdomen DHY8FZZ
  Arm DHY4FZZ
  Back DHY7FZZ
  Buttock DHY9FZZ
  Chest DHY6FZZ
  Face DHY2FZZ
  Foot DHYCFZZ
  Hand DHY5FZZ
  Leg DHYBFZZ
  Neck DHY3FZZ
Skull DPY0FZZ
Spinal Cord D0Y6FZZ
Spleen D7Y2FZZ
Sternum DPY4FZZ
Stomach DDY1FZZ
Testis DVY1FZZ
Thymus D7Y1FZZ
Thyroid Gland DGY5FZZ
Tibia DPYBFZZ
Tongue D9Y5FZZ
Trachea DBY0FZZ
Ulna DPY7FZZ
Ureter DTY1FZZ
Urethra DTY3FZZ
Uterus DUY2FZZ
Whole Body DWY5FZZ
Plasmapheresis, therapeutic 6A550Z3
Plateletpheresis, therapeutic 6A550Z2
Platysma muscle
  use Muscle, Neck, Left
  use Muscle, Neck, Right
Pleurectomy
  see Excision, Respiratory System 0BB
  see Resection, Respiratory System 0BT
Pleurocentesis *see* Drainage, Anatomical Regions,
  General 0W9
Pleurodesis, pleurosclerosis
  Chemical injection *see* Introduction, Respiratory
    Tract 3E0F
  Surgical *see* Destruction, Respiratory System 0B5
Pleurolysis *see* Release, Respiratory System 0BN
Pleuroscopy 0BJQ4ZZ
Pleurotomy *see* Drainage, Respiratory System 0B9
Plica semilunaris
  use Conjunctiva, Left
  use Conjunctiva, Right
Plication *see* Restriction
Pneumectomy
  see Excision, Respiratory System 0BB
  see Resection, Respiratory System 0BT
Pneumocentesis *see* Drainage, Respiratory System
  0B9
Pneumogastric nerve *use* Nerve, Vagus
Pneumolysis *see* Release, Respiratory System 0BN
Pneumonectomy
  see Resection, Respiratory System 0BT
  see Resection, Respiratory System 0BT
Pneumonolysis *see* Release, Respiratory System 0BN
Pneumonopexy
  see Repair, Respiratory System 0BQ
  see Reposition, Respiratory System 0BS
Pneumonorrhaphy *see* Repair, Respiratory System
  0BQ
Pneumonotomy *see* Drainage, Respiratory System 0B9
Pneumotaxic center *use* Pons

Pneumotomy *see* Drainage, Respiratory System 0B9
Pollicization *see* Transfer, Anatomical Regions, Upper
  Extremities 0XX
Polypectomy, gastrointestinal *see* Excision,
  Gastrointestinal System 0DB
Polysomnogram 4A1ZXQZ
Pontine tegmentum *use* Pons
Popliteal ligament
  use Bursa and Ligament, Knee, Right
  use Bursa and Ligament, Knee, Left
Popliteal lymph node
  use Lymphatic, Lower Extremity, Right
  use Lymphatic, Lower Extremity, Left
Popliteal vein
  use Vein, Femoral, Right
  use Vein, Femoral, Left
Popliteus muscle
  use Muscle, Lower Leg, Right
  use Muscle, Lower Leg, Left
Positive end expiratory pressure *see* Performance,
  Respiratory 5A19
Positron Emission Tomographic (PET) Imaging
  Brain C030
  Bronchi and Lungs CB32
  Central Nervous System C03YYZZ
  Heart C23YYZZ
  Lungs and Bronchi CB32
  Myocardium C23G
  Respiratory System CB3YYZZ
  Whole Body CW3NYZZ
Positron emission tomography *use* Positron Emission
  Tomographic (PET) Imaging
Postauricular (mastoid) lymph node *use* Lymphatic,
  Neck, Right
  use Lymphatic, Neck, Left
Postcava *use* Vena Cava, Inferior
Posterior (subscapular) lymph node
  use Lymphatic, Axillary, Left
  use Lymphatic, Axillary, Right
Posterior auricular artery
  use Artery, External Carotid, Right
  use Artery, External Carotid, Left
Posterior auricular nerve *use* Nerve, Facial
Posterior auricular vein
  use Vein, External Jugular, Left
  use Vein, External Jugular, Right
Posterior cerebral artery *use* Artery, Intracranial
Posterior chamber
  use Eye, Right
  use Eye, Left
Posterior circumflex humeral artery
  use Artery, Axillary, Right
  use Artery, Axillary, Left
Posterior communicating artery *use* Artery,
  Intracranial
Posterior cruciate ligament (PCL)
  use Bursa and Ligament, Knee, Right
  use Bursa and Ligament, Knee, Left
Posterior facial (retromandibular) vein
  use Vein, Face, Right
  use Vein, Face, Left
Posterior femoral cutaneous nerve *use* Nerve, Sacral
  Plexus
Posterior inferior cerebellar artery (PICA) *use*
  Artery, Intracranial
Posterior interosseous nerve *use* Nerve, Radial
Posterior labial nerve *use* Nerve, Pudendal
Posterior scrotal nerve *use* Nerve, Pudendal
Posterior spinal arter
  use Artery, Vertebral, Left
  use Artery, Vertebral, Right
Posterior tibial recurrent artery
  use Artery, Anterior Tibial, Right
  use Artery, Anterior Tibial, Left
Posterior ulnar recurrent artery
  use Artery, Ulnar, Left
  use Artery, Ulnar, Right
Posterior vagal trunk *use* Nerve, Vagus
PPN (peripheral parenteral nutrition) *see* Introduction,
  Nutritional Substance
Preauricular lymph node *use* Lymphatic, Head
Precava *use* Vena Cava, Superior

Prepatellar bursa
  use Bursa and Ligament, Knee, Right
  use Bursa and Ligament, Knee, Left
Preputiotomy *see* Drainage, Male Reproductive
  System 0V9
Pressure Sensor
  Aorta, Thoracic 02HW
  Artery
    Pulmonary
      Left 02HR
      Right 02HQ
    Pulmonary Trunk 02HP
  Atrium
    Left 02H7
    Right 02H6
  Pericardium 02HN
  Vein
    Coronary 02H4
    Pulmonary
      Left 02HT
      Right 02HS
  Vena Cava, Superior 02HV
  Ventricle
    Left 02HL
    Right 02HK
Pressure support ventilation *see* Performance,
  Respiratory 5A19
Pretracheal fascia *use* Subcutaneous Tissue and
  Fascia, Neck, Anterior
Prevertebral fascia *use* Subcutaneous Tissue and
  Fascia, Neck, Posterior
Princeps pollicis artery
  use Artery, Hand, Left
  use Artery, Hand, Right
Probing, duct
  Diagnostic *see* Inspection
  Dilation *see* Dilation
Procerus muscle *use* Muscle, Facial
Proctectomy
  see Excision, Rectum 0DBP
  see Resection, Rectum 0DTP
Proctoclysis *see* Introduction, Gastrointestinal Tract,
  Lower 3E0H
Proctocolectomy
  see Excision, Gastrointestinal System 0DB
  see Resection, Gastrointestinal System 0DT
Proctocolpoplasty
  see Repair, Gastrointestinal System 0DQ
  see Supplement, Gastrointestinal System 0DU
Proctoperineoplasty
  see Repair, Gastrointestinal System 0DQ
  see Supplement, Gastrointestinal System 0DU
Proctoperineorrhaphy *see* Repair, Gastrointestinal
  System 0DQ
Proctopexy
  see Repair, Rectum 0DQP
  see Reposition, Rectum 0DSP
Proctoplasty
  see Repair, Rectum 0DQP
  see Supplement, Rectum 0DUP
Proctorrhaphy *see* Repair, Rectum 0DQP
Proctoscopy 0DJD8ZZ
Proctosigmoidectomy
  see Excision, Gastrointestinal System 0DB
  see Resection, Gastrointestinal System 0DT
Proctosigmoidoscopy 0DJD8ZZ
Proctostomy *see* Drainage, Rectum 0D9P
Proctotomy *see* Drainage, Rectum 0D9P
Production, atrial septal defect *see* Excision, Septum,
  Atrial 02B5
Profunda brachii
  use Artery, Brachial, Right
  use Artery, Brachial, Left
Profunda femoris (deep femoral) vein
  use Vein, Femoral, Right
  use Vein, Femoral, Left
Pronator quadratus muscle
  use Muscle, Lower Arm and Wrist, Left
  use Muscle, Lower Arm and Wrist, Right
Pronator teres muscle
  use Muscle, Lower Arm and Wrist, Right
  use Muscle, Lower Arm and Wrist, Left

Prostatectomy
see Excision, Prostate ØVBØ
see Resection, Prostate ØVTØ
Prostatic urethra use Urethra
Prostatomy, prostatotomy see Drainage, Prostate ØV9Ø
Proximal radioulnar joint
use Joint, Elbow, Left
use Joint, Elbow, Right
Psoas muscle
use Muscle, Hip, Right
use Muscle, Hip, Left
PSV (pressure support ventilation) see Performance, Respiratory 5A19
Psychoanalysis GZ54ZZZ
Psychological Tests
Cognitive Status GZ14ZZZ
Developmental GZ1ØZZZ
Intellectual and Psychoeducational GZ12ZZZ
Neurobehavioral Status GZ14ZZZ
Neuropsychological GZ13ZZZ
Personality and Behavioral GZ11ZZZ
Psychotherapy
Family, Mental Health Services GZ72ZZZ
Group
GZHZZZZ
Mental Health Services GZHZZZZ
Individual
see Psychotherapy, Individual, Mental Health Services
for substance abuse
12-Step HZ53ZZZ
Behavioral HZ51ZZZ
Cognitive HZ5ØZZZ
Cognitive-Behavioral HZ52ZZZ
Confrontational HZ58ZZZ
Interactive HZ55ZZZ
Interpersonal HZ54ZZZ
Motivational Enhancement HZ57ZZZ
Psychoanalysis HZ5BZZZ
Psychodynamic HZ5CZZZ
Psychoeducation HZ56ZZZ
Psychophysiological HZ5DZZZ
Supportive HZ59ZZZ
Mental Health Services
Behavioral GZ51ZZZ
Cognitive GZ52ZZZ
Cognitive-Behavioral GZ58ZZZ
Interactive GZ5ØZZZ
Interpersonal GZ53ZZZ
Psychoanalysis GZ54ZZZ
Psyhodynamic GZ55ZZZ
Psychophysiological GZ59ZZZ
Supportive GZ56ZZZ
PTCA (percutaneous transluminal coronary angioplasty) see Dilation, Heart and Great Vessels Ø27
Pterygoid muscle use Muscle, Head
Pterygoid process
use Bone, Sphenoid, Right
use Bone, Sphenoid, Left
Pterygopalatine (sphenopalatine) ganglion use Nerve, Head and Neck Sympathetic
Pubic ligament
use Bursa and Ligament, Trunk, Right
use Bursa and Ligament, Trunk, Left
Pubis
use Bone, Pelvic, Right
use Bone, Pelvic, Left
Pubofemoral ligament
use Bursa and Ligament, Hip, Left
use Bursa and Ligament, Hip, Right
Pudendal nerve use Nerve, Sacral Plexus
Pull-through, rectal see Resection, Rectum ØDTP
Pulmoaortic canal use Artery, Pulmonary, Left
Pulmonary annulus use Valve, Pulmonary
Pulmonary artery wedge monitoring see Monitoring, Arterial 4A13
Pulmonary plexus
use Nerve, Vagus
use Nerve, Thoracic Sympathetic
Pulmonic valve use Valve, Pulmonary
Pulpectomy see Excision, Mouth and Throat ØCB

Pulverization see Fragmentation
Pulvinar use Thalamus
Punch biopsy see Excision, Diagnostic
Puncture see Drainage
Pyelography
see Plain Radiography, Urinary System BTØ
see Fluoroscopy, Urinary System BT1
Pyeloileostomy, urinary diversion see Bypass, Urinary System ØT1
Pyeloplasty
see Repair, Urinary System ØTQ
see Replacement, Urinary System ØTR
see Supplement, Urinary System ØTU
Pyelorrhaphy see Repair, Urinary System ØTQ
Pyeloscopy ØTJ58ZZ
Pyelostomy
see Drainage, Urinary System ØT9
see Bypass, Urinary System ØT1
Pyelotomy see Drainage, Urinary System ØT9
Pylorectomy
see Excision, Stomach, Pylorus ØDB7
see Resection, Stomach, Pylorus ØDT7
Pyloric antrum use Stomach, Pylorus
Pyloric canal use Stomach, Pylorus
Pyloric sphincter use Stomach, Pylorus
Pylorodiosis see Dilation, Stomach, Pylorus ØD77
Pylorogastrectomy
see Excision, Gastrointestinal System ØDB
see Resection, Gastrointestinal System ØDT
Pyloroplasty
see Repair, Stomach, Pylorus ØDQ7
see Supplement, Stomach, Pylorus ØDU7
Pyloroscopy ØDJ68ZZ
Pylorotomy see Drainage, Stomach, Pylorus ØD97
Pyramidalis muscle
use Muscle, Abdomen, Left
use Muscle, Abdomen, Right

Q

Quadrangular cartilage use Septum, Nasal
Quadrant resection of breast see Excision, Skin and Breast ØHB
Quadrate lobe use Liver
Quadratus femoris muscle
use Muscle, Hip, Left
use Muscle, Hip, Right
Quadratus lumborum muscle
use Muscle, Trunk, Left
use Muscle, Trunk, Right
Quadratus plantae muscle
use Muscle, Foot, Left
use Muscle, Foot, Right
Quadriceps (femoris)
use Muscle, Upper Leg, Left
use Muscle, Upper Leg, Right
Quarantine 8EØZXY6

R

Radial collateral carpal ligament
use Bursa and Ligament, Wrist, Right
use Bursa and Ligament, Wrist, Left
Radial collateral ligament
use Bursa and Ligament, Elbow, Left
use Bursa and Ligament, Elbow, Right
Radial notch
use Ulna, Left
use Ulna, Right
Radial recurrent artery
use Artery, Radial, Right
use Artery, Radial, Left
Radial vein
use Vein, Brachial, Right
use Vein, Brachial, Left
Radialis indicis
use Artery, Hand, Right
use Artery, Hand, Left
Radiation Oncology
use Beam Radiation

Radiation Oncology—continued
see Brachytherapy
Radiation treatment see Radiation Oncology
Radiocarpal joint
use Joint, Wrist, Left
use Joint, Wrist, Right
Radiocarpal ligament
use Bursa and Ligament, Wrist, Left
use Bursa and Ligament, Wrist, Right
Radiography see Plain Radiography
Radiology, analog see Plain Radiography
Radiology, diagnostic see Imaging, Diagnostic
Radioulnar ligament
use Bursa and Ligament, Wrist, Right
use Bursa and Ligament, Wrist, Left
Range of motion testing see Motor Function Assessment, Rehabilitation FØ1
Reattachment
Abdominal Wall ØWMFØZZ
Ampulla of Vater ØFMC
Ankle Region
Left ØYMLØZZ
Right ØYMKØZZ
Arm
Lower
Left ØXMFØZZ
Right ØXMDØZZ
Upper
Left ØXM9ØZZ
Right ØXM8ØZZ
Axilla
Left ØXM5ØZZ
Right ØXM4ØZZ
Back
Lower ØWMLØZZ
Upper ØWMKØZZ
Bladder ØTMB
Bladder Neck ØTMC
Breast
Bilateral ØHMVXZZ
Left ØHMUXZZ
Right ØHMTXZZ
Bronchus
Lingula ØBM9ØZZ
Lower Lobe
Left ØBMBØZZ
Right ØBM6ØZZ
Main
Left ØBM7ØZZ
Right ØBM3ØZZ
Middle Lobe, Right ØBM5ØZZ
Upper Lobe
Left ØBM8ØZZ
Right ØBM4ØZZ
Bursa and Ligament
Abdomen
Left ØMMJ
Right ØMMH
Ankle
Left ØMMR
Right ØMMQ
Elbow
Left ØMM4
Right ØMM3
Foot
Left ØMMT
Right ØMMS
Hand
Left ØMM8
Right ØMM7
Head and Neck ØMMØ
Hip
Left ØMMM
Right ØMML
Knee
Left ØMMP
Right ØMMN
Lower Extremity
Left ØMMW
Right ØMMV
Perineum ØMMK

Reattachment—continued

Skin—continued
    Lower Leg
        Left 0HMLXZZ
        Right 0HMKXZZ
    Neck 0HM4XZZ
    Perineum 0HM9XZZ
    Scalp 0HM0XZZ
    Upper Arm
        Left 0HMCXZZ
        Right 0HMBXZZ
    Upper Leg
        Left 0HMJXZZ
        Right 0HMHXZZ
Stomach 0DM6
Tendon
    Abdomen
        Left 0LMG
        Right 0LMF
    Ankle
        Left 0LMT
        Right 0LMS
    Foot
        Left 0LMW
        Right 0LMV
    Hand
        Left 0LM8
        Right 0LM7
    Head and Neck 0LM0
    Hip
        Left 0LMK
        Right 0LMJ
    Knee
        Left 0LMR
        Right 0LMQ
    Lower Arm and Wrist
        Left 0LM6
        Right 0LM5
    Lower Leg
        Left 0LMP
        Right 0LMN
    Perineum 0LMH
    Shoulder
        Left 0LM2
        Right 0LM1
    Thorax
        Left 0LMD
        Right 0LMC
    Trunk
        Left 0LMB
        Right 0LM9
    Upper Arm
        Left 0LM4
        Right 0LM3
    Upper Leg
        Left 0LMM
        Right 0LML
Testis
    Bilateral 0VMC
    Left 0VMB
    Right 0VM9
Thumb
    Left 0XMM0ZZ
    Right 0XML0ZZ
Thyroid Gland
    Left Lobe 0GMG
    Right Lobe 0GMH
Toe
    1st
        Left 0YMQ0ZZ
        Right 0YMP0ZZ
    2nd
        Left 0YMS0ZZ
        Right 0YMR0ZZ
    3rd
        Left 0YMU0ZZ
        Right 0YMT0ZZ
    4th
        Left 0YMW0ZZ
        Right 0YMV0ZZ
    5th
        Left 0YMY0ZZ
        Right 0YMX0ZZ

Reattachment—continued

Tongue 0CM70ZZ
Tooth
    Lower 0CMX
    Upper 0CMW
Trachea 0BM10ZZ
Tunica Vaginalis
    Left 0VM7
    Right 0VM6
Ureter
    Left 0TM7
    Right 0TM6
Ureters, Bilateral 0TM8
Urethra 0TMD
Uterine Supporting Structure 0UM4
Uterus 0UM9
Uvula 0CMN0ZZ
Vagina 0UMG
Vulva 0UMMXZZ
Wrist Region
    Left 0XMH0ZZ
    Right 0XMG0ZZ

Recession
    see Repair
    see Reposition
Reclosure, disrupted abdominal wall 0WQFXZZ
Reconstruction
    see Repair
    see Replacement
    see Supplement
Rectectomy
    see Excision, Rectum 0DBP
    see Resection, Rectum 0DTP
Rectocele repair
    see Repair, Subcutaneous Tissue and Fascia, Pelvic
        Region 0JQC
    see Repair, Subcutaneous Tissue and Fascia, Pelvic
        Region 0JQC
Rectopexy
    see Repair, Gastrointestinal System 0DQ
    see Reposition, Gastrointestinal System 0DS
Rectoplasty
    see Repair, Gastrointestinal System 0DQ
    see Supplement, Gastrointestinal System 0DU
Rectorrhaphy *see* Repair, Gastrointestinal System 0DQ
Rectoscopy 0DJD8ZZ
Rectosigmoid junction *use* Colon, Sigmoid
Rectosigmoidectomy
    see Excision, Gastrointestinal System 0DB
    see Resection, Gastrointestinal System 0DT
Rectostomy *see* Drainage, Rectum 0D9P
Rectotomy *see* Drainage, Rectum 0D9P
Rectus abdominis muscle
    use Muscle, Abdomen, Left
    use Muscle, Abdomen, Right
Rectus femoris muscle
    use Muscle, Upper Leg, Left
    use Muscle, Upper Leg, Right
Recurrent laryngeal nerve *use* Nerve, Vagus
Reduction
    Dislocation *see* Reposition
    Fracture *see* Reposition
    Intussusception, intestinal *see* Reposition,
        Gastrointestinal System 0DS
    Mammoplasty *see* Excision, Skin and Breast 0HB
    Prolapse *see* Reposition
    Torsion *see* Reposition
    Volvulus, gastrointestinal *see* Reposition,
        Gastrointestinal System 0DS
Refusion *see* Fusion
Reimplantation
    see Reposition
    see Transfer
    see Reattachment
Reinforcement
    see Repair
    see Supplement
Relaxation, scar tissue *see* Release
Release
    Acetabulum
        Left 0QN5
        Right 0QN4
    Adenoids 0CNQ

Release—continued

Ampulla of Vater 0FNC
Anal Sphincter 0DNR
Anterior Chamber
    Left 08N33ZZ
    Right 08N23ZZ
Anus 0DNQ
Aorta
    Abdominal 04N0
    Thoracic 02NW
Aortic Body 0GND
Appendix 0DNJ
Artery
    Anterior Tibial
        Left 04NQ
        Right 04NP
    Axillary
        Left 03N6
        Right 03N5
    Brachial
        Left 03N8
        Right 03N7
    Celiac 04N1
    Colic
        Left 04N7
        Middle 04N8
        Right 04N6
    Common Carotid
        Left 03NJ
        Right 03NH
    Common Iliac
        Left 04ND
        Right 04NC
    External Carotid
        Left 03NN
        Right 03NM
    External Iliac
        Left 04NJ
        Right 04NH
    Face 03NR
    Femoral
        Left 04NL
        Right 04NK
    Foot
        Left 04NW
        Right 04NV
    Gastric 04N2
    Hand
        Left 03NF
        Right 03ND
    Hepatic 04N3
    Inferior Mesenteric 04NB
    Innominate 03N2
    Internal Carotid
        Left 03NL
        Right 03NK
    Internal Iliac
        Left 04NF
        Right 04NE
    Internal Mammary
        Left 03N1
        Right 03N0
    Intracranial 03NG
    Lower 04NY
    Peroneal
        Left 04NU
        Right 04NT
    Popliteal
        Left 04NN
        Right 04NM
    Posterior Tibial
        Left 04NS
        Right 04NR
    Pulmonary
        Left 02NR
        Right 02NQ
    Pulmonary Trunk 02NP
    Radial
        Left 03NC
        Right 03NB
    Renal
        Left 04NA
        Right 04N9

Removal of device from—*continued*
Extremity—*continued*
Upper
Left ØXP7
Right ØXP6
Eye
Left Ø8P1
Right Ø8P0
Face ØWP2
Fallopian Tube ØUP8
Femoral Shaft
Left ØQP9
Right ØQP8
Femur
Lower
Left ØQPC
Right ØQPB
Upper
Left ØQP7
Right ØQP6
Fibula
Left ØQPK
Right ØQPJ
Finger Nail ØHPQX
Gallbladder ØFP4
Gastrointestinal Tract ØWPP
Genitourinary Tract ØWPR
Gland
Adrenal ØGP5
Endocrine ØGPS
Pituitary ØGP0
Salivary ØCPA
Glenoid Cavity
Left ØPP8
Right ØPP7
Great Vessel Ø2PY
Hair ØHPSX
Head ØWP0
Heart Ø2PA
Humeral Head
Left ØPPD
Right ØPPC
Humeral Shaft
Left ØPPG
Right ØPPF
Intestinal Tract
Lower ØDPD
Upper ØDP0
Jaw
Lower ØWP5
Upper ØWP4
Joint
Acromioclavicular
Left ØRPH
Right ØRPG
Ankle
Left ØSPG
Right ØSPF
Carpal
Left ØRPR
Right ØRPQ
Cervical Vertebral ØRP1
Cervicothoracic Vertebral ØRP4
Coccygeal ØSP6
Elbow
Left ØRPM
Right ØRPL
Finger Phalangeal
Left ØRPX
Right ØRPW
Hip
Left ØSPB
Right ØSP9
Knee
Left ØSPD
Right ØSPC
Lumbar Vertebral ØSP0
Lumbosacral ØSP3
Metacarpocarpal
Left ØRPT
Right ØRPS

Removal of device from—*continued*
Joint—*continued*
Metacarpophalangeal
Left ØRPV
Right ØRPU
Metatarsal-Phalangeal
Left ØSPN
Right ØSPM
Metatarsal-Tarsal
Left ØSPL
Right ØSPK
Occipital-cervical ØRP0
Sacrococcygeal ØSP5
Sacroiliac
Left ØSP8
Right ØSP7
Shoulder
Left ØRPK
Right ØRPJ
Sternoclavicular
Left ØRPF
Right ØRPE
Tarsal
Left ØSPJ
Right ØSPH
Temporomandibular
Left ØRPD
Right ØRPC
Thoracic Vertebral ØRP6
Thoracolumbar Vertebral ØRPA
Toe Phalangeal
Left ØSPQ
Right ØSPP
Wrist
Left ØRPP
Right ØRPN
Kidney ØTP5
Larynx ØCPS
Lens
Left Ø8PK3JZ
Right Ø8PJ3JZ
Liver ØFP0
Lung
Left ØBPL
Right ØBPK
Lymphatic Ø7PN
Thoracic Duct Ø7PK
Mediastinum ØWPC
Mesentery ØDPV
Metacarpal
Left ØPPQ
Right ØPPP
Metatarsal
Left ØQPP
Right ØQPN
Mouth and Throat ØCPY
Muscle
Extraocular
Left Ø8PM
Right Ø8PL
Lower ØKPY
Upper ØKPX
Neck ØWP6
Nerve
Cranial Ø0PE
Peripheral Ø1PY
Nose Ø9PK
Omentum ØDPU
Ovary ØUP3
Pancreas ØFPG
Parathyroid Gland ØGPR
Patella
Left ØQPF
Right ØQPD
Pelvic Cavity ØWPJ
Penis ØVPS
Pericardial Cavity ØWPD
Perineum
Female ØWPN
Male ØWPM
Peritoneal Cavity ØWPG
Peritoneum ØDPW

Removal of device from—*continued*
Phalanx
Finger
Left ØPPV
Right ØPPT
Thumb
Left ØPPS
Right ØPPR
Toe
Left ØQPR
Right ØQPQ
Pineal Body ØGP1
Pleura ØBPQ
Pleural Cavity
Left ØWPB
Right ØWP9
Products of Conception 10P0
Prostate and Seminal Vesicles ØVP4
Radius
Left ØPPJ
Right ØPPH
Rectum ØDPP
Respiratory Tract ØWPQ
Retroperitoneum ØWPH
Rib
Left ØPP2
Right ØPP1
Sacrum ØQP1
Scapula
Left ØPP6
Right ØPP5
Scrotum and Tunica Vaginalis ØVP8
Sinus Ø9PY
Skin ØHPPX
Skull ØNP0
Spinal Canal Ø0PU
Spinal Cord Ø0PV
Spleen Ø7PP
Sternum ØPP0
Stomach ØDP6
Subcutaneous Tissue and Fascia
Head and Neck ØJPS
Lower Extremity ØJPW
Trunk ØJPT
Upper Extremity ØJPV
Tarsal
Left ØQPM
Right ØQPL
Tendon
Lower ØLPY
Upper ØLPX
Testis ØVPD
Thymus Ø7PM
Thyroid Gland ØGPK
Tibia
Left ØQPH
Right ØQPG
Toe Nail ØHPRX
Trachea ØBP1
Tracheobronchial Tree ØBP0
Tympanic Membrane
Left Ø9P8
Right Ø9P7
Ulna
Left ØPPL
Right ØPPK
Ureter ØTP9
Urethra ØTPD
Uterus and Cervix ØUPD
Vagina and Cul-de-sac ØUPH
Vas Deferens ØVPR
Vein
Lower Ø6PY
Upper Ø5PY
Vertebra
Cervical ØPP3
Lumbar ØQP0
Thoracic ØPP4
Vulva ØUPM
Renal calyx
use Kidney
use Kidney, Left
use Kidney, Right

Renal calyx—*continued*
  use Kidneys, Bilateral
Renal capsule
  use Kidney
  use Kidney, Left
  use Kidney, Right
  use Kidneys, Bilateral
Renal cortex
  use Kidney
  use Kidney, Left
  use Kidney, Right
  use Kidneys, Bilateral
Renal dialysis *see* Performance, Urinary 5A1D
Renal plexus *use* Nerve, Abdominal Sympathetic
Renal segment
  use Kidney
  use Kidney, Left
  use Kidney, Right
  use Kidneys, Bilateral
Renal segmental artery
  use Artery, Renal, Left
  use Artery, Renal, Right
Reopening, operative site
  Control of bleeding *see* Control postprocedural
    bleeding in
  Inspection only *see* Inspection
Repair
  Abdominal Wall ØWQF
  Acetabulum
    Left ØQQ5
    Right ØQQ4
  Adenoids ØCQQ
  Ampulla of Vater ØFQC
  Anal Sphincter ØDQR
  Ankle Region
    Left ØYQL
    Right ØYQK
  Anterior Chamber
    Left Ø8Q33ZZ
    Right Ø8Q23ZZ
  Anus ØDQQ
  Aorta
    Abdominal Ø4QØ
    Thoracic Ø2QW
  Aortic Body ØGQD
  Appendix ØDQJ
  Arm
    Lower
      Left ØXQF
      Right ØXQD
    Upper
      Left ØXQ9
      Right ØXQ8
  Artery
    Anterior Tibial
      Left Ø4QQ
      Right Ø4QP
    Axillary
      Left Ø3Q6
      Right Ø3Q5
    Brachial
      Left Ø3Q8
      Right Ø3Q7
    Celiac Ø4Q1
    Colic
      Left Ø4Q7
      Middle Ø4Q8
      Right Ø4Q6
    Common Carotid
      Left Ø3QJ
      Right Ø3QH
    Common Iliac
      Left Ø4QD
      Right Ø4QC
    Coronary
      Four or More Sites Ø2Q3
      One Site Ø2QØ
      Three Sites Ø2Q2
      Two Sites Ø2Q1
    External Carotid
      Left Ø3QN
      Right Ø3QM

Repair—*continued*
  Artery—*continued*
    External Iliac
      Left Ø4QJ
      Right Ø4QH
    Face Ø3QR
    Femoral
      Left Ø4QL
      Right Ø4QK
    Foot
      Left Ø4QW
      Right Ø4QV
    Gastric Ø4Q2
    Hand
      Left Ø3QF
      Right Ø3QD
    Hepatic Ø4Q3
    Inferior Mesenteric Ø4QB
    Innominate Ø3Q2
    Internal Carotid
      Left Ø3QL
      Right Ø3QK
    Internal Iliac
      Left Ø4QF
      Right Ø4QE
    Internal Mammary
      Left Ø3Q1
      Right Ø3QØ
    Intracranial Ø3QG
    Lower Ø4QY
    Peroneal
      Left Ø4QU
      Right Ø4QT
    Popliteal
      Left Ø4QN
      Right Ø4QM
    Posterior Tibial
      Left Ø4QS
      Right Ø4QR
    Pulmonary
      Left Ø2QR
      Right Ø2QQ
    Pulmonary Trunk Ø2QP
    Radial
      Left Ø3QC
      Right Ø3QB
    Renal
      Left Ø4QA
      Right Ø4Q9
    Splenic Ø4Q4
    Subclavian
      Left Ø3Q4
      Right Ø3Q3
    Superior Mesenteric Ø4Q5
    Temporal
      Left Ø3QT
      Right Ø3QS
    Thyroid
      Left Ø3QV
      Right Ø3QU
    Ulnar
      Left Ø3QA
      Right Ø3Q9
    Upper Ø3QY
    Vertebral
      Left Ø3QQ
      Right Ø3QP
  Atrium
    Left Ø2Q7
    Right Ø2Q6
  Auditory Ossicle
    Left Ø9QAØZZ
    Right Ø9Q9ØZZ
  Axilla
    Left ØXQ5
    Right ØXQ4
  Back
    Lower ØWQL
    Upper ØWQK
  Basal Ganglia ØØQ8
  Bladder ØTQB
  Bladder Neck ØTQC

Repair—*continued*
  Bone
    Ethmoid
      Left ØNQG
      Right ØNQF
    Frontal
      Left ØNQ2
      Right ØNQ1
    Hyoid ØNQX
    Lacrimal
      Left ØNQJ
      Right ØNQH
    Nasal ØNQB
    Occipital
      Left ØNQ8
      Right ØNQ7
    Palatine
      Left ØNQL
      Right ØNQK
    Parietal
      Left ØNQ4
      Right ØNQ3
    Pelvic
      Left ØQQ3
      Right ØQQ2
    Sphenoid
      Left ØNQD
      Right ØNQC
    Temporal
      Left ØNQ6
      Right ØNQ5
    Zygomatic
      Left ØNQN
      Right ØNQM
  Brain ØØQØ
  Breast
    Bilateral ØHQV
    Left ØHQU
    Right ØHQT
    Supernumerary ØHQY
  Bronchus
    Lingula ØBQ9
    Lower Lobe
      Left ØBQB
      Right ØBQ6
    Main
      Left ØBQ7
      Right ØBQ3
    Middle Lobe, Right ØBQ5
    Upper Lobe
      Left ØBQ8
      Right ØBQ4
  Buccal Mucosa ØCQ4
  Bursa and Ligament
    Abdomen
      Left ØMQJ
      Right ØMQH
    Ankle
      Left ØMQR
      Right ØMQQ
    Elbow
      Left ØMQ4
      Right ØMQ3
    Foot
      Left ØMQT
      Right ØMQS
    Hand
      Left ØMQ8
      Right ØMQ7
    Head and Neck ØMQØ
    Hip
      Left ØMQM
      Right ØMQL
    Knee
      Left ØMQP
      Right ØMQN
    Lower Extremity
      Left ØMQW
      Right ØMQV
    Perineum ØMQK
    Shoulder
      Left ØMQ2
      Right ØMQ1

Repair—continued
Bursa and Ligament—continued
Thorax
Left 0MQG
Right 0MQF
Trunk
Left 0MQD
Right 0MQC
Upper Extremity
Left 0MQB
Right 0MQ9
Wrist
Left 0MQ6
Right 0MQ5
Buttock
Left 0YQ1
Right 0YQ0
Carina 0BQ2
Carotid Bodies, Bilateral 0GQ8
Carotid Body
Left 0GQ6
Right 0GQ7
Carpal
Left 0PQN
Right 0PQM
Cecum 0DQH
Cerebellum 00QC
Cerebral Hemisphere 00Q7
Cerebral Meninges 00Q1
Cerebral Ventricle 00Q6
Cervix 0UQC
Chest Wall 0WQ8
Chordae Tendineae 02Q9
Choroid
Left 08QB
Right 08QA
Cisterna Chyli 07QL
Clavicle
Left 0PQB
Right 0PQ9
Clitoris 0UQJ
Coccygeal Glomus 0GQB
Coccyx 0QQS
Colon
Ascending 0DQK
Descending 0DQM
Sigmoid 0DQN
Transverse 0DQL
Conduction Mechanism 02Q8
Conjunctiva
Left 08QTXZZ
Right 08QSXZZ
Cord
Bilateral 0VQH
Left 0VQG
Right 0VQF
Cornea
Left 08Q9XZZ
Right 08Q8XZZ
Cul-de-sac 0UQF
Diaphragm
Left 0BQS
Right 0BQR
Disc
Cervical Vertebral 0RQ3
Cervicothoracic Vertebral 0RQ5
Lumbar Vertebral 0SQ2
Lumbosacral 0SQ4
Thoracic Vertebral 0RQ9
Thoracolumbar Vertebral 0RQB
Duct
Common Bile 0FQ9
Cystic 0FQ8
Hepatic
Left 0FQ6
Right 0FQ5
Lacrimal
Left 08QY
Right 08QX
Pancreatic 0FQD
Accessory 0FQF

Repair—continued
Duct—continued
Parotid
Left 0CQC
Right 0CQB
Duodenum 0DQ9
Dura Mater 00Q2
Ear
External
Bilateral 09Q2
Left 09Q1
Right 09Q0
External Auditory Canal
Left 09Q4
Right 09Q3
Inner
Left 09QE0ZZ
Right 09QD0ZZ
Middle
Left 09Q60ZZ
Right 09Q50ZZ
Elbow Region
Left 0XQC
Right 0XQB
Epididymis
Bilateral 0VQL
Left 0VQK
Right 0VQJ
Epiglottis 0CQR
Esophagogastric Junction 0DQ4
Esophagus 0DQ5
Lower 0DQ3
Middle 0DQ2
Upper 0DQ1
Eustachian Tube
Left 09QG
Right 09QF
Extremity
Lower
Left 0YQB
Right 0YQ9
Upper
Left 0XQ7
Right 0XQ6
Eye
Left 08Q1XZZ
Right 08Q0XZZ
Eyelid
Lower
Left 08QR
Right 08QQ
Upper
Left 08QP
Right 08QN
Face 0WQ2
Fallopian Tube
Left 0UQ6
Right 0UQ5
Fallopian Tubes, Bilateral 0UQ7
Femoral Region
Bilateral 0YQE
Left 0YQ8
Right 0YQ7
Femoral Shaft
Left 0QQ9
Right 0QQ8
Femur
Lower
Left 0QQC
Right 0QQB
Upper
Left 0QQ7
Right 0QQ6
Fibula
Left 0QQK
Right 0QQJ
Finger
Index
Left 0XQP
Right 0XQN
Little
Left 0XQW
Right 0XQV

Repair—continued
Finger—continued
Middle
Left 0XQR
Right 0XQQ
Ring
Left 0XQT
Right 0XQS
Finger Nail 0HQQXZZ
Foot
Left 0YQN
Right 0YQM
Gallbladder 0FQ4
Gingiva
Lower 0CQ6
Upper 0CQ5
Gland
Adrenal
Bilateral 0GQ4
Left 0GQ2
Right 0GQ3
Lacrimal
Left 08QW
Right 08QV
Minor Salivary 0CQJ
Parotid
Left 0CQ9
Right 0CQ8
Pituitary 0GQ0
Sublingual
Left 0CQF
Right 0CQD
Submaxillary
Left 0CQH
Right 0CQG
Vestibular 0UQL
Glenoid Cavity
Left 0PQ8
Right 0PQ7
Glomus Jugulare 0GQC
Hand
Left 0XQK
Right 0XQJ
Head 0WQ0
Heart 02QA
Left 02QC
Right 02QB
Humeral Head
Left 0PQD
Right 0PQC
Humeral Shaft
Left 0PQG
Right 0PQF
Hymen 0UQK
Hypothalamus 00QA
Ileocecal Valve 0DQC
Ileum 0DQB
Inguinal Region
Bilateral 0YQA
Left 0YQ6
Right 0YQ5
Intestine
Large 0DQE
Left 0DQG
Right 0DQF
Small 0DQ8
Iris
Left 08QD3ZZ
Right 08QC3ZZ
Jaw
Lower 0WQ5
Upper 0WQ4
Jejunum 0DQA
Joint
Acromioclavicular
Left 0RQH
Right 0RQG
Ankle
Left 0SQG
Right 0SQF
Carpal
Left 0RQR
Right 0RQQ

Repair—*continued*
  Joint—*continued*
    Cervical Vertebral ØRQ1
    Cervicothoracic Vertebral ØRQ4
    Coccygeal ØSQ6
    Elbow
      Left ØRQM
      Right ØRQL
    Finger Phalangeal
      Left ØRQX
      Right ØRQW
    Hip
      Left ØSQB
      Right ØSQ9
    Knee
      Left ØSQD
      Right ØSQC
    Lumbar Vertebral ØSQØ
    Lumbosacral ØSQ3
    Metacarpocarpal
      Left ØRQT
      Right ØRQS
    Metacarpophalangeal
      Left ØRQV
      Right ØRQU
    Metatarsal-Phalangeal
      Left ØSQN
      Right ØSQM
    Metatarsal-Tarsal
      Left ØSQL
      Right ØSQK
    Occipital-cervical ØRQØ
    Sacrococcygeal ØSQ5
    Sacroiliac
      Left ØSQ8
      Right ØSQ7
    Shoulder
      Left ØRQK
      Right ØRQJ
    Sternoclavicular
      Left ØRQF
      Right ØRQE
    Tarsal
      Left ØSQJ
      Right ØSQH
    Temporomandibular
      Left ØRQD
      Right ØRQC
    Thoracic Vertebral ØRQ6
    Thoracolumbar Vertebral ØRQA
    Toe Phalangeal
      Left ØSQQ
      Right ØSQP
    Wrist
      Left ØRQP
      Right ØRQN
  Kidney
    Left ØTQ1
    Right ØTQØ
  Kidney Pelvis
    Left ØTQ4
    Right ØTQ3
  Knee Region
    Left ØYQG
    Right ØYQF
  Larynx ØCQS
  Leg
    Lower
      Left ØYQJ
      Right ØYQH
    Upper
      Left ØYQD
      Right ØYQC
  Lens
    Left Ø8QK3ZZ
    Right Ø8QJ3ZZ
  Lip
    Lower ØCQ1
    Upper ØCQØ
  Liver ØFQØ
    Left Lobe ØFQ2
    Right Lobe ØFQ1

Repair—*continued*
  Lung
    Bilateral ØBQM
    Left ØBQL
    Lower Lobe
      Left ØBQJ
      Right ØBQF
    Middle Lobe, Right ØBQD
    Right ØBQK
    Upper Lobe
      Left ØBQG
      Right ØBQC
  Lung Lingula ØBQH
  Lymphatic
    Aortic Ø7QD
    Axillary
      Left Ø7Q6
      Right Ø7Q5
    Head Ø7QØ
    Inguinal
      Left Ø7QJ
      Right Ø7QH
    Internal Mammary
      Left Ø7Q9
      Right Ø7Q8
    Lower Extremity
      Left Ø7QG
      Right Ø7QF
    Mesenteric Ø7QB
    Neck
      Left Ø7Q2
      Right Ø7Q1
    Pelvis Ø7QC
    Thoracic Duct Ø7QK
    Thorax Ø7Q7
    Upper Extremity
      Left Ø7Q4
      Right Ø7Q3
  Mandible
    Left ØNQV
    Right ØNQT
  Maxilla
    Left ØNQS
    Right ØNQR
  Mediastinum ØWQC
  Medulla Oblongata ØØQD
  Mesentery ØDQV
  Metacarpal
    Left ØPQQ
    Right ØPQP
  Metatarsal
    Left ØQQP
    Right ØQQN
  Muscle
    Abdomen
      Left ØKQL
      Right ØKQK
    Extraocular
      Left Ø8QM
      Right Ø8QL
    Facial ØKQ1
    Foot
      Left ØKQW
      Right ØKQV
    Hand
      Left ØKQD
      Right ØKQC
    Head ØKQØ
    Hip
      Left ØKQP
      Right ØKQN
    Lower Arm and Wrist
      Left ØKQB
      Right ØKQ9
    Lower Leg
      Left ØKQT
      Right ØKQS
    Neck
      Left ØKQ3
      Right ØKQ2
    Papillary Ø2QD
    Perineum ØKQM

Repair—*continued*
  Muscle—*continued*
    Shoulder
      Left ØKQ6
      Right ØKQ5
    Thorax
      Left ØKQJ
      Right ØKQH
    Tongue, Palate, Pharynx ØKQ4
    Trunk
      Left ØKQG
      Right ØKQF
    Upper Arm
      Left ØKQ8
      Right ØKQ7
    Upper Leg
      Left ØKQR
      Right ØKQQ
  Nasopharynx Ø9QN
  Neck ØWQ6
  Nerve
    Abdominal Sympathetic Ø1QM
    Abducens ØØQL
    Accessory ØØQR
    Acoustic ØØQN
    Brachial Plexus Ø1Q3
    Cervical Ø1Q1
    Cervical Plexus Ø1QØ
    Facial ØØQM
    Femoral Ø1QD
    Glossopharyngeal ØØQP
    Head and Neck Sympathetic Ø1QK
    Hypoglossal ØØQS
    Lumbar Ø1QB
    Lumbar Plexus Ø1Q9
    Lumbar Sympathetic Ø1QN
    Lumbosacral Plexus Ø1QA
    Median Ø1Q5
    Oculomotor ØØQH
    Olfactory ØØQF
    Optic ØØQG
    Peroneal Ø1QH
    Phrenic Ø1Q2
    Pudendal Ø1QC
    Radial Ø1Q6
    Sacral Ø1QR
    Sacral Plexus Ø1QQ
    Sacral Sympathetic Ø1QP
    Sciatic Ø1QF
    Thoracic Ø1Q8
    Thoracic Sympathetic Ø1QL
    Tibial Ø1QG
    Trigeminal ØØQK
    Trochlear ØØQJ
    Ulnar Ø1Q4
    Vagus ØØQQ
  Nipple
    Left ØHQX
    Right ØHQW
  Nose Ø9QK
  Omentum
    Greater ØDQS
    Lesser ØDQT
  Orbit
    Left ØNQQ
    Right ØNQP
  Ovary
    Bilateral ØUQ2
    Left ØUQ1
    Right ØUQØ
  Palate
    Hard ØCQ2
    Soft ØCQ3
  Pancreas ØFQG
  Para-aortic Body ØGQ9
  Paraganglion Extremity ØGQF
  Parathyroid Gland ØGQR
    Inferior
      Left ØGQP
      Right ØGQN
    Multiple ØGQQ

Index

Repair—Repair

Replacement

Replacement—*continued*
- Bone—*continued*
  - Parietal
    - Left ØNR4
    - Right ØNR3
  - Pelvic
    - Left ØQR3
    - Right ØQR2
  - Sphenoid
    - Left ØNRD
    - Right ØNRC
  - Temporal
    - Left ØNR6
    - Right ØNR5
  - Zygomatic
    - Left ØNRN
    - Right ØNRM
- Breast
  - Bilateral ØHRV
  - Left ØHRU
  - Right ØHRT
- Buccal Mucosa ØCR4
- Carpal
  - Left ØPRN
  - Right ØPRM
- Chordae Tendineae Ø2R9
- Choroid
  - Left Ø8RB
  - Right Ø8RA
- Clavicle
  - Left ØPRB
  - Right ØPR9
- Coccyx ØQRS
- Conjunctiva
  - Left Ø8RTX
  - Right Ø8RSX
- Cornea
  - Left Ø8R9
  - Right Ø8R8
- Disc
  - Cervical Vertebral ØRR3Ø
  - Cervicothoracic Vertebral ØRR5Ø
  - Lumbar Vertebral ØSR2Ø
  - Lumbosacral ØSR4Ø
  - Thoracic Vertebral ØRR9Ø
  - Thoracolumbar Vertebral ØRRBØ
- Duct
  - Common Bile ØFR9
  - Cystic ØFR8
  - Hepatic
    - Left ØFR6
    - Right ØFR5
  - Lacrimal
    - Left Ø8RY
    - Right Ø8RX
  - Pancreatic ØFRD
    - Accessory ØFRF
  - Parotid
    - Left ØCRC
    - Right ØCRB
- Ear
  - External
    - Bilateral Ø9R2
    - Left Ø9R1
    - Right Ø9RØ
  - Inner
    - Left Ø9REØ
    - Right Ø9RDØ
  - Middle
    - Left Ø9R6Ø
    - Right Ø9R5Ø
- Epiglottis ØCRR
- Esophagus ØDR5
- Eye
  - Left Ø8R1
  - Right Ø8RØ
- Eyelid
  - Lower
    - Left Ø8RR
    - Right Ø8RQ
  - Upper
    - Left Ø8RP
    - Right Ø8RN

Replacement—*continued*
- Femoral Shaft
  - Left ØQR9
  - Right ØQR8
- Femur
  - Lower
    - Left ØQRC
    - Right ØQRB
  - Upper
    - Left ØQR7
    - Right ØQR6
- Fibula
  - Left ØQRK
  - Right ØQRJ
- Finger Nail ØHRQX
- Gingiva
  - Lower ØCR6
  - Upper ØCR5
- Glenoid Cavity
  - Left ØPR8
  - Right ØPR7
- Hair ØHRSX
- Humeral Head
  - Left ØPRD
  - Right ØPRC
- Humeral Shaft
  - Left ØPRG
  - Right ØPRF
- Iris
  - Left Ø8RD3
  - Right Ø8RC3
- Joint
  - Acromioclavicular
    - Left ØRRHØ
    - Right ØRRGØ
  - Ankle
    - Left ØSRGØ
    - Right ØSRFØ
  - Carpal
    - Left ØRRRØ
    - Right ØRRQØ
  - Cervical Vertebral ØRR1
  - Cervicothoracic Vertebral ØRR4
  - Coccygeal ØSR6Ø
  - Elbow
    - Left ØRRMØ
    - Right ØRRLØ
  - Finger Phalangeal
    - Left ØRRXØ
    - Right ØRRWØ
  - Hip
    - Left ØSRB
      - Acetabular Surface ØSRE
      - Femoral Surface ØSRS
    - Right ØSR9
      - Acetabular Surface ØSRA
      - Femoral Surface ØSRR
  - Knee
    - Left ØSRDØ
      - Femoral Surface ØSRUØ
      - Tibial Surface ØSRWØ
    - Right ØSRCØ
      - Femoral Surface ØSRTØ
      - Tibial Surface ØSRVØ
  - Lumbar Vertebral ØSRØ
  - Lumbosacral ØSR3
  - Metacarpocarpal
    - Left ØRRTØ
    - Right ØRRSØ
  - Metacarpophalangeal
    - Left ØRRVØ
    - Right ØRRUØ
  - Metatarsal-Phalangeal
    - Left ØSRNØ
    - Right ØSRMØ
  - Metatarsal-Tarsal
    - Left ØSRLØ
    - Right ØSRKØ
  - Occipital-cervical ØRRØ
  - Sacrococcygeal ØSR5Ø
  - Sacroiliac
    - Left ØSR8Ø
    - Right ØSR7Ø

Replacement—*continued*
- Joint—*continued*
  - Shoulder
    - Left ØRRK
    - Right ØRRJ
  - Replacement Joint
    - Shoulder
      - Left ØRRK
      - Right ØRRJ
    - Shoulder
      - Partial *see* Replacement, Upper Joints ØRR Joint
      - Reverse total *see* Replacement, Upper Joints ØRR
  - Sternoclavicular
    - Left ØRRFØ
    - Right ØRREØ
  - Tarsal
    - Left ØSRJØ
    - Right ØSRHØ
  - Temporomandibular
    - Left ØRRDØ
    - Right ØRRCØ
  - Thoracic Vertebral ØRR6
  - Thoracolumbar Vertebral ØRRA
  - Toe Phalangeal
    - Left ØSRQØ
    - Right ØSRPØ
  - Wrist
    - Left ØRRPØ
    - Right ØRRNØ
- Kidney Pelvis
  - Left ØTR4
  - Right ØTR3
- Larynx ØCRS
- Lens
  - Left Ø8RK
  - Right Ø8RJ
- Lip
  - Lower ØCR1
  - Upper ØCRØ
- Mandible
  - Left ØNRV
  - Right ØNRT
- Maxilla
  - Left ØNRS
  - Right ØNRR
- Mesentery ØDRV
- Metacarpal
  - Left ØPRQ
  - Right ØPRP
- Metatarsal
  - Left ØQRP
  - Right ØQRN
- Muscle, Papillary Ø2RD
- Nasopharynx Ø9RN
- Nipple
  - Left ØHRX
  - Right ØHRW
- Nose Ø9RK
- Omentum
  - Greater ØDRS
  - Lesser ØDRT
- Orbit
  - Left ØNRQ
  - Right ØNRP
- Palate
  - Hard ØCR2
  - Soft ØCR3
- Patella
  - Left ØQRF
  - Right ØQRD
- Pericardium Ø2RN
- Peritoneum ØDRW
- Phalanx
  - Finger
    - Left ØPRV
    - Right ØPRT
  - Thumb
    - Left ØPRS
    - Right ØPRR

Replacement—*continued*
  Phalanx—*continued*
    Toe
      Left ØQRR
      Right ØQRQ
  Pharynx ØCRM
  Radius
    Left ØPRJ
    Right ØPRH
  Retinal Vessel
    Left 08RH3
    Right 08RG3
  Rib
    Left ØPR2
    Right ØPR1
  Sacrum ØQR1
  Scapula
    Left ØPR6
    Right ØPR5
  Sclera
    Left 08R7X
    Right 08R6X
  Septum
    Atrial 02R5
    Nasal 09RM
    Ventricular 02RM
  Skin
    Abdomen ØHR7
    Back ØHR6
    Buttock ØHR8
    Chest ØHR5
    Ear
      Left ØHR3
      Right ØHR2
    Face ØHR1
    Foot
      Left ØHRN
      Right ØHRM
    Genitalia ØHRA
    Hand
      Left ØHRG
      Right ØHRF
    Lower Arm
      Left ØHRE
      Right ØHRD
    Lower Leg
      Left ØHRL
      Right ØHRK
    Neck ØHR4
    Perineum ØHR9
    Scalp ØHRØ
    Upper Arm
      Left ØHRC
      Right ØHRB
    Upper Leg
      Left ØHRJ
      Right ØHRH
  Skull ØNRØ
  Sternum ØPRØ
  Subcutaneous Tissue and Fascia
    Abdomen ØJR8
    Back ØJR7
    Buttock ØJR9
    Chest ØJR6
    Face ØJR1
    Foot
      Left ØJRR
      Right ØJRQ
    Hand
      Left ØJRK
      Right ØJRJ
    Lower Arm
      Left ØJRH
      Right ØJRG
    Lower Leg
      Left ØJRP
      Right ØJRN
    Neck
      Anterior ØJR4
      Posterior ØJR5
    Pelvic Region ØJRC
    Perineum ØJRB
    Scalp ØJRØ

Replacement—*continued*
  Subcutaneous Tissue and Fascia—*continued*
    Upper Arm
      Left ØJRF
      Right ØJRD
    Upper Leg
      Left ØJRM
      Right ØJRL
  Tarsal
    Left ØQRM
    Right ØQRL
  Tendon
    Abdomen
      Left ØLRG
      Right ØLRF
    Ankle
      Left ØLRT
      Right ØLRS
    Foot
      Left ØLRW
      Right ØLRV
    Hand
      Left ØLR8
      Right ØLR7
    Head and Neck ØLRØ
    Hip
      Left ØLRK
      Right ØLRJ
    Knee
      Left ØLRR
      Right ØLRQ
    Lower Arm and Wrist
      Left ØLR6
      Right ØLR5
    Lower Leg
      Left ØLRP
      Right ØLRN
    Perineum ØLRH
    Shoulder
      Left ØLR2
      Right ØLR1
    Thorax
      Left ØLRD
      Right ØLRC
    Trunk
      Left ØLRB
      Right ØLR9
    Upper Arm
      Left ØLR4
      Right ØLR3
    Upper Leg
      Left ØLRM
      Right ØLRL
  Testis
    Bilateral ØVRCØJZ
    Left ØVRBØJZ
    Right ØVR9ØJZ
  Thumb
    Left ØXRM
    Right ØXRL
  Tibia
    Left ØQRH
    Right ØQRG
  Toe Nail ØHRRX
  Tongue ØCR7
  Tooth
    Lower ØCRX
    Upper ØCRW
  Turbinate, Nasal 09RL
  Tympanic Membrane
    Left 09R8
    Right 09R7
  Ulna
    Left ØPRL
    Right ØPRK
  Ureter
    Left ØTR7
    Right ØTR6
  Urethra ØTRD
  Uvula ØCRN
  Valve
    Aortic 02RF
    Mitral 02RG

Replacement—*continued*
  Valve—*continued*
    Pulmonary 02RH
    Tricuspid 02RJ
  Vein
    Axillary
      Left 05R8
      Right 05R7
    Azygos 05RØ
    Basilic
      Left 05RC
      Right 05RB
    Brachial
      Left 05RA
      Right 05R9
    Cephalic
      Left 05RF
      Right 05RD
    Colic 06R7
    Common Iliac
      Left 06RD
      Right 06RC
    Esophageal 06R3
    External Iliac
      Left 06RG
      Right 06RF
    External Jugular
      Left 05RQ
      Right 05RP
    Face
      Left 05RV
      Right 05RT
    Femoral
      Left 06RN
      Right 06RM
    Foot
      Left 06RV
      Right 06RT
    Gastric 06R2
    Greater Saphenous
      Left 06RQ
      Right 06RP
    Hand
      Left 05RH
      Right 05RG
    Hemiazygos 05R1
    Hepatic 06R4
    Hypogastric
      Left 06RJ
      Right 06RH
    Inferior Mesenteric 06R6
    Innominate
      Left 05R4
      Right 05R3
    Internal Jugular
      Left 05RN
      Right 05RM
    Intracranial 05RL
    Lesser Saphenous
      Left 06RS
      Right 06RR
    Lower 06RY
    Portal 06R8
    Pulmonary
      Left 02RT
      Right 02RS
    Renal
      Left 06RB
      Right 06R9
    Splenic 06R1
    Subclavian
      Left 05R6
      Right 05R5
    Superior Mesenteric 06R5
    Upper 05RY
    Vertebral
      Left 05RS
      Right 05RR
  Vena Cava
    Inferior 06RØ
    Superior 02RV

Replacement—*continued*
  Ventricle
    Left 02RL
    Right 02RK
  Vertebra
    Cervical 0PR3
    Lumbar 0QR0
    Thoracic 0PR4
  Vitreous
    Left 08R53
    Right 08R43
  Vocal Cord
    Left 0CRV
    Right 0CRT
Replantation *see* Reposition
Replantation, scalp *see* Reattachment, Skin, Scalp
    0HM0
Reposition
  Acetabulum
    Left 0QS5
    Right 0QS4
  Ampulla of Vater 0FSC
  Anus 0DSQ
  Aorta
    Abdominal 04S0
    Thoracic 02SW0ZZ
  Artery
  Anterior Tibial
    Left 04SQ
    Right 04SP
  Axillary
    Left 03S6
    Right 03S5
  Brachial
    Left 03S8
    Right 03S7
  Celiac 04S1
  Colic
    Left 04S7
    Middle 04S8
    Right 04S6
  Common Carotid
    Left 03SJ
    Right 03SH
  Common Iliac
    Left 04SD
    Right 04SC
  External Carotid
    Left 03SN
    Right 03SM
  External Iliac
    Left 04SJ
    Right 04SH
  Face 03SR
  Femoral
    Left 04SL
    Right 04SK
  Foot
    Left 04SW
    Right 04SV
  Gastric 04S2
  Hand
    Left 03SF
    Right 03SD
  Hepatic 04S3
  Inferior Mesenteric 04SB
  Innominate 03S2
  Internal Carotid
    Left 03SL
    Right 03SK
  Internal Iliac
    Left 04SF
    Right 04SE
  Internal Mammary
    Left 03S1
    Right 03S0
  Intracranial 03SG
  Lower 04SY
  Peroneal
    Left 04SU
    Right 04ST

Reposition—*continued*
  Anterior Tibial—*continued*
    Popliteal
      Left 04SN
      Right 04SM
    Posterior Tibial
      Left 04SS
      Right 04SR
    Pulmonary
      Left 02SR0ZZ
      Right 02SQ0ZZ
    Pulmonary Trunk 02SP0ZZ
    Radial
      Left 03SC
      Right 03SB
    Renal
      Left 04SA
      Right 04S9
    Splenic 04S4
    Subclavian
      Left 03S4
      Right 03S3
    Superior Mesenteric 04S5
    Temporal
      Left 03ST
      Right 03SS
    Thyroid
      Left 03SV
      Right 03SU
    Ulnar
      Left 03SA
      Right 03S9
    Upper 03SY
    Vertebral
      Left 03SQ
      Right 03SP
  Auditory Ossicle
    Left 09SA
    Right 09S9
  Bladder 0TSB
  Bladder Neck 0TSC
  Bone
    Ethmoid
      Left 0NSG
      Right 0NSF
    Frontal
      Left 0NS2
      Right 0NS1
    Hyoid 0NSX
    Lacrimal
      Left 0NSJ
      Right 0NSH
    Nasal 0NSB
    Occipital
      Left 0NS8
      Right 0NS7
    Palatine
      Left 0NSL
      Right 0NSK
    Parietal
      Left 0NS4
      Right 0NS3
    Pelvic
      Left 0QS3
      Right 0QS2
    Sphenoid
      Left 0NSD
      Right 0NSC
    Temporal
      Left 0NS6
      Right 0NS5
    Zygomatic
      Left 0NSN
      Right 0NSM
  Breast
    Bilateral 0HSV0ZZ
    Left 0HSU0ZZ
    Right 0HST0ZZ
  Bronchus
    Lingula 0BS90ZZ
    Lower Lobe
      Left 0BSB0ZZ
      Right 0BS60ZZ

Reposition—*continued*
  Bronchus—*continued*
    Main
      Left 0BS70ZZ
      Right 0BS30ZZ
    Middle Lobe, Right 0BS50ZZ
    Upper Lobe
      Left 0BS80ZZ
      Right 0BS40ZZ
  Bursa and Ligament
    Abdomen
      Left 0MSJ
      Right 0MSH
    Ankle
      Left 0MSR
      Right 0MSQ
    Elbow
      Left 0MS4
      Right 0MS3
    Foot
      Left 0MST
      Right 0MSS
    Hand
      Left 0MS8
      Right 0MS7
    Head and Neck 0MS0
    Hip
      Left 0MSM
      Right 0MSL
    Knee
      Left 0MSP
      Right 0MSN
    Lower Extremity
      Left 0MSW
      Right 0MSV
    Perineum 0MSK
    Shoulder
      Left 0MS2
      Right 0MS1
    Thorax
      Left 0MSG
      Right 0MSF
    Trunk
      Left 0MSD
      Right 0MSC
    Upper Extremity
      Left 0MSB
      Right 0MS9
    Wrist
      Left 0MS6
      Right 0MS5
  Carina 0BS20ZZ
  Carpal
    Left 0PSN
    Right 0PSM
  Cecum 0DSH
  Cervix 0USC
  Clavicle
    Left 0PSB
    Right 0PS9
  Coccyx 0QSS
  Colon
    Ascending 0DSK
    Descending 0DSM
    Sigmoid 0DSN
    Transverse 0DSL
  Cord
    Bilateral 0VSH
    Left 0VSG
    Right 0VSF
  Cul-de-sac 0USF
  Diaphragm
    Left 0BSS0ZZ
    Right 0BSR0ZZ
  Duct
    Common Bile 0FS9
    Cystic 0FS8
    Hepatic
      Left 0FS6
      Right 0FS5
    Lacrimal
      Left 08SY
      Right 08SX

Resection—*continued*
Bone—*continued*
Hyoid 0NTX0ZZ
Lacrimal
Left 0NTJ0ZZ
Right 0NTH0ZZ
Nasal 0NTB0ZZ
Occipital
Left 0NT80ZZ
Right 0NT70ZZ
Palatine
Left 0NTL0ZZ
Right 0NTK0ZZ
Parietal
Left 0NT40ZZ
Right 0NT30ZZ
Pelvic
Left 0QT30ZZ
Right 0QT20ZZ
Sphenoid
Left 0NTD0ZZ
Right 0NTC0ZZ
Temporal
Left 0NT60ZZ
Right 0NT50ZZ
Zygomatic
Left 0NTN0ZZ
Right 0NTM0ZZ
Breast
Bilateral 0HTV0ZZ
Left 0HTU0ZZ
Right 0HTT0ZZ
Supernumerary 0HTY0ZZ
Bronchus
Lingula 0BT9
Lower Lobe
Left 0BTB
Right 0BT6
Main
Left 0BT7
Right 0BT3
Middle Lobe, Right 0BT5
Upper Lobe
Left 0BT8
Right 0BT4
Bursa and Ligament
Abdomen
Left 0MTJ
Right 0MTH
Ankle
Left 0MTR
Right 0MTQ
Elbow
Left 0MT4
Right 0MT3
Foot
Left 0MTT
Right 0MTS
Hand
Left 0MT8
Right 0MT7
Head and Neck 0MT0
Hip
Left 0MTM
Right 0MTL
Knee
Left 0MTP
Right 0MTN
Lower Extremity
Left 0MTW
Right 0MTV
Perineum 0MTK
Shoulder
Left 0MT2
Right 0MT1
Thorax
Left 0MTG
Right 0MTF
Trunk
Left 0MTD
Right 0MTC

Resection—*continued*
Bursa and Ligament—*continued*
Upper Extremity
Left 0MTB
Right 0MT9
Wrist
Left 0MT6
Right 0MT5
Carina 0BT2
Carotid Bodies, Bilateral 0GT8
Carotid Body
Left 0GT6
Right 0GT7
Carpal
Left 0PTN0ZZ
Right 0PTM0ZZ
Cecum 0DTH
Cerebral Hemisphere 00T7
Cervix 0UTC
Chordae Tendineae 02T9
Cisterna Chyli 07TL
Clavicle
Left 0PTB0ZZ
Right 0PT90ZZ
Clitoris 0UTJ
Coccygeal Glomus 0GTB
Coccyx 0QTS0ZZ
Colon
Ascending 0DTK
Descending 0DTM
Sigmoid 0DTN
Transverse 0DTL
Conduction Mechanism 02T8
Cord
Bilateral 0VTH
Left 0VTG
Right 0VTF
Cornea
Left 08T9XZZ
Right 08T8XZZ
Cul-de-sac 0UTF
Diaphragm
Left 0BTS
Right 0BTR
Disc
Cervical Vertebral 0RT30ZZ
Cervicothoracic Vertebral 0RT50ZZ
Lumbar Vertebral 0ST20ZZ
Lumbosacral 0ST40ZZ
Thoracic Vertebral 0RT90ZZ
Thoracolumbar Vertebral 0RTB0ZZ
Duct
Common Bile 0FT9
Cystic 0FT8
Hepatic
Left 0FT6
Right 0FT5
Lacrimal
Left 08TY
Right 08TX
Pancreatic 0FTD
Accessory 0FTF
Parotid
Left 0CTC0ZZ
Right 0CTB0ZZ
Duodenum 0DT9
Ear
External
Left 09T1
Right 09T0
Inner
Left 09TE0ZZ
Right 09TD0ZZ
Middle
Left 09T60ZZ
Right 09T50ZZ
Epididymis
Bilateral 0VTL
Left 0VTK
Right 0VTJ
Epiglottis 0CTR
Esophagogastric Junction 0DT4

Resection—*continued*
Esophagus 0DT5
Lower 0DT3
Middle 0DT2
Upper 0DT1
Eustachian Tube
Left 09TG
Right 09TF
Eye
Left 08T1XZZ
Right 08T0XZZ
Eyelid
Lower
Left 08TR
Right 08TQ
Upper
Left 08TP
Right 08TN
Fallopian Tube
Left 0UT6
Right 0UT5
Fallopian Tubes, Bilateral 0UT7
Femoral Shaft
Left 0QT90ZZ
Right 0QT80ZZ
Femur
Lower
Left 0QTC0ZZ
Right 0QTB0ZZ
Upper
Left 0QT70ZZ
Right 0QT60ZZ
Fibula
Left 0QTK0ZZ
Right 0QTJ0ZZ
Finger Nail 0HTQXZZ
Gallbladder 0FT4
Gland
Adrenal
Bilateral 0GT4
Left 0GT2
Right 0GT3
Lacrimal
Left 08TW
Right 08TV
Minor Salivary 0CTJ0ZZ
Parotid
Left 0CT90ZZ
Right 0CT80ZZ
Pituitary 0GT0
Sublingual
Left 0CTF0ZZ
Right 0CTD0ZZ
Submaxillary
Left 0CTH0ZZ
Right 0CTG0ZZ
Vestibular 0UTL
Glenoid Cavity
Left 0PT80ZZ
Right 0PT70ZZ
Glomus Jugulare 0GTC
Humeral Head
Left 0PTD0ZZ
Right 0PTC0ZZ
Humeral Shaft
Left 0PTG0ZZ
Right 0PTF0ZZ
Hymen 0UTK
Ileocecal Valve 0DTC
Ileum 0DTB
Intestine
Large 0DTE
Left 0DTG
Right 0DTF
Small 0DT8
Iris
Left 08TD3ZZ
Right 08TC3ZZ
Jejunum 0DTA
Joint
Acromioclavicular
Left 0RTH0ZZ
Right 0RTG0ZZ

Resection—*continued*
  Sinus—*continued*
    Maxillary
      Left Ø9TR
      Right Ø9TQ
    Sphenoid
      Left Ø9TX
      Right Ø9TW
  Spleen Ø7TP
  Sternum ØPTØØZZ
  Stomach ØDT6
    Pylorus ØDT7
  Tarsal
    Left ØQTMØZZ
    Right ØQTLØZZ
  Tendon
    Abdomen
      Left ØLTG
      Right ØLTF
    Ankle
      Left ØLTT
      Right ØLTS
    Foot
      Left ØLTW
      Right ØLTV
    Hand
      Left ØLT8
      Right ØLT7
    Head and Neck ØLTØ
    Hip
      Left ØLTK
      Right ØLTJ
    Knee
      Left ØLTR
      Right ØLTQ
    Lower Arm and Wrist
      Left ØLT6
      Right ØLT5
    Lower Leg
      Left ØLTP
      Right ØLTN
    Perineum ØLTH
    Shoulder
      Left ØLT2
      Right ØLT1
    Thorax
      Left ØLTD
      Right ØLTC
    Trunk
      Left ØLTB
      Right ØLT9
    Upper Arm
      Left ØLT4
      Right ØLT3
    Upper Leg
      Left ØLTM
      Right ØLTL
  Testis
    Bilateral ØVTC
    Left ØVTB
    Right ØVT9
  Thymus Ø7TM
  Thyroid Gland ØGTK
    Left Lobe ØGTG
    Right Lobe ØGTH
  Tibia
    Left ØQTHØZZ
    Right ØQTGØZZ
  Toe Nail ØHTRXZZ
  Tongue ØCT7
  Tonsils ØCTP
  Tooth
    Lower ØCTXØZ
    Upper ØCTWØZ
  Trachea ØBT1
  Tunica Vaginalis
    Left ØVT7
    Right ØVT6
  Turbinate, Nasal Ø9TL
  Tympanic Membrane
    Left Ø9T8
    Right Ø9T7

Resection—*continued*
  Ulna
    Left ØPTLØZZ
    Right ØPTKØZZ
  Ureter
    Left ØTT7
    Right ØTT6
  Urethra ØTTD
  Uterine Supporting Structure ØUT4
  Uterus ØUT9
  Uvula ØCTN
  Vagina ØUTG
  Valve, Pulmonary Ø2TH
  Vas Deferens
    Bilateral ØVTQ
    Left ØVTP
    Right ØVTN
  Vesicle
    Bilateral ØVT3
    Left ØVT2
    Right ØVT1
  Vitreous
    Left Ø8T53ZZ
    Right Ø8T43ZZ
  Vocal Cord
    Left ØCTV
    Right ØCTT
  Vulva ØUTM
Reservoir
  Insertion of device in
    Abdomen ØJH8
    Chest ØJH6
    Lower Arm
      Left ØJHH
      Right ØJHG
    Lower Leg
      Left ØJHP
      Right ØJHN
    Upper Arm
      Left ØJHF
      Right ØJHD
    Upper Leg
      Left ØJHM
      Right ØJHL
  Removal of device from
    Lower Extremity ØJPW
    Trunk ØJPT
    Upper Extremity ØJPV
  Revision of device in
    Lower Extremity ØJWW
    Trunk ØJWT
    Upper Extremity ØJWV
Restoration, Cardiac, Single, Rhythm 5A22Ø4Z
Restriction
  Ampulla of Vater ØFVC
  Anus ØDVQ
  Aorta
    Abdominal Ø4VØ
    Thoracic Ø2VW
  Artery
    Anterior Tibial
      Left Ø4VQ
      Right Ø4VP
    Axillary
      Left Ø3V6
      Right Ø3V5
    Brachial
      Left Ø3V8
      Right Ø3V7
    Celiac Ø4V1
    Colic
      Left Ø4V7
      Middle Ø4V8
      Right Ø4V6
    Common Carotid
      Left Ø3VJ
      Right Ø3VH
    Common Iliac
      Left Ø4VD
      Right Ø4VC
    External Carotid
      Left Ø3VN
      Right Ø3VM

Restriction—*continued*
  Artery—*continued*
    External Iliac
      Left Ø4VJ
      Right Ø4VH
    Face Ø3VR
    Femoral
      Left Ø4VL
      Right Ø4VK
    Foot
      Left Ø4VW
      Right Ø4VV
    Gastric Ø4V2
    Hand
      Left Ø3VF
      Right Ø3VD
    Hepatic Ø4V3
    Inferior Mesenteric Ø4VB
    Innominate Ø3V2
    Internal Carotid
      Left Ø3VL
      Right Ø3VK
    Internal Iliac
      Left Ø4VF
      Right Ø4VE
    Internal Mammary
      Left Ø3V1
      Right Ø3VØ
    Intracranial Ø3VG
    Lower Ø4VY
    Peroneal
      Left Ø4VU
      Right Ø4VT
    Popliteal
      Left Ø4VN
      Right Ø4VM
    Posterior Tibial
      Left Ø4VS
      Right Ø4VR
    Pulmonary
      Left Ø2VR
      Right Ø2VQ
    Pulmonary Trunk Ø2VP
    Radial
      Left Ø3VC
      Right Ø3VB
    Renal
      Left Ø4VA
      Right Ø4V9
    Splenic Ø4V4
    Subclavian
      Left Ø3V4
      Right Ø3V3
    Superior Mesenteric Ø4V5
    Temporal
      Left Ø3VT
      Right Ø3VS
    Thyroid
      Left Ø3VV
      Right Ø3VU
    Ulnar
      Left Ø3VA
      Right Ø3V9
    Upper Ø3VY
    Vertebral
      Left Ø3VQ
      Right Ø3VP
  Bladder ØTVB
  Bladder Neck ØTVC
  Bronchus
    Lingula ØBV9
    Lower Lobe
      Left ØBVB
      Right ØBV6
    Main
      Left ØBV7
      Right ØBV3
    Middle Lobe, Right ØBV5
    Upper Lobe
      Left ØBV8
      Right ØBV4
  Carina ØBV2
  Cecum ØDVH

Revision of device in—*continued*

Ear
- Inner
    - Left Ø9WE
    - Right Ø9WD
- Left Ø9WJ
- Right Ø9WH

Epididymis and Spermatic Cord ØVWM
Esophagus ØDW5
Extremity
- Lower
    - Left ØYWB
    - Right ØYW9
- Upper
    - Left ØXW7
    - Right ØXW6

Eye
- Left Ø8W1
- Right Ø8WØ

Face ØWW2
Fallopian Tube ØUW8
Femoral Shaft
- Left ØQW9
- Right ØQW8

Femur
- Lower
    - Left ØQWC
    - Right ØQWB
- Upper
    - Left ØQW7
    - Right ØQW6

Fibula
- Left ØQWK
- Right ØQWJ

Finger Nail ØHWQX
Gallbladder ØFW4
Gastrointestinal Tract ØWWP
Genitourinary Tract ØWWR
Gland
- Adrenal ØGW5
- Endocrine ØGWS
- Pituitary ØGWØ
- Salivary ØCWA

Glenoid Cavity
- Left ØPW8
- Right ØPW7

Great Vessel Ø2WY
Hair ØHWSX
Head ØWWØ
Heart Ø2WA
Humeral Head
- Left ØPWD
- Right ØPWC

Humeral Shaft
- Left ØPWG
- Right ØPWF

Intestinal Tract
- Lower ØDWD
- Upper ØDWØ

Intestine
- Large ØDWE
- Small ØDW8

Jaw
- Lower ØWW5
- Upper ØWW4

Joint
- Acromioclavicular
    - Left ØRWH
    - Right ØRWG
- Ankle
    - Left ØSWG
    - Right ØSWF
- Carpal
    - Left ØRWR
    - Right ØRWQ
- Cervical Vertebral ØRW1
- Cervicothoracic Vertebral ØRW4
- Coccygeal ØSW6
- Elbow
    - Left ØRWM
    - Right ØRWL

Revision of device in—*continued*

Joint—*continued*
- Finger Phalangeal
    - Left ØRWX
    - Right ØRWW
- Hip
    - Left ØSWB
    - Right ØSW9
- Knee
    - Left ØSWD
    - Right ØSWC
- Lumbar Vertebral ØSWØ
- Lumbosacral ØSW3
- Metacarpocarpal
    - Left ØRWT
    - Right ØRWS
- Metacarpophalangeal
    - Left ØRWV
    - Right ØRWU
- Metatarsal-Phalangeal
    - Left ØSWN
    - Right ØSWM
- Metatarsal-Tarsal
    - Left ØSWL
    - Right ØSWK
- Occipital-cervical ØRWØ
- Sacrococcygeal ØSW5
- Sacroiliac
    - Left ØSW8
    - Right ØSW7
- Shoulder
    - Left ØRWK
    - Right ØRWJ
- Sternoclavicular
    - Left ØRWF
    - Right ØRWE
- Tarsal
    - Left ØSWJ
    - Right ØSWH
- Temporomandibular
    - Left ØRWD
    - Right ØRWC
- Thoracic Vertebral ØRW6
- Thoracolumbar Vertebral ØRWA
- Toe Phalangeal
    - Left ØSWQ
    - Right ØSWP
- Wrist
    - Left ØRWP
    - Right ØRWN

Kidney ØTW5
Larynx ØCWS
Lens
- Left Ø8WK
- Right Ø8WJ

Liver ØFWØ
Lung
- Left ØBWL
- Right ØBWK

Lymphatic Ø7WN
- Thoracic Duct Ø7WK

Mediastinum ØWWC
Mesentery ØDWV
Metacarpal
- Left ØPWQ
- Right ØPWP

Metatarsal
- Left ØQWP
- Right ØQWN

Mouth and Throat ØCWY
Muscle
- Extraocular
    - Left Ø8WM
    - Right Ø8WL
- Lower ØKWY
- Upper ØKWX

Neck ØWW6
Nerve
- Cranial ØØWE
- Peripheral Ø1WY

Nose Ø9WK
Omentum ØDWU
Ovary ØUW3

Revision of device in—*continued*

Pancreas ØFWG
Parathyroid Gland ØGWR
Patella
- Left ØQWF
- Right ØQWD

Pelvic Cavity ØWWJ
Penis ØVWS
Pericardial Cavity ØWWD
Perineum
- Female ØWWN
- Male ØWWM

Peritoneal Cavity ØWWG
Peritoneum ØDWW
Phalanx
- Finger
    - Left ØPWV
    - Right ØPWT
- Thumb
    - Left ØPWS
    - Right ØPWR
- Toe
    - Left ØQWR
    - Right ØQWQ

Pineal Body ØGW1
Pleura ØBWQ
Pleural Cavity
- Left ØWWB
- Right ØWW9

Prostate and Seminal Vesicles ØVW4
Radius
- Left ØPWJ
- Right ØPWH

Respiratory Tract ØWWQ
Retroperitoneum ØWWH
Rib
- Left ØPW2
- Right ØPW1

Sacrum ØQW1
Scapula
- Left ØPW6
- Right ØPW5

Scrotum and Tunica Vaginalis ØVW8
Septum
- Atrial Ø2W5
- Ventricular Ø2WM

Sinus Ø9WY
Skin ØHWPX
Skull ØNWØ
Spinal Canal ØØWU
Spinal Cord ØØWV
Spleen Ø7WP
Sternum ØPWØ
Stomach ØDW6
Subcutaneous tissue and fascia
- Head and Neck ØJWS
- Lower Extremity ØJWW
- Trunk ØJWT
- Upper Extremity ØJWV

Tarsal
- Left ØQWM
- Right ØQWL

Tendon
- Lower ØLWY
- Upper ØLWX

Testis ØVWD
Thymus Ø7WM
Thyroid Gland ØGWK
Tibia
- Left ØQWH
- Right ØQWG

Toe Nail ØHWRX
Trachea ØBW1
Tracheobronchial Tree ØBWØ
Tympanic membrane
- Left Ø9W8
- Right Ø9W7

Ulna
- Left ØPWL
- Right ØPWK

Ureter ØTW9
Urethra ØTWD
Uterus and Cervix ØUWD

Revision of device in—*continued*
  Vagina and Cul-de-sac 0UWH
  Valve
    Aortic 02WF
    Mitral 02WG
    Pulmonary 02WH
    Tricuspid 02WJ
  Vas Deferens 0VWR
  Vein
    Lower 06WY
    Upper 05WY
  Vertebra
    Cervical 0PW3
    Lumbar 0QW0
    Thoracic 0PW4
  Vulva 0UWM
Rhinopharynx *use* Nasopharynx
Rhinoplasty
  see Alteration, Nose 090K
  see Repair, Nose 09QK
  see Replacement, Nose 09RK
  see Supplement, Nose 09UK
Rhinorrhaphy *see* Repair, Nose 09QK
Rhinoscopy 09JKXZZ
Rhizotomy
  see Division, Central Nervous System 008
  see Division, Peripheral Nervous System 018
Rhomboid major muscle
  use Muscle, Trunk, Left
  use Muscle, Trunk, Right
Rhomboid minor muscle
  use Muscle, Trunk, Right
  use Muscle, Trunk, Left
Rhythm electrocardiogram *see* Measurement,
  Cardiac 4A02
Rhytidectomy *use* Face lift
Right ascending lumbar vein *use* Vein, Azygos
Right atrioventricular valve *use* Valve, Tricuspid
Right auricular appendix *use* Atrium, Right
Right colic vein *use* Vein, Colic
Right coronary sulcus *use* Heart, Right
Right gastric artery *use* Artery, Gastric
Right gastroepiploic vein *use* Vein, Superior
  Mesenteric
Right inferior phrenic vein *use* Vena Cava, Inferior
Right inferior pulmonary vein *use* Vein, Pulmonary,
  Right
Right jugular trunk *use* Lymphatic, Neck, Right
Right lateral ventricle *use* Cerebral Ventricle
Right lymphatic duct *use* Lymphatic, Neck, Right
Right ovarian vein *use* Vena Cava, Inferior
Right second lumbar vein *use* Vena Cava, Inferior
Right subclavian trunk *use* Lymphatic, Neck, Right
Right subcostal vein *use* Vein, Azygos
Right superior pulmonary vein *use* Vein, Pulmonary,
  Right
Right suprarenal vein *use* Vena Cava, Inferior
Right testicular vein *use* Vena Cava, Inferior
Rima glottidis *use* Larynx
Risorius muscle *use* Muscle, Facial
Robotic assisted procedure
  Extremity
    Lower 8E0Y
    Upper 8E0X
  Head and Neck Region 8E09
  Trunk Region 8E0W
Rotation of fetal head
  Forceps 10S07ZZ
  Manual 10S0XZZ
Round ligament of uterus *use* Uterine Supporting
  Structure
Round window
  use Ear, Inner, Right
  use Ear, Inner, Left
Roux-en-Y operation
  see Bypass, Gastrointestinal System 0D1
  see Bypass, Hepatobiliary System and Pancreas 0F1
Rupture
  Adhesions *see* Release
  Fluid collection *see* Drainage

S

Sacral ganglion *use* Nerve, Sacral Sympathetic
Sacral lymph node *use* Lymphatic, Pelvis
Sacral splanchnic nerve *use* Nerve, Sacral
  Sympathetic
Sacrectomy *see* Excision, Lower Bones 0QB
Sacrococcygeal ligament
  use Bursa and Ligament, Trunk, Right
  use Bursa and Ligament, Trunk, Left
Sacrococcygeal symphysis *use* Joint, Sacrococcygeal
Sacroiliac ligament
  use Bursa and Ligament, Trunk, Left
  use Bursa and Ligament, Trunk, Right
Sacrospinous ligament
  use Bursa and Ligament, Trunk, Left
  use Bursa and Ligament, Trunk, Right
Sacrotuberous ligament
  use Bursa and Ligament, Trunk, Left
  use Bursa and Ligament, Trunk, Right
Salpingectomy
  see Excision, Female Reproductive System 0UB
  see Resection, Female Reproductive System 0UT
Salpingolysis *see* Release, Female Reproductive
  System 0UN
Salpingopexy
  see Repair, Female Reproductive System 0UQ
  see Reposition, Female Reproductive System 0US
Salpingopharyngeus muscle *use* Muscle, Tongue,
  Palate, Pharynx
Salpingoplasty
  see Repair, Female Reproductive System 0UQ
  see Supplement, Female Reproductive System 0UU
Salpingorrhaphy *see* Repair, Female Reproductive
  System 0UQ
Salpingoscopy 0UJ88ZZ
Salpingostomy *see* Drainage, Female Reproductive
  System 0U9
Salpingotomy *see* Drainage, Female Reproductive
  System 0U9
Salpinx
  use Fallopian Tube, Left
  use Fallopian Tube, Right
Saphenous nerve *use* Nerve, Femoral
Sartorius muscle
  use Muscle, Upper Leg, Right
  use Muscle, Upper Leg, Left
Scalene muscle
  use Muscle, Neck, Right
  use Muscle, Neck, Left
Scan
  Computerized Tomography (CT) *use* Computerized
    Tomography (CT Scan)
  Radioisotope *use* Planar Nuclear Medicine Imaging
Scaphoid bone
  use Carpal, Left
  use Carpal, Right
Scapholunate ligament
  use Bursa and Ligament, Hand, Right
  use Bursa and Ligament, Hand, Left
Scaphotrapezium ligament
  use Bursa and Ligament, Hand, Right
  use Bursa and Ligament, Hand, Left
Scapulectomy
  see Excision, Upper Bones 0PB
  see Resection, Upper Bones 0PT
Scapulopexy
  see Repair, Upper Bones 0PQ
  see Reposition, Upper Bones 0PS
Scarpa's (vestibular) ganglion *use* Nerve, Acoustic
Sclerectomy *see* Excision, Eye 08B
Sclerotherapy, mechanical *see* Destruction
Sclerotomy *see* Drainage, Eye 089
Scrotectomy
  see Excision, Male Reproductive System 0VB
  see Resection, Male Reproductive System 0VT
Scrotoplasty
  see Repair, Male Reproductive System 0VQ
  see Supplement, Male Reproductive System 0VU
Scrotorrhaphy *see* Repair, Male Reproductive System
  0VQ

Scrototomy *see* Drainage, Male Reproductive System
  0V9
Sebaceous gland *use* Skin
Second cranial nerve *use* Nerve, Optic
Section, cesarean *see* Extraction, Pregnancy 10D
Sella turcica
  use Bone, Sphenoid, Right
  use Bone, Sphenoid, Left
Semicircular canal
  use Ear, Inner, Right
  use Ear, Inner, Left
Semimembranosus muscle
  use Muscle, Upper Leg, Left
  use Muscle, Upper Leg, Right
Semitendinosus muscle
  use Muscle, Upper Leg, Left
  use Muscle, Upper Leg, Right
Septal cartilage *use* Septum, Nasal
Septectomy
  see Excision, Heart and Great Vessels 02B
  see Resection, Heart and Great Vessels 02T
  see Excision, Ear, Nose, Sinus 09B
  see Resection, Ear, Nose, Sinus 09T
Septoplasty
  see Repair, Ear, Nose, Sinus 09Q
  see Replacement, Ear, Nose, Sinus 09R
  see Supplement, Ear, Nose, Sinus 09U
  see Reposition, Ear, Nose, Sinus 09S
  see Repair, Heart and Great Vessels 02Q
  see Replacement, Heart and Great Vessels 02R
  see Supplement, Heart and Great Vessels 02U
Septotomy *see* Drainage, Ear, Nose, Sinus 099
Sequestrectomy, bone *see* Extirpation
Serratus anterior muscle
  use Muscle, Thorax, Left
  use Muscle, Thorax, Right
Serratus posterior muscle
  use Muscle, Trunk, Left
  use Muscle, Trunk, Right
Seventh cranial nerve *use* Nerve, Facial
Shirodkar cervical cerclage 0UVC7ZZ
Shock Wave Therapy, Musculoskeletal 6A93
Short gastric artery *use* Artery, Splenic
Shortening
  see Excision
  see Repair
  see Reposition
Shunt creation *see* Bypass
Sialoadenectomy
  Complete *see* Resection, Mouth and Throat 0CT
  Partial *see* Excision, Mouth and Throat 0CB
Sialodochoplasty
  see Repair, Mouth and Throat 0CQ
  see Replacement, Mouth and Throat 0CR
  see Supplement, Mouth and Throat 0CU
Sialoectomy
  see Excision, Mouth and Throat 0CB
  see Resection, Mouth and Throat 0CT
Sialography *see* Plain Radiography, Ear, Nose, Mouth
  and Throat B90
Sialolithotomy *see* Extirpation, Mouth and Throat 0CC
Sigmoid artery *use* Artery, Inferior Mesenteric
Sigmoid flexure *use* Colon, Sigmoid
Sigmoid vein *use* Vein, Inferior Mesenteric
Sigmoidectomy
  see Excision, Gastrointestinal System 0DB
  see Resection, Gastrointestinal System 0DT
Sigmoidorrhaphy *see* Repair, Gastrointestinal System
  0DQ
Sigmoidoscopy 0DJD8ZZ
Sigmoidotomy *see* Drainage, Gastrointestinal System
  0D9
Sinoatrial node *use* Conduction Mechanism
Sinogram
  Abdominal Wall *see* Fluoroscopy, Abdomen and
    Pelvis BW11
  Chest Wall *see* Plain Radiography, Chest BW03
  Retroperitoneum *see* Fluoroscopy, Abdomen and
    Pelvis BW11
Sinus venosus *use* Atrium, Right
Sinusectomy
  see Excision, Ear, Nose, Sinus 09B
  see Resection, Ear, Nose, Sinus 09T

Sinusoscopy 09JY4ZZ
Sinusotomy *see* Drainage, Ear, Nose, Sinus 099
Sixth cranial nerve *use* Nerve, Abducens
Size reduction, breast *see* Excision, Skin and Breast 0HB
Skene's (paraurethral) gland *use* Gland, Vestibular
Sling
    Fascial, orbicularis muscle (mouth) *see* Supplement, Muscle, Facial 0KU1
    Levator muscle, for urethral suspension *see* Reposition, Bladder Neck 0TSC
    Pubococcygeal, for urethral suspension *see* Reposition, Bladder Neck 0TSC
    Rectum *see* Reposition, Rectum 0DSP
Small bowel series *see* Fluoroscopy, Bowel, Small BD13
Small saphenous vein
    use Vein, Lesser Saphenous, Left
    use Vein, Lesser Saphenous, Right
Snaring, polyp, colon *see* Excision, Gastrointestinal System 0DB
Solar (celiac) plexus *use* Nerve, Abdominal Sympathetic
Soleus muscle
    use Muscle, Lower Leg, Left
    use Muscle, Lower Leg, Right
Spacer
    Insertion of device in
      Disc
        Lumbar Vertebral 0SH2
        Lumbosacral 0SH4
      Joint
        Acromioclavicular
          Left 0RHH
          Right 0RHG
        Ankle
          Left 0SHG
          Right 0SHF
        Carpal
          Left 0RHR
          Right 0RHQ
        Cervical Vertebral 0RH1
        Cervicothoracic Vertebral 0RH4
        Coccygeal 0SH6
        Elbow
          Left 0RHM
          Right 0RHL
        Finger Phalangeal
          Left 0RHX
          Right 0RHW
        Hip
          Left 0SHB
          Right 0SH9
        Knee
          Left 0SHD
          Right 0SHC
        Lumbar Vertebral 0SH0
        Lumbosacral 0SH3
        Metacarpocarpal
          Left 0RHT
          Right 0RHS
        Metacarpophalangeal
          Left 0RHV
          Right 0RHU
        Metatarsal-Phalangeal
          Left 0SHN
          Right 0SHM
        Metatarsal-Tarsal
          Left 0SHL
          Right 0SHK
        Occipital-cervical 0RH0
        Sacrococcygeal 0SH5
        Sacroiliac
          Left 0SH8
          Right 0SH7
        Shoulder
          Left 0RHK
          Right 0RHJ
        Sternoclavicular
          Left 0RHF
          Right 0RHE

Spacer—*continued*
    Insertion of device in—*continued*
      Tarsal
        Left 0SHJ
        Right 0SHH
      Temporomandibular
        Left 0RHD
        Right 0RHC
      Thoracic Vertebral 0RH6
      Thoracolumbar Vertebral 0RHA
      Toe Phalangeal
        Left 0SHQ
        Right 0SHP
      Wrist
        Left 0RHP
        Right 0RHN
    Removal of device from
      Acromioclavicular
        Left 0RPH
        Right 0RPG
      Ankle
        Left 0SPG
        Right 0SPF
      Carpal
        Left 0RPR
        Right 0RPQ
      Cervical Vertebral 0RP1
      Cervicothoracic Vertebral 0RP4
      Coccygeal 0SP6
      Elbow
        Left 0RPM
        Right 0RPL
      Finger Phalangeal
        Left 0RPX
        Right 0RPW
      Hip
        Left 0SPB
        Right 0SP9
      Knee
        Left 0SPD
        Right 0SPC
      Lumbar Vertebral 0SP0
      Lumbosacral 0SP3
      Metacarpocarpal
        Left 0RPT
        Right 0RPS
      Metacarpophalangeal
        Left 0RPV
        Right 0RPU
      Metatarsal-Phalangeal
        Left 0SPN
        Right 0SPM
      Metatarsal-Tarsal
        Left 0SPL
        Right 0SPK
      Occipital-cervical 0RP0
      Sacrococcygeal 0SP5
      Sacroiliac
        Left 0SP8
        Right 0SP7
      Shoulder
        Left 0RPK
        Right 0RPJ
      Sternoclavicular
        Left 0RPF
        Right 0RPE
      Tarsal
        Left 0SPJ
        Right 0SPH
      Temporomandibular
        Left 0RPD
        Right 0RPC
      Thoracic Vertebral 0RP6
      Thoracolumbar Vertebral 0RPA
      Toe Phalangeal
        Left 0SPQ
        Right 0SPP
      Wrist
        Left 0RPP
        Right 0RPN

Spacer—*continued*
    Revision of device in
      Acromioclavicular
        Left 0RWH
        Right 0RWG
      Ankle
        Left 0SWG
        Right 0SWF
      Carpal
        Left 0RWR
        Right 0RWQ
      Cervical Vertebral 0RW1
      Cervicothoracic Vertebral 0RW4
      Coccygeal 0SW6
      Elbow
        Left 0RWM
        Right 0RWL
      Finger Phalangeal
        Left 0RWX
        Right 0RWW
      Hip
        Left 0SWB
        Right 0SW9
      Knee
        Left 0SWD
        Right 0SWC
      Lumbar Vertebral 0SW0
      Lumbosacral 0SW3
      Metacarpocarpal
        Left 0RWT
        Right 0RWS
      Metacarpophalangeal
        Left 0RWV
        Right 0RWU
      Metatarsal-Phalangeal
        Left 0SWN
        Right 0SWM
      Metatarsal-Tarsal
        Left 0SWL
        Right 0SWK
      Occipital-cervical 0RW0
      Sacrococcygeal 0SW5
      Sacroiliac
        Left 0SW8
        Right 0SW7
      Shoulder
        Left 0RWK
        Right 0RWJ
      Sternoclavicular
        Left 0RWF
        Right 0RWE
      Tarsal
        Left 0SWJ
        Right 0SWH
      Temporomandibular
        Left 0RWD
        Right 0RWC
      Thoracic Vertebral 0RW6
      Thoracolumbar Vertebral 0RWA
      Toe Phalangeal
        Left 0SWQ
        Right 0SWP
      Wrist
        Left 0RWP
        Right 0RWN
Spectroscopy
    Intravascular 8E023DZ
    Near infrared 8E023DZ
Speech Assessment F00
Speech therapy *see* Speech Treatment, Rehabilitation F06
Speech Treatment F06
Sphenoidectomy
    see Excision, Ear, Nose, Sinus 09B
    see Resection, Ear, Nose, Sinus 09T
    see Excision, Head and Facial Bones 0NB
    see Resection, Head and Facial Bones 0NT
Sphenoidotomy *see* Drainage, Ear, Nose, Sinus 099
Sphenomandibular ligament *use* Bursa and Ligament, Head and Neck
Sphenopalatine (pterygopalatine) ganglion *use* Nerve, Head and Neck Sympathetic

Sphincterorrhaphy, anal *see* Repair, Anal Sphincter ØDQR
Sphincterotomy, anal
  see Drainage, Anal Sphincter ØD9R
  see Division, Anal Sphincter ØD8R
Spinal dura mater *use* Dura Mater
Spinal epidural space *use* Epidural Space
Spinal subarachnoid space *use* Subarachnoid Space
Spinal subdural space *use* Subdural Space
Spinous process
  use Vertebra, Thoracic
  use Vertebra, Lumbar
  use Vertebra, Cervical
Spiral ganglion *use* Nerve, Acoustic
Splenectomy
  see Excision, Lymphatic and Hemic Systems Ø7B
  see Resection, Lymphatic and Hemic Systems Ø7T
Splenic flexure *use* Colon, Transverse
Splenic plexus *use* Nerve, Abdominal Sympathetic
Splenius capitis muscle *use* Muscle, Head
Splenius cervicis muscle
  use Muscle, Neck, Left
  use Muscle, Neck, Right
Splenolysis *see* Release, Lymphatic and Hemic Systems Ø7N
Splenopexy
  see Repair, Lymphatic and Hemic Systems Ø7Q
  see Reposition, Lymphatic and Hemic Systems Ø7S
Splenoplasty *see* Repair, Lymphatic and Hemic Systems Ø7Q
Splenorrhaphy *see* Repair, Lymphatic and Hemic Systems Ø7Q
Splenotomy *see* Drainage, Lymphatic and Hemic Systems Ø79
Splinting, musculoskeletal *see* Immobilization, Anatomical Regions 2W3
Stapedectomy
  see Excision, Ear, Nose, Sinus Ø9B
  see Resection, Ear, Nose, Sinus Ø9T
Stapediolysis *see* Release, Ear, Nose, Sinus Ø9N
Stapedioplasty
  see Repair, Ear, Nose, Sinus Ø9Q
  see Replacement, Ear, Nose, Sinus Ø9R
  see Supplement, Ear, Nose, Sinus Ø9U
Stapedotomy *see* Drainage, Ear, Nose, Sinus Ø99
Stapes
  use Auditory Ossicle, Right
  use Auditory Ossicle, Left
Stellate ganglion *use* Nerve, Head and Neck Sympathetic
Stensen's duct
  use Duct, Parotid, Right
  use Duct, Parotid, Left
Stereotactic Radiosurgery
  Gamma Beam
    Abdomen DW23JZZ
    Adrenal Gland DG22JZZ
    Bile Ducts DF22JZZ
    Bladder DT22JZZ
    Bone Marrow D720JZZ
    Brain DØ2ØJZZ
    Brain Stem DØ21JZZ
    Breast
      Left DM2ØJZZ
      Right DM21JZZ
    Bronchus DB21JZZ
    Cervix DU21JZZ
    Chest DW22JZZ
    Chest Wall DB27JZZ
    Colon DD25JZZ
    Diaphragm DB28JZZ
    Duodenum DD22JZZ
    Ear D920JZZ
    Esophagus DD2ØJZZ
    Eye D82ØJZZ
    Gallbladder DF21JZZ
    Gland
      Adrenal DG22JZZ
      Parathyroid DG24JZZ
      Pituitary DG2ØJZZ
      Thyroid DG25JZZ
    Glands, Salivary D926JZZ
    Head and Neck DW21JZZ

Stereotactic Radiosurgery—*continued*
  Gamma Beam—*continued*
    Ileum DD24JZZ
    Jejunum DD23JZZ
    Kidney DT2ØJZZ
    Larynx D92BJZZ
    Liver DF2ØJZZ
    Lung DB22JZZ
    Lymphatics
      Abdomen D726JZZ
      Axillary D724JZZ
      Inguinal D728JZZ
      Neck D723JZZ
      Pelvis D727JZZ
      Thorax D725JZZ
    Mediastinum DB26JZZ
    Mouth D924JZZ
    Nasopharynx D92DJZZ
    Neck and Head DW21JZZ
    Nerve, Peripheral DØ27JZZ
    Nose D921JZZ
    Ovary DU2ØJZZ
    Palate
      Hard D928JZZ
      Soft D929JZZ
    Pancreas DF23JZZ
    Parathyroid Gland DG24JZZ
    Pelvic Region DW26JZZ
    Pharynx D92CJZZ
    Pineal Body DG21JZZ
    Pituitary Gland DG2ØJZZ
    Pleura DB25JZZ
    Prostate DV2ØJZZ
    Rectum DD27JZZ
    Sinuses D927JZZ
    Spinal Cord DØ26JZZ
    Spleen D722JZZ
    Stomach DD21JZZ
    Testis DV21JZZ
    Thymus D721JZZ
    Thyroid Gland DG25JZZ
    Tongue D925JZZ
    Trachea DB2ØJZZ
    Ureter DT21JZZ
    Urethra DT23JZZ
    Uterus DU22JZZ
  Other Photon
    Abdomen DW23DZZ
    Adrenal Gland DG22DZZ
    Bile Ducts DF22DZZ
    Bladder DT22DZZ
    Bone Marrow D72ØDZZ
    Brain DØ2ØDZZ
    Brain Stem DØ21DZZ
    Breast
      Left DM2ØDZZ
      Right DM21DZZ
    Bronchus DB21DZZ
    Cervix DU21DZZ
    Chest DW22DZZ
    Chest Wall DB27DZZ
    Colon DD25DZZ
    Diaphragm DB28DZZ
    Duodenum DD22DZZ
    Ear D920DZZ
    Esophagus DD2ØDZZ
    Eye D82ØDZZ
    Gallbladder DF21DZZ
    Gland
      Adrenal DG22DZZ
      Parathyroid DG24DZZ
      Pituitary DG2ØDZZ
      Thyroid DG25DZZ
    Glands, Salivary D926DZZ
    Head and Neck DW21DZZ
    Ileum DD24DZZ
    Jejunum DD23DZZ
    Kidney DT2ØDZZ
    Larynx D92BDZZ
    Liver DF2ØDZZ
    Lung DB22DZZ

Stereotactic Radiosurgery—*continued*
  Other Photon—*continued*
    Lymphatics
      Abdomen D726DZZ
      Axillary D724DZZ
      Inguinal D728DZZ
      Neck D723DZZ
      Pelvis D727DZZ
      Thorax D725DZZ
    Mediastinum DB26DZZ
    Mouth D924DZZ
    Nasopharynx D92DDZZ
    Neck and Head DW21DZZ
    Nerve, Peripheral DØ27DZZ
    Nose D921DZZ
    Ovary DU2ØDZZ
    Palate
      Hard D928DZZ
      Soft D929DZZ
    Pancreas DF23DZZ
    Parathyroid Gland DG24DZZ
    Pelvic Region DW26DZZ
    Pharynx D92CDZZ
    Pineal Body DG21DZZ
    Pituitary Gland DG2ØDZZ
    Pleura DB25DZZ
    Prostate DV2ØDZZ
    Rectum DD27DZZ
    Sinuses D927DZZ
    Spinal Cord DØ26DZZ
    Spleen D722DZZ
    Stomach DD21DZZ
    Testis DV21DZZ
    Thymus D721DZZ
    Thyroid Gland DG25DZZ
    Tongue D925DZZ
    Trachea DB2ØDZZ
    Ureter DT21DZZ
    Urethra DT23DZZ
    Uterus DU22DZZ
  Particulate
    Abdomen DW23HZZ
    Adrenal Gland DG22HZZ
    Bile Ducts DF22HZZ
    Bladder DT22HZZ
    Bone Marrow D72ØHZZ
    Brain DØ2ØHZZ
    Brain Stem DØ21HZZ
    Breast
      Left DM2ØHZZ
      Right DM21HZZ
    Bronchus DB21HZZ
    Cervix DU21HZZ
    Chest DW22HZZ
    Chest Wall DB27HZZ
    Colon DD25HZZ
    Diaphragm DB28HZZ
    Duodenum DD22HZZ
    Ear D920HZZ
    Esophagus DD2ØHZZ
    Eye D82ØHZZ
    Gallbladder DF21HZZ
    Gland
      Adrenal DG22HZZ
      Parathyroid DG24HZZ
      Pituitary DG2ØHZZ
      Thyroid DG25HZZ
    Glands, Salivary D926HZZ
    Head and Neck DW21HZZ
    Ileum DD24HZZ
    Jejunum DD23HZZ
    Kidney DT2ØHZZ
    Larynx D92BHZZ
    Liver DF2ØHZZ
    Lung DB22HZZ
    Lymphatics
      Abdomen D726HZZ
      Axillary D724HZZ
      Inguinal D728HZZ
      Neck D723HZZ
      Pelvis D727HZZ
      Thorax D725HZZ

Stereotactic Radiosurgery—*continued*
  Particulate—*continued*
    Mediastinum DB26HZZ
    Mouth D924HZZ
    Nasopharynx D92DHZZ
    Neck and Head DW21HZZ
    Nerve, Peripheral D027HZZ
    Nose D921HZZ
    Ovary DU20HZZ
    Palate
      Hard D928HZZ
      Soft D929HZZ
    Pancreas DF23HZZ
    Parathyroid Gland DG24HZZ
    Pelvic Region DW26HZZ
    Pharynx D92CHZZ
    Pineal Body DG21HZZ
    Pituitary Gland DG20HZZ
    Pleura DB25HZZ
    Prostate DV20HZZ
    Rectum DD27HZZ
    Sinuses D927HZZ
    Spinal Cord D026HZZ
    Spleen D722HZZ
    Stomach DD21HZZ
    Testis DV21HZZ
    Thymus D721HZZ
    Thyroid Gland DG25HZZ
    Tongue D925HZZ
    Trachea DB20HZZ
    Ureter DT21HZZ
    Urethra DT23HZZ
    Uterus DU22HZZ
Sternoclavicular ligament
  use Bursa and Ligament, Shoulder, Left
  use Bursa and Ligament, Shoulder, Right
Sternocleidomastoid artery
  use Artery, Thyroid, Left
  use Artery, Thyroid, Right
Sternocleidomastoid muscle
  use Muscle, Neck, Left
  use Muscle, Neck, Right
Sternocostal ligament
  use Bursa and Ligament, Thorax, Right
  use Bursa and Ligament, Thorax, Left
Sternotomy
  see Division, Sternum 0P80
  see Drainage, Sternum 0P90
Stimulation, cardiac
  Cardioversion 5A2204Z
  Electrophysiologic testing *see* Measurement,
    Cardiac 4A02
Stimulator Generator
  Insertion of device in
    Abdomen 0JH8
    Back 0JH7
    Chest 0JH6
  Removal of device from, Subcutaneous Tissue and
    Fascia, Trunk 0JPT
  Revision of device in, Subcutaneous Tissue and
    Fascia, Trunk 0JWT
Stimulator Lead
  Insertion of device in
    Anal Sphincter 0DHR
    Artery
      Left 03HL
      Right 03HK
    Bladder 0THB
    Muscle
      Lower 0KHY
      Upper 0KHX
    Stomach 0DH6
    Ureter 0TH9
  Removal of device from
    Anal Sphincter 0DPR
    Artery, Upper 03PY
    Bladder 0TPB
    Muscle
      Lower 0KPY
      Upper 0KPX
    Stomach 0DP6
    Ureter 0TP9

Stimulator Lead—*continued*
  Revision of device in
    Anal Sphincter 0DWR
    Artery, Upper 03WY
    Bladder 0TWB
    Muscle
      Lower 0KWY
      Upper 0KWX
    Stomach 0DW6
    Ureter 0TW9
Stoma
  Excision
    Abdominal Wall 0WBFXZ2
    Neck 0WB6XZ2
  Repair
    Abdominal Wall 0WQFXZ2
    Neck 0WQ6XZ2
Stomatoplasty
  see Repair, Mouth and Throat 0CQ
  see Replacement, Mouth and Throat 0CR
  see Supplement, Mouth and Throat 0CU
Stomatorrhaphy *see* Repair, Mouth and Throat 0CQ
Stress test
  Measurement 4A02XM4
  Monitoring 4A12XM4
Stripping *see* Extraction
Study
  Electrophysiologic stimulation, cardiac *see*
    Measurement, Cardiac 4A02
  Ocular motility 4A07X7Z
  Pulmonary airway flow measurement *see*
    Measurement, Respiratory 4A09
  Visual acuity 4A07X0Z
Styloglossus muscle *use* Muscle, Tongue, Palate,
  Pharynx
Stylomandibular ligament *use* Bursa and Ligament,
  Head and Neck
Stylopharyngeus muscle *use* Muscle, Tongue, Palate,
  Pharynx
Subacromial bursa
  use Bursa and Ligament, Shoulder, Left
  use Bursa and Ligament, Shoulder, Right
Subaortic (common iliac) lymph node *use*
  Lymphatic, Pelvis
Subclavicular (apical) lymph node
  use Lymphatic, Axillary, Left
  use Lymphatic, Axillary, Right
Subclavius muscle
  use Muscle, Thorax, Left
  use Muscle, Thorax, Right
Subclavius nerve *use* Nerve, Brachial Plexus
Subcostal artery *use* Aorta, Thoracic
Subcostal muscle
  use Muscle, Thorax, Left
  use Muscle, Thorax, Right
Subcostal nerve *use* Nerve, Thoracic
Submandibular ganglion
  use Nerve, Head and Neck Sympathetic
  use Nerve, Facial
Submandibular gland
  use Gland, Submaxillary, Left
  use Gland, Submaxillary, Right
Submandibular lymph node *use* Lymphatic, Head
Submaxillary ganglion *use* Nerve, Head and Neck
  Sympathetic
Submaxillary lymph node *use* Lymphatic, Head
Submental artery *use* Artery, Face
Submental lymph node *use* Lymphatic, Head
Submucous (Meissner's) plexus *use* Nerve,
  Abdominal Sympathetic
Suboccipital nerve *use* Nerve, Cervical
Suboccipital venous plexus
  use Vein, Vertebral, Left
  use Vein, Vertebral, Right
Subparotid lymph node *use* Lymphatic, Head
Subscapular (posterior) lymph node
  use Lymphatic, Axillary, Left
  use Lymphatic, Axillary, Right
Subscapular aponeurosis
  use Subcutaneous Tissue and Fascia, Upper Arm,
    Right
  use Subcutaneous Tissue and Fascia, Upper Arm,
    Left

Subscapular artery
  use Artery, Axillary, Left
  use Artery, Axillary, Right
Subscapularis muscle
  use Muscle, Shoulder, Left
  use Muscle, Shoulder, Right
Substance Abuse Treatment
  Counseling
    Family, for substance abuse, Other Family
      Counseling HZ63ZZZ
    Group
      12-Step HZ43ZZZ
      Behavioral HZ41ZZZ
      Cognitive HZ40ZZZ
      Cognitive-Behavioral HZ42ZZZ
      Confrontational HZ48ZZZ
      Continuing Care HZ49ZZZ
      Infectious disease
        Post-Test HZ4CZZZ
        Pre-Test HZ4CZZZ
      Interpersonal HZ44ZZZ
      Motivational Enhancement HZ47ZZZ
      Psychoeducation HZ46ZZZ
      Spiritual HZ4BZZZ
      Vocational HZ45ZZZ
    Individual
      12-Step HZ33ZZZ
      Behavioral HZ31ZZZ
      Cognitive HZ30ZZZ
      Cognitive-Behavioral HZ32ZZZ
      Confrontational HZ38ZZZ
      Continuing Care HZ39ZZZ
      Infectious Disease
        Post-Test HZ3CZZZ
        Pre-Test HZ3CZZZ
      Interpersonal HZ34ZZZ
      Motivational Enhancement HZ37ZZZ
      Psychoeducation HZ36ZZZ
      Spiritual HZ3BZZZ
      Vocational HZ35ZZZ
  Detoxification Services, for substance abuse
    HZ2ZZZZ
  Medication Management
    Antabuse HZ83ZZZ
    Bupropion HZ87ZZZ
    Clonidine HZ86ZZZ
    Levo-alpha-acetyl-methadol (LAAM) HZ82ZZZ
    Methadone Maintenance HZ81ZZZ
    Naloxone HZ85ZZZ
    Naltrexone HZ84ZZZ
    Nicotine Replacement HZ80ZZZ
    Other Replacement Medication HZ89ZZZ
    Psychiatric Medication HZ88ZZZ
  Pharmacotherapy
    Antabuse HZ93ZZZ
    Bupropion HZ97ZZZ
    Clonidine HZ96ZZZ
    Levo-alpha-acetyl-methadol (LAAM) HZ92ZZZ
    Methadone Maintenance HZ91ZZZ
    Naloxone HZ95ZZZ
    Naltrexone HZ94ZZZ
    Nicotine Replacement HZ90ZZZ
    Psychiatric Medication HZ98ZZZ
    Replacement Medication, Other HZ99ZZZ
  Psychotherapy
    12-Step HZ53ZZZ
    Behavioral HZ51ZZZ
    Cognitive HZ50ZZZ
    Cognitive-Behavioral HZ52ZZZ
    Confrontational HZ58ZZZ
    Interactive HZ55ZZZ
    Interpersonal HZ54ZZZ
    Motivational Enhancement HZ57ZZZ
    Psychoanalysis HZ5BZZZ
    Psychodynamic HZ5CZZZ
    Psychoeducation HZ56ZZZ
    Psychophysiological HZ5DZZZ
    Supportive HZ59ZZZ
Substantia nigra *use* Basal Ganglia
Subtalar (talocalcaneal) joint
  use Joint, Tarsal, Right
  use Joint, Tarsal, Left

Supplement—Suprahyoid muscle

Tibialis posterior muscle
  use Muscle, Lower Leg, Right
  use Muscle, Lower Leg, Left
Tissue Expander
  Insertion of device in
    Breast
      Bilateral ØHHV
      Left ØHHU
      Right ØHHT
    Nipple
      Left ØHHX
      Right ØHHW
    Subcutaneous Tissue and Fascia
      Abdomen ØJH8
      Back ØJH7
      Buttock ØJH9
      Chest ØJH6
      Face ØJH1
      Foot
        Left ØJHR
        Right ØJHQ
      Hand
        Left ØJHK
        Right ØJHJ
      Lower Arm
        Left ØJHH
        Right ØJHG
      Lower Leg
        Left ØJHP
        Right ØJHN
      Neck
        Anterior ØJH4
        Posterior ØJH5
      Pelvic Region ØJHC
      Perineum ØJHB
      Scalp ØJHØ
      Upper Arm
        Left ØJHF
        Right ØJHD
      Upper Leg
        Left ØJHM
        Right ØJHL
  Removal of device from
    Breast
      Left ØHPU
      Right ØHPT
    Subcutaneous Tissue and Fascia
      Head and Neck ØJPS
      Lower Extremity ØJPW
      Trunk ØJPT
      Upper Extremity ØJPV
  Revision of device in
    Breast
      Left ØHWU
      Right ØHWT
    Subcutaneous Tissue and Fascia
      Head and Neck ØJWS
      Lower Extremity ØJWW
      Trunk ØJWT
      Upper Extremity ØJWV
Tomographic (Tomo) Nuclear Medicine Imaging
  CP2YYZZ
  Abdomen CW2Ø
  Abdomen and Chest CW24
  Abdomen and Pelvis CW21
  Anatomical Regions, Multiple CW2YYZZ
  Bladder, Kidneys and Ureters CT23
  Brain CØ2Ø
  Breast CH2YYZZ
    Bilateral CH22
    Left CH21
    Right CH2Ø
  Bronchi and Lungs CB22
  Central Nervous System CØ2YYZZ
  Cerebrospinal Fluid CØ25
  Chest CW23
  Chest and Abdomen CW24
  Chest and Neck CW26
  Digestive System CD2YYZZ
  Endocrine System CG2YYZZ
  Extremity
    Lower CW2D
      Bilateral CP2F

Tomographic (Tomo) Nuclear Medicine Imaging—
    continued
  Extremity—*continued*
    Lower—*continued*
      Left CP2D
      Right CP2C
    Upper CW2M
      Bilateral CP2B
      Left CP29
      Right CP28
  Gallbladder CF24
  Gastrointestinal Tract CD27
  Gland, Parathyroid CG21
  Head and Neck CW2B
  Heart C22YYZZ
    Right and Left C226
  Hepatobiliary System and Pancreas CF2YYZZ
  Kidneys, Ureters and Bladder CT23
  Liver CF25
  Liver and Spleen CF26
  Lungs and Bronchi CB22
  Lymphatics and Hematologic System C72YYZZ
  Myocardium C22G
  Neck and Chest CW26
  Neck and Head CW2B
  Pancreas and Hepatobiliary System CF2YYZZ
  Pelvic Region CW2J
  Pelvis CP26
  Pelvis and Abdomen CW21
  Pelvis and Spine CP27
  Respiratory System CB2YYZZ
  Skin CH2YYZZ
  Skull CP21
  Skull and Cervical Spine CP23
  Spine
    Cervical CP22
    Cervical and Skull CP23
    Lumbar CP2H
    Thoracic CP2G
    Thoracolumbar CP2J
  Spine and Pelvis CP27
  Spleen C722
  Spleen and Liver CF26
  Subcutaneous Tissue CH2YYZZ
  Thorax CP24
  Ureters, Kidneys and Bladder CT23
  Urinary System CT2YYZZ
Tomography, computerized see Computerized
    Tomography (CT Scan)
Tonometry 4AØ7XBZ
Tonsillectomy
  see Excision, Mouth and Throat ØCB
  see Resection, Mouth and Throat ØCT
Tonsillotomy see Drainage, Mouth and Throat ØC9
Total parenteral nutrition (TPN) see Introduction,
    Nutritional Substance
Trachectomy
  see Excision, Trachea ØBB1
  see Resection, Trachea ØBT1
Trachelectomy
  see Excision, Cervix ØUBC
  see Resection, Cervix ØUTC
Trachelopexy
  see Repair, Cervix ØUQC
  see Reposition, Cervix ØUSC
Tracheloplasty see Repair, Cervix ØUQC
Trachelorrhaphy see Repair, Cervix ØUQC
Trachelotomy see Drainage, Cervix ØU9C
Tracheobronchial lymph node use Lymphatic, Thorax
Tracheoesophageal fistulization ØB11ØD6
Tracheolysis see Release, Respiratory System ØBN
Tracheoplasty
  see Repair, Respiratory System ØBQ
  see Supplement, Respiratory System ØBU
Tracheorrhaphy see Repair, Respiratory System ØBQ
Tracheoscopy ØBJ18ZZ
Tracheostomy see Bypass, Respiratory System ØB1
Tracheostomy Device
  Bypass, Trachea ØB11
  Change device in, Trachea ØB21XFZ
  Removal of device from, Trachea ØBP1
  Revision of device in, Trachea ØBW1
Tracheotomy see Drainage, Respiratory System ØB9

Traction
  Abdominal Wall 2W63X
  Arm
    Lower
      Left 2W6DX
      Right 2W6CX
    Upper
      Left 2W6BX
      Right 2W6AX
  Back 2W65X
  Chest Wall 2W64X
  Extremity
    Lower
      Left 2W6MX
      Right 2W6LX
    Upper
      Left 2W69X
      Right 2W68X
  Face 2W61X
  Finger
    Left 2W6KX
    Right 2W6JX
  Foot
    Left 2W6TX
    Right 2W6SX
  Hand
    Left 2W6FX
    Right 2W6EX
  Head 2W6ØX
  Inguinal Region
    Left 2W67X
    Right 2W66X
  Leg
    Lower
      Left 2W6RX
      Right 2W6QX
    Upper
      Left 2W6PX
      Right 2W6NX
  Neck 2W62X
  Thumb
    Left 2W6HX
    Right 2W6GX
  Toe
    Left 2W6VX
    Right 2W6UX
Tractotomy see Division, Central Nervous System ØØ8
Tragus
  use Ear, External, Left
  use Ear, External, Right
  use Ear, External, Bilateral
Training, caregiver use Caregiver Training
**TRAM (transverse rectus abdominis
    myocutaneous) flap reconstruction**
  Free see Replacement, Skin and Breast ØHR
  Pedicled see Transfer, Muscles ØKX
Transection see Division
Transfer
  Buccal Mucosa ØCX4
  Bursa and Ligament
    Abdomen
      Left ØMXJ
      Right ØMXH
    Ankle
      Left ØMXR
      Right ØMXQ
    Elbow
      Left ØMX4
      Right ØMX3
    Foot
      Left ØMXT
      Right ØMXS
    Hand
      Left ØMX8
      Right ØMX7
    Head and Neck ØMXØ
    Hip
      Left ØMXM
      Right ØMXL
    Knee
      Left ØMXP
      Right ØMXN

Transfer—continued
  Bursa and Ligament—continued
    Lower Extremity
      Left ØMXW
      Right ØMXV
    Perineum ØMXK
    Shoulder
      Left ØMX2
      Right ØMX1
    Thorax
      Left ØMXG
      Right ØMXF
    Trunk
      Left ØMXD
      Right ØMXC
    Upper Extremity
      Left ØMXB
      Right ØMX9
    Wrist
      Left ØMX6
      Right ØMX5
  Finger
    Left ØXXPØZM
    Right ØXXNØZL
  Gingiva
    Lower ØCX6
    Upper ØCX5
  Intestine
    Large ØDXE
    Small ØDX8
  Lip
    Lower ØCX1
    Upper ØCXØ
  Muscle
    Abdomen
      Left ØKXL
      Right ØKXK
    Extraocular
      Left Ø8XM
      Right Ø8XL
    Facial ØKX1
    Foot
      Left ØKXW
      Right ØKXV
    Hand
      Left ØKXD
      Right ØKXC
    Head ØKXØ
    Hip
      Left ØKXP
      Right ØKXN
    Lower Arm and Wrist
      Left ØKXB
      Right ØKX9
    Lower Leg
      Left ØKXT
      Right ØKXS
    Neck
      Left ØKX3
      Right ØKX2
    Perineum ØKXM
    Shoulder
      Left ØKX6
      Right ØKX5
    Thorax
      Left ØKXJ
      Right ØKXH
    Tongue, Palate, Pharynx ØKX4
    Trunk
      Left ØKXG
      Right ØKXF
    Upper Arm
      Left ØKX8
      Right ØKX7
    Upper Leg
      Left ØKXR
      Right ØKXQ
  Nerve
    Abducens ØØXL
    Accessory ØØXR
    Acoustic ØØXN
    Cervical Ø1X1
    Facial ØØXM

Transfer—continued
  Nerve—continued
    Femoral Ø1XD
    Glossopharyngeal ØØXP
    Hypoglossal ØØXS
    Lumbar Ø1XB
    Median Ø1X5
    Oculomotor ØØXH
    Olfactory ØØXF
    Optic ØØXG
    Peroneal Ø1XH
    Phrenic Ø1X2
    Pudendal Ø1XC
    Radial Ø1X6
    Sciatic Ø1XF
    Thoracic Ø1X8
    Tibial Ø1XG
    Trigeminal ØØXK
    Trochlear ØØXJ
    Ulnar Ø1X4
    Vagus ØØXQ
  Palate, Soft ØCX3
  Skin
    Abdomen ØHX7XZZ
    Back ØHX6XZZ
    Buttock ØHX8XZZ
    Chest ØHX5XZZ
    Ear
      Left ØHX3XZZ
      Right ØHX2XZZ
    Face ØHX1XZZ
    Foot
      Left ØHXNXZZ
      Right ØHXMXZZ
    Genitalia ØHXAXZZ
    Hand
      Left ØHXGXZZ
      Right ØHXFXZZ
    Lower Arm
      Left ØHXEXZZ
      Right ØHXDXZZ
    Lower Leg
      Left ØHXLXZZ
      Right ØHXKXZZ
    Neck ØHX4XZZ
    Perineum ØHX9XZZ
    Scalp ØHXØXZZ
    Upper Arm
      Left ØHXCXZZ
      Right ØHXBXZZ
    Upper Leg
      Left ØHXJXZZ
      Right ØHXHXZZ
  Stomach ØDX6
  Subcutaneous Tissue and Fascia
    Abdomen ØJX8
    Back ØJX7
    Buttock ØJX9
    Chest ØJX6
    Face ØJX1
    Foot
      Left ØJXR
      Right ØJXQ
    Hand
      Left ØJXK
      Right ØJXJ
    Lower Arm
      Left ØJXH
      Right ØJXG
    Lower Leg
      Left ØJXP
      Right ØJXN
    Neck
      Anterior ØJX4
      Posterior ØJX5
    Pelvic Region ØJXC
    Perineum ØJXB
    Scalp ØJXØ
    Upper Arm
      Left ØJXF
      Right ØJXD

Transfer—continued
  Subcutaneous Tissue and Fascia—continued
    Upper Leg
      Left ØJXM
      Right ØJXL
  Tendon
    Abdomen
      Left ØLXG
      Right ØLXF
    Ankle
      Left ØLXT
      Right ØLXS
    Foot
      Left ØLXW
      Right ØLXV
    Hand
      Left ØLX8
      Right ØLX7
    Head and Neck ØLXØ
    Hip
      Left ØLXK
      Right ØLXJ
    Knee
      Left ØLXR
      Right ØLXQ
    Lower Arm and Wrist
      Left ØLX6
      Right ØLX5
    Lower Leg
      Left ØLXP
      Right ØLXN
    Perineum ØLXH
    Shoulder
      Left ØLX2
      Right ØLX1
    Thorax
      Left ØLXD
      Right ØLXC
    Trunk
      Left ØLXB
      Right ØLX9
    Upper Arm
      Left ØLX4
      Right ØLX3
    Upper Leg
      Left ØLXM
      Right ØLXL
  Tongue ØCX7
Transfusion
  Artery
    Central
      Antihemophilic Factors 3Ø26
      Blood
        Platelets 3Ø26
        Red Cells 3Ø26
          Frozen 3Ø26
        White Cells 3Ø26
        Whole 3Ø26
      Bone Marrow 3Ø26
      Factor IX 3Ø26
      Fibrinogen 3Ø26
      Globulin 3Ø26
      Plasma
        Fresh 3Ø26
        Frozen 3Ø26
      Plasma Cryoprecipitate 3Ø26
      Serum Albumin 3Ø26
      Stem Cells
        Cord Blood 3Ø26
        Hematopoietic 3Ø26
    Peripheral
      Antihemophilic Factors 3Ø25
      Blood
        Platelets 3Ø25
        Red Cells 3Ø25
          Frozen 3Ø25
        White Cells 3Ø25
        Whole 3Ø25
      Bone Marrow 3Ø25
      Factor IX 3Ø25
      Fibrinogen 3Ø25
      Globulin 3Ø25

Transfusion—*continued*
  Artery—*continued*
    Plasma
      Fresh 3025
      Frozen 3025
    Plasma Cryoprecipitate 3025
      Serum Albumin 3025
      Stem Cells
        Cord Blood 3025
        Hematopoietic 3025
    Products of Conception
    Antihemophilic Factors 3027
      Blood
        Platelets 3027
        Red Cells 3027
          Frozen 3027
          White Cells 3027
          Whole 3027
      Factor IX 3027
      Fibrinogen 3027
      Globulin 3027
      Plasma
        Fresh 3027
        Frozen 3027
      Plasma Cryoprecipitate 3027
      Serum Albumin 3027
    Vein
      Central
        Antihemophilic Factors 3024
        Blood
          Platelets 3024
          Red Cells 3024
            Frozen 3024
            White Cells 3024
            Whole 3024
        Bone Marrow 3024
        Factor IX 3024
        Fibrinogen 3024
        Globulin 3024
        Plasma
          Fresh 3024
          Frozen 3024
        Plasma Cryoprecipitate 3024
        Serum Albumin 3024
        Stem Cells
          Cord Blood 3024
          Embryonic 3024
          Hematopoietic 3024
      Peripheral
        Antihemophilic Factors 3023
        Blood
          Platelets 3023
          Red Cells 3023
            Frozen 3023
            White Cells 3023
            Whole 3023
        Bone Marrow 3023
        Factor IX 3023
        Fibrinogen 3023
        Globulin 3023
        Plasma
          Fresh 3023
          Frozen 3023
        Plasma Cryoprecipitate 3023
        Serum Albumin 3023
        Stem Cells
          Cord Blood 3023
          Embryonic 3023
          Hematopoietic 3023
Transplantation
  Esophagus 0DY50Z
  Heart 02YA0Z
  Intestine
    Large 0DYE0Z
    Small 0DY80Z
  Kidney
    Left 0TY10Z
    Right 0TY00Z
  Liver 0FY00Z
  Lung
    Bilateral 0BYM0Z
    Left 0BYL0Z
    Lower Lobe

Transplantation—*continued*
  Lung—*continued*
    Lower Lobe—*continued*
      Left 0BYJ0Z
      Right 0BYF0Z
    Middle Lobe, Right 0BYD0Z
    Right 0BYK0Z
    Upper Lobe
      Left 0BYG0Z
      Right 0BYC0Z
  Lung Lingula 0BYH0Z
  Ovary
    Left 0UY10Z
    Right 0UY00Z
  Pancreas 0FYG0Z
  Products of Conception 10Y0
  Spleen 07YP0Z
  Stomach 0DY60Z
  Thymus 07YM0Z
Transposition
  see Reposition
  see Transfer
Transversalis fascia *use* Subcutaneous Tissue and Fascia, Trunk
Transverse (cutaneous) cervical nerve *use* Nerve, Cervical Plexus
Transverse acetabular ligament
  use Bursa and Ligament, Hip, Left
  use Bursa and Ligament, Hip, Right
Transverse facial artery
  use Artery, Temporal, Left
  use Artery, Temporal, Right
Transverse humeral ligament
  use Bursa and Ligament, Shoulder, Left
  use Bursa and Ligament, Shoulder, Right
Transverse ligament of atlas *use* Bursa and Ligament, Head and Neck
Transverse Rectus Abdominis Myocutaneous Flap
  Replacement
    Bilateral 0HRV076
    Left 0HRU076
    Right 0HRT076
  Transfer
    Left 0KXL
    Right 0KXK
Transverse scapular ligament
  use Bursa and Ligament, Shoulder, Left
  use Bursa and Ligament, Shoulder, Right
Transverse thoracis muscle
  use Muscle, Thorax, Right
  use Muscle, Thorax, Left
Transversospinalis muscle
  use Muscle, Trunk, Right
  use Muscle, Trunk, Left
Transversus abdominis muscle
  use Muscle, Abdomen, Left
  use Muscle, Abdomen, Right
Trapezium bone
  use Carpal, Right
  use Carpal, Left
Trapezius muscle
  use Muscle, Trunk, Right
  use Muscle, Trunk, Left
Trapezoid bone
  use Carpal, Right
  use Carpal, Left
Triceps brachii muscle
  use Muscle, Upper Arm, Right
  use Muscle, Upper Arm, Left
Tricuspid annulus *use* Valve, Tricuspid
Trifacial nerve *use* Nerve, Trigeminal
Trigone of bladder *use* Bladder
Trimming, excisional *see* Excision
Triquetral bone
  use Carpal, Right
  use Carpal, Left
Trochanteric bursa
  use Bursa and Ligament, Hip, Right
  use Bursa and Ligament, Hip, Left
TUMT (transurethral microwave thermotherapy of prostate) 0V507ZZ
TUNA (transurethral needle ablation of prostate) 0V507ZZ

Turbinectomy
  see Excision, Ear, Nose, Sinus 09B
  see Resection, Ear, Nose, Sinus 09T
Turbinoplasty
  see Repair, Ear, Nose, Sinus 09Q
  see Replacement, Ear, Nose, Sinus 09R
  see Supplement, Ear, Nose, Sinus 09U
Turbinotomy
  see Drainage, Ear, Nose, Sinus 099
  see Division, Ear, Nose, Sinus 098
TURP (transurethral resection of prostate) 0VB07ZZ
Twelfth cranial nerve *use* Nerve, Hypoglossal
Tympanic cavity
  use Ear, Middle, Left
  use Ear, Middle, Right
Tympanic nerve *use* Nerve, Glossopharyngeal
Tympanic part of temporoal bone
  use Bone, Temporal, Right
  use Bone, Temporal, Left
Tympanogram *see* Hearing Assessment, Diagnostic Audiology F13
Tympanoplasty
  see Repair, Ear, Nose, Sinus 09Q
  see Replacement, Ear, Nose, Sinus 09R
  see Supplement, Ear, Nose, Sinus 09U
Tympanosympathectomy *see* Excision, Nerve, Head and Neck Sympathetic 01BK
Tympanotomy *see* Drainage, Ear, Nose, Sinus 099

U

Ulnar collateral carpal ligament
  use Bursa and Ligament, Wrist, Left
  use Bursa and Ligament, Wrist, Right
Ulnar collateral ligament
  use Bursa and Ligament, Elbow, Right
  use Bursa and Ligament, Elbow, Left
Ulnar notch
  use Radius, Left
  use Radius, Right
Ulnar vein
  use Vein, Brachial, Left
  use Vein, Brachial, Right
Ultrafiltration
  Hemodialysis *see* Performance, Urinary 5A1D
  Therapeutic plasmapheresis *see* Pheresis, Circulatory 6A55
Ultrasonography
  Abdomen BW40ZZZ
  Abdomen and Pelvis BW41ZZZ
  Abdominal Wall BH49ZZZ
  Aorta
    Abdominal, Intravascular B440ZZ3
    Thoracic, Intravascular B340ZZ3
  Appendix BD48ZZZ
  Artery
    Brachiocephalic-Subclavian, Right, Intravascular B341ZZ3
    Celiac and Mesenteric, Intravascular B44KZZ3
    Common Carotid
      Bilateral, Intravascular B345ZZ3
      Left, Intravascular B344ZZ3
      Right, Intravascular B343ZZ3
    Coronary
      Multiple B241YZZ
        Intravascular B241ZZ3
        Transesophageal B241ZZ4
      Single B240YZZ
        Intravascular B240ZZ3
        Transesophageal B240ZZ4
    Femoral, Intravascular B44LZZ3
    Inferior Mesenteric, Intravascular B445ZZ3
    Internal Carotid
      Bilateral, Intravascular B348ZZ3
      Left, Intravascular B347ZZ3
      Right, Intravascular B346ZZ3
    Intra-Abdominal, Other, Intravascular B44BZZ3
    Intracranial, Intravascular B34RZZ3

Urethrorrhaphy *see* Repair, Urethra ØTQD
Urethroscopy ØTJD8ZZ
Urethrotomy *see* Drainage, Urethra ØT9D
Urography *see* Fluoroscopy, Urinary System BT1
Uterine artery
  use Artery, Internal Iliac, Left
  use Artery, Internal Iliac, Right
Uterine cornu *use* Uterus
Uterine tube
  use Fallopian Tube, Left
  use Fallopian Tube, Right
Uterine vein
  use Vein, Hypogastric, Left
  use Vein, Hypogastric, Right
Uvulectomy
  see Excision, Uvula ØCBN
  see Resection, Uvula ØCTN
Uvulorrhaphy *see* Repair, Uvula ØCQN
Uvulotomy *see* Drainage, Uvula ØC9N

V

Vaccination *see* Introduction, Serum, Toxoid, and
  Vaccine
Vacuum extraction, obstetric 10D07Z6
Vaginal artery
  use Artery, Internal Iliac, Right
  use Artery, Internal Iliac, Left
Vaginal vein
  use Vein, Hypogastric, Right
  use Vein, Hypogastric, Left
Vaginectomy
  see Excision, Vagina ØUBG
  see Resection, Vagina ØUTG
Vaginofixation
  see Repair, Vagina ØUQG
  see Reposition, Vagina ØUSG
Vaginoplasty
  see Repair, Vagina ØUQG
  see Supplement, Vagina ØUUG
Vaginorrhaphy *see* Repair, Vagina ØUQG
Vaginoscopy ØUJH8ZZ
Vaginotomy *see* Drainage, Female Reproductive
  System ØU9
Vagotomy *see* Division, Nerve, Vagus ØØ8Q
Valvotomy
  see Division, Heart and Great Vessels Ø28
  see Release, Heart and Great Vessels Ø2N
Valvuloplasty
  see Repair, Heart and Great Vessels Ø2Q
  see Replacement, Heart and Great Vessels Ø2R
  see Supplement, Heart and Great Vessels Ø2U
Valvulotomy
  see Division, Heart and Great Vessels Ø28
  see Release, Heart and Great Vessels Ø2N
Vascular Access Device
  Insertion of device in
    Abdomen ØJH8
    Chest ØJH6
    Lower Arm
      Left ØJHH
      Right ØJHG
    Lower Leg
      Left ØJHP
      Right ØJHN
    Upper Arm
      Left ØJHF
      Right ØJHD
    Upper Leg
      Left ØJHM
      Right ØJHL
  Removal of device from
    Lower Extremity ØJPW
    Trunk ØJPT
    Upper Extremity ØJPV
  Revision of device in
    Lower Extremity ØJWW
    Trunk ØJWT
    Upper Extremity ØJWV
Vasectomy *see* Excision, Male Reproductive System
  ØVB

Vasography
  see Plain Radiography, Male Reproductive System
    BVØ
  see Fluoroscopy, Male Reproductive System BV1
Vasoligation *see* Occlusion, Male Reproductive System
  ØVL
Vasorrhaphy *see* Repair, Male Reproductive System
  ØVQ
Vasostomy *see* Bypass, Male Reproductive System ØV1
Vasotomy
  Drainage *see* Drainage, Male Reproductive System
    ØV9
  With ligation *see* Occlusion, Male Reproductive
    System ØVL
Vasovasostomy *see* Repair, Male Reproductive System
  ØVQ
Vastus intermedius muscle
  use Muscle, Upper Leg, Right
  use Muscle, Upper Leg, Left
Vastus lateralis muscle
  use Muscle, Upper Leg, Left
  use Muscle, Upper Leg, Right
Vastus medialis muscle
  use Muscle, Upper Leg, Right
  use Muscle, Upper Leg, Left
VCG (vectorcardiogram) *see* Measurement, Cardiac 4A02
Venectomy
  see Excision, Upper Veins Ø5B
  see Excision, Lower Veins Ø6B
Venography
  see Plain Radiography, Veins B5Ø
  see Fluoroscopy, Veins B51
Venorrhaphy
  see Repair, Upper Veins Ø5Q
  see Repair, Lower Veins Ø6Q
Venotripsy
  see Occlusion, Upper Veins Ø5L
  see Occlusion, Lower Veins Ø6L
Ventricular fold *use* Larynx
Ventriculoatriostomy *see* Bypass, Central Nervous
  System ØØ1
Ventriculocisternostomy *see* Bypass, Central Nervous
  System ØØ1
Ventriculogram, cardiac
  Combined left and right heart *see* Plain
    Radiography, Heart, Right and Left B2Ø6
  Left ventricle *see* Plain Radiography, Heart, Left B2Ø5
  Right ventricle *see* Plain Radiography, Heart, Right
    B2Ø4
Ventriculopuncture, through previously implanted
  catheter 8CØ1X6J
Ventriculoscopy ØØJØ4ZZ
Ventriculostomy
  see Bypass, Cerebral Ventricle ØØ16
  see Drainage, Cerebral Ventricle ØØ96
Ventriculovenostomy *see* Bypass, Cerebral Ventricle
  ØØ16
VEP (visual evoked potential) 4AØ7XØZ
Vermiform appendix *use* Appendix
Vermilion border
  use Lip, Lower
  use Lip, Upper
Version, obstetric
  External 10SØXZZ
  Internal 10SØ7ZZ
Vertebral arch
  use Vertebra, Thoracic
  use Vertebra, Lumbar
  use Vertebra, Cervical
Vertebral canal *use* Spinal Canal
Vertebral foramen
  use Vertebra, Thoracic
  use Vertebra, Lumbar
  use Vertebra, Cervical
Vertebral lamina
  use Vertebra, Thoracic
  use Vertebra, Cervical
  use Vertebra, Lumbar
Vertebral pedicle
  use Vertebra, Lumbar
  use Vertebra, Thoracic
  use Vertebra, Cervical

Vesical vein
  use Vein, Hypogastric, Left
  use Vein, Hypogastric, Right
Vesicotomy *see* Drainage, Urinary System ØT9
Vesiculectomy
  see Excision, Male Reproductive System ØVB
  see Resection, Male Reproductive System ØVT
Vesiculogram, seminal *see* Plain Radiography, Male
  Reproductive System BVØ
Vesiculotomy *see* Drainage, Male Reproductive
  System ØV9
Vestibular (Scarpa's) ganglion *use* Nerve, Acoustic
Vestibular Assessment F15Z
Vestibular nerve *use* Nerve, Acoustic
Vestibular Treatment FØC
Vestibulocochlear nerve *use* Nerve, Acoustic
Virchow's (supraclavicular) lymph node
  use Lymphatic, Neck, Left
  use Lymphatic, Neck, Right
Vitrectomy
  see Excision, Eye Ø8B
  see Resection, Eye Ø8T
Vitreous body
  use Vitreous, Left
  use Vitreous, Right
Vocal fold
  use Vocal Cord, Left
  use Vocal Cord, Right
Vocational
  Assessment *see* Activities of Daily Living
    Assessment, Rehabilitation FØ2
  Retraining *see* Activities of Daily Living Treatment,
    Rehabilitation FØ8
Volar (palmar) digital vein
  use Vein, Hand, Left
  use Vein, Hand, Right
Volar (palmar) metacarpal vein
  use Vein, Hand, Right
  use Vein, Hand, Left
Vomer bone *use* Septum, Nasal
Vomer of nasal septum *use* Bone, Nasal
Vulvectomy
  see Excision, Female Reproductive System ØUB
  see Resection, Female Reproductive System ØUT

W

Washing *see* Irrigation
Wedge resection, pulmonary *see* Excision,
  Respiratory System ØBB
Window *see* Drainage
Wiring, dental 2W31X9Z

X

X-ray *see* Plain Radiography
Xiphoid process *use* Sternum

Y

Yoga Therapy 8EØZXY4

Z

Z-plasty, skin for scar contracture *see* Release, Skin
  and Breast ØHN
Zonule of Zinn
  use Lens, Left
  use Lens, Right
Zygomatic process of frontal bone
  use Bone, Frontal, Left
  use Bone, Frontal, Right
Zygomatic process of temporal bone
  use Bone, Temporal, Right
  use Bone, Temporal, Left
Zygomaticus muscle *use* Muscle, Facial

Tables

Central Nervous System 001–00X

Ø	**Medical and Surgical**	
Ø	**Central Nervous System**	
1	**Bypass**	Altering the route of passage of the contents of a tubular body part

Body Part Character 4	Approach Character 5	Device Character 6	Qualifier Character 7
6 Cerebral Ventricle	Ø Open	7 Autologous Tissue Substitute J Synthetic Substitute K Nonautologous Tissue Substitute	Ø Nasopharynx 1 Mastoid Sinus 2 Atrium 3 Blood Vessel 4 Pleural Cavity 5 Intestine 6 Peritoneal Cavity 7 Urinary Tract 8 Bone Marrow B Cerebral Cisterns
U Spinal Canal	Ø Open	7 Autologous Tissue Substitute J Synthetic Substitute K Nonautologous Tissue Substitute	4 Pleural Cavity 6 Peritoneal Cavity 7 Urinary Tract 9 Fallopian Tube

Ø	**Medical and Surgical**	
Ø	**Central Nervous System**	
2	**Change**	Taking out or off a device from a body part and putting back an identical or similar device in or on the same body part without cutting or puncturing the skin or a mucous membrane

Body Part Character 4	Approach Character 5	Device Character 6	Qualifier Character 7
Ø Brain E Cranial Nerve U Spinal Canal	X External	Ø Drainage Device Y Other Device	Z No Qualifier

Ø	**Medical and Surgical**	
Ø	**Central Nervous System**	
5	**Destruction**	Physical eradication of all or a portion of a body part by the direct use of energy, force, or a destructive agent

Body Part Character 4	Approach Character 5	Device Character 6	Qualifier Character 7
Ø Brain 1 Cerebral Meninges 2 Dura Mater 6 Cerebral Ventricle 7 Cerebral Hemisphere 8 Basal Ganglia 9 Thalamus A Hypothalamus B Pons C Cerebellum D Medulla Oblongata F Olfactory Nerve G Optic Nerve H Oculomotor Nerve J Trochlear Nerve K Trigeminal Nerve L Abducens Nerve M Facial Nerve N Acoustic Nerve P Glossopharyngeal Nerve Q Vagus Nerve R Accessory Nerve S Hypoglossal Nerve T Spinal Meninges W Cervical Spinal Cord X Thoracic Spinal Cord Y Lumbar Spinal Cord	Ø Open 3 Percutaneous 4 Percutaneous Endoscopic	Z No Device	Z No Qualifier

Ø   **Medical and Surgical**
Ø   **Central Nervous System**
8   **Division**   Cutting into a body part without draining fluids and/or gases from the body part in order to separate or transect a body part

Body Part Character 4	Approach Character 5	Device Character 6	Qualifier Character 7
Ø Brain **7** Cerebral Hemisphere **8** Basal Ganglia **F** Olfactory Nerve **G** Optic Nerve **H** Oculomotor Nerve **J** Trochlear Nerve **K** Trigeminal Nerve **L** Abducens Nerve **M** Facial Nerve **N** Acoustic Nerve **P** Glossopharyngeal Nerve **Q** Vagus Nerve **R** Accessory Nerve **S** Hypoglossal Nerve **W** Cervical Spinal Cord **X** Thoracic Spinal Cord **Y** Lumbar Spinal Cord	**Ø** Open **3** Percutaneous **4** Percutaneous Endoscopic	**Z** No Device	**Z** No Qualifier

Ø   **Medical and Surgical**
Ø   **Central Nervous System**
9   **Drainage**   Taking or letting out fluids and/or gases from a body part

Body Part Character 4	Approach Character 5	Device Character 6	Qualifier Character 7
Ø Brain **1** Cerebral Meninges **2** Dura Mater **3** Epidural Space **4** Subdural Space **5** Subarachnoid Space **6** Cerebral Ventricle **7** Cerebral Hemisphere **8** Basal Ganglia **9** Thalamus **A** Hypothalamus **B** Pons **C** Cerebellum **D** Medulla Oblongata **F** Olfactory Nerve **G** Optic Nerve **H** Oculomotor Nerve **J** Trochlear Nerve **K** Trigeminal Nerve **L** Abducens Nerve **M** Facial Nerve **N** Acoustic Nerve **P** Glossopharyngeal Nerve **Q** Vagus Nerve **R** Accessory Nerve **S** Hypoglossal Nerve **T** Spinal Meninges **U** Spinal Canal **W** Cervical Spinal Cord **X** Thoracic Spinal Cord **Y** Lumbar Spinal Cord	**Ø** Open **3** Percutaneous **4** Percutaneous Endoscopic	**Ø** Drainage Device	**Z** No Qualifier

Ø09 Continued on next page

     Revised Text in **BLUE**

Central Nervous System

009 Continued

0	Medical and Surgical
0	Central Nervous System
9	Drainage

Taking or letting out fluids and/or gases from a body part

Body Part Character 4	Approach Character 5	Device Character 6	Qualifier Character 7
0 Brain	0 Open	Z No Device	X Diagnostic
1 Cerebral Meninges	3 Percutaneous		Z No Qualifier
2 Dura Mater	4 Percutaneous Endoscopic		
3 Epidural Space			
4 Subdural Space			
5 Subarachnoid Space			
6 Cerebral Ventricle			
7 Cerebral Hemisphere			
8 Basal Ganglia			
9 Thalamus			
A Hypothalamus			
B Pons			
C Cerebellum			
D Medulla Oblongata			
F Olfactory Nerve			
G Optic Nerve			
H Oculomotor Nerve			
J Trochlear Nerve			
K Trigeminal Nerve			
L Abducens Nerve			
M Facial Nerve			
N Acoustic Nerve			
P Glossopharyngeal Nerve			
Q Vagus Nerve			
R Accessory Nerve			
S Hypoglossal Nerve			
T Spinal Meninges			
U Spinal Canal			
W Cervical Spinal Cord			
X Thoracic Spinal Cord			
Y Lumbar Spinal Cord			

0	Medical and Surgical
0	Central Nervous System
B	Excision

Cutting out or off, without replacement, a portion of a body part

Body Part Character 4	Approach Character 5	Device Character 6	Qualifier Character 7
0 Brain	0 Open	Z No Device	X Diagnostic
1 Cerebral Meninges	3 Percutaneous		Z No Qualifier
2 Dura Mater	4 Percutaneous Endoscopic		
6 Cerebral Ventricle			
7 Cerebral Hemisphere			
8 Basal Ganglia			
9 Thalamus			
A Hypothalamus			
B Pons			
C Cerebellum			
D Medulla Oblongata			
F Olfactory Nerve			
G Optic Nerve			
H Oculomotor Nerve			
J Trochlear Nerve			
K Trigeminal Nerve			
L Abducens Nerve			
M Facial Nerve			
N Acoustic Nerve			
P Glossopharyngeal Nerve			
Q Vagus Nerve			
R Accessory Nerve			
S Hypoglossal Nerve			
T Spinal Meninges			
W Cervical Spinal Cord			
X Thoracic Spinal Cord			
Y Lumbar Spinal Cord			

Central Nervous System

Ø   **Medical and Surgical**
Ø   **Central Nervous System**
C   **Extirpation**   Taking or cutting out solid matter from a body part

Body Part Character 4	Approach Character 5	Device Character 6	Qualifier Character 7
Ø Brain 1 Cerebral Meninges 2 Dura Mater 3 Epidural Space 4 Subdural Space 5 Subarachnoid Space 6 Cerebral Ventricle 7 Cerebral Hemisphere 8 Basal Ganglia 9 Thalamus A Hypothalamus B Pons C Cerebellum D Medulla Oblongata F Olfactory Nerve G Optic Nerve H Oculomotor Nerve J Trochlear Nerve K Trigeminal Nerve L Abducens Nerve M Facial Nerve N Acoustic Nerve P Glossopharyngeal Nerve Q Vagus Nerve R Accessory Nerve S Hypoglossal Nerve T Spinal Meninges W Cervical Spinal Cord X Thoracic Spinal Cord Y Lumbar Spinal Cord	Ø Open 3 Percutaneous 4 Percutaneous Endoscopic	Z No Device	Z No Qualifier

Ø   **Medical and Surgical**
Ø   **Central Nervous System**
D   **Extraction**   Pulling or stripping out or off all or a portion of a body part by the use of force

Body Part Character 4	Approach Character 5	Device Character 6	Qualifier Character 7
1 Cerebral Meninges 2 Dura Mater F Olfactory Nerve G Optic Nerve H Oculomotor Nerve J Trochlear Nerve K Trigeminal Nerve L Abducens Nerve M Facial Nerve N Acoustic Nerve P Glossopharyngeal Nerve Q Vagus Nerve R Accessory Nerve S Hypoglossal Nerve T Spinal Meninges	Ø Open 3 Percutaneous 4 Percutaneous Endoscopic	Z No Device	Z No Qualifier

Ø   **Medical and Surgical**
Ø   **Central Nervous System**
F   **Fragmentation**   Breaking solid matter in a body part into pieces

Body Part Character 4	Approach Character 5	Device Character 6	Qualifier Character 7
3 Epidural Space 4 Subdural Space 5 Subarachnoid Space 6 Cerebral Ventricle U Spinal Canal	Ø Open 3 Percutaneous 4 Percutaneous Endoscopic X External	Z No Device	Z No Qualifier

       Revised Text in **BLUE**

0   **Medical and Surgical**
0   **Central Nervous System**
H   **Insertion**   Putting in a nonbiological appliance that monitors, assists, performs, or prevents a physiological function but does not physically take the place of a body part

Body Part Character 4	Approach Character 5	Device Character 6	Qualifier Character 7
0 Brain 6 Cerebral Ventricle E Cranial Nerve U Spinal Canal V Spinal Cord	0 Open 3 Percutaneous 4 Percutaneous Endoscopic	2 Monitoring Device 3 Infusion Device M Neurostimulator Lead	Z No Qualifier

0   **Medical and Surgical**
0   **Central Nervous System**
J   **Inspection**   Visually and/or manually exploring a body part

Body Part Character 4	Approach Character 5	Device Character 6	Qualifier Character 7
0 Brain E Cranial Nerve U Spinal Canal V Spinal Cord	0 Open 3 Percutaneous 4 Percutaneous Endoscopic	Z No Device	Z No Qualifier

0   **Medical and Surgical**
0   **Central Nervous System**
K   **Map**   Locating the route of passage of electrical impulses and/or locating functional areas in a body part

Body Part Character 4	Approach Character 5	Device Character 6	Qualifier Character 7
0 Brain 7 Cerebral Hemisphere 8 Basal Ganglia 9 Thalamus A Hypothalamus B Pons C Cerebellum D Medulla Oblongata	0 Open 3 Percutaneous 4 Percutaneous Endoscopic	Z No Device	Z No Qualifier

0   **Medical and Surgical**
0   **Central Nervous System**
N   **Release**   Freeing a body part from an abnormal physical constraint

Body Part Character 4	Approach Character 5	Device Character 6	Qualifier Character 7
0 Brain 1 Cerebral Meninges 2 Dura Mater 6 Cerebral Ventricle 7 Cerebral Hemisphere 8 Basal Ganglia 9 Thalamus A Hypothalamus B Pons C Cerebellum D Medulla Oblongata F Olfactory Nerve G Optic Nerve H Oculomotor Nerve J Trochlear Nerve K Trigeminal Nerve L Abducens Nerve M Facial Nerve N Acoustic Nerve P Glossopharyngeal Nerve Q Vagus Nerve R Accessory Nerve S Hypoglossal Nerve T Spinal Meninges W Cervical Spinal Cord X Thoracic Spinal Cord Y Lumbar Spinal Cord	0 Open 3 Percutaneous 4 Percutaneous Endoscopic	Z No Device	Z No Qualifier

Central Nervous System

0   **Medical and Surgical**
0   **Central Nervous System**
P   **Removal**   Taking out or off a device from a body part

Body Part Character 4	Approach Character 5	Device Character 6	Qualifier Character 7
0 Brain **6** Cerebral Ventricle **E** Cranial Nerve **U** Spinal Canal **V** Spinal Cord	**X** External	**0** Drainage Device **2** Monitoring Device **3** Infusion Device **M** Neurostimulator Lead	**Z** No Qualifier
0 Brain **V** Spinal Cord	**0** Open **3** Percutaneous **4** Percutaneous Endoscopic	**0** Drainage Device **2** Monitoring Device **3** Infusion Device **7** Autologous Tissue Substitute **J** Synthetic Substitute **K** Nonautologous Tissue Substitute **M** Neurostimulator Lead	**Z** No Qualifier
6 Cerebral Ventricle **U** Spinal Canal	**0** Open **3** Percutaneous **4** Percutaneous Endoscopic	**0** Drainage Device **2** Monitoring Device **3** Infusion Device **J** Synthetic Substitute **M** Neurostimulator Lead	**Z** No Qualifier
E Cranial Nerve	**0** Open **3** Percutaneous **4** Percutaneous Endoscopic	**0** Drainage Device **2** Monitoring Device **3** Infusion Device **7** Autologous Tissue Substitute **M** Neurostimulator Lead	**Z** No Qualifier

0   **Medical and Surgical**
0   **Central Nervous System**
Q   **Repair**   Restoring, to the extent possible, a body part to its normal anatomic structure and function

Body Part Character 4	Approach Character 5	Device Character 6	Qualifier Character 7
0 Brain **1** Cerebral Meninges **2** Dura Mater **6** Cerebral Ventricle **7** Cerebral Hemisphere **8** Basal Ganglia **9** Thalamus **A** Hypothalamus **B** Pons **C** Cerebellum **D** Medulla Oblongata **F** Olfactory Nerve **G** Optic Nerve **H** Oculomotor Nerve **J** Trochlear Nerve **K** Trigeminal Nerve **L** Abducens Nerve **M** Facial Nerve **N** Acoustic Nerve **P** Glossopharyngeal Nerve **Q** Vagus Nerve **R** Accessory Nerve **S** Hypoglossal Nerve **T** Spinal Meninges **W** Cervical Spinal Cord **X** Thoracic Spinal Cord **Y** Lumbar Spinal Cord	**0** Open **3** Percutaneous **4** Percutaneous Endoscopic	**Z** No Device	**Z** No Qualifier

Ø   Medical and Surgical
Ø   Central Nervous System
S   Reposition   Moving to its normal location or other suitable location all or a portion of a body part

Body Part Character 4	Approach Character 5	Device Character 6	Qualifier Character 7
F Olfactory Nerve G Optic Nerve H Oculomotor Nerve J Trochlear Nerve K Trigeminal Nerve L Abducens Nerve M Facial Nerve N Acoustic Nerve P Glossopharyngeal Nerve Q Vagus Nerve R Accessory Nerve S Hypoglossal Nerve W Cervical Spinal Cord X Thoracic Spinal Cord Y Lumbar Spinal Cord	Ø Open 3 Percutaneous 4 Percutaneous Endoscopic	Z No Device	Z No Qualifier

Ø   Medical and Surgical
Ø   Central Nervous System
T   Resection   Cutting out or off, without replacement, all of a body part

Body Part Character 4	Approach Character 5	Device Character 6	Qualifier Character 7
7 Cerebral Hemisphere	Ø Open 3 Percutaneous 4 Percutaneous Endoscopic	Z No Device	Z No Qualifier

Ø   Medical and Surgical
Ø   Central Nervous System
U   Supplement   Putting in or on biological or synthetic material that physically reinforces and/or augments the function of a portion of a body part

Body Part Character 4	Approach Character 5	Device Character 6	Qualifier Character 7
1 Cerebral Meninges 2 Dura Mater T Spinal Meninges	Ø Open 3 Percutaneous 4 Percutaneous Endoscopic	7 Autologous Tissue Substitute J Synthetic Substitute K Nonautologous Tissue Substitute	Z No Qualifier
F Olfactory Nerve G Optic Nerve H Oculomotor Nerve J Trochlear Nerve K Trigeminal Nerve L Abducens Nerve M Facial Nerve N Acoustic Nerve P Glossopharyngeal Nerve Q Vagus Nerve R Accessory Nerve S Hypoglossal Nerve	Ø Open 3 Percutaneous 4 Percutaneous Endoscopic	7 Autologous Tissue Substitute	Z No Qualifier

Ø   Medical and Surgical
Ø   Central Nervous System
W   Revision   Correcting, to the extent possible, a portion of a malfunctioning device or the position of a displaced device

Body Part Character 4	Approach Character 5	Device Character 6	Qualifier Character 7
Ø Brain V Spinal Cord	Ø Open 3 Percutaneous 4 Percutaneous Endoscopic X External	Ø Drainage Device 2 Monitoring Device 3 Infusion Device 7 Autologous Tissue Substitute J Synthetic Substitute K Nonautologous Tissue Substitute M Neurostimulator Lead	Z No Qualifier
6 Cerebral Ventricle U Spinal Canal	Ø Open 3 Percutaneous 4 Percutaneous Endoscopic X External	Ø Drainage Device 2 Monitoring Device 3 Infusion Device J Synthetic Substitute M Neurostimulator Lead	Z No Qualifier
E Cranial Nerve	Ø Open 3 Percutaneous 4 Percutaneous Endoscopic X External	Ø Drainage Device 2 Monitoring Device 3 Infusion Device 7 Autologous Tissue Substitute M Neurostimulator Lead	Z No Qualifier

Central Nervous System

0   **Medical and Surgical**
0   **Central Nervous System**
X   **Transfer**   Moving, without taking out, all or a portion of a body part to another location to take over the function of all or a portion of a body part

Body Part Character 4	Approach Character 5	Device Character 6	Qualifier Character 7
F Olfactory Nerve G Optic Nerve H Oculomotor Nerve J Trochlear Nerve K Trigeminal Nerve L Abducens Nerve M Facial Nerve N Acoustic Nerve P Glossopharyngeal Nerve Q Vagus Nerve R Accessory Nerve S Hypoglossal Nerve	0 Open 4 Percutaneous Endoscopic	Z No Device	F Olfactory Nerve G Optic Nerve H Oculomotor Nerve J Trochlear Nerve K Trigeminal Nerve L Abducens Nerve M Facial Nerve N Acoustic Nerve P Glossopharyngeal Nerve Q Vagus Nerve R Accessory Nerve S Hypoglossal Nerve

Peripheral Nervous System Ø12–Ø1X

Ø **Medical and Surgical**
1 **Peripheral Nervous System**
2 **Change** Taking out or off a device from a body part and putting back an identical or similar device in or on the same body part without cutting or puncturing the skin or a mucous membrane

Body Part Character 4	Approach Character 5	Device Character 6	Qualifier Character 7
Y Peripheral Nerve	**X** External	**Ø** Drainage Device **Y** Other Device	**Z** No Qualifier

Ø **Medical and Surgical**
1 **Peripheral Nervous System**
5 **Destruction** Physical eradication of all or a portion of a body part by the direct use of energy, force, or a destructive agent

Body Part Character 4	Approach Character 5	Device Character 6	Qualifier Character 7
Ø Cervical Plexus **1** Cervical Nerve **2** Phrenic Nerve **3** Brachial Plexus **4** Ulnar Nerve **5** Median Nerve **6** Radial Nerve **8** Thoracic Nerve **9** Lumbar Plexus **A** Lumbosacral Plexus **B** Lumbar Nerve **C** Pudendal Nerve **D** Femoral Nerve **F** Sciatic Nerve **G** Tibial Nerve **H** Peroneal Nerve **K** Head and Neck Sympathetic Nerve **L** Thoracic Sympathetic Nerve **M** Abdominal Sympathetic Nerve **N** Lumbar Sympathetic Nerve **P** Sacral Sympathetic Nerve **Q** Sacral Plexus **R** Sacral Nerve	**Ø** Open **3** Percutaneous **4** Percutaneous Endoscopic	**Z** No Device	**Z** No Qualifier

Ø **Medical and Surgical**
1 **Peripheral Nervous System**
8 **Division** Cutting into a body part without draining fluids and/or gases from the body part in order to separate or transect a body part

Body Part Character 4	Approach Character 5	Device Character 6	Qualifier Character 7
Ø Cervical Plexus **1** Cervical Nerve **2** Phrenic Nerve **3** Brachial Plexus **4** Ulnar Nerve **5** Median Nerve **6** Radial Nerve **8** Thoracic Nerve **9** Lumbar Plexus **A** Lumbosacral Plexus **B** Lumbar Nerve **C** Pudendal Nerve **D** Femoral Nerve **F** Sciatic Nerve **G** Tibial Nerve **H** Peroneal Nerve **K** Head and Neck Sympathetic Nerve **L** Thoracic Sympathetic Nerve **M** Abdominal Sympathetic Nerve **N** Lumbar Sympathetic Nerve **P** Sacral Sympathetic Nerve **Q** Sacral Plexus **R** Sacral Nerve	**Ø** Open **3** Percutaneous **4** Percutaneous Endoscopic	**Z** No Device	**Z** No Qualifier

Peripheral Nervous System *(left margin)*

Ø **Medical and Surgical**
1 **Peripheral Nervous System**
9 **Drainage**   Taking or letting out fluids and/or gases from a body part

Body Part Character 4	Approach Character 5	Device Character 6	Qualifier Character 7
Ø Cervical Plexus 1 Cervical Nerve 2 Phrenic Nerve 3 Brachial Plexus 4 Ulnar Nerve 5 Median Nerve 6 Radial Nerve 8 Thoracic Nerve 9 Lumbar Plexus A Lumbosacral Plexus B Lumbar Nerve C Pudendal Nerve D Femoral Nerve F Sciatic Nerve G Tibial Nerve H Peroneal Nerve K Head and Neck Sympathetic Nerve L Thoracic Sympathetic Nerve M Abdominal Sympathetic Nerve N Lumbar Sympathetic Nerve P Sacral Sympathetic Nerve Q Sacral Plexus R Sacral Nerve	Ø Open 3 Percutaneous 4 Percutaneous Endoscopic	Ø Drainage Device	Z No Qualifier
Ø Cervical Plexus 1 Cervical Nerve 2 Phrenic Nerve 3 Brachial Plexus 4 Ulnar Nerve 5 Median Nerve 6 Radial Nerve 8 Thoracic Nerve 9 Lumbar Plexus A Lumbosacral Plexus B Lumbar Nerve C Pudendal Nerve D Femoral Nerve F Sciatic Nerve G Tibial Nerve H Peroneal Nerve K Head and Neck Sympathetic Nerve L Thoracic Sympathetic Nerve M Abdominal Sympathetic Nerve N Lumbar Sympathetic Nerve P Sacral Sympathetic Nerve Q Sacral Plexus R Sacral Nerve	Ø Open 3 Percutaneous 4 Percutaneous Endoscopic	Z No Device	X Diagnostic Z No Qualifier

Ø19–Ø19 (left margin)

Revised Text in **BLUE**

Ø   **Medical and Surgical**
1   **Peripheral Nervous System**
B   **Excision**   Cutting out or off, without replacement, a portion of a body part

Body Part Character 4	Approach Character 5	Device Character 6	Qualifier Character 7
Ø Cervical Plexus 1 Cervical Nerve 2 Phrenic Nerve 3 Brachial Plexus 4 Ulnar Nerve 5 Median Nerve 6 Radial Nerve 8 Thoracic Nerve 9 Lumbar Plexus A Lumbosacral Plexus B Lumbar Nerve C Pudendal Nerve D Femoral Nerve F Sciatic Nerve G Tibial Nerve H Peroneal Nerve K Head and Neck Sympathetic Nerve L Thoracic Sympathetic Nerve M Abdominal Sympathetic Nerve N Lumbar Sympathetic Nerve P Sacral Sympathetic Nerve Q Sacral Plexus R Sacral Nerve	Ø Open 3 Percutaneous 4 Percutaneous Endoscopic	Z No Device	X Diagnostic Z No Qualifier

Ø   **Medical and Surgical**
1   **Peripheral Nervous System**
C   **Extirpation**   Taking or cutting out solid matter from a body part

Body Part Character 4	Approach Character 5	Device Character 6	Qualifier Character 7
Ø Cervical Plexus 1 Cervical Nerve 2 Phrenic Nerve 3 Brachial Plexus 4 Ulnar Nerve 5 Median Nerve 6 Radial Nerve 8 Thoracic Nerve 9 Lumbar Plexus A Lumbosacral Plexus B Lumbar Nerve C Pudendal Nerve D Femoral Nerve F Sciatic Nerve G Tibial Nerve H Peroneal Nerve K Head and Neck Sympathetic Nerve L Thoracic Sympathetic Nerve M Abdominal Sympathetic Nerve N Lumbar Sympathetic Nerve P Sacral Sympathetic Nerve Q Sacral Plexus R Sacral Nerve	Ø Open 3 Percutaneous 4 Percutaneous Endoscopic	Z No Device	Z No Qualifier

Ø   **Medical and Surgical**
1   **Peripheral Nervous System**
D   **Extraction**   Pulling or stripping out or off all or a portion of a body part by the use of force

Body Part Character 4	Approach Character 5	Device Character 6	Qualifier Character 7
Ø Cervical Plexus **1** Cervical Nerve **2** Phrenic Nerve **3** Brachial Plexus **4** Ulnar Nerve **5** Median Nerve **6** Radial Nerve **8** Thoracic Nerve **9** Lumbar Plexus **A** Lumbosacral Plexus **B** Lumbar Nerve **C** Pudendal Nerve **D** Femoral Nerve **F** Sciatic Nerve **G** Tibial Nerve **H** Peroneal Nerve **K** Head and Neck Sympathetic Nerve **L** Thoracic Sympathetic Nerve **M** Abdominal Sympathetic Nerve **N** Lumbar Sympathetic Nerve **P** Sacral Sympathetic Nerve **Q** Sacral Plexus **R** Sacral Nerve	**Ø** Open **3** Percutaneous **4** Percutaneous Endoscopic	**Z** No Device	**Z** No Qualifier

Ø   **Medical and Surgical**
1   **Peripheral Nervous System**
H   **Insertion**   Putting in a nonbiological appliance that monitors, assists, performs, or prevents a physiological function but does not physically take the place of a body part

Body Part Character 4	Approach Character 5	Device Character 6	Qualifier Character 7
Y Peripheral Nerve	**Ø** Open **3** Percutaneous **4** Percutaneous Endoscopic	**2** Monitoring Device **M** Neurostimulator Lead	**Z** No Qualifier

Ø   **Medical and Surgical**
1   **Peripheral Nervous System**
J   **Inspection**   Visually and/or manually exploring a body part

Body Part Character 4	Approach Character 5	Device Character 6	Qualifier Character 7
Y Peripheral Nerve	**Ø** Open **3** Percutaneous **4** Percutaneous Endoscopic	**Z** No Device	**Z** No Qualifier

    Revised Text in **BLUE**

0   Medical and Surgical
1   Peripheral Nervous System
N   Release   Freeing a body part from an abnormal physical constraint

Body Part Character 4	Approach Character 5	Device Character 6	Qualifier Character 7
0 Cervical Plexus 1 Cervical Nerve 2 Phrenic Nerve 3 Brachial Plexus 4 Ulnar Nerve 5 Median Nerve 6 Radial Nerve 8 Thoracic Nerve 9 Lumbar Plexus A Lumbosacral Plexus B Lumbar Nerve C Pudendal Nerve D Femoral Nerve F Sciatic Nerve G Tibial Nerve H Peroneal Nerve K Head and Neck Sympathetic Nerve L Thoracic Sympathetic Nerve M Abdominal Sympathetic Nerve N Lumbar Sympathetic Nerve P Sacral Sympathetic Nerve Q Sacral Plexus R Sacral Nerve	0 Open 3 Percutaneous 4 Percutaneous Endoscopic	Z No Device	Z No Qualifier

0   Medical and Surgical
1   Peripheral Nervous System
P   Removal   Taking out or off a device from a body part

Body Part Character 4	Approach Character 5	Device Character 6	Qualifier Character 7
Y Peripheral Nerve	0 Open 3 Percutaneous 4 Percutaneous Endoscopic	0 Drainage Device 2 Monitoring Device 7 Autologous Tissue Substitute M Neurostimulator Lead	Z No Qualifier
Y Peripheral Nerve	X External	0 Drainage Device 2 Monitoring Device M Neurostimulator Lead	Z No Qualifier

0   Medical and Surgical
1   Peripheral Nervous System
Q   Repair   Restoring, to the extent possible, a body part to its normal anatomic structure and function

Body Part Character 4	Approach Character 5	Device Character 6	Qualifier Character 7
0 Cervical Plexus 1 Cervical Nerve 2 Phrenic Nerve 3 Brachial Plexus 4 Ulnar Nerve 5 Median Nerve 6 Radial Nerve 8 Thoracic Nerve 9 Lumbar Plexus A Lumbosacral Plexus B Lumbar Nerve C Pudendal Nerve D Femoral Nerve F Sciatic Nerve G Tibial Nerve H Peroneal Nerve K Head and Neck Sympathetic Nerve L Thoracic Sympathetic Nerve M Abdominal Sympathetic Nerve N Lumbar Sympathetic Nerve P Sacral Sympathetic Nerve Q Sacral Plexus R Sacral Nerve	0 Open 3 Percutaneous 4 Percutaneous Endoscopic	Z No Device	Z No Qualifier

0   Medical and Surgical
1   Peripheral Nervous System
S   Reposition   Moving to its normal location or other suitable location all or a portion of a body part

Body Part Character 4	Approach Character 5	Device Character 6	Qualifier Character 7
0 Cervical Plexus **1** Cervical Nerve **2** Phrenic Nerve **3** Brachial Plexus **4** Ulnar Nerve **5** Median Nerve **6** Radial Nerve **8** Thoracic Nerve **9** Lumbar Plexus **A** Lumbosacral Plexus **B** Lumbar Nerve **C** Pudendal Nerve **D** Femoral Nerve **F** Sciatic Nerve **G** Tibial Nerve **H** Peroneal Nerve **Q** Sacral Plexus **R** Sacral Nerve	**0** Open **3** Percutaneous **4** Percutaneous Endoscopic	**Z** No Device	**Z** No Qualifier

0   Medical and Surgical
1   Peripheral Nervous System
U   Supplement   Putting in or on biological or synthetic material that physically reinforces and/or augments the function of a portion of a body part

Body Part Character 4	Approach Character 5	Device Character 6	Qualifier Character 7
1 Cervical Nerve **2** Phrenic Nerve **4** Ulnar Nerve **5** Median Nerve **6** Radial Nerve **8** Thoracic Nerve **B** Lumbar Nerve **C** Pudendal Nerve **D** Femoral Nerve **F** Sciatic Nerve **G** Tibial Nerve **H** Peroneal Nerve **R** Sacral Nerve	**0** Open **3** Percutaneous **4** Percutaneous Endoscopic	**7** Autologous Tissue Substitute	**Z** No Qualifier

0   Medical and Surgical
1   Peripheral Nervous System
W   Revision   Correcting, to the extent possible, a portion of a malfunctioning device or the position of a displaced device

Body Part Character 4	Approach Character 5	Device Character 6	Qualifier Character 7
Y Peripheral Nerve	**0** Open **3** Percutaneous **4** Percutaneous Endoscopic **X** External	**0** Drainage Device **2** Monitoring Device **7** Autologous Tissue Substitute **M** Neurostimulator Lead	**Z** No Qualifier

0   Medical and Surgical
1   Peripheral Nervous System
X   Transfer   Moving, without taking out, all or a portion of a body part to another location to take over the function of all or a portion of a body part

Body Part Character 4	Approach Character 5	Device Character 6	Qualifier Character 7
1 Cervical Nerve **2** Phrenic Nerve	**0** Open **4** Percutaneous Endoscopic	**Z** No Device	**1** Cervical Nerve **2** Phrenic Nerve
4 Ulnar Nerve **5** Median Nerve **6** Radial Nerve	**0** Open **4** Percutaneous Endoscopic	**Z** No Device	**4** Ulnar Nerve **5** Median Nerve **6** Radial Nerve
8 Thoracic Nerve	**0** Open **4** Percutaneous Endoscopic	**Z** No Device	**8** Thoracic Nerve
B Lumbar Nerve **C** Pudendal Nerve	**0** Open **4** Percutaneous Endoscopic	**Z** No Device	**B** Lumbar Nerve **C** Perineal Nerve
D Femoral Nerve **F** Sciatic Nerve **G** Tibial Nerve **H** Peroneal Nerve	**0** Open **4** Percutaneous Endoscopic	**Z** No Device	**D** Femoral Nerve **F** Sciatic Nerve **G** Tibial Nerve **H** Peroneal Nerve

Heart and Great Vessels Ø21–Ø2Y

Ø **Medical and Surgical**
2 **Heart and Great Vessels**
1 **Bypass**　　　Altering the route of passage of the contents of a tubular body part

Body Part Character 4	Approach Character 5	Device Character 6	Qualifier Character 7
Ø Coronary Artery, One Site 1 Coronary Artery, Two Sites 2 Coronary Artery, Three Sites 3 Coronary Artery, Four or More Sites	Ø Open 4 Percutaneous Endoscopic	9 Autologous Venous Tissue A Autologous Arterial Tissue J Synthetic Substitute K Nonautologous Tissue Substitute	3 Coronary Artery 8 Internal Mammary, Right 9 Internal Mammary, Left C Thoracic Artery F Abdominal Artery W Aorta
Ø Coronary Artery, One Site 1 Coronary Artery, Two Sites 2 Coronary Artery, Three Sites 3 Coronary Artery, Four or More Sites	Ø Open 4 Percutaneous Endoscopic	Z No Device	3 Coronary Artery 8 Internal Mammary, Right 9 Internal Mammary, Left C Thoracic Artery F Abdominal Artery
Ø Coronary Artery, One Site 1 Coronary Artery, Two Sites 2 Coronary Artery, Three Sites 3 Coronary Artery, Four or More Sites	3 Percutaneous 4 Percutaneous Endoscopic	4 Drug-eluting Intraluminal Device D Intraluminal Device	4 Coronary Vein
6 Atrium, Right	Ø Open 4 Percutaneous Endoscopic	Z No Device	7 Atrium, Left P Pulmonary Trunk Q Pulmonary Artery, Right R Pulmonary Artery, Left
6 Atrium, Right K Ventricle, Right L Ventricle, Left	Ø Open 4 Percutaneous Endoscopic	9 Autologous Venous Tissue A Autologous Arterial Tissue J Synthetic Substitute K Nonautologous Tissue Substitute	P Pulmonary Trunk Q Pulmonary Artery, Right R Pulmonary Artery, Left
7 Atrium, Left V Superior Vena Cava	Ø Open 4 Percutaneous Endoscopic	9 Autologous Venous Tissue A Autologous Arterial Tissue J Synthetic Substitute K Nonautologous Tissue Substitute Z No Device	P Pulmonary Trunk Q Pulmonary Artery, Right R Pulmonary Artery, Left
K Ventricle, Right L Ventricle, Left	Ø Open 4 Percutaneous Endoscopic	Z No Device	5 Coronary Circulation 8 Internal Mammary, Right 9 Internal Mammary, Left C Thoracic Artery F Abdominal Artery P Pulmonary Trunk Q Pulmonary Artery, Right R Pulmonary Artery, Left W Aorta
W Thoracic Aorta	Ø Open 4 Percutaneous Endoscopic	9 Autologous Venous Tissue A Autologous Arterial Tissue J Synthetic Substitute K Nonautologous Tissue Substitute Z No Device	B Subclavian D Carotid P Pulmonary Trunk Q Pulmonary Artery, Right R Pulmonary Artery, Left

Revised Text in **BLUE**

Heart and Great Vessels

025–028

Ø   **Medical and Surgical**
2   **Heart and Great Vessels**
5   **Destruction**   Physical eradication of all or a portion of a body part by the direct use of energy, force, or a destructive agent

Body Part Character 4	Approach Character 5	Device Character 6	Qualifier Character 7
4 Coronary Vein 5 Atrial Septum 6 Atrium, Right 7 Atrium, Left 8 Conduction Mechanism 9 Chordae Tendineae D Papillary Muscle F Aortic Valve G Mitral Valve H Pulmonary Valve J Tricuspid Valve K Ventricle, Right L Ventricle, Left M Ventricular Septum N Pericardium P Pulmonary Trunk Q Pulmonary Artery, Right R Pulmonary Artery, Left S Pulmonary Vein, Right T Pulmonary Vein, Left V Superior Vena Cava W Thoracic Aorta	Ø Open 3 Percutaneous 4 Percutaneous Endoscopic	Z No Device	Z No Qualifier

Ø   **Medical and Surgical**
2   **Heart and Great Vessels**
7   **Dilation**   Expanding an orifice or the lumen of a tubular body part

Body Part Character 4	Approach Character 5	Device Character 6	Qualifier Character 7
Ø Coronary Artery, One Site 1 Coronary Artery, Two Sites 2 Coronary Artery, Three Sites 3 Coronary Artery, Four or More Sites	Ø Open 3 Percutaneous 4 Percutaneous Endoscopic	4 Drug-eluting Intraluminal Device D Intraluminal Device T Radioactive Intraluminal Device Z No Device	6 Bifurcation Z No Qualifier
F Aortic Valve G Mitral Valve H Pulmonary Valve J Tricuspid Valve K Ventricle, Right P Pulmonary Trunk Q Pulmonary Artery, Right S Pulmonary Vein, Right T Pulmonary Vein, Left V Superior Vena Cava W Thoracic Aorta	Ø Open 3 Percutaneous 4 Percutaneous Endoscopic	4 Drug-eluting Intraluminal Device D Intraluminal Device Z No Device	Z No Qualifier
R Pulmonary Artery, Left	Ø Open 3 Percutaneous 4 Percutaneous Endoscopic	4 Drug-eluting Intraluminal Device D Intraluminal Device Z No Device	T Ductus Arteriosus Z No Qualifier

Ø   **Medical and Surgical**
2   **Heart and Great Vessels**
8   **Division**   Cutting into a body part without draining fluids and/or gases from the body part in order to separate or transect a body part

Body Part Character 4	Approach Character 5	Device Character 6	Qualifier Character 7
8 Conduction Mechanism 9 Chordae Tendineae D Papillary Muscle	Ø Open 3 Percutaneous 4 Percutaneous Endoscopic	Z No Device	Z No Qualifier

Revised Text in **BLUE**

0　Medical and Surgical
2　Heart and Great Vessels
B　Excision　　Cutting out or off, without replacement, a portion of a body part

Body Part Character 4	Approach Character 5	Device Character 6	Qualifier Character 7
4 Coronary Vein 5 Atrial Septum 6 Atrium, Right 7 Atrium, Left 8 Conduction Mechanism 9 Chordae Tendineae D Papillary Muscle F Aortic Valve G Mitral Valve H Pulmonary Valve J Tricuspid Valve K Ventricle, Right L Ventricle, Left M Ventricular Septum N Pericardium P Pulmonary Trunk Q Pulmonary Artery, Right R Pulmonary Artery, Left S Pulmonary Vein, Right T Pulmonary Vein, Left V Superior Vena Cava W Thoracic Aorta	0 Open 3 Percutaneous 4 Percutaneous Endoscopic	Z No Device	X Diagnostic Z No Qualifier

0　Medical and Surgical
2　Heart and Great Vessels
C　Extirpation　　Taking or cutting out solid matter from a body part

Body Part Character 4	Approach Character 5	Device Character 6	Qualifier Character 7
0 Coronary Artery, One Site 1 Coronary Artery, Two Sites 2 Coronary Artery, Three Sites 3 Coronary Artery, Four or More Sites 4 Coronary Vein 5 Atrial Septum 6 Atrium, Right 7 Atrium, Left 8 Conduction Mechanism 9 Chordae Tendineae D Papillary Muscle F Aortic Valve G Mitral Valve H Pulmonary Valve J Tricuspid Valve K Ventricle, Right L Ventricle, Left M Ventricular Septum N Pericardium P Pulmonary Trunk Q Pulmonary Artery, Right R Pulmonary Artery, Left S Pulmonary Vein, Right T Pulmonary Vein, Left V Superior Vena Cava W Thoracic Aorta	0 Open 3 Percutaneous 4 Percutaneous Endoscopic	Z No Device	Z No Qualifier

0　Medical and Surgical
2　Heart and Great Vessels
F　Fragmentation　　Breaking solid matter in a body part into pieces

Body Part Character 4	Approach Character 5	Device Character 6	Qualifier Character 7
N Pericardium	0 Open 3 Percutaneous 4 Percutaneous Endoscopic X External	Z No Device	Z No Qualifier

Ø Medical and Surgical
2 Heart and Great Vessels
H Insertion Putting in a nonbiological appliance that monitors, assists, performs, or prevents a physiological function but does not physically take the place of a body part

Body Part Character 4	Approach Character 5	Device Character 6	Qualifier Character 7
4 Coronary Vein **6** Atrium, Right **7** Atrium, Left **K** Ventricle, Right **L** Ventricle, Left **N** Pericardium	**Ø** Open **3** Percutaneous **4** Percutaneous Endoscopic	**M** Cardiac Lead	**A** Pacemaker Lead **E** Defibrillator Lead **Z** No Qualifier
4 Coronary Vein **6** Atrium, Right **7** Atrium, Left **K** Ventricle, Right **L** Ventricle, Left **N** Pericardium **P** Pulmonary Trunk **Q** Pulmonary Artery, Right **R** Pulmonary Artery, Left **S** Pulmonary Vein, Right **T** Pulmonary Vein, Left **V** Superior Vena Cava **W** Thoracic Aorta	**Ø** Open **3** Percutaneous **4** Percutaneous Endoscopic	**2** Monitoring Device	**G** Pressure Sensor **Z** No Qualifier
4 Coronary Vein **6** Atrium, Right **7** Atrium, Left **K** Ventricle, Right **L** Ventricle, Left **P** Pulmonary Trunk **Q** Pulmonary Artery, Right **R** Pulmonary Artery, Left **S** Pulmonary Vein, Right **T** Pulmonary Vein, Left **V** Superior Vena Cava **W** Thoracic Aorta	**Ø** Open **3** Percutaneous **4** Percutaneous Endoscopic	**3** Infusion Device **D** Intraluminal Device	**Z** No Qualifier
A Heart	**Ø** Open **3** Percutaneous **4** Percutaneous Endoscopic	**Q** Implantable Heart Assist System	**Z** No Qualifier
A Heart	**Ø** Open **3** Percutaneous **4** Percutaneous Endoscopic	**R** External Heart Assist System	**S** Biventricular **Z** No Qualifier

Ø Medical and Surgical
2 Heart and Great Vessels
J Inspection Visually and/or manually exploring a body part

Body Part Character 4	Approach Character 5	Device Character 6	Qualifier Character 7
A Heart **Y** Great Vessel	**Ø** Open **3** Percutaneous **4** Percutaneous Endoscopic	**Z** No Device	**Z** No Qualifier

Ø Medical and Surgical
2 Heart and Great Vessels
K Map Locating the route of passage of electrical impulses and/or locating functional areas in a body part

Body Part Character 4	Approach Character 5	Device Character 6	Qualifier Character 7
8 Conduction Mechanism	**Ø** Open **3** Percutaneous **4** Percutaneous Endoscopic	**Z** No Device	**Z** No Qualifier

Ø Medical and Surgical
2 Heart and Great Vessels
L Occlusion   Completely closing an orifice or the lumen of a tubular body part

Body Part Character 4	Approach Character 5	Device Character 6	Qualifier Character 7
R Pulmonary Artery, Left	**Ø** Open **3** Percutaneous **4** Percutaneous Endoscopic	**C** Extraluminal Device **D** Intraluminal Device **Z** No Device	**T** Ductus Arteriosus
S Pulmonary Vein, Right **T** Pulmonary Vein, Left **V** Superior Vena Cava	**Ø** Open **3** Percutaneous **4** Percutaneous Endoscopic	**C** Extraluminal Device **D** Intraluminal Device **Z** No Device	**Z** No Qualifier

Ø Medical and Surgical
2 Heart and Great Vessels
N Release   Freeing a body part from an abnormal physical constraint

Body Part Character 4	Approach Character 5	Device Character 6	Qualifier Character 7
4 Coronary Vein **5** Atrial Septum **6** Atrium, Right **7** Atrium, Left **8** Conduction Mechanism **9** Chordae Tendineae **D** Papillary Muscle **F** Aortic Valve **G** Mitral Valve **H** Pulmonary Valve **J** Tricuspid Valve **K** Ventricle, Right **L** Ventricle, Left **M** Ventricular Septum **N** Pericardium **P** Pulmonary Trunk **Q** Pulmonary Artery, Right **R** Pulmonary Artery, Left **S** Pulmonary Vein, Right **T** Pulmonary Vein, Left **V** Superior Vena Cava **W** Thoracic Aorta	**Ø** Open **3** Percutaneous **4** Percutaneous Endoscopic	**Z** No Device	**Z** No Qualifier

Ø Medical and Surgical
2 Heart and Great Vessels
P Removal   Taking out or off a device from a body part

Body Part Character 4	Approach Character 5	Device Character 6	Qualifier Character 7
A Heart	**Ø** Open **3** Percutaneous **4** Percutaneous Endoscopic	**2** Monitoring Device **3** Infusion Device **4** Drug-eluting Intraluminal Device **7** Autologous Tissue Substitute **8** Zooplastic Tissue **9** Autologous Venous Tissue **A** Autologous Arterial Tissue **C** Extraluminal Device **D** Intraluminal Device **J** Synthetic Substitute **K** Nonautologous Tissue Substitute **M** Cardiac Lead **Q** Implantable Heart Assist System **R** External Heart Assist System **T** Radioactive Intraluminal Device	**Z** No Qualifier
A Heart	**X** External	**2** Monitoring Device **3** Infusion Device **4** Drug-eluting Intraluminal Device **D** Intraluminal Device **M** Cardiac Lead **T** Radioactive Intraluminal Device	**Z** No Qualifier

02P Continued on next page

02P Continued

0   Medical and Surgical
2   Heart and Great Vessels
P   Removal   Taking out or off a device from a body part

Body Part Character 4	Approach Character 5	Device Character 6	Qualifier Character 7
Y Great Vessel	**0** Open **3** Percutaneous **4** Percutaneous Endoscopic	**2** Monitoring Device **3** Infusion Device **4** Drug-eluting Intraluminal Device **7** Autologous Tissue Substitute **8** Zooplastic Tissue **9** Autologous Venous Tissue **A** Autologous Arterial Tissue **C** Extraluminal Device **D** Intraluminal Device **J** Synthetic Substitute **K** Nonautologous Tissue Substitute	**Z** No Qualifier
Y Great Vessel	**X** External	**2** Monitoring Device **3** Infusion Device **4** Drug-eluting Intraluminal Device **D** Intraluminal Device	**Z** No Qualifier

0   Medical and Surgical
2   Heart and Great Vessels
Q   Repair   Restoring, to the extent possible, a body part to its normal anatomic structure and function

Body Part Character 4	Approach Character 5	Device Character 6	Qualifier Character 7
0 Coronary Artery, One Site **1** Coronary Artery, Two Sites **2** Coronary Artery, Three Sites **3** Coronary Artery, Four or More Sites **4** Coronary Vein **5** Atrial Septum **6** Atrium, Right **7** Atrium, Left **8** Conduction Mechanism **9** Chordae Tendineae **A** Heart **B** Heart, Right **C** Heart, Left **D** Papillary Muscle **F** Aortic Valve **G** Mitral Valve **H** Pulmonary Valve **J** Tricuspid Valve **K** Ventricle, Right **L** Ventricle, Left **M** Ventricular Septum **N** Pericardium **P** Pulmonary Trunk **Q** Pulmonary Artery, Right **R** Pulmonary Artery, Left **S** Pulmonary Vein, Right **T** Pulmonary Vein, Left **V** Superior Vena Cava **W** Thoracic Aorta	**0** Open **3** Percutaneous **4** Percutaneous Endoscopic	**Z** No Device	**Z** No Qualifier

0　**Medical and Surgical**
2　**Heart and Great Vessels**
R　**Replacement**　　Putting in or on biological or synthetic material that physically takes the place and/or function of all or a portion of a body part

Body Part Character 4	Approach Character 5	Device Character 6	Qualifier Character 7
5 Atrial Septum **6** Atrium, Right **7** Atrium, Left **9** Chordae Tendineae **D** Papillary Muscle **J** Tricuspid Valve **K** Ventricle, Right **L** Ventricle, Left **M** Ventricular Septum **N** Pericardium **P** Pulmonary Trunk **Q** Pulmonary Artery, Right **R** Pulmonary Artery, Left **S** Pulmonary Vein, Right **T** Pulmonary Vein, Left **V** Superior Vena Cava **W** Thoracic Aorta	**0** Open **4** Percutaneous Endoscopic	**7** Autologous Tissue Substitute **8** Zooplastic Tissue **J** Synthetic Substitute **K** Nonautologous Tissue Substitute	**Z** No Qualifier
F Aortic Valve **G** Mitral Valve **H** Pulmonary Valve	**0** Open **3** Percutaneous **4** Percutaneous Endoscopic	**7** Autologous Tissue Substitute **8** Zooplastic Tissue **J** Synthetic Substitute **K** Nonautologous Tissue Substitute	**Z** No Qualifier

0　**Medical and Surgical**
2　**Heart and Great Vessels**
S　**Reposition**　　Moving to its normal location or other suitable location all or a portion of a body part

Body Part Character 4	Approach Character 5	Device Character 6	Qualifier Character 7
P Pulmonary Trunk **Q** Pulmonary Artery, Right **R** Pulmonary Artery, Left **S** Pulmonary Vein, Right **T** Pulmonary Vein, Left **V** Superior Vena Cava **W** Thoracic Aorta	**0** Open	**Z** No Device	**Z** No Qualifier

0　**Medical and Surgical**
2　**Heart and Great Vessels**
T　**Resection**　　Cutting out or off, without replacement, all of a body part

Body Part Character 4	Approach Character 5	Device Character 6	Qualifier Character 7
5 Atrial Septum **8** Conduction Mechanism **9** Chordae Tendineae **D** Papillary Muscle **H** Pulmonary Valve **M** Ventricular Septum **N** Pericardium	**0** Open **3** Percutaneous **4** Percutaneous Endoscopic	**Z** No Device	**Z** No Qualifier

Ø Medical and Surgical
2 Heart and Great Vessels
U Supplement   Putting in or on biological or synthetic material that physically reinforces and/or augments the function of a portion of a body part

Body Part Character 4	Approach Character 5	Device Character 6	Qualifier Character 7
5 Atrial Septum 6 Atrium, Right 7 Atrium, Left 9 Chordae Tendineae A Heart D Papillary Muscle F Aortic Valve G Mitral Valve H Pulmonary Valve J Tricuspid Valve K Ventricle, Right L Ventricle, Left M Ventricular Septum N Pericardium P Pulmonary Trunk Q Pulmonary Artery, Right R Pulmonary Artery, Left S Pulmonary Vein, Right T Pulmonary Vein, Left V Superior Vena Cava W Thoracic Aorta	Ø Open 3 Percutaneous 4 Percutaneous Endoscopic	7 Autologous Tissue Substitute 8 Zooplastic Tissue J Synthetic Substitute K Nonautologous Tissue Substitute	Z No Qualifier

Ø Medical and Surgical
2 Heart and Great Vessels
V Restriction   Partially closing an orifice or the lumen of a tubular body part

Body Part Character 4	Approach Character 5	Device Character 6	Qualifier Character 7
A Heart	Ø Open 3 Percutaneous 4 Percutaneous Endoscopic	C Extraluminal Device Z No Device	Z No Qualifier
P Pulmonary Trunk Q Pulmonary Artery, Right S Pulmonary Vein, Right T Pulmonary Vein, Left V Superior Vena Cava W Thoracic Aorta	Ø Open 3 Percutaneous 4 Percutaneous Endoscopic	C Extraluminal Device D Intraluminal Device Z No Device	Z No Qualifier
R Pulmonary Artery, Left	Ø Open 3 Percutaneous 4 Percutaneous Endoscopic	C Extraluminal Device D Intraluminal Device Z No Device	T Ductus Arteriosus Z No Qualifier

Ø　**Medical and Surgical**
2　**Heart and Great Vessels**
W　**Revision**　　Correcting, to the extent possible, a portion of a malfunctioning device or the position of a displaced device

Body Part Character 4	Approach Character 5	Device Character 6	Qualifier Character 7
5　Atrial Septum M　Ventricular Septum	Ø　Open 4　Percutaneous Endoscopic	J　Synthetic Substitute	Z　No Qualifier
A　Heart	Ø　Open 3　Percutaneous 4　Percutaneous Endoscopic X　External	2　Monitoring Device 3　Infusion Device 4　Drug-eluting Intraluminal Device 7　Autologous Tissue Substitute 8　Zooplastic Tissue 9　Autologous Venous Tissue A　Autologous Arterial Tissue C　Extraluminal Device D　Intraluminal Device J　Synthetic Substitute K　Nonautologous Tissue Substitute M　Cardiac Lead Q　Implantable Heart Assist System R　External Heart Assist System T　Radioactive Intraluminal Device	Z　No Qualifier
F　Aortic Valve G　Mitral Valve H　Pulmonary Valve J　Tricuspid Valve	Ø　Open 4　Percutaneous Endoscopic	7　Autologous Tissue Substitute 8　Zooplastic Tissue J　Synthetic Substitute K　Nonautologous Tissue Substitute	Z　No Qualifier
Y　Great Vessel	Ø　Open 3　Percutaneous 4　Percutaneous Endoscopic X　External	2　Monitoring Device 3　Infusion Device 4　Drug-eluting Intraluminal Device 7　Autologous Tissue Substitute 8　Zooplastic Tissue 9　Autologous Venous Tissue A　Autologous Arterial Tissue C　Extraluminal Device D　Intraluminal Device J　Synthetic Substitute K　Nonautologous Tissue Substitute	Z　No Qualifier

Ø　**Medical and Surgical**
2　**Heart and Great Vessels**
Y　**Transplantation**　Putting in or on all or a portion of a living body part taken from another individual or animal to physically take the place and/or function of all or a portion of a similar body part

Body Part Character 4	Approach Character 5	Device Character 6	Qualifier Character 7
A　Heart	Ø　Open	Z　No Device	Ø　Allogeneic 1　Syngeneic 2　Zooplastic

Upper Arteries Ø31–Ø3W

Ø   **Medical and Surgical**
3   **Upper Arteries**
1   **Bypass**   Altering the route of passage of the contents of a tubular body part

Body Part Character 4	Approach Character 5	Device Character 6	Qualifier Character 7
2 Innominate Artery 5 Axillary Artery, Right 6 Axillary Artery, Left	Ø Open	9 Autologous Venous Tissue A Autologous Arterial Tissue J Synthetic Substitute K Nonautologous Tissue Substitute Z No Device	Ø Upper Arm Artery, Right 1 Upper Arm Artery, Left 2 Upper Arm Artery, Bilateral 3 Lower Arm Artery, Right 4 Lower Arm Artery, Left 5 Lower Arm Artery, Bilateral 6 Upper Leg Artery, Right 7 Upper Leg Artery, Left 8 Upper Leg Artery, Bilateral 9 Lower Leg Artery, Right B Lower Leg Artery, Left C Lower Leg Artery, Bilateral D Upper Arm Vein F Lower Arm Vein J Extracranial Artery, Right K Extracranial Artery, Left
3 Subclavian Artery, Right 4 Subclavian Artery, Left	Ø Open	9 Autologous Venous Tissue A Autologous Arterial Tissue J Synthetic Substitute K Nonautologous Tissue Substitute Z No Device	Ø Upper Arm Artery, Right 1 Upper Arm Artery, Left 2 Upper Arm Artery, Bilateral 3 Lower Arm Artery, Right 4 Lower Arm Artery, Left 5 Lower Arm Artery, Bilateral 6 Upper Leg Artery, Right 7 Upper Leg Artery, Left 8 Upper Leg Artery, Bilateral 9 Lower Leg Artery, Right B Lower Leg Artery, Left C Lower Leg Artery, Bilateral D Upper Arm Vein F Lower Arm Vein J Extracranial Artery, Right K Extracranial Artery, Left M Pulmonary Artery, Right N Pulmonary Artery, Left
7 Brachial Artery, Right	Ø Open	9 Autologous Venous Tissue A Autologous Arterial Tissue J Synthetic Substitute K Nonautologous Tissue Substitute Z No Device	Ø Upper Arm Artery, Right 3 Lower Arm Artery, Right D Upper Arm Vein F Lower Arm Vein
8 Brachial Artery, Left	Ø Open	9 Autologous Venous Tissue A Autologous Arterial Tissue J Synthetic Substitute K Nonautologous Tissue Substitute Z No Device	1 Upper Arm Artery, Left 4 Lower Arm Artery, Left D Upper Arm Vein F Lower Arm Vein
9 Ulnar Artery, Right B Radial Artery, Right	Ø Open	9 Autologous Venous Tissue A Autologous Arterial Tissue J Synthetic Substitute K Nonautologous Tissue Substitute Z No Device	3 Lower Arm Artery, Right F Lower Arm Vein
A Ulnar Artery, Left C Radial Artery, Left	Ø Open	9 Autologous Venous Tissue A Autologous Arterial Tissue J Synthetic Substitute K Nonautologous Tissue Substitute Z No Device	4 Lower Arm Artery, Left F Lower Arm Vein
G Intracranial Artery S Temporal Artery, Right T Temporal Artery, Left	Ø Open	9 Autologous Venous Tissue A Autologous Arterial Tissue J Synthetic Substitute K Nonautologous Tissue Substitute Z No Device	G Intracranial Artery
H Common Carotid Artery, Right K Internal Carotid Artery, Right M External Carotid Artery, Right	Ø Open	9 Autologous Venous Tissue A Autologous Arterial Tissue J Synthetic Substitute K Nonautologous Tissue Substitute Z No Device	J Extracranial Artery, Right
J Common Carotid Artery, Left L Internal Carotid Artery, Left N External Carotid Artery, Left	Ø Open	9 Autologous Venous Tissue A Autologous Arterial Tissue J Synthetic Substitute K Nonautologous Tissue Substitute Z No Device	K Extracranial Artery, Left

     Revised Text in **BLUE**   © 2011 Ingenix, Inc

Ø **Medical and Surgical**
3 **Upper Arteries**
5 **Destruction**　　　Physical eradication of all or a portion of a body part by the direct use of energy, force, or a destructive agent

Body Part Character 4	Approach Character 5	Device Character 6	Qualifier Character 7
Ø Internal Mammary Artery, Right **1** Internal Mammary Artery, Left **2** Innominate Artery **3** Subclavian Artery, Right **4** Subclavian Artery, Left **5** Axillary Artery, Right **6** Axillary Artery, Left **7** Brachial Artery, Right **8** Brachial Artery, Left **9** Ulnar Artery, Right **A** Ulnar Artery, Left **B** Radial Artery, Right **C** Radial Artery, Left **D** Hand Artery, Right **F** Hand Artery, Left **G** Intracranial Artery **H** Common Carotid Artery, Right **J** Common Carotid Artery, Left **K** Internal Carotid Artery, Right **L** Internal Carotid Artery, Left **M** External Carotid Artery, Right **N** External Carotid Artery, Left **P** Vertebral Artery, Right **Q** Vertebral Artery, Left **R** Face Artery **S** Temporal Artery, Right **T** Temporal Artery, Left **U** Thyroid Artery, Right **V** Thyroid Artery, Left **Y** Upper Artery	**Ø** Open **3** Percutaneous **4** Percutaneous Endoscopic	**Z** No Device	**Z** No Qualifier

Ø **Medical and Surgical**
3 **Upper Arteries**
7 **Dilation**　　　Expanding an orifice or the lumen of a tubular body part

Body Part Character 4	Approach Character 5	Device Character 6	Qualifier Character 7
Ø Internal Mammary Artery, Right **1** Internal Mammary Artery, Left **2** Innominate Artery **3** Subclavian Artery, Right **4** Subclavian Artery, Left **5** Axillary Artery, Right **6** Axillary Artery, Left **7** Brachial Artery, Right **8** Brachial Artery, Left **9** Ulnar Artery, Right **A** Ulnar Artery, Left **B** Radial Artery, Right **C** Radial Artery, Left **D** Hand Artery, Right **F** Hand Artery, Left **G** Intracranial Artery **H** Common Carotid Artery, Right **J** Common Carotid Artery, Left **K** Internal Carotid Artery, Right **L** Internal Carotid Artery, Left **M** External Carotid Artery, Right **N** External Carotid Artery, Left **P** Vertebral Artery, Right **Q** Vertebral Artery, Left **R** Face Artery **S** Temporal Artery, Right **T** Temporal Artery, Left **U** Thyroid Artery, Right **V** Thyroid Artery, Left **Y** Upper Artery	**Ø** Open **3** Percutaneous **4** Percutaneous Endoscopic	**4** Drug-eluting Intraluminal Device **D** Intraluminal Device **Z** No Device	**Z** No Qualifier

Ø   Medical and Surgical
3   Upper Arteries
9   Drainage   Taking or letting out fluids and/or gases from a body part

Body Part Character 4	Approach Character 5	Device Character 6	Qualifier Character 7
Ø Internal Mammary Artery, Right 1 Internal Mammary Artery, Left 2 Innominate Artery 3 Subclavian Artery, Right 4 Subclavian Artery, Left 5 Axillary Artery, Right 6 Axillary Artery, Left 7 Brachial Artery, Right 8 Brachial Artery, Left 9 Ulnar Artery, Right A Ulnar Artery, Left B Radial Artery, Right C Radial Artery, Left D Hand Artery, Right F Hand Artery, Left G Intracranial Artery H Common Carotid Artery, Right J Common Carotid Artery, Left K Internal Carotid Artery, Right L Internal Carotid Artery, Left M External Carotid Artery, Right N External Carotid Artery, Left P Vertebral Artery, Right Q Vertebral Artery, Left R Face Artery S Temporal Artery, Right T Temporal Artery, Left U Thyroid Artery, Right V Thyroid Artery, Left Y Upper Artery	Ø Open 3 Percutaneous 4 Percutaneous Endoscopic	Ø Drainage Device	Z No Qualifier
Ø Internal Mammary Artery, Right 1 Internal Mammary Artery, Left 2 Innominate Artery 3 Subclavian Artery, Right 4 Subclavian Artery, Left 5 Axillary Artery, Right 6 Axillary Artery, Left 7 Brachial Artery, Right 8 Brachial Artery, Left 9 Ulnar Artery, Right A Ulnar Artery, Left B Radial Artery, Right C Radial Artery, Left D Hand Artery, Right F Hand Artery, Left G Intracranial Artery H Common Carotid Artery, Right J Common Carotid Artery, Left K Internal Carotid Artery, Right L Internal Carotid Artery, Left M External Carotid Artery, Right N External Carotid Artery, Left P Vertebral Artery, Right Q Vertebral Artery, Left R Face Artery S Temporal Artery, Right T Temporal Artery, Left U Thyroid Artery, Right V Thyroid Artery, Left Y Upper Artery	Ø Open 3 Percutaneous 4 Percutaneous Endoscopic	Z No Device	X Diagnostic Z No Qualifier

Revised Text in **BLUE**

0　Medical and Surgical
3　Upper Arteries
B　Excision　　　Cutting out or off, without replacement, a portion of a body part

Body Part Character 4	Approach Character 5	Device Character 6	Qualifier Character 7
0　Internal Mammary Artery, Right 1　Internal Mammary Artery, Left 2　Innominate Artery 3　Subclavian Artery, Right 4　Subclavian Artery, Left 5　Axillary Artery, Right 6　Axillary Artery, Left 7　Brachial Artery, Right 8　Brachial Artery, Left 9　Ulnar Artery, Right A　Ulnar Artery, Left B　Radial Artery, Right C　Radial Artery, Left D　Hand Artery, Right F　Hand Artery, Left G　Intracranial Artery H　Common Carotid Artery, Right J　Common Carotid Artery, Left K　Internal Carotid Artery, Right L　Internal Carotid Artery, Left M　External Carotid Artery, Right N　External Carotid Artery, Left P　Vertebral Artery, Right Q　Vertebral Artery, Left R　Face Artery S　Temporal Artery, Right T　Temporal Artery, Left U　Thyroid Artery, Right V　Thyroid Artery, Left Y　Upper Artery	0　Open 3　Percutaneous 4　Percutaneous Endoscopic	Z　No Device	X　Diagnostic Z　No Qualifier

0　Medical and Surgical
3　Upper Arteries
C　Extirpation　　　Taking or cutting out solid matter from a body part

Body Part Character 4	Approach Character 5	Device Character 6	Qualifier Character 7
0　Internal Mammary Artery, Right 1　Internal Mammary Artery, Left 2　Innominate Artery 3　Subclavian Artery, Right 4　Subclavian Artery, Left 5　Axillary Artery, Right 6　Axillary Artery, Left 7　Brachial Artery, Right 8　Brachial Artery, Left 9　Ulnar Artery, Right A　Ulnar Artery, Left B　Radial Artery, Right C　Radial Artery, Left D　Hand Artery, Right F　Hand Artery, Left G　Intracranial Artery H　Common Carotid Artery, Right J　Common Carotid Artery, Left K　Internal Carotid Artery, Right L　Internal Carotid Artery, Left M　External Carotid Artery, Right N　External Carotid Artery, Left P　Vertebral Artery, Right Q　Vertebral Artery, Left R　Face Artery S　Temporal Artery, Right T　Temporal Artery, Left U　Thyroid Artery, Right V　Thyroid Artery, Left Y　Upper Artery	0　Open 3　Percutaneous 4　Percutaneous Endoscopic	Z　No Device	Z　No Qualifier

Upper Arteries

0   Medical and Surgical
3   Upper Arteries
H   Insertion   Putting in a nonbiological appliance that monitors, assists, performs, or prevents a physiological function but does not physically take the place of a body part

Body Part Character 4	Approach Character 5	Device Character 6	Qualifier Character 7
0 Internal Mammary Artery, Right 1 Internal Mammary Artery, Left 2 Innominate Artery 3 Subclavian Artery, Right 4 Subclavian Artery, Left 5 Axillary Artery, Right 6 Axillary Artery, Left 7 Brachial Artery, Right 8 Brachial Artery, Left 9 Ulnar Artery, Right A Ulnar Artery, Left B Radial Artery, Right C Radial Artery, Left D Hand Artery, Right F Hand Artery, Left G Intracranial Artery H Common Carotid Artery, Right J Common Carotid Artery, Left M External Carotid Artery, Right N External Carotid Artery, Left P Vertebral Artery, Right Q Vertebral Artery, Left R Face Artery S Temporal Artery, Right T Temporal Artery, Left U Thyroid Artery, Right V Thyroid Artery, Left	0 Open 3 Percutaneous 4 Percutaneous Endoscopic	3 Infusion Device D Intraluminal Device	Z No Qualifier
K Internal Carotid Artery, Right L Internal Carotid Artery, Left	0 Open 3 Percutaneous 4 Percutaneous Endoscope	3 Infusion Device D Intraluminal Device **M Stimulator Lead**	Z No Qualifier
Y Upper Artery	0 Open 3 Percutaneous 4 Percutaneous Endoscopic	2 Monitoring Device 3 Infusion Device D Intraluminal Device	Z No Qualifier

0   Medical and Surgical
3   Upper Arteries
J   Inspection   Visually and/or manually exploring a body part

Body Part Character 4	Approach Character 5	Device Character 6	Qualifier Character 7
Y Upper Artery	0 Open 3 Percutaneous 4 Percutaneous Endoscopic X External	Z No Device	Z No Qualifier

0   Medical and Surgical
3   Upper Arteries
L   Occlusion   Completely closing an orifice or the lumen of a tubular body part

Body Part Character 4	Approach Character 5	Device Character 6	Qualifier Character 7
0 Internal Mammary Artery, Right 1 Internal Mammary Artery, Left 2 Innominate Artery 3 Subclavian Artery, Right 4 Subclavian Artery, Left 5 Axillary Artery, Right 6 Axillary Artery, Left 7 Brachial Artery, Right 8 Brachial Artery, Left 9 Ulnar Artery, Right A Ulnar Artery, Left B Radial Artery, Right C Radial Artery, Left D Hand Artery, Right F Hand Artery, Left R Face Artery S Temporal Artery, Right T Temporal Artery, Left U Thyroid Artery, Right V Thyroid Artery, Left Y Upper Artery	0 Open 3 Percutaneous 4 Percutaneous Endoscopic	C Extraluminal Device D Intraluminal Device Z No Device	Z No Qualifier

03L Continued on next page

Ø Medical and Surgical
3 Upper Arteries   *03L Continued*
L Occlusion   Completely closing an orifice or the lumen of a tubular body part

Body Part Character 4	Approach Character 5	Device Character 6	Qualifier Character 7
G Intracranial Artery **H** Common Carotid Artery, Right **J** Common Carotid Artery, Left **K** Internal Carotid Artery, Right **L** Internal Carotid Artery, Left **M** External Carotid Artery, Right **N** External Carotid Artery, Left **P** Vertebral Artery, Right **Q** Vertebral Artery, Left	**Ø** Open **3** Percutaneous **4** Percutaneous Endoscopic	**B** Bioactive Intraluminal Device **C** Extraluminal Device **D** Intraluminal Device **Z** No Device	**Z** No Qualifier

Ø Medical and Surgical
3 Upper Arteries
N Release   Freeing a body part from an abnormal physical constraint

Body Part Character 4	Approach Character 5	Device Character 6	Qualifier Character 7
Ø Internal Mammary Artery, Right **1** Internal Mammary Artery, Left **2** Innominate Artery **3** Subclavian Artery, Right **4** Subclavian Artery, Left **5** Axillary Artery, Right **6** Axillary Artery, Left **7** Brachial Artery, Right **8** Brachial Artery, Left **9** Ulnar Artery, Right **A** Ulnar Artery, Left **B** Radial Artery, Right **C** Radial Artery, Left **D** Hand Artery, Right **F** Hand Artery, Left **G** Intracranial Artery **H** Common Carotid Artery, Right **J** Common Carotid Artery, Left **K** Internal Carotid Artery, Right **L** Internal Carotid Artery, Left **M** External Carotid Artery, Right **N** External Carotid Artery, Left **P** Vertebral Artery, Right **Q** Vertebral Artery, Left **R** Face Artery **S** Temporal Artery, Right **T** Temporal Artery, Left **U** Thyroid Artery, Right **V** Thyroid Artery, Left **Y** Upper Artery	**Ø** Open **3** Percutaneous **4** Percutaneous Endoscopic	**Z** No Device	**Z** No Qualifier

Ø Medical and Surgical
3 Upper Arteries
P Removal   Taking out or off a device from a body part

Body Part Character 4	Approach Character 5	Device Character 6	Qualifier Character 7
Y Upper Artery	**Ø** Open **3** Percutaneous **4** Percutaneous Endoscopic	**Ø** Drainage Device **2** Monitoring Device **3** Infusion Device **4** Drug-eluting Intraluminal Device **7** Autologous Tissue Substitute **9** Autologous Venous Tissue **A** Autologous Arterial Tissue **B** Bioactive Intraluminal Device **C** Extraluminal Device **D** Intraluminal Device **J** Synthetic Substitute **K** Nonautologous Tissue Substitute **M** **Stimulator Lead**	**Z** No Qualifier
Y Upper Artery	**X** External	**Ø** Drainage Device **2** Monitoring Device **3** Infusion Device **4** Drug-eluting Intraluminal Device **B** Bioactive Intraluminal Device **D** Intraluminal Device **M** **Stimulator Lead**	**Z** No Qualifier

Upper Arteries

0   **Medical and Surgical**
3   **Upper Arteries**
Q   **Repair**   Restoring, to the extent possible, a body part to its normal anatomic structure and function

Body Part Character 4	Approach Character 5	Device Character 6	Qualifier Character 7
0 Internal Mammary Artery, Right **1** Internal Mammary Artery, Left **2** Innominate Artery **3** Subclavian Artery, Right **4** Subclavian Artery, Left **5** Axillary Artery, Right **6** Axillary Artery, Left **7** Brachial Artery, Right **8** Brachial Artery, Left **9** Ulnar Artery, Right **A** Ulnar Artery, Left **B** Radial Artery, Right **C** Radial Artery, Left **D** Hand Artery, Right **F** Hand Artery, Left **G** Intracranial Artery **H** Common Carotid Artery, Right **J** Common Carotid Artery, Left **K** Internal Carotid Artery, Right **L** Internal Carotid Artery, Left **M** External Carotid Artery, Right **N** External Carotid Artery, Left **P** Vertebral Artery, Right **Q** Vertebral Artery, Left **R** Face Artery **S** Temporal Artery, Right **T** Temporal Artery, Left **U** Thyroid Artery, Right **V** Thyroid Artery, Left **Y** Upper Artery	**0** Open **3** Percutaneous **4** Percutaneous Endoscopic	**Z** No Device	**Z** No Qualifier

0   **Medical and Surgical**
3   **Upper Arteries**
R   **Replacement**   Putting in or on biological or synthetic material that physically takes the place and/or function of all or a portion of a body part

Body Part Character 4	Approach Character 5	Device Character 6	Qualifier Character 7
0 Internal Mammary Artery, Right **1** Internal Mammary Artery, Left **2** Innominate Artery **3** Subclavian Artery, Right **4** Subclavian Artery, Left **5** Axillary Artery, Right **6** Axillary Artery, Left **7** Brachial Artery, Right **8** Brachial Artery, Left **9** Ulnar Artery, Right **A** Ulnar Artery, Left **B** Radial Artery, Right **C** Radial Artery, Left **D** Hand Artery, Right **F** Hand Artery, Left **G** Intracranial Artery **H** Common Carotid Artery, Right **J** Common Carotid Artery, Left **K** Internal Carotid Artery, Right **L** Internal Carotid Artery, Left **M** External Carotid Artery, Right **N** External Carotid Artery, Left **P** Vertebral Artery, Right **Q** Vertebral Artery, Left **R** Face Artery **S** Temporal Artery, Right **T** Temporal Artery, Left **U** Thyroid Artery, Right **V** Thyroid Artery, Left **Y** Upper Artery	**0** Open **4** Percutaneous Endoscopic	**7** Autologous Tissue Substitute **J** Synthetic Substitute **K** Nonautologous Tissue Substitute	**Z** No Qualifier

0　Medical and Surgical
3　Upper Arteries
S　Reposition　　Moving to its normal location or other suitable location all or a portion of a body part

Body Part Character 4	Approach Character 5	Device Character 6	Qualifier Character 7
0　Internal Mammary Artery, Right	0　Open	Z　No Device	Z　No Qualifier
1　Internal Mammary Artery, Left	3　Percutaneous		
2　Innominate Artery	4　Percutaneous Endoscopic		
3　Subclavian Artery, Right			
4　Subclavian Artery, Left			
5　Axillary Artery, Right			
6　Axillary Artery, Left			
7　Brachial Artery, Right			
8　Brachial Artery, Left			
9　Ulnar Artery, Right			
A　Ulnar Artery, Left			
B　Radial Artery, Right			
C　Radial Artery, Left			
D　Hand Artery, Right			
F　Hand Artery, Left			
G　Intracranial Artery			
H　Common Carotid Artery, Right			
J　Common Carotid Artery, Left			
K　Internal Carotid Artery, Right			
L　Internal Carotid Artery, Left			
M　External Carotid Artery, Right			
N　External Carotid Artery, Left			
P　Vertebral Artery, Right			
Q　Vertebral Artery, Left			
R　Face Artery			
S　Temporal Artery, Right			
T　Temporal Artery, Left			
U　Thyroid Artery, Right			
V　Thyroid Artery, Left			
Y　Upper Artery			

0　Medical and Surgical
3　Upper Arteries
U　Supplement　　Putting in or on biological or synthetic material that physically reinforces and/or augments the function of a portion of a body part

Body Part Character 4	Approach Character 5	Device Character 6	Qualifier Character 7
0　Internal Mammary Artery, Right	0　Open	7　Autologous Tissue Substitute	Z　No Qualifier
1　Internal Mammary Artery, Left	3　Percutaneous	J　Synthetic Substitute	
2　Innominate Artery	4　Percutaneous Endoscopic	K　Nonautologous Tissue Substitute	
3　Subclavian Artery, Right			
4　Subclavian Artery, Left			
5　Axillary Artery, Right			
6　Axillary Artery, Left			
7　Brachial Artery, Right			
8　Brachial Artery, Left			
9　Ulnar Artery, Right			
A　Ulnar Artery, Left			
B　Radial Artery, Right			
C　Radial Artery, Left			
D　Hand Artery, Right			
F　Hand Artery, Left			
G　Intracranial Artery			
H　Common Carotid Artery, Right			
J　Common Carotid Artery, Left			
K　Internal Carotid Artery, Right			
L　Internal Carotid Artery, Left			
M　External Carotid Artery, Right			
N　External Carotid Artery, Left			
P　Vertebral Artery, Right			
Q　Vertebral Artery, Left			
R　Face Artery			
S　Temporal Artery, Right			
T　Temporal Artery, Left			
U　Thyroid Artery, Right			
V　Thyroid Artery, Left			
Y　Upper Artery			

0 Medical and Surgical
3 Upper Arteries
V Restriction   Partially closing an orifice or the lumen of a tubular body part

Body Part Character 4	Approach Character 5	Device Character 6	Qualifier Character 7
0 Internal Mammary Artery, Right 1 Internal Mammary Artery, Left 2 Innominate Artery 3 Subclavian Artery, Right 4 Subclavian Artery, Left 5 Axillary Artery, Right 6 Axillary Artery, Left 7 Brachial Artery, Right 8 Brachial Artery, Left 9 Ulnar Artery, Right A Ulnar Artery, Left B Radial Artery, Right C Radial Artery, Left D Hand Artery, Right F Hand Artery, Left R Face Artery S Temporal Artery, Right T Temporal Artery, Left U Thyroid Artery, Right V Thyroid Artery, Left Y Upper Artery	0 Open 3 Percutaneous 4 Percutaneous Endoscopic	C Extraluminal Device D Intraluminal Device Z No Device	Z No Qualifier
G Intracranial Artery H Common Carotid Artery, Right J Common Carotid Artery, Left K Internal Carotid Artery, Right L Internal Carotid Artery, Left M External Carotid Artery, Right N External Carotid Artery, Left P Vertebral Artery, Right Q Vertebral Artery, Left	0 Open 3 Percutaneous 4 Percutaneous Endoscopic	B Bioactive Intraluminal Device C Extraluminal Device D Intraluminal Device Z No Device	Z No Qualifier

0 Medical and Surgical
3 Upper Arteries
W Revision   Correcting, to the extent possible, a portion of a malfunctioning device or the position of a displaced device

Body Part Character 4	Approach Character 5	Device Character 6	Qualifier Character 7
Y Upper Artery	0 Open 3 Percutaneous 4 Percutaneous Endoscopic X External	0 Drainage Device 2 Monitoring Device 3 Infusion Device 4 Drug-eluting Intraluminal Device 7 Autologous Tissue Substitute 9 Autologous Venous Tissue A Autologous Arterial Tissue B Bioactive Intraluminal Device C Extraluminal Device D Intraluminal Device J Synthetic Substitute K Nonautologous Tissue Substitute **M Stimulator Lead**	Z No Qualifier

Lower Arteries 041–04W

0   **Medical and Surgical**
4   **Lower Arteries**
1   **Bypass**   Altering the route of passage of the contents of a tubular body part

Body Part Character 4	Approach Character 5	Device Character 6	Qualifier Character 7
0 Abdominal Aorta **C** Common Iliac Artery, Right **D** Common Iliac Artery, Left	**0** Open **4** Percutaneous Endoscopic	**9** Autologous Venous Tissue **A** Autologous Arterial Tissue **J** Synthetic Substitute **K** Nonautologous Tissue Substitute **Z** No Device	**0** Abdominal Aorta **1** Celiac Artery **2** Mesenteric Artery **3** Renal Artery, Right **4** Renal Artery, Left **5** Renal Artery, Bilateral **6** Common Iliac Artery, Right **7** Common Iliac Artery, Left **8** Common Iliac Arteries, Bilateral **9** Internal Iliac Artery, Right **B** Internal Iliac Artery, Left **C** Internal Iliac Arteries, Bilateral **D** External Iliac Artery, Right **F** External Iliac Artery, Left **G** External Iliac Arteries, Bilateral **H** Femoral Artery, Right **J** Femoral Artery, Left **K** Femoral Arteries, Bilateral **Q** Lower Extremity Artery **R** Lower Artery
4 Splenic Artery	**0** Open **4** Percutaneous Endoscopic	**9** Autologous Venous Tissue **A** Autologous Arterial Tissue **J** Synthetic Substitute **K** Nonautologous Tissue Substitute **Z** No Device	**3** Renal Artery, Right **4** Renal Artery, Left **5** Renal Artery, Bilateral
E Internal Iliac Artery, Right **F** Internal Iliac Artery, Left **H** External Iliac Artery, Right **J** External Iliac Artery, Left	**0** Open **4** Percutaneous Endoscopic	**9** Autologous Venous Tissue **A** Autologous Arterial Tissue **J** Synthetic Substitute **K** Nonautologous Tissue Substitute **Z** No Device	**9** Internal Iliac Artery, Right **B** Internal Iliac Artery, Left **C** Internal Iliac Arteries, Bilateral **D** External Iliac Artery, Right **F** External Iliac Artery, Left **G** External Iliac Arteries, Bilateral **H** Femoral Artery, Right **J** Femoral Artery, Left **K** Femoral Arteries, Bilateral **P** Foot Artery **Q** Lower Extremity Artery
K Femoral Artery, Right **L** Femoral Artery, Left	**0** Open **4** Percutaneous Endoscopic	**9** Autologous Venous Tissue **A** Autologous Arterial Tissue **J** Synthetic Substitute **K** Nonautologous Tissue Substitute **Z** No Device	**H** Femoral Artery, Right **J** Femoral Artery, Left **K** Femoral Arteries, Bilateral **L** Popliteal Artery **M** Peroneal Artery **N** Posterior Tibial Artery **P** Foot Artery **Q** Lower Extremity Artery **S** Lower Extremity Vein
M Popliteal Artery, Right **N** Popliteal Artery, Left	**0** Open **4** Percutaneous Endoscopic	**9** Autologous Venous Tissue **A** Autologous Arterial Tissue **J** Synthetic Substitute **K** Nonautologous Tissue Substitute **Z** No Device	**L** Popliteal Artery **M** Peroneal Artery **P** Foot Artery **Q** Lower Extremity Artery **S** Lower Extremity Vein

0   Medical and Surgical
4   Lower Arteries
5   Destruction   Physical eradication of all or a portion of a body part by the direct use of energy, force, or a destructive agent

Body Part Character 4	Approach Character 5	Device Character 6	Qualifier Character 7
0 Abdominal Aorta **1** Celiac Artery **2** Gastric Artery **3** Hepatic Artery **4** Splenic Artery **5** Superior Mesenteric Artery **6** Colic Artery, Right **7** Colic Artery, Left **8** Colic Artery, Middle **9** Renal Artery, Right **A** Renal Artery, Left **B** Inferior Mesenteric Artery **C** Common Iliac Artery, Right **D** Common Iliac Artery, Left **E** Internal Iliac Artery, Right **F** Internal Iliac Artery, Left **H** External Iliac Artery, Right **J** External Iliac Artery, Left **K** Femoral Artery, Right **L** Femoral Artery, Left **M** Popliteal Artery, Right **N** Popliteal Artery, Left **P** Anterior Tibial Artery, Right **Q** Anterior Tibial Artery, Left **R** Posterior Tibial Artery, Right **S** Posterior Tibial Artery, Left **T** Peroneal Artery, Right **U** Peroneal Artery, Left **V** Foot Artery, Right **W** Foot Artery, Left **Y** Lower Artery	**0** Open **3** Percutaneous **4** Percutaneous Endoscopic	**Z** No Device	**Z** No Qualifier

0   Medical and Surgical
4   Lower Arteries
7   Dilation   Expanding an orifice or the lumen of a tubular body part

Body Part Character 4	Approach Character 5	Device Character 6	Qualifier Character 7
0 Abdominal Aorta **1** Celiac Artery **2** Gastric Artery **3** Hepatic Artery **4** Splenic Artery **5** Superior Mesenteric Artery **6** Colic Artery, Right **7** Colic Artery, Left **8** Colic Artery, Middle **9** Renal Artery, Right **A** Renal Artery, Left **B** Inferior Mesenteric Artery **C** Common Iliac Artery, Right **D** Common Iliac Artery, Left **E** Internal Iliac Artery, Right **F** Internal Iliac Artery, Left **H** External Iliac Artery, Right **J** External Iliac Artery, Left **K** Femoral Artery, Right **L** Femoral Artery, Left **M** Popliteal Artery, Right **N** Popliteal Artery, Left **P** Anterior Tibial Artery, Right **Q** Anterior Tibial Artery, Left **R** Posterior Tibial Artery, Right **S** Posterior Tibial Artery, Left **T** Peroneal Artery, Right **U** Peroneal Artery, Left **V** Foot Artery, Right **W** Foot Artery, Left **Y** Lower Artery	**0** Open **3** Percutaneous **4** Percutaneous Endoscopic	**4** Drug-eluting Intraluminal Device **D** Intraluminal Device **Z** No Device	**Z** No Qualifier

0 Medical and Surgical
4 Lower Arteries
9 Drainage   Taking or letting out fluids and/or gases from a body part

Body Part Character 4	Approach Character 5	Device Character 6	Qualifier Character 7
0 Abdominal Aorta **1** Celiac Artery **2** Gastric Artery **3** Hepatic Artery **4** Splenic Artery **5** Superior Mesenteric Artery **6** Colic Artery, Right **7** Colic Artery, Left **8** Colic Artery, Middle **9** Renal Artery, Right **A** Renal Artery, Left **B** Inferior Mesenteric Artery **C** Common Iliac Artery, Right **D** Common Iliac Artery, Left **E** Internal Iliac Artery, Right **F** Internal Iliac Artery, Left **H** External Iliac Artery, Right **J** External Iliac Artery, Left **K** Femoral Artery, Right **L** Femoral Artery, Left **M** Popliteal Artery, Right **N** Popliteal Artery, Left **P** Anterior Tibial Artery, Right **Q** Anterior Tibial Artery, Left **R** Posterior Tibial Artery, Right **S** Posterior Tibial Artery, Left **T** Peroneal Artery, Right **U** Peroneal Artery, Left **V** Foot Artery, Right **W** Foot Artery, Left **Y** Lower Artery	**0** Open **3** Percutaneous **4** Percutaneous Endoscopic	**0** Drainage Device	**Z** No Qualifier
0 Abdominal Aorta **1** Celiac Artery **2** Gastric Artery **3** Hepatic Artery **4** Splenic Artery **5** Superior Mesenteric Artery **6** Colic Artery, Right **7** Colic Artery, Left **8** Colic Artery, Middle **9** Renal Artery, Right **A** Renal Artery, Left **B** Inferior Mesenteric Artery **C** Common Iliac Artery, Right **D** Common Iliac Artery, Left **E** Internal Iliac Artery, Right **F** Internal Iliac Artery, Left **H** External Iliac Artery, Right **J** External Iliac Artery, Left **K** Femoral Artery, Right **L** Femoral Artery, Left **M** Popliteal Artery, Right **N** Popliteal Artery, Left **P** Anterior Tibial Artery, Right **Q** Anterior Tibial Artery, Left **R** Posterior Tibial Artery, Right **S** Posterior Tibial Artery, Left **T** Peroneal Artery, Right **U** Peroneal Artery, Left **V** Foot Artery, Right **W** Foot Artery, Left **Y** Lower Artery	**0** Open **3** Percutaneous **4** Percutaneous Endoscopic	**Z** No Device	**X** Diagnostic **Z** No Qualifier

Lower Arteries *(side tab)*

0　Medical and Surgical
4　Lower Arteries
B　Excision　　Cutting out or off, without replacement, a portion of a body part

Body Part Character 4	Approach Character 5	Device Character 6	Qualifier Character 7
0　Abdominal Aorta 1　Celiac Artery 2　Gastric Artery 3　Hepatic Artery 4　Splenic Artery 5　Superior Mesenteric Artery 6　Colic Artery, Right 7　Colic Artery, Left 8　Colic Artery, Middle 9　Renal Artery, Right A　Renal Artery, Left B　Inferior Mesenteric Artery C　Common Iliac Artery, Right D　Common Iliac Artery, Left E　Internal Iliac Artery, Right F　Internal Iliac Artery, Left H　External Iliac Artery, Right J　External Iliac Artery, Left K　Femoral Artery, Right L　Femoral Artery, Left M　Popliteal Artery, Right N　Popliteal Artery, Left P　Anterior Tibial Artery, Right Q　Anterior Tibial Artery, Left R　Posterior Tibial Artery, Right S　Posterior Tibial Artery, Left T　Peroneal Artery, Right U　Peroneal Artery, Left V　Foot Artery, Right W　Foot Artery, Left Y　Lower Artery	0　Open 3　Percutaneous 4　Percutaneous Endoscopic	Z　No Device	X　Diagnostic Z　No Qualifier

0　Medical and Surgical
4　Lower Arteries
C　Extirpation　　Taking or cutting out solid matter from a body part

Body Part Character 4	Approach Character 5	Device Character 6	Qualifier Character 7
0　Abdominal Aorta 1　Celiac Artery 2　Gastric Artery 3　Hepatic Artery 4　Splenic Artery 5　Superior Mesenteric Artery 6　Colic Artery, Right 7　Colic Artery, Left 8　Colic Artery, Middle 9　Renal Artery, Right A　Renal Artery, Left B　Inferior Mesenteric Artery C　Common Iliac Artery, Right D　Common Iliac Artery, Left E　Internal Iliac Artery, Right F　Internal Iliac Artery, Left H　External Iliac Artery, Right J　External Iliac Artery, Left K　Femoral Artery, Right L　Femoral Artery, Left M　Popliteal Artery, Right N　Popliteal Artery, Left P　Anterior Tibial Artery, Right Q　Anterior Tibial Artery, Left R　Posterior Tibial Artery, Right S　Posterior Tibial Artery, Left T　Peroneal Artery, Right U　Peroneal Artery, Left V　Foot Artery, Right W　Foot Artery, Left Y　Lower Artery	0　Open 3　Percutaneous 4　Percutaneous Endoscopic	Z　No Device	Z　No Qualifier

Revised Text in **BLUE**

0　Medical and Surgical
4　Lower Arteries
H　Insertion　　Putting in a nonbiological appliance that monitors, assists, performs, or prevents a physiological function but does not physically take the place of a body part

Body Part Character 4	Approach Character 5	Device Character 6	Qualifier Character 7
0　Abdominal Aorta	0　Open 3　Percutaneous 4　Percutaneous Endoscopic	2　Monitoring Device 3　Infusion Device D　Intraluminal Device	Z　No Qualifier
1　Celiac Artery 2　Gastric Artery 3　Hepatic Artery 4　Splenic Artery 5　Superior Mesenteric Artery 6　Colic Artery, Right 7　Colic Artery, Left 8　Colic Artery, Middle 9　Renal Artery, Right A　Renal Artery, Left B　Inferior Mesenteric Artery C　Common Iliac Artery, Right D　Common Iliac Artery, Left E　Internal Iliac Artery, Right F　Internal Iliac Artery, Left H　External Iliac Artery, Right J　External Iliac Artery, Left K　Femoral Artery, Right L　Femoral Artery, Left M　Popliteal Artery, Right N　Popliteal Artery, Left P　Anterior Tibial Artery, Right Q　Anterior Tibial Artery, Left R　Posterior Tibial Artery, Right S　Posterior Tibial Artery, Left T　Peroneal Artery, Right U　Peroneal Artery, Left V　Foot Artery, Right W　Foot Artery, Left	0　Open 3　Percutaneous 4　Percutaneous Endoscopic	3　Infusion Device	Z　No Qualifier
Y　Lower Artery	0　Open 3　Percutaneous 4　Percutaneous Endoscopic	2　Monitoring Device 3　Infusion Device	Z　No Qualifier

0　Medical and Surgical
4　Lower Arteries
J　Inspection　　Visually and/or manually exploring a body part

Body Part Character 4	Approach Character 5	Device Character 6	Qualifier Character 7
Y　Lower Artery	0　Open 3　Percutaneous 4　Percutaneous Endoscopic X　External	Z　No Device	Z　No Qualifier

　　　　　　　Revised Text in **BLUE**

Ø   Medical and Surgical
4   Lower Arteries
L   Occlusion   Completely closing an orifice or the lumen of a tubular body part

Body Part Character 4	Approach Character 5	Device Character 6	Qualifier Character 7
Ø Abdominal Aorta 1 Celiac Artery 2 Gastric Artery 3 Hepatic Artery 4 Splenic Artery 5 Superior Mesenteric Artery 6 Colic Artery, Right 7 Colic Artery, Left 8 Colic Artery, Middle 9 Renal Artery, Right A Renal Artery, Left B Inferior Mesenteric Artery C Common Iliac Artery, Right D Common Iliac Artery, Left E Internal Iliac Artery, Right F Internal Iliac Artery, Left H External Iliac Artery, Right J External Iliac Artery, Left K Femoral Artery, Right L Femoral Artery, Left M Popliteal Artery, Right N Popliteal Artery, Left P Anterior Tibial Artery, Right Q Anterior Tibial Artery, Left R Posterior Tibial Artery, Right S Posterior Tibial Artery, Left T Peroneal Artery, Right U Peroneal Artery, Left V Foot Artery, Right W Foot Artery, Left Y Lower Artery	Ø Open 3 Percutaneous 4 Percutaneous Endoscopic	C Extraluminal Device D Intraluminal Device Z No Device	Z No Qualifier

Ø   Medical and Surgical
4   Lower Arteries
N   Release   Freeing a body part from an abnormal physical constraint

Body Part Character 4	Approach Character 5	Device Character 6	Qualifier Character 7
Ø Abdominal Aorta 1 Celiac Artery 2 Gastric Artery 3 Hepatic Artery 4 Splenic Artery 5 Superior Mesenteric Artery 6 Colic Artery, Right 7 Colic Artery, Left 8 Colic Artery, Middle 9 Renal Artery, Right A Renal Artery, Left B Inferior Mesenteric Artery C Common Iliac Artery, Right D Common Iliac Artery, Left E Internal Iliac Artery, Right F Internal Iliac Artery, Left H External Iliac Artery, Right J External Iliac Artery, Left K Femoral Artery, Right L Femoral Artery, Left M Popliteal Artery, Right N Popliteal Artery, Left P Anterior Tibial Artery, Right Q Anterior Tibial Artery, Left R Posterior Tibial Artery, Right S Posterior Tibial Artery, Left T Peroneal Artery, Right U Peroneal Artery, Left V Foot Artery, Right W Foot Artery, Left Y Lower Artery	Ø Open 3 Percutaneous 4 Percutaneous Endoscopic	Z No Device	Z No Qualifier

0   **Medical and Surgical**
4   **Lower Arteries**
P   **Removal**   Taking out or off a device from a body part

Body Part Character 4	Approach Character 5	Device Character 6	Qualifier Character 7
Y Lower Artery	**0** Open **3** Percutaneous **4** Percutaneous Endoscopic	**0** Drainage Device **2** Monitoring Device **3** Infusion Device **4** Drug-eluting Intraluminal Device **7** Autologous Tissue Substitute **9** Autologous Venous Tissue **A** Autologous Arterial Tissue **C** Extraluminal Device **D** Intraluminal Device **J** Synthetic Substitute **K** Nonautologous Tissue Substitute	**Z** No Qualifier
Y Lower Artery	**X** External	**0** Drainage Device **1** Radioactive Element **2** Monitoring Device **3** Infusion Device **4** Drug-eluting Intraluminal Device **D** Intraluminal Device	**Z** No Qualifier

0   **Medical and Surgical**
4   **Lower Arteries**
Q   **Repair**   Restoring, to the extent possible, a body part to its normal anatomic structure and function

Body Part Character 4	Approach Character 5	Device Character 6	Qualifier Character 7
0 Abdominal Aorta **1** Celiac Artery **2** Gastric Artery **3** Hepatic Artery **4** Splenic Artery **5** Superior Mesenteric Artery **6** Colic Artery, Right **7** Colic Artery, Left **8** Colic Artery, Middle **9** Renal Artery, Right **A** Renal Artery, Left **B** Inferior Mesenteric Artery **C** Common Iliac Artery, Right **D** Common Iliac Artery, Left **E** Internal Iliac Artery, Right **F** Internal Iliac Artery, Left **H** External Iliac Artery, Right **J** External Iliac Artery, Left **K** Femoral Artery, Right **L** Femoral Artery, Left **M** Popliteal Artery, Right **N** Popliteal Artery, Left **P** Anterior Tibial Artery, Right **Q** Anterior Tibial Artery, Left **R** Posterior Tibial Artery, Right **S** Posterior Tibial Artery, Left **T** Peroneal Artery, Right **U** Peroneal Artery, Left **V** Foot Artery, Right **W** Foot Artery, Left **Y** Lower Artery	**0** Open **3** Percutaneous **4** Percutaneous Endoscopic	**Z** No Device	**Z** No Qualifier

0   **Medical and Surgical**
4   **Lower Arteries**
R   **Replacement**   Putting in or on biological or synthetic material that physically takes the place and/or function of all or a portion of a body part

Body Part Character 4	Approach Character 5	Device Character 6	Qualifier Character 7
0 Abdominal Aorta **1** Celiac Artery **2** Gastric Artery **3** Hepatic Artery **4** Splenic Artery **5** Superior Mesenteric Artery **6** Colic Artery, Right **7** Colic Artery, Left **8** Colic Artery, Middle **9** Renal Artery, Right **A** Renal Artery, Left **B** Inferior Mesenteric Artery **C** Common Iliac Artery, Right **D** Common Iliac Artery, Left **E** Internal Iliac Artery, Right **F** Internal Iliac Artery, Left **H** External Iliac Artery, Right **J** External Iliac Artery, Left **K** Femoral Artery, Right **L** Femoral Artery, Left **M** Popliteal Artery, Right **N** Popliteal Artery, Left **P** Anterior Tibial Artery, Right **Q** Anterior Tibial Artery, Left **R** Posterior Tibial Artery, Right **S** Posterior Tibial Artery, Left **T** Peroneal Artery, Right **U** Peroneal Artery, Left **V** Foot Artery, Right **W** Foot Artery, Left **Y** Lower Artery	**0** Open **4** Percutaneous Endoscopic	**7** Autologous Tissue Substitute **J** Synthetic Substitute **K** Nonautologous Tissue Substitute	**Z** No Qualifier

0   **Medical and Surgical**
4   **Lower Arteries**
S   **Reposition**   Moving to its normal location or other suitable location all or a portion of a body part

Body Part Character 4	Approach Character 5	Device Character 6	Qualifier Character 7
0 Abdominal Aorta **1** Celiac Artery **2** Gastric Artery **3** Hepatic Artery **4** Splenic Artery **5** Superior Mesenteric Artery **6** Colic Artery, Right **7** Colic Artery, Left **8** Colic Artery, Middle **9** Renal Artery, Right **A** Renal Artery, Left **B** Inferior Mesenteric Artery **C** Common Iliac Artery, Right **D** Common Iliac Artery, Left **E** Internal Iliac Artery, Right **F** Internal Iliac Artery, Left **H** External Iliac Artery, Right **J** External Iliac Artery, Left **K** Femoral Artery, Right **L** Femoral Artery, Left **M** Popliteal Artery, Right **N** Popliteal Artery, Left **P** Anterior Tibial Artery, Right **Q** Anterior Tibial Artery, Left **R** Posterior Tibial Artery, Right **S** Posterior Tibial Artery, Left **T** Peroneal Artery, Right **U** Peroneal Artery, Left **V** Foot Artery, Right **W** Foot Artery, Left **Y** Lower Artery	**0** Open **3** Percutaneous **4** Percutaneous Endoscopic	**Z** No Device	**Z** No Qualifier

Revised Text in **BLUE**   © 2011 Ingenix, Inc

Ø Medical and Surgical
4 Lower Arteries
U Supplement   Putting in or on biological or synthetic material that physically reinforces and/or augments the function of a portion of a body part

Body Part Character 4	Approach Character 5	Device Character 6	Qualifier Character 7
Ø Abdominal Aorta 1 Celiac Artery 2 Gastric Artery 3 Hepatic Artery 4 Splenic Artery 5 Superior Mesenteric Artery 6 Colic Artery, Right 7 Colic Artery, Left 8 Colic Artery, Middle 9 Renal Artery, Right A Renal Artery, Left B Inferior Mesenteric Artery C Common Iliac Artery, Right D Common Iliac Artery, Left E Internal Iliac Artery, Right F Internal Iliac Artery, Left H External Iliac Artery, Right J External Iliac Artery, Left K Femoral Artery, Right L Femoral Artery, Left M Popliteal Artery, Right N Popliteal Artery, Left P Anterior Tibial Artery, Right Q Anterior Tibial Artery, Left R Posterior Tibial Artery, Right S Posterior Tibial Artery, Left T Peroneal Artery, Right U Peroneal Artery, Left V Foot Artery, Right W Foot Artery, Left Y Lower Artery	Ø Open 3 Percutaneous 4 Percutaneous Endoscopic	7 Autologous Tissue Substitute J Synthetic Substitute K Nonautologous Tissue Substitute	Z No Qualifier

Ø Medical and Surgical
4 Lower Arteries
V Restriction   Partially closing an orifice or the lumen of a tubular body part

Body Part Character 4	Approach Character 5	Device Character 6	Qualifier Character 7
Ø Abdominal Aorta 1 Celiac Artery 2 Gastric Artery 3 Hepatic Artery 4 Splenic Artery 5 Superior Mesenteric Artery 6 Colic Artery, Right 7 Colic Artery, Left 8 Colic Artery, Middle 9 Renal Artery, Right A Renal Artery, Left B Inferior Mesenteric Artery C Common Iliac Artery, Right D Common Iliac Artery, Left E Internal Iliac Artery, Right F Internal Iliac Artery, Left H External Iliac Artery, Right J External Iliac Artery, Left K Femoral Artery, Right L Femoral Artery, Left M Popliteal Artery, Right N Popliteal Artery, Left P Anterior Tibial Artery, Right Q Anterior Tibial Artery, Left R Posterior Tibial Artery, Right S Posterior Tibial Artery, Left T Peroneal Artery, Right U Peroneal Artery, Left V Foot Artery, Right W Foot Artery, Left Y Lower Artery	Ø Open 3 Percutaneous 4 Percutaneous Endoscopic	C Extraluminal Device D Intraluminal Device Z No Device	Z No Qualifier

Ø Medical and Surgical
4 Lower Arteries
W Revision   Correcting, to the extent possible, a portion of a malfunctioning device or the position of a displaced device

Body Part Character 4	Approach Character 5	Device Character 6	Qualifier Character 7
Y Lower Artery	Ø Open 3 Percutaneous 4 Percutaneous Endoscopic X External	Ø Drainage Device 2 Monitoring Device 3 Infusion Device 4 Drug-eluting Intraluminal Device 7 Autologous Tissue Substitute 9 Autologous Venous Tissue A Autologous Arterial Tissue C Extraluminal Device D Intraluminal Device J Synthetic Substitute K Nonautologous Tissue Substitute	Z No Qualifier

Upper Veins Ø51–Ø5W

Ø **Medical and Surgical**
5 **Upper Veins**
1 **Bypass**　　　Altering the route of passage of the contents of a tubular body part

Body Part Character 4	Approach Character 5	Device Character 6	Qualifier Character 7
Ø Azygos Vein	**Ø** Open	**7** Autologous Tissue Substitute	**Y** Upper Vein
1 Hemiazygos Vein	**4** Percutaneous Endoscopic	**9** Autologous Venous Tissue	
3 Innominate Vein, Right		**A** Autologous Arterial Tissue	
4 Innominate Vein, Left		**J** Synthetic Substitute	
5 Subclavian Vein, Right		**K** Nonautologous Tissue Substitute	
6 Subclavian Vein, Left		**Z** No Device	
7 Axillary Vein, Right			
8 Axillary Vein, Left			
9 Brachial Vein, Right			
A Brachial Vein, Left			
B Basilic Vein, Right			
C Basilic Vein, Left			
D Cephalic Vein, Right			
F Cephalic Vein, Left			
G Hand Vein, Right			
H Hand Vein, Left			
L Intracranial Vein			
M Internal Jugular Vein, Right			
N Internal Jugular Vein, Left			
P External Jugular Vein, Right			
Q External Jugular Vein, Left			
R Vertebral Vein, Right			
S Vertebral Vein, Left			
T Face Vein, Right			
V Face Vein, Left			

Ø **Medical and Surgical**
5 **Upper Veins**
5 **Destruction**　　　Physical eradication of all or a portion of a body part by the direct use of energy, force, or a destructive agent

Body Part Character 4	Approach Character 5	Device Character 6	Qualifier Character 7
Ø Azygos Vein	**Ø** Open	**Z** No Device	**Z** No Qualifier
1 Hemiazygos Vein	**3** Percutaneous		
3 Innominate Vein, Right	**4** Percutaneous Endoscopic		
4 Innominate Vein, Left			
5 Subclavian Vein, Right			
6 Subclavian Vein, Left			
7 Axillary Vein, Right			
8 Axillary Vein, Left			
9 Brachial Vein, Right			
A Brachial Vein, Left			
B Basilic Vein, Right			
C Basilic Vein, Left			
D Cephalic Vein, Right			
F Cephalic Vein, Left			
G Hand Vein, Right			
H Hand Vein, Left			
L Intracranial Vein			
M Internal Jugular Vein, Right			
N Internal Jugular Vein, Left			
P External Jugular Vein, Right			
Q External Jugular Vein, Left			
R Vertebral Vein, Right			
S Vertebral Vein, Left			
T Face Vein, Right			
V Face Vein, Left			
Y Upper Vein			

0   **Medical and Surgical**
5   **Upper Veins**
7   **Dilation**   Expanding an orifice or the lumen of a tubular body part

Body Part Character 4	Approach Character 5	Device Character 6	Qualifier Character 7
0 Azygos Vein	0 Open	D Intraluminal Device	Z No Qualifier
1 Hemiazygos Vein	3 Percutaneous	Z No Device	
3 Innominate Vein, Right	4 Percutaneous Endoscopic		
4 Innominate Vein, Left			
5 Subclavian Vein, Right			
6 Subclavian Vein, Left			
7 Axillary Vein, Right			
8 Axillary Vein, Left			
9 Brachial Vein, Right			
A Brachial Vein, Left			
B Basilic Vein, Right			
C Basilic Vein, Left			
D Cephalic Vein, Right			
F Cephalic Vein, Left			
G Hand Vein, Right			
H Hand Vein, Left			
L Intracranial Vein			
M Internal Jugular Vein, Right			
N Internal Jugular Vein, Left			
P External Jugular Vein, Right			
Q External Jugular Vein, Left			
R Vertebral Vein, Right			
S Vertebral Vein, Left			
T Face Vein, Right			
V Face Vein, Left			
Y Upper Vein			

0   **Medical and Surgical**
5   **Upper Veins**
9   **Drainage**   Taking or letting out fluids and/or gases from a body part

Body Part Character 4	Approach Character 5	Device Character 6	Qualifier Character 7
0 Azygos Vein	0 Open	0 Drainage Device	Z No Qualifier
1 Hemiazygos Vein	3 Percutaneous		
3 Innominate Vein, Right	4 Percutaneous Endoscopic		
4 Innominate Vein, Left			
5 Subclavian Vein, Right			
6 Subclavian Vein, Left			
7 Axillary Vein, Right			
8 Axillary Vein, Left			
9 Brachial Vein, Right			
A Brachial Vein, Left			
B Basilic Vein, Right			
C Basilic Vein, Left			
D Cephalic Vein, Right			
F Cephalic Vein, Left			
G Hand Vein, Right			
H Hand Vein, Left			
L Intracranial Vein			
M Internal Jugular Vein, Right			
N Internal Jugular Vein, Left			
P External Jugular Vein, Right			
Q External Jugular Vein, Left			
R Vertebral Vein, Right			
S Vertebral Vein, Left			
T Face Vein, Right			
V Face Vein, Left			
Y Upper Vein			

059 Continued on next page

    Revised Text in **BLUE**   © 2011 Ingenix, Inc

Ø   **Medical and Surgical**   *059 Continued*
5   **Upper Veins**
9   **Drainage**   Taking or letting out fluids and/or gases from a body part

Body Part Character 4	Approach Character 5	Device Character 6	Qualifier Character 7
Ø Azygos Vein 1 Hemiazygos Vein 3 Innominate Vein, Right 4 Innominate Vein, Left 5 Subclavian Vein, Right 6 Subclavian Vein, Left 7 Axillary Vein, Right 8 Axillary Vein, Left 9 Brachial Vein, Right A Brachial Vein, Left B Basilic Vein, Right C Basilic Vein, Left D Cephalic Vein, Right F Cephalic Vein, Left G Hand Vein, Right H Hand Vein, Left L Intracranial Vein M Internal Jugular Vein, Right N Internal Jugular Vein, Left P External Jugular Vein, Right Q External Jugular Vein, Left R Vertebral Vein, Right S Vertebral Vein, Left T Face Vein, Right V Face Vein, Left Y Upper Vein	Ø Open 3 Percutaneous 4 Percutaneous Endoscopic	Z No Device	X Diagnostic Z No Qualifier

Ø   **Medical and Surgical**
5   **Upper Veins**
B   **Excision**   Cutting out or off, without replacement, a portion of a body part

Body Part Character 4	Approach Character 5	Device Character 6	Qualifier Character 7
Ø Azygos Vein 1 Hemiazygos Vein 3 Innominate Vein, Right 4 Innominate Vein, Left 5 Subclavian Vein, Right 6 Subclavian Vein, Left 7 Axillary Vein, Right 8 Axillary Vein, Left 9 Brachial Vein, Right A Brachial Vein, Left B Basilic Vein, Right C Basilic Vein, Left D Cephalic Vein, Right F Cephalic Vein, Left G Hand Vein, Right H Hand Vein, Left L Intracranial Vein M Internal Jugular Vein, Right N Internal Jugular Vein, Left P External Jugular Vein, Right Q External Jugular Vein, Left R Vertebral Vein, Right S Vertebral Vein, Left T Face Vein, Right V Face Vein, Left Y Upper Vein	Ø Open 3 Percutaneous 4 Percutaneous Endoscopic	Z No Device	X Diagnostic Z No Qualifier

0   **Medical and Surgical**
5   **Upper Veins**
C   **Extirpation**   Taking or cutting out solid matter from a body part

Body Part Character 4	Approach Character 5	Device Character 6	Qualifier Character 7
0 Azygos Vein **1** Hemiazygos Vein **3** Innominate Vein, Right **4** Innominate Vein, Left **5** Subclavian Vein, Right **6** Subclavian Vein, Left **7** Axillary Vein, Right **8** Axillary Vein, Left **9** Brachial Vein, Right **A** Brachial Vein, Left **B** Basilic Vein, Right **C** Basilic Vein, Left **D** Cephalic Vein, Right **F** Cephalic Vein, Left **G** Hand Vein, Right **H** Hand Vein, Left **L** Intracranial Vein **M** Internal Jugular Vein, Right **N** Internal Jugular Vein, Left **P** External Jugular Vein, Right **Q** External Jugular Vein, Left **R** Vertebral Vein, Right **S** Vertebral Vein, Left **T** Face Vein, Right **V** Face Vein, Left **Y** Upper Vein	**0** Open **3** Percutaneous **4** Percutaneous Endoscopic	**Z** No Device	**Z** No Qualifier

0   **Medical and Surgical**
5   **Upper Veins**
D   **Extraction**   Pulling or stripping out or off all or a portion of a body part by the use of force

Body Part Character 4	Approach Character 5	Device Character 6	Qualifier Character 7
9 Brachial Vein, Right **A** Brachial Vein, Left **B** Basilic Vein, Right **C** Basilic Vein, Left **D** Cephalic Vein, Right **F** Cephalic Vein, Left **G** Hand Vein, Right **H** Hand Vein, Left **Y** Upper Vein	**0** Open **3** Percutaneous	**Z** No Device	**Z** No Qualifier

0   Medical and Surgical
5   Upper Veins
H   Insertion   Putting in a nonbiological appliance that monitors, assists, performs, or prevents a physiological function but does not physically take the place of a body part

Body Part Character 4	Approach Character 5	Device Character 6	Qualifier Character 7
0 Azygos Vein 1 Hemiazygos Vein 3 Innominate Vein, Right 4 Innominate Vein, Left 5 Subclavian Vein, Right 6 Subclavian Vein, Left 7 Axillary Vein, Right 8 Axillary Vein, Left 9 Brachial Vein, Right A Brachial Vein, Left B Basilic Vein, Right C Basilic Vein, Left D Cephalic Vein, Right F Cephalic Vein, Left G Hand Vein, Right H Hand Vein, Left L Intracranial Vein M Internal Jugular Vein, Right N Internal Jugular Vein, Left P External Jugular Vein, Right Q External Jugular Vein, Left R Vertebral Vein, Right S Vertebral Vein, Left T Face Vein, Right V Face Vein, Left	0 Open 3 Percutaneous 4 Percutaneous Endoscopic	3 Infusion Device D Intraluminal Device	Z No Qualifier
Y Upper Vein	0 Open 3 Percutaneous 4 Percutaneous Endoscopic	2 Monitoring Device 3 Infusion Device D Intraluminal Device	Z No Qualifier

0   Medical and Surgical
5   Upper Veins
J   Inspection   Visually and/or manually exploring a body part

Body Part Character 4	Approach Character 5	Device Character 6	Qualifier Character 7
Y Upper Vein	0 Open 3 Percutaneous 4 Percutaneous Endoscopic X External	Z No Device	Z No Qualifier

0   Medical and Surgical
5   Upper Veins
L   Occlusion   Completely closing an orifice or the lumen of a tubular body part

Body Part Character 4	Approach Character 5	Device Character 6	Qualifier Character 7
0 Azygos Vein 1 Hemiazygos Vein 3 Innominate Vein, Right 4 Innominate Vein, Left 5 Subclavian Vein, Right 6 Subclavian Vein, Left 7 Axillary Vein, Right 8 Axillary Vein, Left 9 Brachial Vein, Right A Brachial Vein, Left B Basilic Vein, Right C Basilic Vein, Left D Cephalic Vein, Right F Cephalic Vein, Left G Hand Vein, Right H Hand Vein, Left L Intracranial Vein M Internal Jugular Vein, Right N Internal Jugular Vein, Left P External Jugular Vein, Right Q External Jugular Vein, Left R Vertebral Vein, Right S Vertebral Vein, Left T Face Vein, Right V Face Vein, Left Y Upper Vein	0 Open 3 Percutaneous 4 Percutaneous Endoscopic	C Extraluminal Device D Intraluminal Device Z No Device	Z No Qualifier

Upper Veins

05N–05P   Upper Veins   ICD-10-PCS (2011 Draft)

0   Medical and Surgical
5   Upper Veins
N   Release   Freeing a body part from an abnormal physical constraint

Body Part Character 4	Approach Character 5	Device Character 6	Qualifier Character 7
0 Azygos Vein 1 Hemiazygos Vein 3 Innominate Vein, Right 4 Innominate Vein, Left 5 Subclavian Vein, Right 6 Subclavian Vein, Left 7 Axillary Vein, Right 8 Axillary Vein, Left 9 Brachial Vein, Right A Brachial Vein, Left B Basilic Vein, Right C Basilic Vein, Left D Cephalic Vein, Right F Cephalic Vein, Left G Hand Vein, Right H Hand Vein, Left L Intracranial Vein M Internal Jugular Vein, Right N Internal Jugular Vein, Left P External Jugular Vein, Right Q External Jugular Vein, Left R Vertebral Vein, Right S Vertebral Vein, Left T Face Vein, Right V Face Vein, Left Y Upper Vein	0 Open 3 Percutaneous 4 Percutaneous Endoscopic	Z No Device	Z No Qualifier

0   Medical and Surgical
5   Upper Veins
P   Removal   Taking out or off a device from a body part

Body Part Character 4	Approach Character 5	Device Character 6	Qualifier Character 7
Y Upper Vein	0 Open 3 Percutaneous 4 Percutaneous Endoscopic	0 Drainage Device 2 Monitoring Device 3 Infusion Device 7 Autologous Tissue Substitute 9 Autologous Venous Tissue A Autologous Arterial Tissue C Extraluminal Device D Intraluminal Device J Synthetic Substitute K Nonautologous Tissue Substitute	Z No Qualifier
Y Upper Vein	X External	0 Drainage Device 2 Monitoring Device 3 Infusion Device D Intraluminal Device	Z No Qualifier

174   Revised Text in **BLUE**   © 2011 Ingenix, Inc

Ø   **Medical and Surgical**
5   **Upper Veins**
Q   **Repair**   Restoring, to the extent possible, a body part to its normal anatomic structure and function

Body Part Character 4	Approach Character 5	Device Character 6	Qualifier Character 7
Ø Azygos Vein 1 Hemiazygos Vein 3 Innominate Vein, Right 4 Innominate Vein, Left 5 Subclavian Vein, Right 6 Subclavian Vein, Left 7 Axillary Vein, Right 8 Axillary Vein, Left 9 Brachial Vein, Right A Brachial Vein, Left B Basilic Vein, Right C Basilic Vein, Left D Cephalic Vein, Right F Cephalic Vein, Left G Hand Vein, Right H Hand Vein, Left L Intracranial Vein M Internal Jugular Vein, Right N Internal Jugular Vein, Left P External Jugular Vein, Right Q External Jugular Vein, Left R Vertebral Vein, Right S Vertebral Vein, Left T Face Vein, Right V Face Vein, Left Y Upper Vein	Ø Open 3 Percutaneous 4 Percutaneous Endoscopic	Z No Device	Z No Qualifier

Ø   **Medical and Surgical**
5   **Upper Veins**
R   **Replacement**   Putting in or on biological or synthetic material that physically takes the place and/or function of all or a portion of a body part

Body Part Character 4	Approach Character 5	Device Character 6	Qualifier Character 7
Ø Azygos Vein 1 Hemiazygos Vein 3 Innominate Vein, Right 4 Innominate Vein, Left 5 Subclavian Vein, Right 6 Subclavian Vein, Left 7 Axillary Vein, Right 8 Axillary Vein, Left 9 Brachial Vein, Right A Brachial Vein, Left B Basilic Vein, Right C Basilic Vein, Left D Cephalic Vein, Right F Cephalic Vein, Left G Hand Vein, Right H Hand Vein, Left L Intracranial Vein M Internal Jugular Vein, Right N Internal Jugular Vein, Left P External Jugular Vein, Right Q External Jugular Vein, Left R Vertebral Vein, Right S Vertebral Vein, Left T Face Vein, Right V Face Vein, Left Y Upper Vein	Ø Open 4 Percutaneous Endoscopic	7 Autologous Tissue Substitute J Synthetic Substitute K Nonautologous Tissue Substitute	Z No Qualifier

Ø   **Medical and Surgical**
5   **Upper Veins**
S   **Reposition**   Moving to its normal location or other suitable location all or a portion of a body part

Body Part Character 4	Approach Character 5	Device Character 6	Qualifier Character 7
Ø Azygos Vein 1 Hemiazygos Vein 3 Innominate Vein, Right 4 Innominate Vein, Left 5 Subclavian Vein, Right 6 Subclavian Vein, Left 7 Axillary Vein, Right 8 Axillary Vein, Left 9 Brachial Vein, Right A Brachial Vein, Left B Basilic Vein, Right C Basilic Vein, Left D Cephalic Vein, Right F Cephalic Vein, Left G Hand Vein, Right H Hand Vein, Left L Intracranial Vein M Internal Jugular Vein, Right N Internal Jugular Vein, Left P External Jugular Vein, Right Q External Jugular Vein, Left R Vertebral Vein, Right S Vertebral Vein, Left T Face Vein, Right V Face Vein, Left Y Upper Vein	Ø Open 3 Percutaneous 4 Percutaneous Endoscopic	Z No Device	Z No Qualifier

Ø   **Medical and Surgical**
5   **Upper Veins**
U   **Supplement**   Putting in or on biological or synthetic material that physically reinforces and/or augments the function of a portion of a body part

Body Part Character 4	Approach Character 5	Device Character 6	Qualifier Character 7
Ø Azygos Vein 1 Hemiazygos Vein 3 Innominate Vein, Right 4 Innominate Vein, Left 5 Subclavian Vein, Right 6 Subclavian Vein, Left 7 Axillary Vein, Right 8 Axillary Vein, Left 9 Brachial Vein, Right A Brachial Vein, Left B Basilic Vein, Right C Basilic Vein, Left D Cephalic Vein, Right F Cephalic Vein, Left G Hand Vein, Right H Hand Vein, Left L Intracranial Vein M Internal Jugular Vein, Right N Internal Jugular Vein, Left P External Jugular Vein, Right Q External Jugular Vein, Left R Vertebral Vein, Right S Vertebral Vein, Left T Face Vein, Right V Face Vein, Left Y Upper Vein	Ø Open 3 Percutaneous 4 Percutaneous Endoscopic	7 Autologous Tissue Substitute J Synthetic Substitute K Nonautologous Tissue Substitute	Z No Qualifier

0   **Medical and Surgical**
5   **Upper Veins**
V   **Restriction**   Partially closing an orifice or the lumen of a tubular body part

Body Part Character 4	Approach Character 5	Device Character 6	Qualifier Character 7
0 Azygos Vein **1** Hemiazygos Vein **3** Innominate Vein, Right **4** Innominate Vein, Left **5** Subclavian Vein, Right **6** Subclavian Vein, Left **7** Axillary Vein, Right **8** Axillary Vein, Left **9** Brachial Vein, Right **A** Brachial Vein, Left **B** Basilic Vein, Right **C** Basilic Vein, Left **D** Cephalic Vein, Right **F** Cephalic Vein, Left **G** Hand Vein, Right **H** Hand Vein, Left **L** Intracranial Vein **M** Internal Jugular Vein, Right **N** Internal Jugular Vein, Left **P** External Jugular Vein, Right **Q** External Jugular Vein, Left **R** Vertebral Vein, Right **S** Vertebral Vein, Left **T** Face Vein, Right **V** Face Vein, Left **Y** Upper Vein	**0** Open **3** Percutaneous **4** Percutaneous Endoscopic	**C** Extraluminal Device **D** Intraluminal Device **Z** No Device	**Z** No Qualifier

0   **Medical and Surgical**
5   **Upper Veins**
W   **Revision**   Correcting, to the extent possible, a portion of a malfunctioning device or the position of a displaced device

Body Part Character 4	Approach Character 5	Device Character 6	Qualifier Character 7
Y Upper Vein	**0** Open **3** Percutaneous **4** Percutaneous Endoscopic **X** External	**0** Drainage Device **2** Monitoring Device **3** Infusion Device **7** Autologous Tissue Substitute **9** Autologous Venous Tissue **A** Autologous Arterial Tissue **C** Extraluminal Device **D** Intraluminal Device **J** Synthetic Substitute **K** Nonautologous Tissue Substitute	**Z** No Qualifier

Lower Veins Ø61–Ø6W

Ø **Medical and Surgical**
6 **Lower Veins**
1 **Bypass**   Altering the route of passage of the contents of a tubular body part

Body Part Character 4	Approach Character 5	Device Character 6	Qualifier Character 7
Ø Inferior Vena Cava	Ø Open 4 Percutaneous Endoscopic	7 Autologous Tissue Substitute 9 Autologous Venous Tissue A Autologous Arterial Tissue J Synthetic Substitute K Nonautologous Tissue Substitute Z No Device	5 Superior Mesenteric Vein 6 Inferior Mesenteric Vein Y Lower Vein
1 Splenic Vein 8 Portal Vein	Ø Open 4 Percutaneous Endoscopic	7 Autologous Tissue Substitute 9 Autologous Venous Tissue A Autologous Arterial Tissue J Synthetic Substitute K Nonautologous Tissue Substitute Z No Device	9 Renal Vein, Right B Renal Vein, Left Y Lower Vein
2 Gastric Vein 3 Esophageal Vein 4 Hepatic Vein 5 Superior Mesenteric Vein 6 Inferior Mesenteric Vein 7 Colic Vein 9 Renal Vein, Right B Renal Vein, Left C Common Iliac Vein, Right D Common Iliac Vein, Left F External Iliac Vein, Right G External Iliac Vein, Left H Hypogastric Vein, Right J Hypogastric Vein, Left M Femoral Vein, Right N Femoral Vein, Left P Greater Saphenous Vein, Right Q Greater Saphenous Vein, Left R Lesser Saphenous Vein, Right S Lesser Saphenous Vein, Left T Foot Vein, Right V Foot Vein, Left	Ø Open 4 Percutaneous Endoscopic	7 Autologous Tissue Substitute 9 Autologous Venous Tissue A Autologous Arterial Tissue J Synthetic Substitute K Nonautologous Tissue Substitute Z No Device	Y Lower Vein
8 Portal Vein	3 Percutaneous 4 Percutaneous Endoscopic	D Intraluminal Device	Y Lower Vein

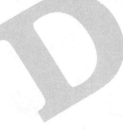

Ø　Medical and Surgical
6　Lower Veins
5　Destruction　　Physical eradication of all or a portion of a body part by the direct use of energy, force, or a destructive agent

Body Part Character 4	Approach Character 5	Device Character 6	Qualifier Character 7
Ø　Inferior Vena Cava 1　Splenic Vein 2　Gastric Vein 3　Esophageal Vein 4　Hepatic Vein 5　Superior Mesenteric Vein 6　Inferior Mesenteric Vein 7　Colic Vein 8　Portal Vein 9　Renal Vein, Right B　Renal Vein, Left C　Common Iliac Vein, Right D　Common Iliac Vein, Left F　External Iliac Vein, Right G　External Iliac Vein, Left H　Hypogastric Vein, Right J　Hypogastric Vein, Left M　Femoral Vein, Right N　Femoral Vein, Left P　Greater Saphenous Vein, Right Q　Greater Saphenous Vein, Left R　Lesser Saphenous Vein, Right S　Lesser Saphenous Vein, Left T　Foot Vein, Right V　Foot Vein, Left	Ø　Open 3　Percutaneous 4　Percutaneous Endoscopic	Z　No Device	Z　No Qualifier
Y　Lower Vein	Ø　Open 3　Percutaneous 4　Percutaneous Endoscopic	Z　No Device	**C　Hemorrhoidal Plexus** Z　No Qualifier

Ø　Medical and Surgical
6　Lower Veins
7　Dilation　　Expanding an orifice or the lumen of a tubular body part

Body Part Character 4	Approach Character 5	Device Character 6	Qualifier Character 7
Ø　Inferior Vena Cava 1　Splenic Vein 2　Gastric Vein 3　Esophageal Vein 4　Hepatic Vein 5　Superior Mesenteric Vein 6　Inferior Mesenteric Vein 7　Colic Vein 8　Portal Vein 9　Renal Vein, Right B　Renal Vein, Left C　Common Iliac Vein, Right D　Common Iliac Vein, Left F　External Iliac Vein, Right G　External Iliac Vein, Left H　Hypogastric Vein, Right J　Hypogastric Vein, Left M　Femoral Vein, Right N　Femoral Vein, Left P　Greater Saphenous Vein, Right Q　Greater Saphenous Vein, Left R　Lesser Saphenous Vein, Right S　Lesser Saphenous Vein, Left T　Foot Vein, Right V　Foot Vein, Left Y　Lower Vein	Ø　Open 3　Percutaneous 4　Percutaneous Endoscopic	D　Intraluminal Device Z　No Device	Z　No Qualifier

Ø   Medical and Surgical
6   Lower Veins
9   Drainage   Taking or letting out fluids and/or gases from a body part

Body Part Character 4	Approach Character 5	Device Character 6	Qualifier Character 7
Ø Inferior Vena Cava 1 Splenic Vein 2 Gastric Vein 3 Esophageal Vein 4 Hepatic Vein 5 Superior Mesenteric Vein 6 Inferior Mesenteric Vein 7 Colic Vein 8 Portal Vein 9 Renal Vein, Right B Renal Vein, Left C Common Iliac Vein, Right D Common Iliac Vein, Left F External Iliac Vein, Right G External Iliac Vein, Left H Hypogastric Vein, Right J Hypogastric Vein, Left M Femoral Vein, Right N Femoral Vein, Left P Greater Saphenous Vein, Right Q Greater Saphenous Vein, Left R Lesser Saphenous Vein, Right S Lesser Saphenous Vein, Left T Foot Vein, Right V Foot Vein, Left Y Lower Vein	Ø Open 3 Percutaneous 4 Percutaneous Endoscopic	Ø Drainage Device	Z No Qualifier
Ø Inferior Vena Cava 1 Splenic Vein 2 Gastric Vein 3 Esophageal Vein 4 Hepatic Vein 5 Superior Mesenteric Vein 6 Inferior Mesenteric Vein 7 Colic Vein 8 Portal Vein 9 Renal Vein, Right B Renal Vein, Left C Common Iliac Vein, Right D Common Iliac Vein, Left F External Iliac Vein, Right G External Iliac Vein, Left H Hypogastric Vein, Right J Hypogastric Vein, Left M Femoral Vein, Right N Femoral Vein, Left P Greater Saphenous Vein, Right Q Greater Saphenous Vein, Left R Lesser Saphenous Vein, Right S Lesser Saphenous Vein, Left T Foot Vein, Right V Foot Vein, Left Y Lower Vein	Ø Open 3 Percutaneous 4 Percutaneous Endoscopic	Z No Device	X Diagnostic Z No Qualifier

0　　Medical and Surgical
6　　Lower Veins
B　　Excision　　　Cutting out or off, without replacement, a portion of a body part

Body Part Character 4	Approach Character 5	Device Character 6	Qualifier Character 7
0 Inferior Vena Cava 1 Splenic Vein 2 Gastric Vein 3 Esophageal Vein 4 Hepatic Vein 5 Superior Mesenteric Vein 6 Inferior Mesenteric Vein 7 Colic Vein 8 Portal Vein 9 Renal Vein, Right B Renal Vein, Left C Common Iliac Vein, Right D Common Iliac Vein, Left F External Iliac Vein, Right G External Iliac Vein, Left H Hypogastric Vein, Right J Hypogastric Vein, Left M Femoral Vein, Right N Femoral Vein, Left P Greater Saphenous Vein, Right Q Greater Saphenous Vein, Left R Lesser Saphenous Vein, Right S Lesser Saphenous Vein, Left T Foot Vein, Right V Foot Vein, Left	0 Open 3 Percutaneous 4 Percutaneous Endoscopic	Z No Device	X Diagnostic Z No Qualifier
Y Lower Vein	0 Open 3 Percutaneous 4 Percutaneous Endoscopic	Z No Device	**C Hemorrhoidal Plexus** X Diagnostic Z No Qualifier

0　　Medical and Surgical
6　　Lower Veins
C　　Extirpation　　　Taking or cutting out solid matter from a body part

Body Part Character 4	Approach Character 5	Device Character 6	Qualifier Character 7
0 Inferior Vena Cava 1 Splenic Vein 2 Gastric Vein 3 Esophageal Vein 4 Hepatic Vein 5 Superior Mesenteric Vein 6 Inferior Mesenteric Vein 7 Colic Vein 8 Portal Vein 9 Renal Vein, Right B Renal Vein, Left C Common Iliac Vein, Right D Common Iliac Vein, Left F External Iliac Vein, Right G External Iliac Vein, Left H Hypogastric Vein, Right J Hypogastric Vein, Left M Femoral Vein, Right N Femoral Vein, Left P Greater Saphenous Vein, Right Q Greater Saphenous Vein, Left R Lesser Saphenous Vein, Right S Lesser Saphenous Vein, Left T Foot Vein, Right V Foot Vein, Left Y Lower Vein	0 Open 3 Percutaneous 4 Percutaneous Endoscopic	Z No Device	Z No Qualifier

Ø   Medical and Surgical
6   Lower Veins
D   Extraction   Pulling or stripping out or off all or a portion of a body part by the use of force

Body Part Character 4	Approach Character 5	Device Character 6	Qualifier Character 7
M Femoral Vein, Right **N** Femoral Vein, Left **P** Greater Saphenous Vein, Right **Q** Greater Saphenous Vein, Left **R** Lesser Saphenous Vein, Right **S** Lesser Saphenous Vein, Left **T** Foot Vein, Right **V** Foot Vein, Left **Y** Lower Vein	**Ø** Open **3** Percutaneous **4** Percutaneous Endoscopic	**Z** No Device	**Z** No Qualifier

Ø   Medical and Surgical
6   Lower Veins
H   Insertion   Putting in a nonbiological appliance that monitors, assists, performs, or prevents a physiological function but does not physically take the place of a body part

Body Part Character 4	Approach Character 5	Device Character 6	Qualifier Character 7
Ø Inferior Vena Cava	**Ø** Open **3** Percutaneous	**3** Infusion Device	**T** Via Umbilical Vein **Z** No Qualifier
Ø Inferior Vena Cava	**Ø** Open **3** Percutaneous	**D** Intraluminal Device	**Z** No Qualifier
Ø Inferior Vena Cava	**4** Percutaneous Endoscopic	**3** Infusion Device **D** Intraluminal Device	**Z** No Qualifier
1 Splenic Vein **2** Gastric Vein **3** Esophageal Vein **4** Hepatic Vein **5** Superior Mesenteric Vein **6** Inferior Mesenteric Vein **7** Colic Vein **8** Portal Vein **9** Renal Vein, Right **B** Renal Vein, Left **C** Common Iliac Vein, Right **D** Common Iliac Vein, Left **F** External Iliac Vein, Right **G** External Iliac Vein, Left **H** Hypogastric Vein, Right **J** Hypogastric Vein, Left **M** Femoral Vein, Right **N** Femoral Vein, Left **P** Greater Saphenous Vein, Right **Q** Greater Saphenous Vein, Left **R** Lesser Saphenous Vein, Right **S** Lesser Saphenous Vein, Left **T** Foot Vein, Right **V** Foot Vein, Left	**Ø** Open **3** Percutaneous **4** Percutaneous Endoscopic	**3** Infusion Device **D** Intraluminal Device	**Z** No Qualifier
Y Lower Vein	**Ø** Open **3** Percutaneous **4** Percutaneous Endoscopic	**2** Monitoring Device **3** Infusion Device **D** Intraluminal Device	**Z** No Qualifier

Ø   Medical and Surgical
6   Lower Veins
J   Inspection   Visually and/or manually exploring a body part

Body Part Character 4	Approach Character 5	Device Character 6	Qualifier Character 7
Y Lower Vein	**Ø** Open **3** Percutaneous **4** Percutaneous Endoscopic **X** External	**Z** No Device	**Z** No Qualifier

Revised Text in **BLUE**   © 2011 Ingenix, Inc

0   Medical and Surgical
6   Lower Veins
L   Occlusion   Completely closing an orifice or the lumen of a tubular body part

Body Part Character 4	Approach Character 5	Device Character 6	Qualifier Character 7
0 Inferior Vena Cava 1 Splenic Vein 2 Gastric Vein 3 Esophageal Vein 4 Hepatic Vein 5 Superior Mesenteric Vein 6 Inferior Mesenteric Vein 7 Colic Vein 8 Portal Vein 9 Renal Vein, Right B Renal Vein, Left C Common Iliac Vein, Right D Common Iliac Vein, Left F External Iliac Vein, Right G External Iliac Vein, Left H Hypogastric Vein, Right J Hypogastric Vein, Left M Femoral Vein, Right N Femoral Vein, Left P Greater Saphenous Vein, Right Q Greater Saphenous Vein, Left R Lesser Saphenous Vein, Right S Lesser Saphenous Vein, Left T Foot Vein, Right V Foot Vein, Left	0 Open 3 Percutaneous 4 Percutaneous Endoscopic	C Extraluminal Device D Intraluminal Device Z No Device	Z No Qualifier
Y Lower Vein	0 Open 3 Percutaneous 4 Percutaneous Endoscopic	C Extraluminal Device D Intraluminal Device Z No Device	C Hemorrhoidal Plexus Z No Qualifier

0   Medical and Surgical
6   Lower Veins
N   Release   Freeing a body part from an abnormal physical constraint

Body Part Character 4	Approach Character 5	Device Character 6	Qualifier Character 7
0 Inferior Vena Cava 1 Splenic Vein 2 Gastric Vein 3 Esophageal Vein 4 Hepatic Vein 5 Superior Mesenteric Vein 6 Inferior Mesenteric Vein 7 Colic Vein 8 Portal Vein 9 Renal Vein, Right B Renal Vein, Left C Common Iliac Vein, Right D Common Iliac Vein, Left F External Iliac Vein, Right G External Iliac Vein, Left H Hypogastric Vein, Right J Hypogastric Vein, Left M Femoral Vein, Right N Femoral Vein, Left P Greater Saphenous Vein, Right Q Greater Saphenous Vein, Left R Lesser Saphenous Vein, Right S Lesser Saphenous Vein, Left T Foot Vein, Right V Foot Vein, Left Y Lower Vein	0 Open 3 Percutaneous 4 Percutaneous Endoscopic	Z No Device	Z No Qualifier

Ø Medical and Surgical
6 Lower Veins
P Removal Taking out or off a device from a body part

Body Part Character 4	Approach Character 5	Device Character 6	Qualifier Character 7
Y Lower Vein	Ø Open 3 Percutaneous 4 Percutaneous Endoscopic	Ø Drainage Device 2 Monitoring Device 3 Infusion Device 7 Autologous Tissue Substitute 9 Autologous Venous Tissue A Autologous Arterial Tissue C Extraluminal Device D Intraluminal Device J Synthetic Substitute K Nonautologous Tissue Substitute	Z No Qualifier
Y Lower Vein	X External	Ø Drainage Device 2 Monitoring Device 3 Infusion Device D Intraluminal Device	Z No Qualifier

Ø Medical and Surgical
6 Lower Veins
Q Repair Restoring, to the extent possible, a body part to its normal anatomic structure and function

Body Part Character 4	Approach Character 5	Device Character 6	Qualifier Character 7
Ø Inferior Vena Cava 1 Splenic Vein 2 Gastric Vein 3 Esophageal Vein 4 Hepatic Vein 5 Superior Mesenteric Vein 6 Inferior Mesenteric Vein 7 Colic Vein 8 Portal Vein 9 Renal Vein, Right B Renal Vein, Left C Common Iliac Vein, Right D Common Iliac Vein, Left F External Iliac Vein, Right G External Iliac Vein, Left H Hypogastric Vein, Right J Hypogastric Vein, Left M Femoral Vein, Right N Femoral Vein, Left P Greater Saphenous Vein, Right Q Greater Saphenous Vein, Left R Lesser Saphenous Vein, Right S Lesser Saphenous Vein, Left T Foot Vein, Right V Foot Vein, Left Y Lower Vein	Ø Open 3 Percutaneous 4 Percutaneous Endoscopic	Z No Device	Z No Qualifier

Ø Medical and Surgical
6 Lower Veins
R Replacement   Putting in or on biological or synthetic material that physically takes the place and/or function of all or a portion of a body part

Body Part Character 4	Approach Character 5	Device Character 6	Qualifier Character 7
Ø Inferior Vena Cava 1 Splenic Vein 2 Gastric Vein 3 Esophageal Vein 4 Hepatic Vein 5 Superior Mesenteric Vein 6 Inferior Mesenteric Vein 7 Colic Vein 8 Portal Vein 9 Renal Vein, Right B Renal Vein, Left C Common Iliac Vein, Right D Common Iliac Vein, Left F External Iliac Vein, Right G External Iliac Vein, Left H Hypogastric Vein, Right J Hypogastric Vein, Left M Femoral Vein, Right N Femoral Vein, Left P Greater Saphenous Vein, Right Q Greater Saphenous Vein, Left R Lesser Saphenous Vein, Right S Lesser Saphenous Vein, Left T Foot Vein, Right V Foot Vein, Left Y Lower Vein	Ø Open 4 Percutaneous Endoscopic	7 Autologous Tissue Substitute J Synthetic Substitute K Nonautologous Tissue Substitute	Z No Qualifier

Ø Medical and Surgical
6 Lower Veins
S Reposition   Moving to its normal location or other suitable location all or a portion of a body part

Body Part Character 4	Approach Character 5	Device Character 6	Qualifier Character 7
Ø Inferior Vena Cava 1 Splenic Vein 2 Gastric Vein 3 Esophageal Vein 4 Hepatic Vein 5 Superior Mesenteric Vein 6 Inferior Mesenteric Vein 7 Colic Vein 8 Portal Vein 9 Renal Vein, Right B Renal Vein, Left C Common Iliac Vein, Right D Common Iliac Vein, Left F External Iliac Vein, Right G External Iliac Vein, Left H Hypogastric Vein, Right J Hypogastric Vein, Left M Femoral Vein, Right N Femoral Vein, Left P Greater Saphenous Vein, Right Q Greater Saphenous Vein, Left R Lesser Saphenous Vein, Right S Lesser Saphenous Vein, Left T Foot Vein, Right V Foot Vein, Left Y Lower Vein	Ø Open 3 Percutaneous 4 Percutaneous Endoscopic	Z No Device	Z No Qualifier

0   Medical and Surgical
6   Lower Veins
U   Supplement   Putting in or on biological or synthetic material that physically reinforces and/or augments the function of a portion of a body part

Body Part Character 4	Approach Character 5	Device Character 6	Qualifier Character 7
0 Inferior Vena Cava **1** Splenic Vein **2** Gastric Vein **3** Esophageal Vein **4** Hepatic Vein **5** Superior Mesenteric Vein **6** Inferior Mesenteric Vein **7** Colic Vein **8** Portal Vein **9** Renal Vein, Right **B** Renal Vein, Left **C** Common Iliac Vein, Right **D** Common Iliac Vein, Left **F** External Iliac Vein, Right **G** External Iliac Vein, Left **H** Hypogastric Vein, Right **J** Hypogastric Vein, Left **M** Femoral Vein, Right **N** Femoral Vein, Left **P** Greater Saphenous Vein, Right **Q** Greater Saphenous Vein, Left **R** Lesser Saphenous Vein, Right **S** Lesser Saphenous Vein, Left **T** Foot Vein, Right **V** Foot Vein, Left **Y** Lower Vein	**0** Open **3** Percutaneous **4** Percutaneous Endoscopic	**7** Autologous Tissue Substitute **J** Synthetic Substitute **K** Nonautologous Tissue Substitute	**Z** No Qualifier

0   Medical and Surgical
6   Lower Veins
V   Restriction   Partially closing an orifice or the lumen of a tubular body part

Body Part Character 4	Approach Character 5	Device Character 6	Qualifier Character 7
0 Inferior Vena Cava **1** Splenic Vein **2** Gastric Vein **3** Esophageal Vein **4** Hepatic Vein **5** Superior Mesenteric Vein **6** Inferior Mesenteric Vein **7** Colic Vein **8** Portal Vein **9** Renal Vein, Right **B** Renal Vein, Left **C** Common Iliac Vein, Right **D** Common Iliac Vein, Left **F** External Iliac Vein, Right **G** External Iliac Vein, Left **H** Hypogastric Vein, Right **J** Hypogastric Vein, Left **M** Femoral Vein, Right **N** Femoral Vein, Left **P** Greater Saphenous Vein, Right **Q** Greater Saphenous Vein, Left **R** Lesser Saphenous Vein, Right **S** Lesser Saphenous Vein, Left **T** Foot Vein, Right **V** Foot Vein, Left **Y** Lower Vein	**0** Open **3** Percutaneous **4** Percutaneous Endoscopic	**C** Extraluminal Device **D** Intraluminal Device **Z** No Device	**Z** No Qualifier

06U–06V

0   Medical and Surgical
6   Lower Veins
W   Revision   Correcting, to the extent possible, a portion of a malfunctioning device or the position of a displaced device

Body Part Character 4	Approach Character 5	Device Character 6	Qualifier Character 7
Y Lower Vein	0 Open 3 Percutaneous 4 Percutaneous Endoscopic X External	0 Drainage Device 2 Monitoring Device 3 Infusion Device 7 Autologous Tissue Substitute 9 Autologous Venous Tissue A Autologous Arterial Tissue C Extraluminal Device D Intraluminal Device J Synthetic Substitute K Nonautologous Tissue Substitute	Z No Qualifier

Lymphatic and Hemic Systems Ø72–Ø7Y

Ø   Medical and Surgical
7   Lymphatic and Hemic Systems
2   Change   Taking out or off a device from a body part and putting back an identical or similar device in or on the same body part without cutting or puncturing the skin or a mucous membrane

Body Part Character 4	Approach Character 5	Device Character 6	Qualifier Character 7
K Thoracic Duct **L** Cisterna Chyli **M** Thymus **N** Lymphatic **P** Spleen **T** Bone Marrow	**X** External	**Ø** Drainage Device **Y** Other Device	**Z** No Qualifier

Ø   Medical and Surgical
7   Lymphatic and Hemic Systems
5   Destruction   Physical eradication of all or a portion of a body part by the direct use of energy, force, or a destructive agent

Body Part Character 4	Approach Character 5	Device Character 6	Qualifier Character 7
Ø Lymphatic, Head **1** Lymphatic, Right Neck **2** Lymphatic, Left Neck **3** Lymphatic, Right Upper Extremity **4** Lymphatic, Left Upper Extremity **5** Lymphatic, Right Axillary **6** Lymphatic, Left Axillary **7** Lymphatic, Thorax **8** Lymphatic, Internal Mammary, Right **9** Lymphatic, Internal Mammary, Left **B** Lymphatic, Mesenteric **C** Lymphatic, Pelvis **D** Lymphatic, Aortic **F** Lymphatic, Right Lower Extremity **G** Lymphatic, Left Lower Extremity **H** Lymphatic, Right Inguinal **J** Lymphatic, Left Inguinal **K** Thoracic Duct **L** Cisterna Chyli **M** Thymus **P** Spleen	**Ø** Open **3** Percutaneous **4** Percutaneous Endoscopic	**Z** No Device	**Z** No Qualifier

Ø   Medical and Surgical
7   Lymphatic and Hemic Systems
9   Drainage   Taking or letting out fluids and/or gases from a body part

Body Part Character 4	Approach Character 5	Device Character 6	Qualifier Character 7
Ø Lymphatic, Head **1** Lymphatic, Right Neck **2** Lymphatic, Left Neck **3** Lymphatic, Right Upper Extremity **4** Lymphatic, Left Upper Extremity **5** Lymphatic, Right Axillary **6** Lymphatic, Left Axillary **7** Lymphatic, Thorax **8** Lymphatic, Internal Mammary, Right **9** Lymphatic, Internal Mammary, Left **B** Lymphatic, Mesenteric **C** Lymphatic, Pelvis **D** Lymphatic, Aortic **F** Lymphatic, Right Lower Extremity **G** Lymphatic, Left Lower Extremity **H** Lymphatic, Right Inguinal **J** Lymphatic, Left Inguinal **K** Thoracic Duct **L** Cisterna Chyli **M** Thymus **P** Spleen **T** Bone Marrow	**Ø** Open **3** Percutaneous **4** Percutaneous Endoscopic	**Ø** Drainage Device	**Z** No Qualifier

Ø79 Continued on next page

    Revised Text in **BLUE**   © 2011 Ingenix, Inc

Ø **Medical and Surgical**

7 **Lymphatic and Hemic Systems**　　　　　　　　　　　　　　　　　　　*079 Continued*

9 **Drainage**　　　Taking or letting out fluids and/or gases from a body part

Body Part Character 4	Approach Character 5	Device Character 6	Qualifier Character 7
Ø Lymphatic, Head **1** Lymphatic, Right Neck **2** Lymphatic, Left Neck **3** Lymphatic, Right Upper Extremity **4** Lymphatic, Left Upper Extremity **5** Lymphatic, Right Axillary **6** Lymphatic, Left Axillary **7** Lymphatic, Thorax **8** Lymphatic, Internal Mammary, 　　Right **9** Lymphatic, Internal Mammary, Left **B** Lymphatic, Mesenteric **C** Lymphatic, Pelvis **D** Lymphatic, Aortic **F** Lymphatic, Right Lower Extremity **G** Lymphatic, Left Lower Extremity **H** Lymphatic, Right Inguinal **J** Lymphatic, Left Inguinal **K** Thoracic Duct **L** Cisterna Chyli **M** Thymus **P** Spleen **T** Bone Marrow	**Ø** Open **3** Percutaneous **4** Percutaneous Endoscopic	**Z** No Device	**X** Diagnostic **Z** No Qualifier

Ø **Medical and Surgical**

7 **Lymphatic and Hemic Systems**

B **Excision**　　　Cutting out or off, without replacement, a portion of a body part

Body Part Character 4	Approach Character 5	Device Character 6	Qualifier Character 7
Ø Lymphatic, Head **1** Lymphatic, Right Neck **2** Lymphatic, Left Neck **3** Lymphatic, Right Upper Extremity **4** Lymphatic, Left Upper Extremity **5** Lymphatic, Right Axillary **6** Lymphatic, Left Axillary **7** Lymphatic, Thorax **8** Lymphatic, Internal Mammary, 　　Right **9** Lymphatic, Internal Mammary, Left **B** Lymphatic, Mesenteric **C** Lymphatic, Pelvis **D** Lymphatic, Aortic **F** Lymphatic, Right Lower Extremity **G** Lymphatic, Left Lower Extremity **H** Lymphatic, Right Inguinal **J** Lymphatic, Left Inguinal **K** Thoracic Duct **L** Cisterna Chyli **M** Thymus **P** Spleen	**Ø** Open **3** Percutaneous **4** Percutaneous Endoscopic	**Z** No Device	**X** Diagnostic **Z** No Qualifier

Lymphatic and Hemic Systems

07C–07J

0   **Medical and Surgical**
7   **Lymphatic and Hemic Systems**
C   **Extirpation**   Taking or cutting out solid matter from a body part

Body Part Character 4	Approach Character 5	Device Character 6	Qualifier Character 7
0 Lymphatic, Head **1** Lymphatic, Right Neck **2** Lymphatic, Left Neck **3** Lymphatic, Right Upper Extremity **4** Lymphatic, Left Upper Extremity **5** Lymphatic, Right Axillary **6** Lymphatic, Left Axillary **7** Lymphatic, Thorax **8** Lymphatic, Internal Mammary, Right **9** Lymphatic, Internal Mammary, Left **B** Lymphatic, Mesenteric **C** Lymphatic, Pelvis **D** Lymphatic, Aortic **F** Lymphatic, Right Lower Extremity **G** Lymphatic, Left Lower Extremity **H** Lymphatic, Right Inguinal **J** Lymphatic, Left Inguinal **K** Thoracic Duct **L** Cisterna Chyli **M** Thymus **P** Spleen	**0** Open **3** Percutaneous **4** Percutaneous Endoscopic	**Z** No Device	**Z** No Qualifier

0   **Medical and Surgical**
7   **Lymphatic and Hemic Systems**
D   **Extraction**   Pulling or stripping out or off all or a portion of a body part by the use of force

Body Part Character 4	Approach Character 5	Device Character 6	Qualifier Character 7
Q Bone Marrow, Sternum **R** Bone Marrow, Iliac **S** Bone Marrow, Vertebral	**0** Open **3** Percutaneous	**Z** No Device	**X** Diagnostic **Z** No Qualifier

0   **Medical and Surgical**
7   **Lymphatic and Hemic Systems**
H   **Insertion**   Putting in a nonbiological appliance that monitors, assists, performs, or prevents a physiological function but does not physically take the place of a body part

Body Part Character 4	Approach Character 5	Device Character 6	Qualifier Character 7
K Thoracic Duct **L** Cisterna Chyli **M** Thymus **N** Lymphatic **P** Spleen	**0** Open **3** Percutaneous **4** Percutaneous Endoscopic	**3** Infusion Device	**Z** No Qualifier

0   **Medical and Surgical**
7   **Lymphatic and Hemic Systems**
J   **Inspection**   Visually and/or manually exploring a body part

Body Part Character 4	Approach Character 5	Device Character 6	Qualifier Character 7
K Thoracic Duct **L** Cisterna Chyli **M** Thymus **T** Bone Marrow	**0** Open **3** Percutaneous **4** Percutaneous Endoscopic	**Z** No Device	**Z** No Qualifier
N Lymphatic **P** Spleen	**0** Open **3** Percutaneous **4** Percutaneous Endoscopic **X** External	**Z** No Device	**Z** No Qualifier

Lymphatic and Hemic Systems

0 **Medical and Surgical**
7 **Lymphatic and Hemic Systems**
L **Occlusion**   Completely closing an orifice or the lumen of a tubular body part

Body Part Character 4	Approach Character 5	Device Character 6	Qualifier Character 7
0 Lymphatic, Head **1** Lymphatic, Right Neck **2** Lymphatic, Left Neck **3** Lymphatic, Right Upper Extremity **4** Lymphatic, Left Upper Extremity **5** Lymphatic, Right Axillary **6** Lymphatic, Left Axillary **7** Lymphatic, Thorax **8** Lymphatic, Internal Mammary, Right **9** Lymphatic, Internal Mammary, Left **B** Lymphatic, Mesenteric **C** Lymphatic, Pelvis **D** Lymphatic, Aortic **F** Lymphatic, Right Lower Extremity **G** Lymphatic, Left Lower Extremity **H** Lymphatic, Right Inguinal **J** Lymphatic, Left Inguinal **K** Thoracic Duct **L** Cisterna Chyli	**0** Open **3** Percutaneous **4** Percutaneous Endoscopic	**C** Extraluminal Device **D** Intraluminal Device **Z** No Device	**Z** No Qualifier

0 **Medical and Surgical**
7 **Lymphatic and Hemic Systems**
N **Release**   Freeing a body part from an abnormal physical constraint

Body Part Character 4	Approach Character 5	Device Character 6	Qualifier Character 7
0 Lymphatic, Head **1** Lymphatic, Right Neck **2** Lymphatic, Left Neck **3** Lymphatic, Right Upper Extremity **4** Lymphatic, Left Upper Extremity **5** Lymphatic, Right Axillary **6** Lymphatic, Left Axillary **7** Lymphatic, Thorax **8** Lymphatic, Internal Mammary, Right **9** Lymphatic, Internal Mammary, Left **B** Lymphatic, Mesenteric **C** Lymphatic, Pelvis **D** Lymphatic, Aortic **F** Lymphatic, Right Lower Extremity **G** Lymphatic, Left Lower Extremity **H** Lymphatic, Right Inguinal **J** Lymphatic, Left Inguinal **K** Thoracic Duct **L** Cisterna Chyli **M** Thymus **P** Spleen	**0** Open **3** Percutaneous **4** Percutaneous Endoscopic	**Z** No Device	**Z** No Qualifier

0 **Medical and Surgical**
7 **Lymphatic and Hemic Systems**
P **Removal**   Taking out or off a device from a body part

Body Part Character 4	Approach Character 5	Device Character 6	Qualifier Character 7
K Thoracic Duct **L** Cisterna Chyli **N** Lymphatic	**0** Open **3** Percutaneous **4** Percutaneous Endoscopic	**0** Drainage Device **3** Infusion Device **7** Autologous Tissue Substitute **C** Extraluminal Device **D** Intraluminal Device **J** Synthetic Substitute **K** Nonautologous Tissue Substitute	**Z** No Qualifier
K Thoracic Duct **L** Cisterna Chyli **N** Lymphatic	**X** External	**0** Drainage Device **3** Infusion Device **D** Intraluminal Device	**Z** No Qualifier
M Thymus **P** Spleen	**0** Open **3** Percutaneous **4** Percutaneous Endoscopic **X** External	**0** Drainage Device **3** Infusion Device	**Z** No Qualifier

07P Continued on next page

Lymphatic and Hemic Systems *(side margin)*

07P–07T *(side margin)*

07P Continued

0　Medical and Surgical
7　Lymphatic and Hemic Systems
P　Removal　　　Taking out or off a device from a body part

Body Part Character 4	Approach Character 5	Device Character 6	Qualifier Character 7
T　Bone Marrow	0　Open 3　Percutaneous 4　Percutaneous Endoscopic X　External	0　Drainage Device	Z　No Qualifier

0　Medical and Surgical
7　Lymphatic and Hemic Systems
Q　Repair　　　Restoring, to the extent possible, a body part to its normal anatomic structure and function

Body Part Character 4	Approach Character 5	Device Character 6	Qualifier Character 7
0　Lymphatic, Head 1　Lymphatic, Right Neck 2　Lymphatic, Left Neck 3　Lymphatic, Right Upper Extremity 4　Lymphatic, Left Upper Extremity 5　Lymphatic, Right Axillary 6　Lymphatic, Left Axillary 7　Lymphatic, Thorax 8　Lymphatic, Internal Mammary, Right 9　Lymphatic, Internal Mammary, Left B　Lymphatic, Mesenteric C　Lymphatic, Pelvis D　Lymphatic, Aortic F　Lymphatic, Right Lower Extremity G　Lymphatic, Left Lower Extremity H　Lymphatic, Right Inguinal J　Lymphatic, Left Inguinal K　Thoracic Duct L　Cisterna Chyli M　Thymus P　Spleen	0　Open 3　Percutaneous 4　Percutaneous Endoscopic	Z　No Device	Z　No Qualifier

0　Medical and Surgical
7　Lymphatic and Hemic Systems
S　Reposition　　　Moving to its normal location or other suitable location all or a portion of a body part

Body Part Character 4	Approach Character 5	Device Character 6	Qualifier Character 7
M　Thymus P　Spleen	0　Open	Z　No Device	Z　No Qualifier

0　Medical and Surgical
7　Lymphatic and Hemic Systems
T　Resection　　　Cutting out or off, without replacement, all of a body part

Body Part Character 4	Approach Character 5	Device Character 6	Qualifier Character 7
0　Lymphatic, Head 1　Lymphatic, Right Neck 2　Lymphatic, Left Neck 3　Lymphatic, Right Upper Extremity 4　Lymphatic, Left Upper Extremity 5　Lymphatic, Right Axillary 6　Lymphatic, Left Axillary 7　Lymphatic, Thorax 8　Lymphatic, Internal Mammary, Right 9　Lymphatic, Internal Mammary, Left B　Lymphatic, Mesenteric C　Lymphatic, Pelvis D　Lymphatic, Aortic F　Lymphatic, Right Lower Extremity G　Lymphatic, Left Lower Extremity H　Lymphatic, Right Inguinal J　Lymphatic, Left Inguinal K　Thoracic Duct L　Cisterna Chyli M　Thymus P　Spleen	0　Open 4　Percutaneous Endoscopic	Z　No Device	Z　No Qualifier

Revised Text in **BLUE**　　　© 2011 Ingenix, Inc

0　Medical and Surgical
7　Lymphatic and Hemic Systems
U　Supplement　　Putting in or on biological or synthetic material that physically reinforces and/or augments the function of a portion of a body part

Body Part Character 4	Approach Character 5	Device Character 6	Qualifier Character 7
0　Lymphatic, Head 1　Lymphatic, Right Neck 2　Lymphatic, Left Neck 3　Lymphatic, Right Upper Extremity 4　Lymphatic, Left Upper Extremity 5　Lymphatic, Right Axillary 6　Lymphatic, Left Axillary 7　Lymphatic, Thorax 8　Lymphatic, Internal Mammary, Right 9　Lymphatic, Internal Mammary, Left B　Lymphatic, Mesenteric C　Lymphatic, Pelvis D　Lymphatic, Aortic F　Lymphatic, Right Lower Extremity G　Lymphatic, Left Lower Extremity H　Lymphatic, Right Inguinal J　Lymphatic, Left Inguinal K　Thoracic Duct L　Cisterna Chyli	0　Open 4　Percutaneous Endoscopic	7　Autologous Tissue Substitute J　Synthetic Substitute K　Nonautologous Tissue Substitute	Z　No Qualifier

0　Medical and Surgical
7　Lymphatic and Hemic Systems
V　Restriction　　Partially closing an orifice or the lumen of a tubular body part

Body Part Character 4	Approach Character 5	Device Character 6	Qualifier Character 7
0　Lymphatic, Head 1　Lymphatic, Right Neck 2　Lymphatic, Left Neck 3　Lymphatic, Right Upper Extremity 4　Lymphatic, Left Upper Extremity 5　Lymphatic, Right Axillary 6　Lymphatic, Left Axillary 7　Lymphatic, Thorax 8　Lymphatic, Internal Mammary, Right 9　Lymphatic, Internal Mammary, Left B　Lymphatic, Mesenteric C　Lymphatic, Pelvis D　Lymphatic, Aortic F　Lymphatic, Right Lower Extremity G　Lymphatic, Left Lower Extremity H　Lymphatic, Right Inguinal J　Lymphatic, Left Inguinal K　Thoracic Duct L　Cisterna Chyli	0　Open 3　Percutaneous 4　Percutaneous Endoscopic	C　Extraluminal Device D　Intraluminal Device Z　No Device	Z　No Qualifier

0　Medical and Surgical
7　Lymphatic and Hemic Systems
W　Revision　　Correcting, to the extent possible, a portion of a malfunctioning device or the position of a displaced device

Body Part Character 4	Approach Character 5	Device Character 6	Qualifier Character 7
K　Thoracic Duct L　Cisterna Chyli N　Lymphatic	0　Open 3　Percutaneous 4　Percutaneous Endoscopic X　External	0　Drainage Device 3　Infusion Device 7　Autologous Tissue Substitute C　Extraluminal Device D　Intraluminal Device J　Synthetic Substitute K　Nonautologous Tissue Substitute	Z　No Qualifier
M　Thymus P　Spleen	0　Open 3　Percutaneous 4　Percutaneous Endoscopic X　External	0　Drainage Device 3　Infusion Device	Z　No Qualifier
T　Bone Marrow	0　Open 3　Percutaneous 4　Percutaneous Endoscopic X　External	0　Drainage Device	Z　No Qualifier

Lymphatic and Hemic Systems

07U—07W

Ø Medical and Surgical
7 Lymphatic and Hemic Systems
Y Transplantation Putting in or on all or a portion of a living body part taken from another individual or animal to physically take the place and/or function of all or a portion of a similar body part

Body Part Character 4	Approach Character 5	Device Character 6	Qualifier Character 7
M Thymus P Spleen	Ø Open	Z No Device	Ø Allogeneic 1 Syngeneic 2 Zooplastic

Eye Ø8Ø–Ø8X

Ø Medical and Surgical
8 Eye
Ø Alteration   Modifying the anatomic structure of a body part without affecting the function of the body part

Body Part Character 4	Approach Character 5	Device Character 6	Qualifier Character 7
N Upper Eyelid, Right P Upper Eyelid, Left Q Lower Eyelid, Right R Lower Eyelid, Left	Ø Open 3 Percutaneous X External	7 Autologous Tissue Substitute J Synthetic Substitute K Nonautologous Tissue Substitute Z No Device	Z No Qualifier

Ø Medical and Surgical
8 Eye
1 Bypass   Altering the route of passage of the contents of a tubular body part

Body Part Character 4	Approach Character 5	Device Character 6	Qualifier Character 7
2 Anterior Chamber, Right 3 Anterior Chamber, Left	3 Percutaneous	J Synthetic Substitute K Nonautologous Tissue Substitute Z No Device	4 Sclera
X Lacrimal Duct, Right Y Lacrimal Duct, Left	Ø Open 3 Percutaneous	J Synthetic Substitute K Nonautologous Tissue Substitute Z No Device	3 Nasal Cavity

Ø Medical and Surgical
8 Eye
2 Change   Taking out or off a device from a body part and putting back an identical or similar device in or on the same body part without cutting or puncturing the skin or a mucous membrane

Body Part Character 4	Approach Character 5	Device Character 6	Qualifier Character 7
Ø Eye, Right 1 Eye, Left	X External	Ø Drainage Device Y Other Device	Z No Qualifier

Ø Medical and Surgical
8 Eye
5 Destruction   Physical eradication of all or a portion of a body part by the direct use of energy, force, or a destructive agent

Body Part Character 4	Approach Character 5	Device Character 6	Qualifier Character 7
Ø Eye, Right 1 Eye, Left 6 Sclera, Right 7 Sclera, Left 8 Cornea, Right 9 Cornea, Left S Conjunctiva, Right T Conjunctiva, Left	X External	Z No Device	Z No Qualifier
2 Anterior Chamber, Right 3 Anterior Chamber, Left 4 Vitreous, Right 5 Vitreous, Left C Iris, Right D Iris, Left E Retina, Right F Retina, Left G Retinal Vessel, Right H Retinal Vessel, Left J Lens, Right K Lens, Left	3 Percutaneous	Z No Device	Z No Qualifier
A Choroid, Right B Choroid, Left L Extraocular Muscle, Right M Extraocular Muscle, Left V Lacrimal Gland, Right W Lacrimal Gland, Left	Ø Open 3 Percutaneous	Z No Device	Z No Qualifier
N Upper Eyelid, Right P Upper Eyelid, Left Q Lower Eyelid, Right R Lower Eyelid, Left	Ø Open 3 Percutaneous X External	Z No Device	Z No Qualifier

Ø85 Continued on next page

    Revised Text in **BLUE**

085 Continued

0 Medical and Surgical
8 Eye
5 Destruction   Physical eradication of all or a portion of a body part by the direct use of energy, force, or a destructive agent

Body Part Character 4	Approach Character 5	Device Character 6	Qualifier Character 7
X Lacrimal Duct, Right **Y** Lacrimal Duct, Left	**0** Open **3** Percutaneous **7** Via Natural or Artificial Opening **8** Via Natural or Artificial Opening Endoscopic	**Z** No Device	**Z** No Qualifier

0 Medical and Surgical
8 Eye
7 Dilation   Expanding an orifice or the lumen of a tubular body part

Body Part Character 4	Approach Character 5	Device Character 6	Qualifier Character 7
X Lacrimal Duct, Right **Y** Lacrimal Duct, Left	**0** Open **3** Percutaneous **7** Via Natural or Artificial Opening **8** Via Natural or Artificial Opening Endoscopic	**D** Intraluminal Device **Z** No Device	**Z** No Qualifier

0 Medical and Surgical
8 Eye
9 Drainage   Taking or letting out fluids and/or gases from a body part

Body Part Character 4	Approach Character 5	Device Character 6	Qualifier Character 7
0 Eye, Right **1** Eye, Left **6** Sclera, Right **7** Sclera, Left **8** Cornea, Right **9** Cornea, Left **S** Conjunctiva, Right **T** Conjunctiva, Left	**X** External	**0** Drainage Device	**Z** No Qualifier
0 Eye, Right **1** Eye, Left **6** Sclera, Right **7** Sclera, Left **8** Cornea, Right **9** Cornea, Left **S** Conjunctiva, Right **T** Conjunctiva, Left	**X** External	**Z** No Device	**X** Diagnostic **Z** No Qualifier
2 Anterior Chamber, Right **3** Anterior Chamber, Left **4** Vitreous, Right **5** Vitreous, Left **C** Iris, Right **D** Iris, Left **E** Retina, Right **F** Retina, Left **G** Retinal Vessel, Right **H** Retinal Vessel, Left **J** Lens, Right **K** Lens, Left	**3** Percutaneous	**0** Drainage Device	**Z** No Qualifier
2 Anterior Chamber, Right **3** Anterior Chamber, Left **4** Vitreous, Right **5** Vitreous, Left **C** Iris, Right **D** Iris, Left **E** Retina, Right **F** Retina, Left **G** Retinal Vessel, Right **H** Retinal Vessel, Left **J** Lens, Right **K** Lens, Left	**3** Percutaneous	**Z** No Device	**X** Diagnostic **Z** No Qualifier
A Choroid, Right **B** Choroid, Left **L** Extraocular Muscle, Right **M** Extraocular Muscle, Left **V** Lacrimal Gland, Right **W** Lacrimal Gland, Left	**0** Open **3** Percutaneous	**0** Drainage Device	**Z** No Qualifier

089 Continued on next page

Ø   **Medical and Surgical**   *Ø89 Continued*
8   **Eye**
9   **Drainage**   Taking or letting out fluids and/or gases from a body part

Body Part Character 4	Approach Character 5	Device Character 6	Qualifier Character 7
A Choroid, Right **B** Choroid, Left **L** Extraocular Muscle, Right **M** Extraocular Muscle, Left **V** Lacrimal Gland, Right **W** Lacrimal Gland, Left	**Ø** Open **3** Percutaneous	**Z** No Device	**X** Diagnostic **Z** No Qualifier
N Upper Eyelid, Right **P** Upper Eyelid, Left **Q** Lower Eyelid, Right **R** Lower Eyelid, Left	**Ø** Open **3** Percutaneous **X** External	**Ø** Drainage Device	**Z** No Qualifier
N Upper Eyelid, Right **P** Upper Eyelid, Left **Q** Lower Eyelid, Right **R** Lower Eyelid, Left	**Ø** Open **3** Percutaneous **X** External	**Z** No Device	**X** Diagnostic **Z** No Qualifier
X Lacrimal Duct, Right **Y** Lacrimal Duct, Left	**Ø** Open **3** Percutaneous **7** Via Natural or Artificial Opening **8** Via Natural or Artificial Opening Endoscopic	**Ø** Drainage Device	**Z** No Qualifier
X Lacrimal Duct, Right **Y** Lacrimal Duct, Left	**Ø** Open **3** Percutaneous **7** Via Natural or Artificial Opening **8** Via Natural or Artificial Opening Endoscopic	**Z** No Device	**X** Diagnostic **Z** No Qualifier

Ø   **Medical and Surgical**
8   **Eye**
B   **Excision**   Cutting out or off, without replacement, a portion of a body part

Body Part Character 4	Approach Character 5	Device Character 6	Qualifier Character 7
Ø Eye, Right **1** Eye, Left **N** Upper Eyelid, Right **P** Upper Eyelid, Left **Q** Lower Eyelid, Right **R** Lower Eyelid, Left	**Ø** Open **3** Percutaneous **X** External	**Z** No Device	**X** Diagnostic **Z** No Qualifier
4 Vitreous, Right **5** Vitreous, Left **C** Iris, Right **D** Iris, Left **E** Retina, Right **F** Retina, Left **J** Lens, Right **K** Lens, Left	**3** Percutaneous	**Z** No Device	**X** Diagnostic **Z** No Qualifier
6 Sclera, Right **7** Sclera, Left **8** Cornea, Right **9** Cornea, Left **S** Conjunctiva, Right **T** Conjunctiva, Left	**X** External	**Z** No Device	**X** Diagnostic **Z** No Qualifier
A Choroid, Right **B** Choroid, Left **L** Extraocular Muscle, Right **M** Extraocular Muscle, Left **V** Lacrimal Gland, Right **W** Lacrimal Gland, Left	**Ø** Open **3** Percutaneous	**Z** No Device	**X** Diagnostic **Z** No Qualifier
X Lacrimal Duct, Right **Y** Lacrimal Duct, Left	**Ø** Open **3** Percutaneous **7** Via Natural or Artificial Opening **8** Via Natural or Artificial Opening Endoscopic	**Z** No Device	**X** Diagnostic **Z** No Qualifier

Ø   **Medical and Surgical**
8   **Eye**
C   **Extirpation**   Taking or cutting out solid matter from a body part

Body Part Character 4	Approach Character 5	Device Character 6	Qualifier Character 7
Ø Eye, Right 1 Eye, Left 6 Sclera, Right 7 Sclera, Left 8 Cornea, Right 9 Cornea, Left S Conjunctiva, Right T Conjunctiva, Left	X External	Z No Device	Z No Qualifier
2 Anterior Chamber, Right 3 Anterior Chamber, Left 4 Vitreous, Right 5 Vitreous, Left C Iris, Right D Iris, Left E Retina, Right F Retina, Left G Retinal Vessel, Right H Retinal Vessel, Left J Lens, Right K Lens, Left	3 Percutaneous X External	Z No Device	Z No Qualifier
A Choroid, Right B Choroid, Left L Extraocular Muscle, Right M Extraocular Muscle, Left N Upper Eyelid, Right P Upper Eyelid, Left Q Lower Eyelid, Right R Lower Eyelid, Left V Lacrimal Gland, Right W Lacrimal Gland, Left	Ø Open 3 Percutaneous X External	Z No Device	Z No Qualifier
X Lacrimal Duct, Right Y Lacrimal Duct, Left	Ø Open 3 Percutaneous 7 Via Natural or Artificial Opening 8 Via Natural or Artificial Opening Endoscopic	Z No Device	Z No Qualifier

Ø   **Medical and Surgical**
8   **Eye**
D   **Extraction**   Pulling or stripping out or off all or a portion of a body part by the use of force

Body Part Character 4	Approach Character 5	Device Character 6	Qualifier Character 7
8 Cornea, Right 9 Cornea, Left	X External	Z No Device	X Diagnostic Z No Qualifier
J Lens, Right K Lens, Left	3 Percutaneous	Z No Device	Z No Qualifier

Ø   **Medical and Surgical**
8   **Eye**
F   **Fragmentation**   Breaking solid matter in a body part into pieces

Body Part Character 4	Approach Character 5	Device Character 6	Qualifier Character 7
4 Vitreous, Right 5 Vitreous, Left	3 Percutaneous X External	Z No Device	Z No Qualifier

Ø   **Medical and Surgical**
8   **Eye**
H   **Insertion**   Putting in a nonbiological appliance that monitors, assists, performs, or prevents a physiological function but does not physically take the place of a body part

Body Part Character 4	Approach Character 5	Device Character 6	Qualifier Character 7
Ø Eye, Right 1 Eye, Left	3 Percutaneous X External	1 Radioactive Element 3 Infusion Device	Z No Qualifier

0   Medical and Surgical
8   Eye
J   Inspection   Visually and/or manually exploring a body part

Body Part Character 4	Approach Character 5	Device Character 6	Qualifier Character 7
0 Eye, Right 1 Eye, Left J Lens, Right K Lens, Left	X External	Z No Device	Z No Qualifier
L Extraocular Muscle, Right M Extraocular Muscle, Left	0 Open X External	Z No Device	Z No Qualifier

0   Medical and Surgical
8   Eye
L   Occlusion   Completely closing an orifice or the lumen of a tubular body part

Body Part Character 4	Approach Character 5	Device Character 6	Qualifier Character 7
X Lacrimal Duct, Right Y Lacrimal Duct, Left	0 Open 3 Percutaneous	C Extraluminal Device D Intraluminal Device Z No Device	Z No Qualifier
X Lacrimal Duct, Right Y Lacrimal Duct, Left	7 Via Natural or Artificial Opening 8 Via Natural or Artificial Opening Endoscopic	D Intraluminal Device Z No Device	Z No Qualifier

0   Medical and Surgical
8   Eye
M   Reattachment   Putting back in or on all or a portion of a separated body part to its normal location or other suitable location

Body Part Character 4	Approach Character 5	Device Character 6	Qualifier Character 7
N Upper Eyelid, Right P Upper Eyelid, Left Q Lower Eyelid, Right R Lower Eyelid, Left	X External	Z No Device	Z No Qualifier

0   Medical and Surgical
8   Eye
N   Release   Freeing a body part from an abnormal physical constraint

Body Part Character 4	Approach Character 5	Device Character 6	Qualifier Character 7
0 Eye, Right 1 Eye, Left 6 Sclera, Right 7 Sclera, Left 8 Cornea, Right 9 Cornea, Left S Conjunctiva, Right T Conjunctiva, Left	X External	Z No Device	Z No Qualifier
2 Anterior Chamber, Right 3 Anterior Chamber, Left 4 Vitreous, Right 5 Vitreous, Left C Iris, Right D Iris, Left E Retina, Right F Retina, Left G Retinal Vessel, Right H Retinal Vessel, Left J Lens, Right K Lens, Left	3 Percutaneous	Z No Device	Z No Qualifier
A Choroid, Right B Choroid, Left L Extraocular Muscle, Right M Extraocular Muscle, Left V Lacrimal Gland, Right W Lacrimal Gland, Left	0 Open 3 Percutaneous	Z No Device	Z No Qualifier
N Upper Eyelid, Right P Upper Eyelid, Left Q Lower Eyelid, Right R Lower Eyelid, Left	0 Open 3 Percutaneous X External	Z No Device	Z No Qualifier

08N Continued on next page

0   Medical and Surgical   *08N Continued*
8   Eye
N   Release   Freeing a body part from an abnormal physical constraint

Body Part Character 4	Approach Character 5	Device Character 6	Qualifier Character 7
X Lacrimal Duct, Right **Y** Lacrimal Duct, Left	**0** Open **3** Percutaneous **7** Via Natural or Artificial Opening **8** Via Natural or Artificial Opening Endoscopic	**Z** No Device	**Z** No Qualifier

0   Medical and Surgical
8   Eye
P   Removal   Taking out or off a device from a body part

Body Part Character 4	Approach Character 5	Device Character 6	Qualifier Character 7
0 Eye, Right **1** Eye, Left	**0** Open **3** Percutaneous **7** Via Natural or Artificial Opening **8** Via Natural or Artificial Opening Endoscopic **X** External	**0** Drainage Device **1** Radioactive Element **3** Infusion Device **7** Autologous Tissue Substitute **C** Extraluminal Device **D** Intraluminal Device **J** Synthetic Substitute **K** Nonautologous Tissue Substitute	**Z** No Qualifier
J Lens, Right **K** Lens, Left	**3** Percutaneous	**J** Synthetic Substitute	**Z** No Qualifier
L Extraocular Muscle, Right **M** Extraocular Muscle, Left	**0** Open **3** Percutaneous	**0** Drainage Device **7** Autologous Tissue Substitute **J** Synthetic Substitute **K** Nonautologous Tissue Substitute	**Z** No Qualifier

0   Medical and Surgical
8   Eye
Q   Repair   Restoring, to the extent possible, a body part to its normal anatomic structure and function

Body Part Character 4	Approach Character 5	Device Character 6	Qualifier Character 7
0 Eye, Right **1** Eye, Left **6** Sclera, Right **7** Sclera, Left **8** Cornea, Right **9** Cornea, Left **S** Conjunctiva, Right **T** Conjunctiva, Left	**X** External	**Z** No Device	**Z** No Qualifier
2 Anterior Chamber, Right **3** Anterior Chamber, Left **4** Vitreous, Right **5** Vitreous, Left **C** Iris, Right **D** Iris, Left **E** Retina, Right **F** Retina, Left **G** Retinal Vessel, Right **H** Retinal Vessel, Left **J** Lens, Right **K** Lens, Left	**3** Percutaneous	**Z** No Device	**Z** No Qualifier
A Choroid, Right **B** Choroid, Left **L** Extraocular Muscle, Right **M** Extraocular Muscle, Left **V** Lacrimal Gland, Right **W** Lacrimal Gland, Left	**0** Open **3** Percutaneous	**Z** No Device	**Z** No Qualifier
N Upper Eyelid, Right **P** Upper Eyelid, Left **Q** Lower Eyelid, Right **R** Lower Eyelid, Left	**0** Open **3** Percutaneous **X** External	**Z** No Device	**Z** No Qualifier
X Lacrimal Duct, Right **Y** Lacrimal Duct, Left	**0** Open **3** Percutaneous **7** Via Natural or Artificial Opening **8** Via Natural or Artificial Opening Endoscopic	**Z** No Device	**Z** No Qualifier

0 Medical and Surgical
8 Eye
R Replacement — Putting in or on biological or synthetic material that physically takes the place and/or function of all or a portion of a body part

Body Part Character 4	Approach Character 5	Device Character 6	Qualifier Character 7
0 Eye, Right **1** Eye, Left **A** Choroid, Right **B** Choroid, Left	**0** Open **3** Percutaneous	**7** Autologous Tissue Substitute **J** Synthetic Substitute **K** Nonautologous Tissue Substitute	**Z** No Qualifier
4 Vitreous, Right **5** Vitreous, Left **C** Iris, Right **D** Iris, Left **G** Retinal Vessel, Right **H** Retinal Vessel, Left	**3** Percutaneous	**7** Autologous Tissue Substitute **J** Synthetic Substitute **K** Nonautologous Tissue Substitute	**Z** No Qualifier
6 Sclera, Right **7** Sclera, Left **S** Conjunctiva, Right **T** Conjunctiva, Left	**X** External	**7** Autologous Tissue Substitute **J** Synthetic Substitute **K** Nonautologous Tissue Substitute	**Z** No Qualifier
8 Cornea, Right **9** Cornea, Left	**3** Percutaneous **X** External	**7** Autologous Tissue Substitute **J** Synthetic Substitute **K** Nonautologous Tissue Substitute	**Z** No Qualifier
J Lens, Right **K** Lens, Left	**3** Percutaneous	**7** Autologous Tissue Substitute **K** Nonautologous Tissue Substitute	**Z** No Qualifier
J Lens, Right **K** Lens, Left	**3** Percutaneous	**J** Synthetic Substitute	**5** Intraocular Telescope **Z** No Qualifier
N Upper Eyelid, Right **P** Upper Eyelid, Left **Q** Lower Eyelid, Right **R** Lower Eyelid, Left	**0** Open **3** Percutaneous **X** External	**7** Autologous Tissue Substitute **J** Synthetic Substitute **K** Nonautologous Tissue Substitute	**Z** No Qualifier
X Lacrimal Duct, Right **Y** Lacrimal Duct, Left	**0** Open **3** Percutaneous **7** Via Natural or Artificial Opening **8** Via Natural or Artificial Opening Endoscopic	**7** Autologous Tissue Substitute **J** Synthetic Substitute **K** Nonautologous Tissue Substitute	**Z** No Qualifier

0 Medical and Surgical
8 Eye
S Reposition — Moving to its normal location or other suitable location all or a portion of a body part

Body Part Character 4	Approach Character 5	Device Character 6	Qualifier Character 7
C Iris, Right **D** Iris, Left **G** Retinal Vessel, Right **H** Retinal Vessel, Left **J** Lens, Right **K** Lens, Left	**3** Percutaneous	**Z** No Device	**Z** No Qualifier
L Extraocular Muscle, Right **M** Extraocular Muscle, Left **V** Lacrimal Gland, Right **W** Lacrimal Gland, Left	**0** Open **3** Percutaneous	**Z** No Device	**Z** No Qualifier
N Upper Eyelid, Right **P** Upper Eyelid, Left **Q** Lower Eyelid, Right **R** Lower Eyelid, Left	**0** Open **3** Percutaneous **X** External	**Z** No Device	**Z** No Qualifier
X Lacrimal Duct, Right **Y** Lacrimal Duct, Left	**0** Open **3** Percutaneous **7** Via Natural or Artificial Opening **8** Via Natural or Artificial Opening Endoscopic	**Z** No Device	**Z** No Qualifier

Ø   **Medical and Surgical**
8   **Eye**
T   **Resection**   Cutting out or off, without replacement, all of a body part

Body Part Character 4	Approach Character 5	Device Character 6	Qualifier Character 7
Ø Eye, Right **1** Eye, Left **8** Cornea, Right **9** Cornea, Left	**X** External	**Z** No Device	**Z** No Qualifier
4 Vitreous, Right **5** Vitreous, Left **C** Iris, Right **D** Iris, Left **J** Lens, Right **K** Lens, Left	**3** Percutaneous	**Z** No Device	**Z** No Qualifier
L Extraocular Muscle, Right **M** Extraocular Muscle, Left **V** Lacrimal Gland, Right **W** Lacrimal Gland, Left	**Ø** Open **3** Percutaneous	**Z** No Device	**Z** No Qualifier
N Upper Eyelid, Right **P** Upper Eyelid, Left **Q** Lower Eyelid, Right **R** Lower Eyelid, Left	**Ø** Open **X** External	**Z** No Device	**Z** No Qualifier
X Lacrimal Duct, Right **Y** Lacrimal Duct, Left	**Ø** Open **3** Percutaneous **7** Via Natural or Artificial Opening **8** Via Natural or Artificial Opening Endoscopic	**Z** No Device	**Z** No Qualifier

Ø   **Medical and Surgical**
8   **Eye**
U   **Supplement**   Putting in or on biological or synthetic material that physically reinforces and/or augments the function of a portion of a body part

Body Part Character 4	Approach Character 5	Device Character 6	Qualifier Character 7
Ø Eye, Right **1** Eye, Left **C** Iris, Right **D** Iris, Left **E** Retina, Right **F** Retina, Left **G** Retinal Vessel, Right **H** Retinal Vessel, Left **L** Extraocular Muscle, Right **M** Extraocular Muscle, Left	**Ø** Open **3** Percutaneous	**7** Autologous Tissue Substitute **J** Synthetic Substitute **K** Nonautologous Tissue Substitute	**Z** No Qualifier
8 Cornea, Right **9** Cornea, Left **N** Upper Eyelid, Right **P** Upper Eyelid, Left **Q** Lower Eyelid, Right **R** Lower Eyelid, Left	**Ø** Open **3** Percutaneous **X** External	**7** Autologous Tissue Substitute **J** Synthetic Substitute **K** Nonautologous Tissue Substitute	**Z** No Qualifier
X Lacrimal Duct, Right **Y** Lacrimal Duct, Left	**Ø** Open **3** Percutaneous **7** Via Natural or Artificial Opening **8** Via Natural or Artificial Opening Endoscopic	**7** Autologous Tissue Substitute **J** Synthetic Substitute **K** Nonautologous Tissue Substitute	**Z** No Qualifier

Ø   **Medical and Surgical**
8   **Eye**
V   **Restriction**   Partially closing an orifice or the lumen of a tubular body part

Body Part Character 4	Approach Character 5	Device Character 6	Qualifier Character 7
X Lacrimal Duct, Right **Y** Lacrimal Duct, Left	**Ø** Open **3** Percutaneous	**C** Extraluminal Device **D** Intraluminal Device **Z** No Device	**Z** No Qualifier
X Lacrimal Duct, Right **Y** Lacrimal Duct, Left	**7** Via Natural or Artificial Opening **8** Via Natural or Artificial Opening Endoscopic	**D** Intraluminal Device **Z** No Device	**Z** No Qualifier

0　Medical and Surgical
8　Eye
W　Revision　　　Correcting, to the extent possible, a portion of a malfunctioning device or the position of a displaced device

Body Part Character 4	Approach Character 5	Device Character 6	Qualifier Character 7
0 Eye, Right **1** Eye, Left	**0** Open **3** Percutaneous **7** Via Natural or Artificial Opening **8** Via Natural or Artificial Opening Endoscopic **X** External	**0** Drainage Device **3** Infusion Device **7** Autologous Tissue Substitute **C** Extraluminal Device **D** Intraluminal Device **J** Synthetic Substitute **K** Nonautologous Tissue Substitute	**Z** No Qualifier
J Lens, Right **K** Lens, Left	**3** Percutaneous **X** External	**J** Synthetic Substitute	**Z** No Qualifier
L Extraocular Muscle, Right **M** Extraocular Muscle, Left	**0** Open **3** Percutaneous	**0** Drainage Device **7** Autologous Tissue Substitute **J** Synthetic Substitute **K** Nonautologous Tissue Substitute	**Z** No Qualifier

0　Medical and Surgical
8　Eye
X　Transfer　　　Moving, without taking out, all or a portion of a body part to another location to take over the function of all or a portion of a body part

Body Part Character 4	Approach Character 5	Device Character 6	Qualifier Character 7
L Extraocular Muscle, Right **M** Extraocular Muscle, Left	**0** Open **3** Percutaneous	**Z** No Device	**Z** No Qualifier

Ear, Nose, Sinus 090–09W

0   **Medical and Surgical**
9   **Ear, Nose, Sinus**
0   **Alteration**   Modifying the anatomic structure of a body part without affecting the function of the body part

Body Part Character 4	Approach Character 5	Device Character 6	Qualifier Character 7
0 External Ear, Right 1 External Ear, Left 2 External Ear, Bilateral K Nose	0 Open 3 Percutaneous 4 Percutaneous Endoscopic X External	7 Autologous Tissue Substitute J Synthetic Substitute K Nonautologous Tissue Substitute Z No Device	Z No Qualifier

0   **Medical and Surgical**
9   **Ear, Nose, Sinus**
1   **Bypass**   Altering the route of passage of the contents of a tubular body part

Body Part Character 4	Approach Character 5	Device Character 6	Qualifier Character 7
D Inner Ear, Right E Inner Ear, Left	0 Open	7 Autologous Tissue Substitute J Synthetic Substitute K Nonautologous Tissue Substitute Z No Device	0 Endolymphatic

0   **Medical and Surgical**
9   **Ear, Nose, Sinus**
2   **Change**   Taking out or off a device from a body part and putting back an identical or similar device in or on the same body part without cutting or puncturing the skin or a mucous membrane

Body Part Character 4	Approach Character 5	Device Character 6	Qualifier Character 7
H Ear, Right J Ear, Left K Nose Y Sinus	X External	0 Drainage Device Y Other Device	Z No Qualifier

0   **Medical and Surgical**
9   **Ear, Nose, Sinus**
5   **Destruction**   Physical eradication of all or a portion of a body part by the direct use of energy, force, or a destructive agent

Body Part Character 4	Approach Character 5	Device Character 6	Qualifier Character 7
0 External Ear, Right 1 External Ear, Left K Nose	0 Open 3 Percutaneous 4 Percutaneous Endoscopic X External	Z No Device	Z No Qualifier
3 External Auditory Canal, Right 4 External Auditory Canal, Left	0 Open 3 Percutaneous 4 Percutaneous Endoscopic 7 Via Natural or Artificial Opening 8 Via Natural or Artificial Opening Endoscopic X External	Z No Device	Z No Qualifier
5 Middle Ear, Right 6 Middle Ear, Left 9 Auditory Ossicle, Right A Auditory Ossicle, Left D Inner Ear, Right E Inner Ear, Left	0 Open	Z No Device	Z No Qualifier
7 Tympanic Membrane, Right 8 Tympanic Membrane, Left F Eustachian Tube, Right G Eustachian Tube, Left L Nasal Turbinate N Nasopharynx	0 Open 3 Percutaneous 4 Percutaneous Endoscopic 7 Via Natural or Artificial Opening 8 Via Natural or Artificial Opening Endoscopic	Z No Device	Z No Qualifier

095 Continued on next page

Ø Medical and Surgical
9 Ear, Nose, Sinus
5 Destruction   Physical eradication of all or a portion of a body part by the direct use of energy, force, or a destructive agent

095 Continued

Body Part Character 4	Approach Character 5	Device Character 6	Qualifier Character 7
B Mastoid Sinus, Right **C** Mastoid Sinus, Left **M** Nasal Septum **P** Accessory Sinus **Q** Maxillary Sinus, Right **R** Maxillary Sinus, Left **S** Frontal Sinus, Right **T** Frontal Sinus, Left **U** Ethmoid Sinus, Right **V** Ethmoid Sinus, Left **W** Sphenoid Sinus, Right **X** Sphenoid Sinus, Left	**Ø** Open **3** Percutaneous **4** Percutaneous Endoscopic	**Z** No Device	**Z** No Qualifier

Ø Medical and Surgical
9 Ear, Nose, Sinus
7 Dilation   Expanding an orifice or the lumen of a tubular body part

Body Part Character 4	Approach Character 5	Device Character 6	Qualifier Character 7
F Eustachian Tube, Right **G** Eustachian Tube, Left	**Ø** Open **7** Via Natural or Artificial Opening **8** Via Natural or Artificial Opening Endoscopic	**D** Intraluminal Device **Z** No Device	**Z** No Qualifier
F Eustachian Tube, Right **G** Eustachian Tube, Left	**3** Percutaneous **4** Percutaneous Endoscopic	**Z** No Device	**Z** No Qualifier

Ø Medical and Surgical
9 Ear, Nose, Sinus
8 Division   Cutting into a body part without draining fluids and/or gases from the body part in order to separate or transect a body part

Body Part Character 4	Approach Character 5	Device Character 6	Qualifier Character 7
L Nasal Turbinate	**Ø** Open **3** Percutaneous **4** Percutaneous Endoscopic **7** Via Natural or Artificial Opening **8** Via Natural or Artificial Opening Endoscopic	**Z** No Device	**Z** No Qualifier

Ø Medical and Surgical
9 Ear, Nose, Sinus
9 Drainage   Taking or letting out fluids and/or gases from a body part

Body Part Character 4	Approach Character 5	Device Character 6	Qualifier Character 7
Ø External Ear, Right **1** External Ear, Left **K** Nose	**Ø** Open **3** Percutaneous **4** Percutaneous Endoscopic **X** External	**Ø** Drainage Device	**Z** No Qualifier
Ø External Ear, Right **1** External Ear, Left **K** Nose	**Ø** Open **3** Percutaneous **4** Percutaneous Endoscopic **X** External	**Z** No Device	**X** Diagnostic **Z** No Qualifier
3 External Auditory Canal, Right **4** External Auditory Canal, Left	**Ø** Open **3** Percutaneous **4** Percutaneous Endoscopic **7** Via Natural or Artificial Opening **8** Via Natural or Artificial Opening Endoscopic **X** External	**Ø** Drainage Device	**Z** No Qualifier
3 External Auditory Canal, Right **4** External Auditory Canal, Left	**Ø** Open **3** Percutaneous **4** Percutaneous Endoscopic **7** Via Natural or Artificial Opening **8** Via Natural or Artificial Opening Endoscopic **X** External	**Z** No Device	**X** Diagnostic **Z** No Qualifier

099 Continued on next page

099 Continued

0   Medical and Surgical
9   Ear, Nose, Sinus
9   Drainage   Taking or letting out fluids and/or gases from a body part

Body Part Character 4	Approach Character 5	Device Character 6	Qualifier Character 7
5 Middle Ear, Right 6 Middle Ear, Left 9 Auditory Ossicle, Right A Auditory Ossicle, Left D Inner Ear, Right E Inner Ear, Left	0 Open	0 Drainage Device	Z No Qualifier
5 Middle Ear, Right 6 Middle Ear, Left 9 Auditory Ossicle, Right A Auditory Ossicle, Left D Inner Ear, Right E Inner Ear, Left	0 Open	Z No Device	X Diagnostic Z No Qualifier
7 Tympanic Membrane, Right 8 Tympanic Membrane, Left F Eustachian Tube, Right G Eustachian Tube, Left L Nasal Turbinate N Nasopharynx	0 Open 3 Percutaneous 4 Percutaneous Endoscopic 7 Via Natural or Artificial Opening 8 Via Natural or Artificial Opening Endoscopic	0 Drainage Device	Z No Qualifier
7 Tympanic Membrane, Right 8 Tympanic Membrane, Left F Eustachian Tube, Right G Eustachian Tube, Left L Nasal Turbinate N Nasopharynx	0 Open 3 Percutaneous 4 Percutaneous Endoscopic 7 Via Natural or Artificial Opening 8 Via Natural or Artificial Opening Endoscopic	Z No Device	X Diagnostic Z No Qualifier
B Mastoid Sinus, Right C Mastoid Sinus, Left M Nasal Septum P Accessory Sinus Q Maxillary Sinus, Right R Maxillary Sinus, Left S Frontal Sinus, Right T Frontal Sinus, Left U Ethmoid Sinus, Right V Ethmoid Sinus, Left W Sphenoid Sinus, Right X Sphenoid Sinus, Left	0 Open 3 Percutaneous 4 Percutaneous Endoscopic	0 Drainage Device	Z No Qualifier
B Mastoid Sinus, Right C Mastoid Sinus, Left M Nasal Septum P Accessory Sinus Q Maxillary Sinus, Right R Maxillary Sinus, Left S Frontal Sinus, Right T Frontal Sinus, Left U Ethmoid Sinus, Right V Ethmoid Sinus, Left W Sphenoid Sinus, Right X Sphenoid Sinus, Left	0 Open 3 Percutaneous 4 Percutaneous Endoscopic	Z No Device	X Diagnostic Z No Qualifier

0   Medical and Surgical
9   Ear, Nose, Sinus
B   Excision   Cutting out or off, without replacement, a portion of a body part

Body Part Character 4	Approach Character 5	Device Character 6	Qualifier Character 7
0 External Ear, Right 1 External Ear, Left K Nose	0 Open 3 Percutaneous 4 Percutaneous Endoscopic X External	Z No Device	X Diagnostic Z No Qualifier
3 External Auditory Canal, Right 4 External Auditory Canal, Left	0 Open 3 Percutaneous 4 Percutaneous Endoscopic 7 Via Natural or Artificial Opening 8 Via Natural or Artificial Opening Endoscopic X External	Z No Device	X Diagnostic Z No Qualifier
5 Middle Ear, Right 6 Middle Ear, Left 9 Auditory Ossicle, Right A Auditory Ossicle, Left D Inner Ear, Right E Inner Ear, Left	0 Open	Z No Device	X Diagnostic Z No Qualifier

09B Continued on next page

Ø　**Medical and Surgical**　　　　　　　　　　　　　　　　　*Ø9B Continued*
9　**Ear, Nose, Sinus**
B　**Excision**　　Cutting out or off, without replacement, a portion of a body part

Body Part Character 4	Approach Character 5	Device Character 6	Qualifier Character 7
7 Tympanic Membrane, Right 8 Tympanic Membrane, Left F Eustachian Tube, Right G Eustachian Tube, Left L Nasal Turbinate N Nasopharynx	Ø Open 3 Percutaneous 4 Percutaneous Endoscopic 7 Via Natural or Artificial Opening 8 Via Natural or Artificial Opening Endoscopic	Z No Device	X Diagnostic Z No Qualifier
B Mastoid Sinus, Right C Mastoid Sinus, Left M Nasal Septum P Accessory Sinus Q Maxillary Sinus, Right R Maxillary Sinus, Left S Frontal Sinus, Right T Frontal Sinus, Left U Ethmoid Sinus, Right V Ethmoid Sinus, Left W Sphenoid Sinus, Right X Sphenoid Sinus, Left	Ø Open 3 Percutaneous 4 Percutaneous Endoscopic	Z No Device	X Diagnostic Z No Qualifier

Ø　**Medical and Surgical**
9　**Ear, Nose, Sinus**
C　**Extirpation**　　Taking or cutting out solid matter from a body part

Body Part Character 4	Approach Character 5	Device Character 6	Qualifier Character 7
Ø External Ear, Right 1 External Ear, Left K Nose	Ø Open 3 Percutaneous 4 Percutaneous Endoscopic X External	Z No Device	Z No Qualifier
3 External Auditory Canal, Right 4 External Auditory Canal, Left	Ø Open 3 Percutaneous 4 Percutaneous Endoscopic 7 Via Natural or Artificial Opening 8 Via Natural or Artificial Opening Endoscopic X External	Z No Device	Z No Qualifier
5 Middle Ear, Right 6 Middle Ear, Left 9 Auditory Ossicle, Right A Auditory Ossicle, Left D Inner Ear, Right E Inner Ear, Left	Ø Open	Z No Device	Z No Qualifier
7 Tympanic Membrane, Right 8 Tympanic Membrane, Left F Eustachian Tube, Right G Eustachian Tube, Left L Nasal Turbinate N Nasopharynx	Ø Open 3 Percutaneous 4 Percutaneous Endoscopic 7 Via Natural or Artificial Opening 8 Via Natural or Artificial Opening Endoscopic	Z No Device	Z No Qualifier
B Mastoid Sinus, Right C Mastoid Sinus, Left M Nasal Septum P Accessory Sinus Q Maxillary Sinus, Right R Maxillary Sinus, Left S Frontal Sinus, Right T Frontal Sinus, Left U Ethmoid Sinus, Right V Ethmoid Sinus, Left W Sphenoid Sinus, Right X Sphenoid Sinus, Left	Ø Open 3 Percutaneous 4 Percutaneous Endoscopic	Z No Device	Z No Qualifier

0 Medical and Surgical
9 Ear, Nose, Sinus
D Extraction   Pulling or stripping out or off all or a portion of a body part by the use of force

Body Part Character 4	Approach Character 5	Device Character 6	Qualifier Character 7
7 Tympanic Membrane, Right 8 Tympanic Membrane, Left L Nasal Turbinate	0 Open 3 Percutaneous 4 Percutaneous Endoscopic 7 Via Natural or Artificial Opening 8 Via Natural or Artificial Opening Endoscopic	Z No Device	Z No Qualifier
9 Auditory Ossicle, Right A Auditory Ossicle, Left	0 Open	Z No Device	Z No Qualifier
B Mastoid Sinus, Right C Mastoid Sinus, Left M Nasal Septum P Accessory Sinus Q Maxillary Sinus, Right R Maxillary Sinus, Left S Frontal Sinus, Right T Frontal Sinus, Left U Ethmoid Sinus, Right V Ethmoid Sinus, Left W Sphenoid Sinus, Right X Sphenoid Sinus, Left	0 Open 3 Percutaneous 4 Percutaneous Endoscopic	Z No Device	Z No Qualifier

0 Medical and Surgical
9 Ear, Nose, Sinus
H Insertion   Putting in a nonbiological appliance that monitors, assists, performs, or prevents a physiological function but does not physically take the place of a body part

Body Part Character 4	Approach Character 5	Device Character 6	Qualifier Character 7
D Inner Ear, Right E Inner Ear, Left	0 Open	S Hearing Device	1 Bone Conduction 2 Cochlear Prosthesis, Single Channel 3 Cochlear Prosthesis, Multiple Channel Y Other Hearing Device
N Nasopharynx	7 Via Natural or Artificial Opening 8 Via Natural or Artificial Opening Endoscopic	B Airway	Z No Qualifier

0 Medical and Surgical
9 Ear, Nose, Sinus
J Inspection   Visually and/or manually exploring a body part

Body Part Character 4	Approach Character 5	Device Character 6	Qualifier Character 7
7 Tympanic Membrane, Right 8 Tympanic Membrane, Left H Ear, Right J Ear, Left	0 Open 3 Percutaneous 4 Percutaneous Endoscopic 7 Via Natural or Artificial Opening 8 Via Natural or Artificial Opening Endoscopic X External	Z No Device	Z No Qualifier
D Inner Ear, Right E Inner Ear, Left K Nose Y Sinus	0 Open 3 Percutaneous 4 Percutaneous Endoscopic X External	Z No Device	Z No Qualifier

0 Medical and Surgical
9 Ear, Nose, Sinus
M Reattachment   Putting back in or on all or a portion of a separated body part to its normal location or other suitable location

Body Part Character 4	Approach Character 5	Device Character 6	Qualifier Character 7
0 External Ear, Right 1 External Ear, Left K Nose	X External	Z No Device	Z No Qualifier

Ø   **Medical and Surgical**
9   **Ear, Nose, Sinus**
N   **Release**   Freeing a body part from an abnormal physical constraint

Body Part Character 4	Approach Character 5	Device Character 6	Qualifier Character 7
Ø External Ear, Right 1 External Ear, Left K Nose	Ø Open 3 Percutaneous 4 Percutaneous Endoscopic X External	Z No Device	Z No Qualifier
3 External Auditory Canal, Right 4 External Auditory Canal, Left	Ø Open 3 Percutaneous 4 Percutaneous Endoscopic 7 Via Natural or Artificial Opening 8 Via Natural or Artificial Opening Endoscopic X External	Z No Device	Z No Qualifier
5 Middle Ear, Right 6 Middle Ear, Left 9 Auditory Ossicle, Right A Auditory Ossicle, Left D Inner Ear, Right E Inner Ear, Left	Ø Open	Z No Device	Z No Qualifier
7 Tympanic Membrane, Right 8 Tympanic Membrane, Left F Eustachian Tube, Right G Eustachian Tube, Left L Nasal Turbinate N Nasopharynx	Ø Open 3 Percutaneous 4 Percutaneous Endoscopic 7 Via Natural or Artificial Opening 8 Via Natural or Artificial Opening Endoscopic	Z No Device	Z No Qualifier
B Mastoid Sinus, Right C Mastoid Sinus, Left M Nasal Septum P Accessory Sinus Q Maxillary Sinus, Right R Maxillary Sinus, Left S Frontal Sinus, Right T Frontal Sinus, Left U Ethmoid Sinus, Right V Ethmoid Sinus, Left W Sphenoid Sinus, Right X Sphenoid Sinus, Left	Ø Open 3 Percutaneous 4 Percutaneous Endoscopic	Z No Device	Z No Qualifier

Ø   **Medical and Surgical**
9   **Ear, Nose, Sinus**
P   **Removal**   Taking out or off a device from a body part

Body Part Character 4	Approach Character 5	Device Character 6	Qualifier Character 7
7 Tympanic Membrane, Right 8 Tympanic Membrane, Left	Ø Open 7 Via Natural or Artificial Opening 8 Via Natural or Artificial Opening Endoscopic X External	Ø Drainage Device	Z No Qualifier
D Inner Ear, Right E Inner Ear, Left	Ø Open 7 Via Natural or Artificial Opening 8 Via Natural or Artificial Opening Endoscopic	S Hearing Device	Z No Qualifier
H Ear, Right J Ear, Left	Ø Open 3 Percutaneous 4 Percutaneous Endoscopic 7 Via Natural or Artificial Opening 8 Via Natural or Artificial Opening Endoscopic X External	Ø Drainage Device 7 Autologous Tissue Substitute D Intraluminal Device J Synthetic Substitute K Nonautologous Tissue Substitute	Z No Qualifier
K Nose	Ø Open 3 Percutaneous 4 Percutaneous Endoscopic 7 Via Natural or Artificial Opening 8 Via Natural or Artificial Opening Endoscopic X External	Ø Drainage Device 7 Autologous Tissue Substitute B Airway J Synthetic Substitute K Nonautologous Tissue Substitute	Z No Qualifier
Y Sinus	Ø Open 3 Percutaneous 4 Percutaneous Endoscopic X External	Ø Drainage Device	Z No Qualifier

Ear, Nose, Sinus

0   Medical and Surgical
9   Ear, Nose, Sinus
Q   Repair   Restoring, to the extent possible, a body part to its normal anatomic structure and function

Body Part Character 4	Approach Character 5	Device Character 6	Qualifier Character 7
0 External Ear, Right 1 External Ear, Left 2 External Ear, Bilateral K Nose	0 Open 3 Percutaneous 4 Percutaneous Endoscopic X External	Z No Device	Z No Qualifier
3 External Auditory Canal, Right 4 External Auditory Canal, Left F Eustachian Tube, Right G Eustachian Tube, Left	0 Open 3 Percutaneous 4 Percutaneous Endoscopic 7 Via Natural or Artificial Opening 8 Via Natural or Artificial Opening Endoscopic X External	Z No Device	Z No Qualifier
5 Middle Ear, Right 6 Middle Ear, Left 9 Auditory Ossicle, Right A Auditory Ossicle, Left D Inner Ear, Right E Inner Ear, Left	0 Open	Z No Device	Z No Qualifier
7 Tympanic Membrane, Right 8 Tympanic Membrane, Left L Nasal Turbinate N Nasopharynx	0 Open 3 Percutaneous 4 Percutaneous Endoscopic 7 Via Natural or Artificial Opening 8 Via Natural or Artificial Opening Endoscopic	Z No Device	Z No Qualifier
B Mastoid Sinus, Right C Mastoid Sinus, Left M Nasal Septum P Accessory Sinus Q Maxillary Sinus, Right R Maxillary Sinus, Left S Frontal Sinus, Right T Frontal Sinus, Left U Ethmoid Sinus, Right V Ethmoid Sinus, Left W Sphenoid Sinus, Right X Sphenoid Sinus, Left	0 Open 3 Percutaneous 4 Percutaneous Endoscopic	Z No Device	Z No Qualifier

0   Medical and Surgical
9   Ear, Nose, Sinus
R   Replacement   Putting in or on biological or synthetic material that physically takes the place and/or function of all or a portion of a body part

Body Part Character 4	Approach Character 5	Device Character 6	Qualifier Character 7
0 External Ear, Right 1 External Ear, Left 2 External Ear, Bilateral K Nose	0 Open X External	7 Autologous Tissue Substitute J Synthetic Substitute K Nonautologous Tissue Substitute	Z No Qualifier
5 Middle Ear, Right 6 Middle Ear, Left 9 Auditory Ossicle, Right A Auditory Ossicle, Left D Inner Ear, Right E Inner Ear, Left	0 Open	7 Autologous Tissue Substitute J Synthetic Substitute K Nonautologous Tissue Substitute	Z No Qualifier
7 Tympanic Membrane, Right 8 Tympanic Membrane, Left N Nasopharynx	0 Open 7 Via Natural or Artificial Opening 8 Via Natural or Artificial Opening Endoscopic	7 Autologous Tissue Substitute J Synthetic Substitute K Nonautologous Tissue Substitute	Z No Qualifier
L Nasal Turbinate	0 Open 3 Percutaneous 4 Percutaneous Endoscopic 7 Via Natural or Artificial Opening 8 Via Natural or Artificial Opening Endoscopic	7 Autologous Tissue Substitute J Synthetic Substitute K Nonautologous Tissue Substitute	Z No Qualifier
M Nasal Septum	0 Open 3 Percutaneous 4 Percutaneous Endoscopic	7 Autologous Tissue Substitute J Synthetic Substitute K Nonautologous Tissue Substitute	Z No Qualifier

   Revised Text in **BLUE**   © 2011 Ingenix, Inc

Ø　**Medical and Surgical**
9　**Ear, Nose, Sinus**
S　**Reposition**　　Moving to its normal location or other suitable location all or a portion of a body part

Body Part Character 4	Approach Character 5	Device Character 6	Qualifier Character 7
Ø External Ear, Right 1 External Ear, Left 2 External Ear, Bilateral K Nose	Ø Open 4 Percutaneous Endoscopic X External	Z No Device	Z No Qualifier
7 Tympanic Membrane, Right 8 Tympanic Membrane, Left F Eustachian Tube, Right G Eustachian Tube, Left L Nasal Turbinate	Ø Open 4 Percutaneous Endoscopic 7 Via Natural or Artificial Opening 8 Via Natural or Artificial Opening Endoscopic	Z No Device	Z No Qualifier
9 Auditory Ossicle, Right A Auditory Ossicle, Left M Nasal Septum	Ø Open 4 Percutaneous Endoscopic	Z No Device	Z No Qualifier

Ø　**Medical and Surgical**
9　**Ear, Nose, Sinus**
T　**Resection**　　Cutting out or off, without replacement, all of a body part

Body Part Character 4	Approach Character 5	Device Character 6	Qualifier Character 7
Ø External Ear, Right 1 External Ear, Left K Nose	Ø Open 4 Percutaneous Endoscopic X External	Z No Device	Z No Qualifier
5 Middle Ear, Right 6 Middle Ear, Left 9 Auditory Ossicle, Right A Auditory Ossicle, Left D Inner Ear, Right E Inner Ear, Left	Ø Open	Z No Device	Z No Qualifier
7 Tympanic Membrane, Right 8 Tympanic Membrane, Left F Eustachian Tube, Right G Eustachian Tube, Left L Nasal Turbinate N Nasopharynx	Ø Open 4 Percutaneous Endoscopic 7 Via Natural or Artificial Opening 8 Via Natural or Artificial Opening Endoscopic	Z No Device	Z No Qualifier
B Mastoid Sinus, Right C Mastoid Sinus, Left M Nasal Septum P Accessory Sinus Q Maxillary Sinus, Right R Maxillary Sinus, Left S Frontal Sinus, Right T Frontal Sinus, Left U Ethmoid Sinus, Right V Ethmoid Sinus, Left W Sphenoid Sinus, Right X Sphenoid Sinus, Left	Ø Open 4 Percutaneous Endoscopic	Z No Device	Z No Qualifier

Ø   **Medical and Surgical**
9   **Ear, Nose, Sinus**
U   **Supplement**   Putting in or on biological or synthetic material that physically reinforces and/or augments the function of a portion of a body part

Body Part Character 4	Approach Character 5	Device Character 6	Qualifier Character 7
Ø External Ear, Right **1** External Ear, Left **2** External Ear, Bilateral **K** Nose	**Ø** Open **X** External	**7** Autologous Tissue Substitute **J** Synthetic Substitute **K** Nonautologous Tissue Substitute	**Z** No Qualifier
5 Middle Ear, Right **6** Middle Ear, Left **9** Auditory Ossicle, Right **A** Auditory Ossicle, Left **D** Inner Ear, Right **E** Inner Ear, Left	**Ø** Open	**7** Autologous Tissue Substitute **J** Synthetic Substitute **K** Nonautologous Tissue Substitute	**Z** No Qualifier
7 Tympanic Membrane, Right **8** Tympanic Membrane, Left **N** Nasopharynx	**Ø** Open **7** Via Natural or Artificial Opening **8** Via Natural or Artificial Opening Endoscopic	**7** Autologous Tissue Substitute **J** Synthetic Substitute **K** Nonautologous Tissue Substitute	**Z** No Qualifier
L Nasal Turbinate	**Ø** Open **3** Percutaneous **4** Percutaneous Endoscopic **7** Via Natural or Artificial Opening **8** Via Natural or Artificial Opening Endoscopic	**7** Autologous Tissue Substitute **J** Synthetic Substitute **K** Nonautologous Tissue Substitute	**Z** No Qualifier
M Nasal Septum	**Ø** Open **3** Percutaneous **4** Percutaneous Endoscopic	**7** Autologous Tissue Substitute **J** Synthetic Substitute **K** Nonautologous Tissue Substitute	**Z** No Qualifier

Ø   **Medical and Surgical**
9   **Ear, Nose, Sinus**
W   **Revision**   Correcting, to the extent possible, a portion of a malfunctioning device or the position of a displaced device

Body Part Character 4	Approach Character 5	Device Character 6	Qualifier Character 7
7 Tympanic Membrane, Right **8** Tympanic Membrane, Left **9** Auditory Ossicle, Right **A** Auditory Ossicle, Left	**Ø** Open **7** Via Natural or Artificial Opening **8** Via Natural or Artificial Opening Endoscopic	**7** Autologous Tissue Substitute **J** Synthetic Substitute **K** Nonautologous Tissue Substitute	**Z** No Qualifier
D Inner Ear, Right **E** Inner Ear, Left	**Ø** Open **7** Via Natural or Artificial Opening **8** Via Natural or Artificial Opening Endoscopic	**S** Hearing Device	**Z** No Qualifier
H Ear, Right **J** Ear, Left	**Ø** Open **3** Percutaneous **4** Percutaneous Endoscopic **7** Via Natural or Artificial Opening **8** Via Natural or Artificial Opening Endoscopic **X** External	**Ø** Drainage Device **7** Autologous Tissue Substitute **D** Intraluminal Device **J** Synthetic Substitute **K** Nonautologous Tissue Substitute	**Z** No Qualifier
K Nose	**Ø** Open **3** Percutaneous **4** Percutaneous Endoscopic **7** Via Natural or Artificial Opening **8** Via Natural or Artificial Opening Endoscopic **X** External	**Ø** Drainage Device **7** Autologous Tissue Substitute **B** Airway **J** Synthetic Substitute **K** Nonautologous Tissue Substitute	**Z** No Qualifier
Y Sinus	**Ø** Open **3** Percutaneous **4** Percutaneous Endoscopic **X** External	**Ø** Drainage Device	**Z** No Qualifier

Respiratory System 0B1–0BY

0   Medical and Surgical
B   Respiratory System
1   Bypass   Altering the route of passage of the contents of a tubular body part

Body Part Character 4	Approach Character 5	Device Character 6	Qualifier Character 7
1 Trachea	**0** Open	**D** Intraluminal Device	**6** Esophagus
1 Trachea	**0** Open **3** Percutaneous **4** Percutaneous Endoscopic	**F** Tracheostomy Device **Z** No Device	**4** Cutaneous

0   Medical and Surgical
B   Respiratory System
2   Change   Taking out or off a device from a body part and putting back an identical or similar device in or on the same body part without cutting or puncturing the skin or a mucous membrane

Body Part Character 4	Approach Character 5	Device Character 6	Qualifier Character 7
0 Tracheobronchial Tree **K** Lung, Right **L** Lung, Left **Q** Pleura **T** Diaphragm	**X** External	**0** Drainage Device **Y** Other Device	**Z** No Qualifier
1 Trachea	**X** External	**0** Drainage Device **E** Endotracheal Airway **F** Tracheostomy Device **Y** Other Device	**Z** No Qualifier

0   Medical and Surgical
B   Respiratory System
5   Destruction   Physical eradication of all or a portion of a body part by the direct use of energy, force, or a destructive agent

Body Part Character 4	Approach Character 5	Device Character 6	Qualifier Character 7
1 Trachea **2** Carina **3** Main Bronchus, Right **4** Upper Lobe Bronchus, Right **5** Middle Lobe Bronchus, Right **6** Lower Lobe Bronchus, Right **7** Main Bronchus, Left **8** Upper Lobe Bronchus, Left **9** Lingula Bronchus **B** Lower Lobe Bronchus, Left **C** Upper Lung Lobe, Right **D** Middle Lung Lobe, Right **F** Lower Lung Lobe, Right **G** Upper Lung Lobe, Left **H** Lung Lingula **J** Lower Lung Lobe, Left **K** Lung, Right **L** Lung, Left **M** Lungs, Bilateral	**0** Open **3** Percutaneous **4** Percutaneous Endoscopic **7** Via Natural or Artificial Opening **8** Via Natural or Artificial Opening Endoscopic	**Z** No Device	**Z** No Qualifier
N Pleura, Right **P** Pleura, Left **R** Diaphragm, Right **S** Diaphragm, Left	**0** Open **3** Percutaneous **4** Percutaneous Endoscopic	**Z** No Device	**Z** No Qualifier

Ø   **Medical and Surgical**
B   **Respiratory System**
7   **Dilation**   Expanding an orifice or the lumen of a tubular body part

Body Part Character 4	Approach Character 5	Device Character 6	Qualifier Character 7
1 Trachea 2 Carina 3 Main Bronchus, Right 4 Upper Lobe Bronchus, Right 5 Middle Lobe Bronchus, Right 6 Lower Lobe Bronchus, Right 7 Main Bronchus, Left 8 Upper Lobe Bronchus, Left 9 Lingula Bronchus B Lower Lobe Bronchus, Left	Ø Open 3 Percutaneous 4 Percutaneous Endoscopic 7 Via Natural or Artificial Opening 8 Via Natural or Artificial Opening Endoscopic	D Intraluminal Device Z No Device	Z No Qualifier

Ø   **Medical and Surgical**
B   **Respiratory System**
9   **Drainage**   Taking or letting out fluids and/or gases from a body part

Body Part Character 4	Approach Character 5	Device Character 6	Qualifier Character 7
1 Trachea 2 Carina 3 Main Bronchus, Right 4 Upper Lobe Bronchus, Right 5 Middle Lobe Bronchus, Right 6 Lower Lobe Bronchus, Right 7 Main Bronchus, Left 8 Upper Lobe Bronchus, Left 9 Lingula Bronchus B Lower Lobe Bronchus, Left C Upper Lung Lobe, Right D Middle Lung Lobe, Right F Lower Lung Lobe, Right G Upper Lung Lobe, Left H Lung Lingula J Lower Lung Lobe, Left K Lung, Right L Lung, Left M Lungs, Bilateral	Ø Open 3 Percutaneous 4 Percutaneous Endoscopic 7 Via Natural or Artificial Opening 8 Via Natural or Artificial Opening Endoscopic	Ø Drainage Device	Z No Qualifier
1 Trachea 2 Carina 3 Main Bronchus, Right 4 Upper Lobe Bronchus, Right 5 Middle Lobe Bronchus, Right 6 Lower Lobe Bronchus, Right 7 Main Bronchus, Left 8 Upper Lobe Bronchus, Left 9 Lingula Bronchus B Lower Lobe Bronchus, Left C Upper Lung Lobe, Right D Middle Lung Lobe, Right F Lower Lung Lobe, Right G Upper Lung Lobe, Left H Lung Lingula J Lower Lung Lobe, Left K Lung, Right L Lung, Left M Lungs, Bilateral	Ø Open 3 Percutaneous 4 Percutaneous Endoscopic 7 Via Natural or Artificial Opening 8 Via Natural or Artificial Opening Endoscopic	Z No Device	X Diagnostic Z No Qualifier
N Pleura, Right P Pleura, Left R Diaphragm, Right S Diaphragm, Left	Ø Open 3 Percutaneous 4 Percutaneous Endoscopic	Ø Drainage Device	Z No Qualifier
N Pleura, Right P Pleura, Left R Diaphragm, Right S Diaphragm, Left	Ø Open 3 Percutaneous 4 Percutaneous Endoscopic	Z No Device	X Diagnostic Z No Qualifier

Revised Text in **BLUE**

Ø   **Medical and Surgical**
B   **Respiratory System**
B   **Excision**   Cutting out or off, without replacement, a portion of a body part

Body Part Character 4	Approach Character 5	Device Character 6	Qualifier Character 7
1 Trachea 2 Carina 3 Main Bronchus, Right 4 Upper Lobe Bronchus, Right 5 Middle Lobe Bronchus, Right 6 Lower Lobe Bronchus, Right 7 Main Bronchus, Left 8 Upper Lobe Bronchus, Left 9 Lingula Bronchus B Lower Lobe Bronchus, Left C Upper Lung Lobe, Right D Middle Lung Lobe, Right F Lower Lung Lobe, Right G Upper Lung Lobe, Left H Lung Lingula J Lower Lung Lobe, Left K Lung, Right L Lung, Left M Lungs, Bilateral	Ø Open 3 Percutaneous 4 Percutaneous Endoscopic 7 Via Natural or Artificial Opening 8 Via Natural or Artificial Opening Endoscopic	Z No Device	X Diagnostic Z No Qualifier
N Pleura, Right P Pleura, Left R Diaphragm, Right S Diaphragm, Left	Ø Open 3 Percutaneous 4 Percutaneous Endoscopic	Z No Device	X Diagnostic Z No Qualifier

Ø   **Medical and Surgical**
B   **Respiratory System**
C   **Extirpation**   Taking or cutting out solid matter from a body part

Body Part Character 4	Approach Character 5	Device Character 6	Qualifier Character 7
1 Trachea 2 Carina 3 Main Bronchus, Right 4 Upper Lobe Bronchus, Right 5 Middle Lobe Bronchus, Right 6 Lower Lobe Bronchus, Right 7 Main Bronchus, Left 8 Upper Lobe Bronchus, Left 9 Lingula Bronchus B Lower Lobe Bronchus, Left C Upper Lung Lobe, Right D Middle Lung Lobe, Right F Lower Lung Lobe, Right G Upper Lung Lobe, Left H Lung Lingula J Lower Lung Lobe, Left K Lung, Right L Lung, Left M Lungs, Bilateral	Ø Open 3 Percutaneous 4 Percutaneous Endoscopic 7 Via Natural or Artificial Opening 8 Via Natural or Artificial Opening Endoscopic	Z No Device	Z No Qualifier
N Pleura, Right P Pleura, Left R Diaphragm, Right S Diaphragm, Left	Ø Open 3 Percutaneous 4 Percutaneous Endoscopic	Z No Device	Z No Qualifier

Ø   **Medical and Surgical**
B   **Respiratory System**
D   **Extraction**   Pulling or stripping out or off all or a portion of a body part by the use of force

Body Part Character 4	Approach Character 5	Device Character 6	Qualifier Character 7
N Pleura, Right P Pleura, Left	Ø Open 3 Percutaneous 4 Percutaneous Endoscopic	Z No Device	X Diagnostic Z No Qualifier

Respiratory System

ØBF–ØBJ

Ø   **Medical and Surgical**
B   **Respiratory System**
F   **Fragmentation**   Breaking solid matter in a body part into pieces

Body Part Character 4	Approach Character 5	Device Character 6	Qualifier Character 7
1 Trachea **2** Carina **3** Main Bronchus, Right **4** Upper Lobe Bronchus, Right **5** Middle Lobe Bronchus, Right **6** Lower Lobe Bronchus, Right **7** Main Bronchus, Left **8** Upper Lobe Bronchus, Left **9** Lingula Bronchus **B** Lower Lobe Bronchus, Left	**Ø** Open **3** Percutaneous **4** Percutaneous Endoscopic **7** Via Natural or Artificial Opening **8** Via Natural or Artificial Opening Endoscopic **X** External	**Z** No Device	**Z** No Qualifier

Ø   **Medical and Surgical**
B   **Respiratory System**
H   **Insertion**   Putting in a nonbiological appliance that monitors, assists, performs, or prevents a physiological function but does not physically take the place of a body part

Body Part Character 4	Approach Character 5	Device Character 6	Qualifier Character 7
Ø Tracheobronchial Tree	**Ø** Open **3** Percutaneous **4** Percutaneous Endoscopic **7** Via Natural or Artificial Opening **8** Via Natural or Artificial Opening Endoscopic	**1** Radioactive Element **2** Monitoring Device **3** Infusion Device **D** Intraluminal Device	**Z** No Qualifier
1 Trachea	**Ø** Open	**2** Monitoring Device **D** Intraluminal Device	**Z** No Qualifier
1 Trachea	**3** Percutaneous	**D** Intraluminal Device **E** Endotracheal Airway	**Z** No Qualifier
1 Trachea	**4** Percutaneous Endoscopic	**D** Intraluminal Device	**Z** No Qualifier
1 Trachea	**7** Via Natural or Artificial Opening **8** Via Natural or Artificial Opening Endoscopic	**2** Monitoring Device **D** Intraluminal Device **E** Endotracheal Airway	**Z** No Qualifier
3 Main Bronchus, Right **4** Upper Lobe Bronchus, Right **5** Middle Lobe Bronchus, Right **6** Lower Lobe Bronchus, Right **7** Main Bronchus, Left **8** Upper Lobe Bronchus, Left **9** Lingula Bronchus **B** Lower Lobe Bronchus, Left	**Ø** Open **3** Percutaneous **4** Percutaneous Endoscopic **7** Via Natural or Artificial Opening **8** Via Natural or Artificial Opening Endoscopic	**G** Endobronchial Valve	**Z** No Qualifier
K Lung, Right **L** Lung, Left	**Ø** Open **3** Percutaneous **4** Percutaneous Endoscopic **7** Via Natural or Artificial Opening **8** Via Natural or Artificial Opening Endoscopic	**1** Radioactive Element **2** Monitoring Device **3** Infusion Device	**Z** No Qualifier
R Diaphragm, Right **S** Diaphragm, Left	**Ø** Open **3** Percutaneous **4** Percutaneous Endoscopic	**2** Monitoring Device **M** Diaphragmatic Pacemaker Lead	**Z** No Qualifier

Ø   **Medical and Surgical**
B   **Respiratory System**
J   **Inspection**   Visually and/or manually exploring a body part

Body Part Character 4	Approach Character 5	Device Character 6	Qualifier Character 7
Ø Tracheobronchial Tree **1** Trachea **K** Lung, Right **L** Lung, Left **Q** Pleura **T** Diaphragm	**Ø** Open **3** Percutaneous **4** Percutaneous Endoscopic **7** Via Natural or Artificial Opening **8** Via Natural or Artificial Opening Endoscopic **X** External	**Z** No Device	**Z** No Qualifier

            Revised Text in **BLUE**

Ø **Medical and Surgical**
B **Respiratory System**
L **Occlusion**　　　　　Completely closing an orifice or the lumen of a tubular body part

Body Part Character 4	Approach Character 5	Device Character 6	Qualifier Character 7
1 Trachea **2** Carina **3** Main Bronchus, Right **4** Upper Lobe Bronchus, Right **5** Middle Lobe Bronchus, Right **6** Lower Lobe Bronchus, Right **7** Main Bronchus, Left **8** Upper Lobe Bronchus, Left **9** Lingula Bronchus **B** Lower Lobe Bronchus, Left	**Ø** Open **3** Percutaneous **4** Percutaneous Endoscopic	**C** Extraluminal Device **D** Intraluminal Device **Z** No Device	**Z** No Qualifier
1 Trachea **2** Carina **3** Main Bronchus, Right **4** Upper Lobe Bronchus, Right **5** Middle Lobe Bronchus, Right **6** Lower Lobe Bronchus, Right **7** Main Bronchus, Left **8** Upper Lobe Bronchus, Left **9** Lingula Bronchus **B** Lower Lobe Bronchus, Left	**7** Via Natural or Artificial Opening **8** Via Natural or Artificial Opening Endoscopic	**D** Intraluminal Device **Z** No Device	**Z** No Qualifier

Ø **Medical and Surgical**
B **Respiratory System**
M **Reattachment**　　　　Putting back in or on all or a portion of a separated body part to its normal location or other suitable location

Body Part Character 4	Approach Character 5	Device Character 6	Qualifier Character 7
1 Trachea **2** Carina **3** Main Bronchus, Right **4** Upper Lobe Bronchus, Right **5** Middle Lobe Bronchus, Right **6** Lower Lobe Bronchus, Right **7** Main Bronchus, Left **8** Upper Lobe Bronchus, Left **9** Lingula Bronchus **B** Lower Lobe Bronchus, Left **C** Upper Lung Lobe, Right **D** Middle Lung Lobe, Right **F** Lower Lung Lobe, Right **G** Upper Lung Lobe, Left **H** Lung Lingula **J** Lower Lung Lobe, Left **K** Lung, Right **L** Lung, Left **R** Diaphragm, Right **S** Diaphragm, Left	**Ø** Open	**Z** No Device	**Z** No Qualifier

Ø **Medical and Surgical**
B **Respiratory System**
N **Release**　　　　Freeing a body part from an abnormal physical constraint

Body Part Character 4	Approach Character 5	Device Character 6	Qualifier Character 7
1 Trachea **2** Carina **3** Main Bronchus, Right **4** Upper Lobe Bronchus, Right **5** Middle Lobe Bronchus, Right **6** Lower Lobe Bronchus, Right **7** Main Bronchus, Left **8** Upper Lobe Bronchus, Left **9** Lingula Bronchus **B** Lower Lobe Bronchus, Left **C** Upper Lung Lobe, Right **D** Middle Lung Lobe, Right **F** Lower Lung Lobe, Right **G** Upper Lung Lobe, Left **H** Lung Lingula **J** Lower Lung Lobe, Left **K** Lung, Right **L** Lung, Left **M** Lungs, Bilateral	**Ø** Open **3** Percutaneous **4** Percutaneous Endoscopic **7** Via Natural or Artificial Opening **8** Via Natural or Artificial Opening Endoscopic	**Z** No Device	**Z** No Qualifier

ØBN Continued on next page

ØBN Continued

Ø   **Medical and Surgical**
B   **Respiratory System**
N   **Release**   Freeing a body part from an abnormal physical constraint

Body Part Character 4	Approach Character 5	Device Character 6	Qualifier Character 7
N Pleura, Right P Pleura, Left R Diaphragm, Right S Diaphragm, Left	Ø Open 3 Percutaneous 4 Percutaneous Endoscopic	Z No Device	Z No Qualifier

Ø   **Medical and Surgical**
B   **Respiratory System**
P   **Removal**   Taking out or off a device from a body part

Body Part Character 4	Approach Character 5	Device Character 6	Qualifier Character 7
Ø Tracheobronchial Tree	Ø Open 3 Percutaneous 4 Percutaneous Endoscopic 7 Via Natural or Artificial Opening 8 Via Natural or Artificial Opening Endoscopic	Ø Drainage Device 1 Radioactive Element 2 Monitoring Device 3 Infusion Device 7 Autologous Tissue Substitute C Extraluminal Device D Intraluminal Device G Endobronchial Valve J Synthetic Substitute K Nonautologous Tissue Substitute	Z No Qualifier
Ø Tracheobronchial Tree	X External	Ø Drainage Device 1 Radioactive Element 2 Monitoring Device 3 Infusion Device D Intraluminal Device	Z No Qualifier
1 Trachea	Ø Open 3 Percutaneous 4 Percutaneous Endoscopic 7 Via Natural or Artificial Opening 8 Via Natural or Artificial Opening Endoscopic	Ø Drainage Device 2 Monitoring Device 7 Autologous Tissue Substitute C Extraluminal Device D Intraluminal Device E Endotracheal Airway F Tracheostomy Device J Synthetic Substitute K Nonautologous Tissue Substitute	Z No Qualifier
1 Trachea	X External	Ø Drainage Device 2 Monitoring Device D Intraluminal Device E Endotracheal Airway F Tracheostomy Device	Z No Qualifier
K Lung, Right L Lung, Left	Ø Open 3 Percutaneous 4 Percutaneous Endoscopic 7 Via Natural or Artificial Opening 8 Via Natural or Artificial Opening Endoscopic X External	Ø Drainage Device 1 Radioactive Element 2 Monitoring Device 3 Infusion Device	Z No Qualifier
Q Pleura	Ø Open 3 Percutaneous 4 Percutaneous Endoscopic 7 Via Natural or Artificial Opening 8 Via Natural or Artificial Opening Endoscopic X External	Ø Drainage Device 1 Radioactive Element 2 Monitoring Device	Z No Qualifier
T Diaphragm	Ø Open 3 Percutaneous 4 Percutaneous Endoscopic 7 Via Natural or Artificial Opening 8 Via Natural or Artificial Opening Endoscopic	Ø Drainage Device 2 Monitoring Device 7 Autologous Tissue Substitute J Synthetic Substitute K Nonautologous Tissue Substitute M Diaphragmatic Pacemaker Lead	Z No Qualifier
T Diaphragm	X External	Ø Drainage Device 2 Monitoring Device M Diaphragmatic Pacemaker Lead	Z No Qualifier

Ø   Medical and Surgical
B   Respiratory System
Q   Repair   Restoring, to the extent possible, a body part to its normal anatomic structure and function

Body Part Character 4	Approach Character 5	Device Character 6	Qualifier Character 7
1 Trachea **2** Carina **3** Main Bronchus, Right **4** Upper Lobe Bronchus, Right **5** Middle Lobe Bronchus, Right **6** Lower Lobe Bronchus, Right **7** Main Bronchus, Left **8** Upper Lobe Bronchus, Left **9** Lingula Bronchus **B** Lower Lobe Bronchus, Left **C** Upper Lung Lobe, Right **D** Middle Lung Lobe, Right **F** Lower Lung Lobe, Right **G** Upper Lung Lobe, Left **H** Lung Lingula **J** Lower Lung Lobe, Left **K** Lung, Right **L** Lung, Left **M** Lungs, Bilateral	**Ø** Open **3** Percutaneous **4** Percutaneous Endoscopic **7** Via Natural or Artificial Opening **8** Via Natural or Artificial Opening Endoscopic	**Z** No Device	**Z** No Qualifier
N Pleura, Right **P** Pleura, Left **R** Diaphragm, Right **S** Diaphragm, Left	**Ø** Open **3** Percutaneous **4** Percutaneous Endoscopic	**Z** No Device	**Z** No Qualifier

Ø   Medical and Surgical
B   Respiratory System
S   Reposition   Moving to its normal location or other suitable location all or a portion of a body part

Body Part Character 4	Approach Character 5	Device Character 6	Qualifier Character 7
1 Trachea **2** Carina **3** Main Bronchus, Right **4** Upper Lobe Bronchus, Right **5** Middle Lobe Bronchus, Right **6** Lower Lobe Bronchus, Right **7** Main Bronchus, Left **8** Upper Lobe Bronchus, Left **9** Lingula Bronchus **B** Lower Lobe Bronchus, Left **C** Upper Lung Lobe, Right **D** Middle Lung Lobe, Right **F** Lower Lung Lobe, Right **G** Upper Lung Lobe, Left **H** Lung Lingula **J** Lower Lung Lobe, Left **K** Lung, Right **L** Lung, Left **R** Diaphragm, Right **S** Diaphragm, Left	**Ø** Open	**Z** No Device	**Z** No Qualifier

Ø Medical and Surgical
B Respiratory System
T Resection   Cutting out or off, without replacement, all of a body part

Body Part Character 4	Approach Character 5	Device Character 6	Qualifier Character 7
1 Trachea **2** Carina **3** Main Bronchus, Right **4** Upper Lobe Bronchus, Right **5** Middle Lobe Bronchus, Right **6** Lower Lobe Bronchus, Right **7** Main Bronchus, Left **8** Upper Lobe Bronchus, Left **9** Lingula Bronchus **B** Lower Lobe Bronchus, Left **C** Upper Lung Lobe, Right **D** Middle Lung Lobe, Right **F** Lower Lung Lobe, Right **G** Upper Lung Lobe, Left **H** Lung Lingula **J** Lower Lung Lobe, Left **K** Lung, Right **L** Lung, Left **M** Lungs, Bilateral **R** Diaphragm, Right **S** Diaphragm, Left	**Ø** Open **4** Percutaneous Endoscopic	**Z** No Device	**Z** No Qualifier

Ø Medical and Surgical
B Respiratory System
U Supplement   Putting in or on biological or synthetic material that physically reinforces and/or augments the function of a portion of a body part

Body Part Character 4	Approach Character 5	Device Character 6	Qualifier Character 7
1 Trachea **2** Carina **3** Main Bronchus, Right **4** Upper Lobe Bronchus, Right **5** Middle Lobe Bronchus, Right **6** Lower Lobe Bronchus, Right **7** Main Bronchus, Left **8** Upper Lobe Bronchus, Left **9** Lingula Bronchus **B** Lower Lobe Bronchus, Left **R** Diaphragm, Right **S** Diaphragm, Left	**Ø** Open **4** Percutaneous Endoscopic	**7** Autologous Tissue Substitute **J** Synthetic Substitute **K** Nonautologous Tissue Substitute	**Z** No Qualifier

Ø Medical and Surgical
B Respiratory System
V Restriction   Partially closing an orifice or the lumen of a tubular body part

Body Part Character 4	Approach Character 5	Device Character 6	Qualifier Character 7
1 Trachea **2** Carina **3** Main Bronchus, Right **4** Upper Lobe Bronchus, Right **5** Middle Lobe Bronchus, Right **6** Lower Lobe Bronchus, Right **7** Main Bronchus, Left **8** Upper Lobe Bronchus, Left **9** Lingula Bronchus **B** Lower Lobe Bronchus, Left	**Ø** Open **3** Percutaneous **4** Percutaneous Endoscopic	**C** Extraluminal Device **D** Intraluminal Device **Z** No Device	**Z** No Qualifier
1 Trachea **2** Carina **3** Main Bronchus, Right **4** Upper Lobe Bronchus, Right **5** Middle Lobe Bronchus, Right **6** Lower Lobe Bronchus, Right **7** Main Bronchus, Left **8** Upper Lobe Bronchus, Left **9** Lingula Bronchus **B** Lower Lobe Bronchus, Left	**7** Via Natural or Artificial Opening **8** Via Natural or Artificial Opening Endoscopic	**D** Intraluminal Device **Z** No Device	**Z** No Qualifier

Ø   **Medical and Surgical**
B   **Respiratory System**
W   **Revision**   Correcting, to the extent possible, a portion of a malfunctioning device or the position of a displaced device

Body Part Character 4	Approach Character 5	Device Character 6	Qualifier Character 7
Ø Tracheobronchial Tree	Ø Open 3 Percutaneous 4 Percutaneous Endoscopic 7 Via Natural or Artificial Opening 8 Via Natural or Artificial Opening Endoscopic X External	Ø Drainage Device 2 Monitoring Device 3 Infusion Device 7 Autologous Tissue Substitute C Extraluminal Device D Intraluminal Device G Endobronchial Valve J Synthetic Substitute K Nonautologous Tissue Substitute	Z No Qualifier
1 Trachea	Ø Open 3 Percutaneous 4 Percutaneous Endoscopic 7 Via Natural or Artificial Opening 8 Via Natural or Artificial Opening Endoscopic X External	Ø Drainage Device 2 Monitoring Device 7 Autologous Tissue Substitute C Extraluminal Device D Intraluminal Device E Endotracheal Airway F Tracheostomy Device J Synthetic Substitute K Nonautologous Tissue Substitute	Z No Qualifier
K Lung, Right L Lung, Left	Ø Open 3 Percutaneous 4 Percutaneous Endoscopic 7 Via Natural or Artificial Opening 8 Via Natural or Artificial Opening Endoscopic X External	Ø Drainage Device 2 Monitoring Device 3 Infusion Device	Z No Qualifier
Q Pleura	Ø Open 3 Percutaneous 4 Percutaneous Endoscopic 7 Via Natural or Artificial Opening 8 Via Natural or Artificial Opening Endoscopic X External	Ø Drainage Device 2 Monitoring Device	Z No Qualifier
T Diaphragm	Ø Open 3 Percutaneous 4 Percutaneous Endoscopic 7 Via Natural or Artificial Opening 8 Via Natural or Artificial Opening Endoscopic X External	Ø Drainage Device 2 Monitoring Device 7 Autologous Tissue Substitute J Synthetic Substitute K Nonautologous Tissue Substitute M Diaphragmatic Pacemaker Lead	Z No Qualifier

Ø   **Medical and Surgical**
B   **Respiratory System**
Y   **Transplantation**   Putting in or on all or a portion of a living body part taken from another individual or animal to physically take the place and/or function of all or a portion of a similar body part

Body Part Character 4	Approach Character 5	Device Character 6	Qualifier Character 7
C Upper Lung Lobe, Right D Middle Lung Lobe, Right F Lower Lung Lobe, Right G Upper Lung Lobe, Left H Lung Lingula J Lower Lung Lobe, Left K Lung, Right L Lung, Left M Lungs, Bilateral	Ø Open	Z No Device	Ø Allogeneic 1 Syngeneic 2 Zooplastic

Mouth and Throat 0C0–0CX

0   **Medical and Surgical**
C   **Mouth and Throat**
0   **Alteration**   Modifying the anatomic structure of a body part without affecting the function of the body part

Body Part Character 4	Approach Character 5	Device Character 6	Qualifier Character 7
0 Upper Lip 1 Lower Lip	X External	7 Autologous Tissue Substitute J Synthetic Substitute K Nonautologous Tissue Substitute Z No Device	Z No Qualifier

0   **Medical and Surgical**
C   **Mouth and Throat**
2   **Change**   Taking out or off a device from a body part and putting back an identical or similar device in or on the same body part without cutting or puncturing the skin or a mucous membrane

Body Part Character 4	Approach Character 5	Device Character 6	Qualifier Character 7
A Salivary Gland S Larynx Y Mouth and Throat	X External	0 Drainage Device Y Other Device	Z No Qualifier

0   **Medical and Surgical**
C   **Mouth and Throat**
5   **Destruction**   Physical eradication of all or a portion of a body part by the direct use of energy, force, or a destructive agent

Body Part Character 4	Approach Character 5	Device Character 6	Qualifier Character 7
0 Upper Lip 1 Lower Lip 2 Hard Palate 3 Soft Palate 4 Buccal Mucosa 5 Upper Gingiva 6 Lower Gingiva 7 Tongue N Uvula P Tonsils Q Adenoids	0 Open 3 Percutaneous X External	Z No Device	Z No Qualifier
8 Parotid Gland, Right 9 Parotid Gland, Left B Parotid Duct, Right C Parotid Duct, Left D Sublingual Gland, Right F Sublingual Gland, Left G Submaxillary Gland, Right H Submaxillary Gland, Left J Minor Salivary Gland	0 Open 3 Percutaneous	Z No Device	Z No Qualifier
M Pharynx R Epiglottis S Larynx T Vocal Cord, Right V Vocal Cord, Left	0 Open 3 Percutaneous 4 Percutaneous Endoscopic 7 Via Natural or Artificial Opening 8 Via Natural or Artificial Opening Endoscopic	Z No Device	Z No Qualifier
W Upper Tooth X Lower Tooth	0 Open X External	Z No Device	0 Single 1 Multiple 2 All

0   Medical and Surgical
C   Mouth and Throat
7   Dilation   Expanding an orifice or the lumen of a tubular body part

Body Part Character 4	Approach Character 5	Device Character 6	Qualifier Character 7
B Parotid Duct, Right C Parotid Duct, Left	0 Open 3 Percutaneous 7 Via Natural or Artificial Opening	D Intraluminal Device Z No Device	Z No Qualifier
M Pharynx	7 Via Natural or Artificial Opening 8 Via Natural or Artificial Opening Endoscopic	D Intraluminal Device Z No Device	Z No Qualifier
S Larynx	0 Open 3 Percutaneous 4 Percutaneous Endoscopic 7 Via Natural or Artificial Opening 8 Via Natural or Artificial Opening Endoscopic	D Intraluminal Device Z No Device	Z No Qualifier

0   Medical and Surgical
C   Mouth and Throat
9   Drainage   Taking or letting out fluids and/or gases from a body part

Body Part Character 4	Approach Character 5	Device Character 6	Qualifier Character 7
0 Upper Lip 1 Lower Lip 2 Hard Palate 3 Soft Palate 4 Buccal Mucosa 5 Upper Gingiva 6 Lower Gingiva 7 Tongue N Uvula P Tonsils Q Adenoids	0 Open 3 Percutaneous X External	0 Drainage Device	Z No Qualifier
0 Upper Lip 1 Lower Lip 2 Hard Palate 3 Soft Palate 4 Buccal Mucosa 5 Upper Gingiva 6 Lower Gingiva 7 Tongue N Uvula P Tonsils Q Adenoids	0 Open 3 Percutaneous X External	Z No Device	X Diagnostic Z No Qualifier
8 Parotid Gland, Right 9 Parotid Gland, Left B Parotid Duct, Right C Parotid Duct, Left D Sublingual Gland, Right F Sublingual Gland, Left G Submaxillary Gland, Right H Submaxillary Gland, Left J Minor Salivary Gland	0 Open 3 Percutaneous	0 Drainage Device	Z No Qualifier
8 Parotid Gland, Right 9 Parotid Gland, Left B Parotid Duct, Right C Parotid Duct, Left D Sublingual Gland, Right F Sublingual Gland, Left G Submaxillary Gland, Right H Submaxillary Gland, Left J Minor Salivary Gland	0 Open 3 Percutaneous	Z No Device	X Diagnostic Z No Qualifier
M Pharynx R Epiglottis S Larynx T Vocal Cord, Right V Vocal Cord, Left	0 Open 3 Percutaneous 4 Percutaneous Endoscopic 7 Via Natural or Artificial Opening 8 Via Natural or Artificial Opening Endoscopic	0 Drainage Device	Z No Qualifier

0C9 Continued on next page

Mouth and Throat

0C9 Continued

0　**Medical and Surgical**
C　**Mouth and Throat**
9　**Drainage**　　Taking or letting out fluids and/or gases from a body part

Body Part Character 4	Approach Character 5	Device Character 6	Qualifier Character 7
M Pharynx R Epiglottis S Larynx T Vocal Cord, Right V Vocal Cord, Left	0 Open 3 Percutaneous 4 Percutaneous Endoscopic 7 Via Natural or Artificial Opening 8 Via Natural or Artificial Opening 　 Endoscopic	Z No Device	X Diagnostic Z No Qualifier
W Upper Tooth X Lower Tooth	0 Open X External	0 Drainage Device Z No Device	0 Single 1 Multiple 2 All

0　**Medical and Surgical**
C　**Mouth and Throat**
B　**Excision**　　Cutting out or off, without replacement, a portion of a body part

Body Part Character 4	Approach Character 5	Device Character 6	Qualifier Character 7
0 Upper Lip 1 Lower Lip 2 Hard Palate 3 Soft Palate 4 Buccal Mucosa 5 Upper Gingiva 6 Lower Gingiva 7 Tongue N Uvula P Tonsils Q Adenoids	0 Open 3 Percutaneous X External	Z No Device	X Diagnostic Z No Qualifier
8 Parotid Gland, Right 9 Parotid Gland, Left B Parotid Duct, Right C Parotid Duct, Left D Sublingual Gland, Right F Sublingual Gland, Left G Submaxillary Gland, Right H Submaxillary Gland, Left J Minor Salivary Gland	0 Open 3 Percutaneous	Z No Device	X Diagnostic Z No Qualifier
M Pharynx R Epiglottis S Larynx T Vocal Cord, Right V Vocal Cord, Left	0 Open 3 Percutaneous 4 Percutaneous Endoscopic 7 Via Natural or Artificial Opening 8 Via Natural or Artificial Opening 　 Endoscopic	Z No Device	X Diagnostic Z No Qualifier
W Upper Tooth X Lower Tooth	0 Open X External	Z No Device	0 Single 1 Multiple 2 All

0   **Medical and Surgical**
C   **Mouth and Throat**
C   **Extirpation**   Taking or cutting out solid matter from a body part

Body Part Character 4	Approach Character 5	Device Character 6	Qualifier Character 7
0 Upper Lip **1** Lower Lip **2** Hard Palate **3** Soft Palate **4** Buccal Mucosa **5** Upper Gingiva **6** Lower Gingiva **7** Tongue **N** Uvula **P** Tonsils **Q** Adenoids	**0** Open **3** Percutaneous **X** External	**Z** No Device	**Z** No Qualifier
8 Parotid Gland, Right **9** Parotid Gland, Left **B** Parotid Duct, Right **C** Parotid Duct, Left **D** Sublingual Gland, Right **F** Sublingual Gland, Left **G** Submaxillary Gland, Right **H** Submaxillary Gland, Left **J** Minor Salivary Gland	**0** Open **3** Percutaneous	**Z** No Device	**Z** No Qualifier
M Pharynx **R** Epiglottis **S** Larynx **T** Vocal Cord, Right **V** Vocal Cord, Left	**0** Open **3** Percutaneous **4** Percutaneous Endoscopic **7** Via Natural or Artificial Opening **8** Via Natural or Artificial Opening Endoscopic	**Z** No Device	**Z** No Qualifier
W Upper Tooth **X** Lower Tooth	**0** Open **X** External	**Z** No Device	**0** Single **1** Multiple **2** All

0   **Medical and Surgical**
C   **Mouth and Throat**
D   **Extraction**   Pulling or stripping out or off all or a portion of a body part by the use of force

Body Part Character 4	Approach Character 5	Device Character 6	Qualifier Character 7
T Vocal Cord, Right **V** Vocal Cord, Left	**0** Open **3** Percutaneous **4** Percutaneous Endoscopic **7** Via Natural or Artificial Opening **8** Via Natural or Artificial Opening Endoscopic	**Z** No Device	**Z** No Qualifier
W Upper Tooth **X** Lower Tooth	**X** External	**Z** No Device	**0** Single **1** Multiple **2** All

0   **Medical and Surgical**
C   **Mouth and Throat**
F   **Fragmentation**   Breaking solid matter in a body part into pieces

Body Part Character 4	Approach Character 5	Device Character 6	Qualifier Character 7
B Parotid Duct, Right **C** Parotid Duct, Left	**0** Open **3** Percutaneous **7** Via Natural or Artificial Opening **X** External	**Z** No Device	**Z** No Qualifier

0   **Medical and Surgical**
C   **Mouth and Throat**
H   **Insertion**   Putting in a nonbiological appliance that monitors, assists, performs, or prevents a physiological function but does not physically take the place of a body part

Body Part Character 4	Approach Character 5	Device Character 6	Qualifier Character 7
7 Tongue	**0** Open **3** Percutaneous **X** External	**1** Radioactive Element	**Z** No Qualifier
Y Mouth and Throat	**7** Via Natural or Artificial Opening **8** Via Natural or Artificial Opening Endoscopic	**B** Airway	**Z** No Qualifier

ØCJ–ØCN

Ø Medical and Surgical
C Mouth and Throat
J Inspection   Visually and/or manually exploring a body part

Body Part Character 4	Approach Character 5	Device Character 6	Qualifier Character 7
A Salivary Gland	Ø Open 3 Percutaneous X External	Z No Device	Z No Qualifier
S Larynx Y Mouth and Throat	Ø Open 3 Percutaneous 4 Percutaneous Endoscopic 7 Via Natural or Artificial Opening 8 Via Natural or Artificial Opening Endoscopic X External	Z No Device	Z No Qualifier

Ø Medical and Surgical
C Mouth and Throat
L Occlusion   Completely closing an orifice or the lumen of a tubular body part

Body Part Character 4	Approach Character 5	Device Character 6	Qualifier Character 7
B Parotid Duct, Right C Parotid Duct, Left	Ø Open 3 Percutaneous 4 Percutaneous Endoscopic	C Extraluminal Device D Intraluminal Device Z No Device	Z No Qualifier
B Parotid Duct, Right C Parotid Duct, Left	7 Via Natural or Artificial Opening 8 Via Natural or Artificial Opening Endoscopic	D Intraluminal Device Z No Device	Z No Qualifier

Ø Medical and Surgical
C Mouth and Throat
M Reattachment   Putting back in or on all or a portion of a separated body part to its normal location or other suitable location

Body Part Character 4	Approach Character 5	Device Character 6	Qualifier Character 7
Ø Upper Lip 1 Lower Lip 3 Soft Palate 7 Tongue N Uvula	Ø Open	Z No Device	Z No Qualifier
W Upper Tooth X Lower Tooth	Ø Open X External	Z No Device	Ø Single 1 Multiple 2 All

Ø Medical and Surgical
C Mouth and Throat
N Release   Freeing a body part from an abnormal physical constraint

Body Part Character 4	Approach Character 5	Device Character 6	Qualifier Character 7
Ø Upper Lip 1 Lower Lip 2 Hard Palate 3 Soft Palate 4 Buccal Mucosa 5 Upper Gingiva 6 Lower Gingiva 7 Tongue N Uvula P Tonsils Q Adenoids	Ø Open 3 Percutaneous X External	Z No Device	Z No Qualifier
8 Parotid Gland, Right 9 Parotid Gland, Left B Parotid Duct, Right C Parotid Duct, Left D Sublingual Gland, Right F Sublingual Gland, Left G Submaxillary Gland, Right H Submaxillary Gland, Left J Minor Salivary Gland	Ø Open 3 Percutaneous	Z No Device	Z No Qualifier

ØCN Continued on next page

0 Medical and Surgical
C Mouth and Throat
N Release　　　Freeing a body part from an abnormal physical constraint

0CN Continued

Body Part Character 4	Approach Character 5	Device Character 6	Qualifier Character 7
W Upper Tooth **X** Lower Tooth	**0** Open **X** External	**Z** No Device	**0** Single **1** Multiple **2** All
M Pharynx **R** Epiglottis **S** Larynx **T** Vocal Cord, Right **V** Vocal Cord, Left	**0** Open **3** Percutaneous **4** Percutaneous Endoscopic **7** Via Natural or Artificial Opening **8** Via Natural or Artificial Opening 　　Endoscopic	**Z** No Device	**Z** No Qualifier

0 Medical and Surgical
C Mouth and Throat
P Removal　　　Taking out or off a device from a body part

Body Part Character 4	Approach Character 5	Device Character 6	Qualifier Character 7
A Salivary Gland	**0** Open **3** Percutaneous	**0** Drainage Device **C** Extraluminal Device	**Z** No Qualifier
S Larynx	**0** Open **3** Percutaneous **7** Via Natural or Artificial Opening **8** Via Natural or Artificial Opening 　　Endoscopic **X** External	**0** Drainage Device **7** Autologous Tissue Substitute **D** Intraluminal Device **J** Synthetic Substitute **K** Nonautologous Tissue Substitute	**Z** No Qualifier
Y Mouth and Throat	**0** Open **3** Percutaneous **X** External	**0** Drainage Device **1** Radioactive Element **7** Autologous Tissue Substitute **D** Intraluminal Device **J** Synthetic Substitute **K** Nonautologous Tissue Substitute	**Z** No Qualifier
Y Mouth and Throat	**7** Via Natural or Artificial Opening **8** Via Natural or Artificial Opening 　　Endoscopic	**0** Drainage Device **1** Radioactive Element **7** Autologous Tissue Substitute **B** Airway **D** Intraluminal Device **J** Synthetic Substitute **K** Nonautologous Tissue Substitute	**Z** No Qualifier

0 Medical and Surgical
C Mouth and Throat
Q Repair　　　Restoring, to the extent possible, a body part to its normal anatomic structure and function

Body Part Character 4	Approach Character 5	Device Character 6	Qualifier Character 7
0 Upper Lip **1** Lower Lip **2** Hard Palate **3** Soft Palate **4** Buccal Mucosa **5** Upper Gingiva **6** Lower Gingiva **7** Tongue **N** Uvula **P** Tonsils **Q** Adenoids	**0** Open **3** Percutaneous **X** External	**Z** No Device	**Z** No Qualifier
8 Parotid Gland, Right **9** Parotid Gland, Left **B** Parotid Duct, Right **C** Parotid Duct, Left **D** Sublingual Gland, Right **F** Sublingual Gland, Left **G** Submaxillary Gland, Right **H** Submaxillary Gland, Left **J** Minor Salivary Gland	**0** Open **3** Percutaneous	**Z** No Device	**Z** No Qualifier
M Pharynx **R** Epiglottis **S** Larynx **T** Vocal Cord, Right **V** Vocal Cord, Left	**0** Open **3** Percutaneous **4** Percutaneous Endoscopic **7** Via Natural or Artificial Opening **8** Via Natural or Artificial Opening 　　Endoscopic	**Z** No Device	**Z** No Qualifier
W Upper Tooth **X** Lower Tooth	**0** Open **X** External	**Z** No Device	**0** Single **1** Multiple **2** All

Ø Medical and Surgical
C Mouth and Throat
R Replacement   Putting in or on biological or synthetic material that physically takes the place and/or function of all or a portion of a body part

Body Part Character 4	Approach Character 5	Device Character 6	Qualifier Character 7
Ø Upper Lip 1 Lower Lip 2 Hard Palate 3 Soft Palate 4 Buccal Mucosa 5 Upper Gingiva 6 Lower Gingiva 7 Tongue N Uvula	Ø Open 3 Percutaneous X External	7 Autologous Tissue Substitute J Synthetic Substitute K Nonautologous Tissue Substitute	Z No Qualifier
B Parotid Duct, Right C Parotid Duct, Left	Ø Open 3 Percutaneous	7 Autologous Tissue Substitute J Synthetic Substitute K Nonautologous Tissue Substitute	Z No Qualifier
M Pharynx R Epiglottis S Larynx T Vocal Cord, Right V Vocal Cord, Left	Ø Open 7 Via Natural or Artificial Opening 8 Via Natural or Artificial Opening Endoscopic	7 Autologous Tissue Substitute J Synthetic Substitute K Nonautologous Tissue Substitute	Z No Qualifier
W Upper Tooth X Lower Tooth	Ø Open X External	7 Autologous Tissue Substitute J Synthetic Substitute K Nonautologous Tissue Substitute	Ø Single 1 Multiple 2 All

Ø Medical and Surgical
C Mouth and Throat
S Reposition   Moving to its normal location or other suitable location all or a portion of a body part

Body Part Character 4	Approach Character 5	Device Character 6	Qualifier Character 7
Ø Upper Lip 1 Lower Lip 2 Hard Palate 3 Soft Palate 7 Tongue N Uvula	Ø Open X External	Z No Device	Z No Qualifier
B Parotid Duct, Right C Parotid Duct, Left	Ø Open 3 Percutaneous	Z No Device	Z No Qualifier
R Epiglottis T Vocal Cord, Right V Vocal Cord, Left	Ø Open 7 Via Natural or Artificial Opening 8 Via Natural or Artificial Opening Endoscopic	Z No Device	Z No Qualifier
W Upper Tooth X Lower Tooth	Ø Open X External	5 External Fixation Device Z No Device	Ø Single 1 Multiple 2 All

Ø Medical and Surgical
C Mouth and Throat
T Resection   Cutting out or off, without replacement, all of a body part

Body Part Character 4	Approach Character 5	Device Character 6	Qualifier Character 7
Ø Upper Lip 1 Lower Lip 2 Hard Palate 3 Soft Palate 7 Tongue N Uvula P Tonsils Q Adenoids	Ø Open X External	Z No Device	Z No Qualifier
8 Parotid Gland, Right 9 Parotid Gland, Left B Parotid Duct, Right C Parotid Duct, Left D Sublingual Gland, Right F Sublingual Gland, Left G Submaxillary Gland, Right H Submaxillary Gland, Left J Minor Salivary Gland	Ø Open	Z No Device	Z No Qualifier

ØCT Continued on next page

0 Medical and Surgical   *0CT Continued*
C Mouth and Throat
T Resection   Cutting out or off, without replacement, all of a body part

Body Part Character 4	Approach Character 5	Device Character 6	Qualifier Character 7
M Pharynx **R** Epiglottis **S** Larynx **T** Vocal Cord, Right **V** Vocal Cord, Left	**0** Open **4** Percutaneous Endoscopic **7** Via Natural or Artificial Opening **8** Via Natural or Artificial Opening Endoscopic	**Z** No Device	**Z** No Qualifier
W Upper Tooth **X** Lower Tooth	**0** Open	**Z** No Device	**0** Single **1** Multiple **2** All

0 Medical and Surgical
C Mouth and Throat
U Supplement   Putting in or on biological or synthetic material that physically reinforces and/or augments the function of a portion of a body part

Body Part Character 4	Approach Character 5	Device Character 6	Qualifier Character 7
0 Upper Lip **1** Lower Lip **2** Hard Palate **3** Soft Palate **4** Buccal Mucosa **5** Upper Gingiva **6** Lower Gingiva **7** Tongue **N** Uvula	**0** Open **3** Percutaneous **X** External	**7** Autologous Tissue Substitute **J** Synthetic Substitute **K** Nonautologous Tissue Substitute	**Z** No Qualifier
M Pharynx **R** Epiglottis **S** Larynx **T** Vocal Cord, Right **V** Vocal Cord, Left	**0** Open **7** Via Natural or Artificial Opening **8** Via Natural or Artificial Opening Endoscopic	**7** Autologous Tissue Substitute **J** Synthetic Substitute **K** Nonautologous Tissue Substitute	**Z** No Qualifier

0 Medical and Surgical
C Mouth and Throat
V Restriction   Partially closing an orifice or the lumen of a tubular body part

Body Part Character 4	Approach Character 5	Device Character 6	Qualifier Character 7
B Parotid Duct, Right **C** Parotid Duct, Left	**0** Open **3** Percutaneous	**C** Extraluminal Device **D** Intraluminal Device **Z** No Device	**Z** No Qualifier
B Parotid Duct, Right **C** Parotid Duct, Left	**7** Via Natural or Artificial Opening **8** Via Natural or Artificial Opening Endoscopic	**D** Intraluminal Device **Z** No Device	**Z** No Qualifier

Mouth and Throat

ØCW–ØCX

Ø   **Medical and Surgical**
C   **Mouth and Throat**
W   **Revision**   Correcting, to the extent possible, a portion of a malfunctioning device or the position of a displaced device

Body Part Character 4	Approach Character 5	Device Character 6	Qualifier Character 7
A Salivary Gland	Ø Open 3 Percutaneous X External	Ø Drainage Device C Extraluminal Device	Z No Qualifier
S Larynx	Ø Open 3 Percutaneous 7 Via Natural or Artificial Opening 8 Via Natural or Artificial Opening Endoscopic X External	Ø Drainage Device 7 Autologous Tissue Substitute D Intraluminal Device J Synthetic Substitute K Nonautologous Tissue Substitute	Z No Qualifier
Y Mouth and Throat	Ø Open 3 Percutaneous X External	Ø Drainage Device 1 Radioactive Element 7 Autologous Tissue Substitute D Intraluminal Device J Synthetic Substitute K Nonautologous Tissue Substitute	Z No Qualifier
Y Mouth and Throat	7 Via Natural or Artificial Opening 8 Via Natural or Artificial Opening Endoscopic	Ø Drainage Device 1 Radioactive Element 7 Autologous Tissue Substitute B Airway D Intraluminal Device J Synthetic Substitute K Nonautologous Tissue Substitute	Z No Qualifier

Ø   **Medical and Surgical**
C   **Mouth and Throat**
X   **Transfer**   Moving, without taking out, all or a portion of a body part to another location to take over the function of all or a portion of a body part

Body Part Character 4	Approach Character 5	Device Character 6	Qualifier Character 7
Ø Upper Lip 1 Lower Lip 3 Soft Palate 4 Buccal Mucosa 5 Upper Gingiva 6 Lower Gingiva 7 Tongue	Ø Open X External	Z No Device	Z No Qualifier

Revised Text in **BLUE**

Gastrointestinal System 0D1–0DY

0   **Medical and Surgical**
D   **Gastrointestinal System**
1   **Bypass**   Altering the route of passage of the contents of a tubular body part

Body Part Character 4	Approach Character 5	Device Character 6	Qualifier Character 7
1 Esophagus, Upper 2 Esophagus, Middle 3 Esophagus, Lower 5 Esophagus	0 Open 4 Percutaneous Endoscopic 8 Via Natural or Artificial Opening Endoscopic	7 Autologous Tissue Substitute J Synthetic Substitute K Nonautologous Tissue Substitute Z No Device	4 Cutaneous 6 Stomach 9 Duodenum A Jejunum B Ileum
1 Esophagus, Upper 2 Esophagus, Middle 3 Esophagus, Lower 5 Esophagus 6 Stomach 9 Duodenum A Jejunum B Ileum H Cecum K Ascending Colon L Transverse Colon M Descending Colon N Sigmoid Colon	3 Percutaneous	J Synthetic Substitute	4 Cutaneous
6 Stomach 9 Duodenum	0 Open 4 Percutaneous Endoscopic 8 Via Natural or Artificial Opening Endoscopic	7 Autologous Tissue Substitute J Synthetic Substitute K Nonautologous Tissue Substitute Z No Device	4 Cutaneous 9 Duodenum A Jejunum B Ileum L Transverse Colon
A Jejunum	0 Open 4 Percutaneous Endoscopic 8 Via Natural or Artificial Opening Endoscopic	7 Autologous Tissue Substitute J Synthetic Substitute K Nonautologous Tissue Substitute Z No Device	4 Cutaneous A Jejunum B Ileum H Cecum K Ascending Colon L Transverse Colon M Descending Colon N Sigmoid Colon P Rectum Q Anus
B Ileum	0 Open 4 Percutaneous Endoscopic 8 Via Natural or Artificial Opening Endoscopic	7 Autologous Tissue Substitute J Synthetic Substitute K Nonautologous Tissue Substitute Z No Device	4 Cutaneous B Ileum H Cecum K Ascending Colon L Transverse Colon M Descending Colon N Sigmoid Colon P Rectum Q Anus
H Cecum	0 Open 4 Percutaneous Endoscopic 8 Via Natural or Artificial Opening Endoscopic	7 Autologous Tissue Substitute J Synthetic Substitute K Nonautologous Tissue Substitute Z No Device	4 Cutaneous H Cecum K Ascending Colon L Transverse Colon M Descending Colon N Sigmoid Colon P Rectum
K Ascending Colon	0 Open 4 Percutaneous Endoscopic 8 Via Natural or Artificial Opening Endoscopic	7 Autologous Tissue Substitute J Synthetic Substitute K Nonautologous Tissue Substitute Z No Device	4 Cutaneous K Ascending Colon L Transverse Colon M Descending Colon N Sigmoid Colon P Rectum
L Transverse Colon	0 Open 4 Percutaneous Endoscopic 8 Via Natural or Artificial Opening Endoscopic	7 Autologous Tissue Substitute J Synthetic Substitute K Nonautologous Tissue Substitute Z No Device	4 Cutaneous L Transverse Colon M Descending Colon N Sigmoid Colon P Rectum
M Descending Colon	0 Open 4 Percutaneous Endoscopic 8 Via Natural or Artificial Opening Endoscopic	7 Autologous Tissue Substitute J Synthetic Substitute K Nonautologous Tissue Substitute Z No Device	4 Cutaneous M Descending Colon N Sigmoid Colon P Rectum
N Sigmoid Colon	0 Open 4 Percutaneous Endoscopic 8 Via Natural or Artificial Opening Endoscopic	7 Autologous Tissue Substitute J Synthetic Substitute K Nonautologous Tissue Substitute Z No Device	4 Cutaneous N Sigmoid Colon P Rectum

Ø   Medical and Surgical
D   Gastrointestinal System
2   Change   Taking out or off a device from a body part and putting back an identical or similar device in or on the same body part without cutting or puncturing the skin or a mucous membrane

Body Part Character 4	Approach Character 5	Device Character 6	Qualifier Character 7
Ø Upper Intestinal Tract D Lower Intestinal Tract	X External	Ø Drainage Device U Feeding Device Y Other Device	Z No Qualifier
U Omentum V Mesentery W Peritoneum	X External	Ø Drainage Device Y Other Device	Z No Qualifier

Ø   Medical and Surgical
D   Gastrointestinal System
5   Destruction   Physical eradication of all or a portion of a body part by the direct use of energy, force, or a destructive agent

Body Part Character 4	Approach Character 5	Device Character 6	Qualifier Character 7
1 Esophagus, Upper 2 Esophagus, Middle 3 Esophagus, Lower 4 Esophagogastric Junction 5 Esophagus 6 Stomach 7 Stomach, Pylorus 8 Small Intestine 9 Duodenum A Jejunum B Ileum C Ileocecal Valve E Large Intestine F Large Intestine, Right G Large Intestine, Left H Cecum J Appendix K Ascending Colon L Transverse Colon M Descending Colon N Sigmoid Colon P Rectum	Ø Open 3 Percutaneous 4 Percutaneous Endoscopic 7 Via Natural or Artificial Opening 8 Via Natural or Artificial Opening Endoscopic	Z No Device	Z No Qualifier
Q Anus	Ø Open 3 Percutaneous 4 Percutaneous Endoscopic 7 Via Natural or Artificial Opening 8 Via Natural or Artificial Opening Endoscopic X External	Z No Device	Z No Qualifier
R Anal Sphincter S Greater Omentum T Lesser Omentum V Mesentery W Peritoneum	Ø Open 3 Percutaneous 4 Percutaneous Endoscopic	Z No Device	Z No Qualifier

Revised Text in **BLUE**

0 **Medical and Surgical**
D **Gastrointestinal System**
7 **Dilation** Expanding an orifice or the lumen of a tubular body part

Body Part Character 4	Approach Character 5	Device Character 6	Qualifier Character 7
1 Esophagus, Upper **2** Esophagus, Middle **3** Esophagus, Lower **4** Esophagogastric Junction **5** Esophagus **6** Stomach **7** Stomach, Pylorus **8** Small Intestine **9** Duodenum **A** Jejunum **B** Ileum **C** Ileocecal Valve **E** Large Intestine **F** Large Intestine, Right **G** Large Intestine, Left **H** Cecum **K** Ascending Colon **L** Transverse Colon **M** Descending Colon **N** Sigmoid Colon **P** Rectum **Q** Anus	**0** Open **3** Percutaneous **4** Percutaneous Endoscopic **7** Via Natural or Artificial Opening **8** Via Natural or Artificial Opening Endoscopic	**D** Intraluminal Device **Z** No Device	**Z** No Qualifier

0 **Medical and Surgical**
D **Gastrointestinal System**
8 **Division** Cutting into a body part without draining fluids and/or gases from the body part in order to separate or transect a body part

Body Part Character 4	Approach Character 5	Device Character 6	Qualifier Character 7
4 Esophagogastric Junction	**0** Open **3** Percutaneous **4** Percutaneous Endoscopic **7** Via Natural or Artificial Opening **8** Via Natural or Artificial Opening Endoscopic	**Z** No Device	**Z** No Qualifier
R Anal Sphincter	**0** Open **3** Percutaneous	**Z** No Device	**Z** No Qualifier

0 **Medical and Surgical**
D **Gastrointestinal System**
9 **Drainage** Taking or letting out fluids and/or gases from a body part

Body Part Character 4	Approach Character 5	Device Character 6	Qualifier Character 7
1 Esophagus, Upper **2** Esophagus, Middle **3** Esophagus, Lower **4** Esophagogastric Junction **5** Esophagus **6** Stomach **7** Stomach, Pylorus **8** Small Intestine **9** Duodenum **A** Jejunum **B** Ileum **C** Ileocecal Valve **E** Large Intestine **F** Large Intestine, Right **G** Large Intestine, Left **H** Cecum **J** Appendix **K** Ascending Colon **L** Transverse Colon **M** Descending Colon **N** Sigmoid Colon **P** Rectum	**0** Open **3** Percutaneous **4** Percutaneous Endoscopic **7** Via Natural or Artificial Opening **8** Via Natural or Artificial Opening Endoscopic	**0** Drainage Device	**Z** No Qualifier

0D9 Continued on next page

Ø **Medical and Surgical**
D **Gastrointestinal System**
9 **Drainage**   Taking or letting out fluids and/or gases from a body part

Body Part Character 4	Approach Character 5	Device Character 6	Qualifier Character 7
1 Esophagus, Upper **2** Esophagus, Middle **3** Esophagus, Lower **4** Esophagogastric Junction **5** Esophagus **6** Stomach **7** Stomach, Pylorus **8** Small Intestine **9** Duodenum **A** Jejunum **B** Ileum **C** Ileocecal Valve **E** Large Intestine **F** Large Intestine, Right **G** Large Intestine, Left **H** Cecum **J** Appendix **K** Ascending Colon **L** Transverse Colon **M** Descending Colon **N** Sigmoid Colon **P** Rectum	**Ø** Open **3** Percutaneous **4** Percutaneous Endoscopic **7** Via Natural or Artificial Opening **8** Via Natural or Artificial Opening Endoscopic	**Z** No Device	**X** Diagnostic **Z** No Qualifier
Q Anus	**Ø** Open **3** Percutaneous **4** Percutaneous Endoscopic **7** Via Natural or Artificial Opening **8** Via Natural or Artificial Opening Endoscopic **X** External	**Ø** Drainage Device	**Z** No Qualifier
Q Anus	**Ø** Open **3** Percutaneous **4** Percutaneous Endoscopic **7** Via Natural or Artificial Opening **8** Via Natural or Artificial Opening Endoscopic **X** External	**Z** No Device	**X** Diagnostic **Z** No Qualifier
R Anal Sphincter **S** Greater Omentum **T** Lesser Omentum **V** Mesentery **W** Peritoneum	**Ø** Open **3** Percutaneous **4** Percutaneous Endoscopic	**Ø** Drainage Device	**Z** No Qualifier
R Anal Sphincter **S** Greater Omentum **T** Lesser Omentum **V** Mesentery **W** Peritoneum	**Ø** Open **3** Percutaneous **4** Percutaneous Endoscopic	**Z** No Device	**X** Diagnostic **Z** No Qualifier

Ø **Medical and Surgical**
D **Gastrointestinal System**
B **Excision**   Cutting out or off, without replacement, a portion of a body part

Body Part Character 4	Approach Character 5	Device Character 6	Qualifier Character 7
1 Esophagus, Upper **2** Esophagus, Middle **3** Esophagus, Lower **4** Esophagogastric Junction **5** Esophagus **6** Stomach **7** Stomach, Pylorus **8** Small Intestine **9** Duodenum **A** Jejunum **B** Ileum **C** Ileocecal Valve **E** Large Intestine **F** Large Intestine, Right **G** Large Intestine, Left **H** Cecum **J** Appendix **K** Ascending Colon **L** Transverse Colon **M** Descending Colon **N** Sigmoid Colon **P** Rectum	**Ø** Open **3** Percutaneous **4** Percutaneous Endoscopic **7** Via Natural or Artificial Opening **8** Via Natural or Artificial Opening Endoscopic	**Z** No Device	**X** Diagnostic **Z** No Qualifier

ØDB Continued on next page

Ø **Medical and Surgical**
D **Gastrointestinal System**
B **Excision**   Cutting out or off, without replacement, a portion of a body part

ØDB Continued

Body Part Character 4	Approach Character 5	Device Character 6	Qualifier Character 7
Q Anus	**Ø** Open **3** Percutaneous **4** Percutaneous Endoscopic **7** Via Natural or Artificial Opening **8** Via Natural or Artificial Opening Endoscopic **X** External	**Z** No Device	**X** Diagnostic **Z** No Qualifier
R Anal Sphincter **S** Greater Omentum **T** Lesser Omentum **V** Mesentery **W** Peritoneum	**Ø** Open **3** Percutaneous **4** Percutaneous Endoscopic	**Z** No Device	**X** Diagnostic **Z** No Qualifier

Ø **Medical and Surgical**
D **Gastrointestinal System**
C **Extirpation**   Taking or cutting out solid matter from a body part

Body Part Character 4	Approach Character 5	Device Character 6	Qualifier Character 7
1 Esophagus, Upper **2** Esophagus, Middle **3** Esophagus, Lower **4** Esophagogastric Junction **5** Esophagus **6** Stomach **7** Stomach, Pylorus **8** Small Intestine **9** Duodenum **A** Jejunum **B** Ileum **C** Ileocecal Valve **E** Large Intestine **F** Large Intestine, Right **G** Large Intestine, Left **H** Cecum **J** Appendix **K** Ascending Colon **L** Transverse Colon **M** Descending Colon **N** Sigmoid Colon **P** Rectum	**Ø** Open **3** Percutaneous **4** Percutaneous Endoscopic **7** Via Natural or Artificial Opening **8** Via Natural or Artificial Opening Endoscopic	**Z** No Device	**Z** No Qualifier
Q Anus	**Ø** Open **3** Percutaneous **4** Percutaneous Endoscopic **7** Via Natural or Artificial Opening **8** Via Natural or Artificial Opening Endoscopic **X** External	**Z** No Device	**Z** No Qualifier
R Anal Sphincter **S** Greater Omentum **T** Lesser Omentum **V** Mesentery **W** Peritoneum	**Ø** Open **3** Percutaneous **4** Percutaneous Endoscopic	**Z** No Device	**Z** No Qualifier

Gastrointestinal System (left margin)

ØDF–ØDH (left margin)

Ø   Medical and Surgical
D   Gastrointestinal System
F   Fragmentation   Breaking solid matter in a body part into pieces

Body Part Character 4	Approach Character 5	Device Character 6	Qualifier Character 7
5 Esophagus 6 Stomach 8 Small Intestine 9 Duodenum A Jejunum B Ileum E Large Intestine F Large Intestine, Right G Large Intestine, Left H Cecum J Appendix K Ascending Colon L Transverse Colon M Descending Colon N Sigmoid Colon P Rectum Q Anus	Ø Open 3 Percutaneous 4 Percutaneous Endoscopic 7 Via Natural or Artificial Opening 8 Via Natural or Artificial Opening Endoscopic X External	Z No Device	Z No Qualifier

Ø   Medical and Surgical
D   Gastrointestinal System
H   Insertion   Putting in a nonbiological appliance that monitors, assists, performs, or prevents a physiological function but does not physically take the place of a body part

Body Part Character 4	Approach Character 5	Device Character 6	Qualifier Character 7
5 Esophagus	Ø Open 3 Percutaneous 4 Percutaneous Endoscopic	1 Radioactive Element 2 Monitoring Device 3 Infusion Device U Feeding Device	Z No Qualifier
5 Esophagus	7 Via Natural or Artificial Opening 8 Via Natural or Artificial Opening Endoscopic	1 Radioactive Element 2 Monitoring Device 3 Infusion Device B Airway U Feeding Device	Z No Qualifier
6 Stomach	Ø Open 3 Percutaneous 4 Percutaneous Endoscopic	2 Monitoring Device 3 Infusion Device M Stimulator Lead U Feeding Device	Z No Qualifier
6 Stomach	7 Via Natural or Artificial Opening 8 Via Natural or Artificial Opening Endoscopic	2 Monitoring Device 3 Infusion Device U Feeding Device	Z No Qualifier
8 Small Intestine 9 Duodenum A Jejunum B Ileum	Ø Open 3 Percutaneous 4 Percutaneous Endoscopic 7 Via Natural or Artificial Opening 8 Via Natural or Artificial Opening Endoscopic	2 Monitoring Device 3 Infusion Device U Feeding Device	Z No Qualifier
P Rectum	Ø Open 3 Percutaneous 4 Percutaneous Endoscopic 7 Via Natural or Artificial Opening 8 Via Natural or Artificial Opening Endoscopic	1 Radioactive Element	Z No Qualifier
Q Anus	Ø Open 3 Percutaneous 4 Percutaneous Endoscopic	L Artificial Sphincter	Z No Qualifier
R Anal Sphincter	Ø Open 3 Percutaneous 4 Percutaneous Endoscopic	M Stimulator Lead	Z No Qualifier

Ø　Medical and Surgical
D　Gastrointestinal System
J　Inspection　　　Visually and/or manually exploring a body part

Body Part Character 4	Approach Character 5	Device Character 6	Qualifier Character 7
Ø Upper Intestinal Tract **6** Stomach **D** Lower Intestinal Tract	**Ø** Open **3** Percutaneous **4** Percutaneous Endoscopic **7** Via Natural or Artificial Opening **8** Via Natural or Artificial Opening Endoscopic **X** External	**Z** No Device	**Z** No Qualifier
U Omentum **V** Mesentery **W** Peritoneum	**Ø** Open **3** Percutaneous **4** Percutaneous Endoscopic **X** External	**Z** No Device	**Z** No Qualifier

Ø　Medical and Surgical
D　Gastrointestinal System
L　Occlusion　　　Completely closing an orifice or the lumen of a tubular body part

Body Part Character 4	Approach Character 5	Device Character 6	Qualifier Character 7
1 Esophagus, Upper **2** Esophagus, Middle **3** Esophagus, Lower **4** Esophagogastric Junction **5** Esophagus **6** Stomach **7** Stomach, Pylorus **8** Small Intestine **9** Duodenum **A** Jejunum **B** Ileum **C** Ileocecal Valve **E** Large Intestine **F** Large Intestine, Right **G** Large Intestine, Left **H** Cecum **K** Ascending Colon **L** Transverse Colon **M** Descending Colon **N** Sigmoid Colon **P** Rectum	**Ø** Open **3** Percutaneous **4** Percutaneous Endoscopic	**C** Extraluminal Device **D** Intraluminal Device **Z** No Device	**Z** No Qualifier
1 Esophagus, Upper **2** Esophagus, Middle **3** Esophagus, Lower **4** Esophagogastric Junction **5** Esophagus **6** Stomach **7** Stomach, Pylorus **8** Small Intestine **9** Duodenum **A** Jejunum **B** Ileum **C** Ileocecal Valve **E** Large Intestine **F** Large Intestine, Right **G** Large Intestine, Left **H** Cecum **K** Ascending Colon **L** Transverse Colon **M** Descending Colon **N** Sigmoid Colon **P** Rectum **Q** Anus	**7** Via Natural or Artificial Opening **8** Via Natural or Artificial Opening Endoscopic	**D** Intraluminal Device **Z** No Device	**Z** No Qualifier
Q Anus	**Ø** Open **3** Percutaneous **4** Percutaneous Endoscopic **X** External	**C** Extraluminal Device **D** Intraluminal Device **Z** No Device	**Z** No Qualifier

Ø   Medical and Surgical
D   Gastrointestinal System
M   Reattachment   Putting back in or on all or a portion of a separated body part to its normal location or other suitable location

Body Part Character 4	Approach Character 5	Device Character 6	Qualifier Character 7
5 Esophagus 6 Stomach 8 Small Intestine 9 Duodenum A Jejunum B Ileum E Large Intestine F Large Intestine, Right G Large Intestine, Left H Cecum K Ascending Colon L Transverse Colon M Descending Colon N Sigmoid Colon P Rectum	Ø Open 4 Percutaneous Endoscopic	Z No Device	Z No Qualifier

Ø   Medical and Surgical
D   Gastrointestinal System
N   Release   Freeing a body part from an abnormal physical constraint

Body Part Character 4	Approach Character 5	Device Character 6	Qualifier Character 7
1 Esophagus, Upper 2 Esophagus, Middle 3 Esophagus, Lower 4 Esophagogastric Junction 5 Esophagus 6 Stomach 7 Stomach, Pylorus 8 Small Intestine 9 Duodenum A Jejunum B Ileum C Ileocecal Valve E Large Intestine F Large Intestine, Right G Large Intestine, Left H Cecum J Appendix K Ascending Colon L Transverse Colon M Descending Colon N Sigmoid Colon P Rectum	Ø Open 3 Percutaneous 4 Percutaneous Endoscopic 7 Via Natural or Artificial Opening 8 Via Natural or Artificial Opening Endoscopic	Z No Device	Z No Qualifier
Q Anus	Ø Open 3 Percutaneous 4 Percutaneous Endoscopic 7 Via Natural or Artificial Opening 8 Via Natural or Artificial Opening Endoscopic X External	Z No Device	Z No Qualifier
R Anal Sphincter S Greater Omentum T Lesser Omentum V Mesentery W Peritoneum	Ø Open 3 Percutaneous 4 Percutaneous Endoscopic	Z No Device	Z No Qualifier

Revised Text in **BLUE**

Ø **Medical and Surgical**
D **Gastrointestinal System**
P **Removal** Taking out or off a device from a body part

Body Part Character 4	Approach Character 5	Device Character 6	Qualifier Character 7
Ø Upper Intestinal Tract **6** Stomach **D** Lower Intestinal Tract	**X** External	**Ø** Drainage Device **2** Monitoring Device **3** Infusion Device **D** Intraluminal Device **U** Feeding Device	**Z** No Qualifier
Ø Upper Intestinal Tract **D** Lower Intestinal Tract	**Ø** Open **3** Percutaneous **4** Percutaneous Endoscopic **7** Via Natural or Artificial Opening **8** Via Natural or Artificial Opening Endoscopic	**Ø** Drainage Device **2** Monitoring Device **3** Infusion Device **7** Autologous Tissue Substitute **C** Extraluminal Device **D** Intraluminal Device **J** Synthetic Substitute **K** Nonautologous Tissue Substitute **U** Feeding Device	**Z** No Qualifier
5 Esophagus	**Ø** Open **3** Percutaneous **4** Percutaneous Endoscopic	**1** Radioactive Element **2** Monitoring Device **3** Infusion Device **U** Feeding Device	**Z** No Qualifier
5 Esophagus	**7** Via Natural or Artificial Opening **8** Via Natural or Artificial Opening Endoscopic	**1** Radioactive Element **B** Airway	**Z** No Qualifier
5 Esophagus	**X** External	**1** Radioactive Element **2** Monitoring Device **3** Infusion Device **B** Airway **U** Feeding Device	**Z** No Qualifier
6 Stomach	**Ø** Open **3** Percutaneous **4** Percutaneous Endoscopic	**Ø** Drainage Device **2** Monitoring Device **3** Infusion Device **7** Autologous Tissue Substitute **C** Extraluminal Device **D** Intraluminal Device **J** Synthetic Substitute **K** Nonautologous Tissue Substitute **M** Stimulator Lead **U** Feeding Device	**Z** No Qualifier
6 Stomach	**7** Via Natural or Artificial Opening **8** Via Natural or Artificial Opening Endoscopic	**Ø** Drainage Device **2** Monitoring Device **3** Infusion Device **7** Autologous Tissue Substitute **C** Extraluminal Device **D** Intraluminal Device **J** Synthetic Substitute **K** Nonautologous Tissue Substitute **U** Feeding Device	**Z** No Qualifier
P Rectum	**Ø** Open **3** Percutaneous **4** Percutaneous Endoscopic **7** Via Natural or Artificial Opening **8** Via Natural or Artificial Opening Endoscopic **X** External	**1** Radioactive Element	**Z** No Qualifier
Q Anus	**Ø** Open **3** Percutaneous **4** Percutaneous Endoscopic **7** Via Natural or Artificial Opening **8** Via Natural or Artificial Opening Endoscopic	**L** Artificial Sphincter	**Z** No Qualifier
R Anal Sphincter	**Ø** Open **3** Percutaneous **4** Percutaneous Endoscopic	**M** Stimulator Lead	**Z** No Qualifier
U Omentum **V** Mesentery **W** Peritoneum	**Ø** Open **3** Percutaneous **4** Percutaneous Endoscopic	**Ø** Drainage Device **1** Radioactive Element **7** Autologous Tissue Substitute **J** Synthetic Substitute **K** Nonautologous Tissue Substitute	**Z** No Qualifier

Revised Text in **BLUE**

Ø   **Medical and Surgical**
D   **Gastrointestinal System**
Q   **Repair**   Restoring, to the extent possible, a body part to its normal anatomic structure and function

Body Part Character 4	Approach Character 5	Device Character 6	Qualifier Character 7
1 Esophagus, Upper **2** Esophagus, Middle **3** Esophagus, Lower **4** Esophagogastric Junction **5** Esophagus **6** Stomach **7** Stomach, Pylorus **8** Small Intestine **9** Duodenum **A** Jejunum **B** Ileum **C** Ileocecal Valve **E** Large Intestine **F** Large Intestine, Right **G** Large Intestine, Left **H** Cecum **J** Appendix **K** Ascending Colon **L** Transverse Colon **M** Descending Colon **N** Sigmoid Colon **P** Rectum	**Ø** Open **3** Percutaneous **4** Percutaneous Endoscopic **7** Via Natural or Artificial Opening **8** Via Natural or Artificial Opening Endoscopic	**Z** No Device	**Z** No Qualifier
Q Anus	**Ø** Open **3** Percutaneous **4** Percutaneous Endoscopic **7** Via Natural or Artificial Opening **8** Via Natural or Artificial Opening Endoscopic **X** External	**Z** No Device	**Z** No Qualifier
R Anal Sphincter **S** Greater Omentum **T** Lesser Omentum **V** Mesentery **W** Peritoneum	**Ø** Open **3** Percutaneous **4** Percutaneous Endoscopic	**Z** No Device	**Z** No Qualifier

Ø   **Medical and Surgical**
D   **Gastrointestinal System**
R   **Replacement**   Putting in or on biological or synthetic material that physically takes the place and/or function of all or a portion of a body part

Body Part Character 4	Approach Character 5	Device Character 6	Qualifier Character 7
5 Esophagus	**Ø** Open **4** Percutaneous Endoscopic **7** Via Natural or Artificial Opening **8** Via Natural or Artificial Opening Endoscopic	**7** Autologous Tissue Substitute **J** Synthetic Substitute **K** Nonautologous Tissue Substitute	**Z** No Qualifier
R Anal Sphincter **S** Greater Omentum **T** Lesser Omentum **V** Mesentery **W** Peritoneum	**Ø** Open **4** Percutaneous Endoscopic	**7** Autologous Tissue Substitute **J** Synthetic Substitute **K** Nonautologous Tissue Substitute	**Z** No Qualifier

Ø   **Medical and Surgical**
D   **Gastrointestinal System**
S   **Reposition**   Moving to its normal location or other suitable location all or a portion of a body part

Body Part Character 4	Approach Character 5	Device Character 6	Qualifier Character 7
5 Esophagus **6** Stomach **9** Duodenum **A** Jejunum **B** Ileum **H** Cecum **K** Ascending Colon **L** Transverse Colon **M** Descending Colon **N** Sigmoid Colon **P** Rectum **Q** Anus	**Ø** Open **4** Percutaneous Endoscopic **7** Via Natural or Artificial Opening **8** Via Natural or Artificial Opening Endoscopic **X** External	**Z** No Device	**Z** No Qualifier

     Revised Text in **BLUE**   © 2Ø11 Ingenix, Inc

0   **Medical and Surgical**
D   **Gastrointestinal System**
T   **Resection**   Cutting out or off, without replacement, all of a body part

Body Part Character 4	Approach Character 5	Device Character 6	Qualifier Character 7
1 Esophagus, Upper **2** Esophagus, Middle **3** Esophagus, Lower **4** Esophagogastric Junction **5** Esophagus **6** Stomach **7** Stomach, Pylorus **8** Small Intestine **9** Duodenum **A** Jejunum **B** Ileum **C** Ileocecal Valve **E** Large Intestine **F** Large Intestine, Right **G** Large Intestine, Left **H** Cecum **J** Appendix **K** Ascending Colon **L** Transverse Colon **M** Descending Colon **N** Sigmoid Colon **P** Rectum **Q** Anus	**0** Open **4** Percutaneous Endoscopic **7** Via Natural or Artificial Opening **8** Via Natural or Artificial Opening Endoscopic	**Z** No Device	**Z** No Qualifier
R Anal Sphincter **S** Greater Omentum **T** Lesser Omentum	**0** Open **4** Percutaneous Endoscopic	**Z** No Device	**Z** No Qualifier

0   **Medical and Surgical**
D   **Gastrointestinal System**
U   **Supplement**   Putting in or on biological or synthetic material that physically reinforces and/or augments the function of a portion of a body part

Body Part Character 4	Approach Character 5	Device Character 6	Qualifier Character 7
1 Esophagus, Upper **2** Esophagus, Middle **3** Esophagus, Lower **4** Esophagogastric Junction **5** Esophagus **6** Stomach **7** Stomach, Pylorus **8** Small Intestine **9** Duodenum **A** Jejunum **B** Ileum **C** Ileocecal Valve **E** Large Intestine **F** Large Intestine, Right **G** Large Intestine, Left **H** Cecum **K** Ascending Colon **L** Transverse Colon **M** Descending Colon **N** Sigmoid Colon **P** Rectum	**0** Open **4** Percutaneous Endoscopic **7** Via Natural or Artificial Opening **8** Via Natural or Artificial Opening Endoscopic	**7** Autologous Tissue Substitute **J** Synthetic Substitute **K** Nonautologous Tissue Substitute	**Z** No Qualifier
Q Anus	**0** Open **4** Percutaneous Endoscopic **7** Via Natural or Artificial Opening **8** Via Natural or Artificial Opening Endoscopic **X** External	**7** Autologous Tissue Substitute **J** Synthetic Substitute **K** Nonautologous Tissue Substitute	**Z** No Qualifier
R Anal Sphincter **S** Greater Omentum **T** Lesser Omentum **V** Mesentery **W** Peritoneum	**0** Open **4** Percutaneous Endoscopic	**7** Autologous Tissue Substitute **J** Synthetic Substitute **K** Nonautologous Tissue Substitute	**Z** No Qualifier

Ø Medical and Surgical
D Gastrointestinal System
V Restriction Partially closing an orifice or the lumen of a tubular body part

Body Part Character 4	Approach Character 5	Device Character 6	Qualifier Character 7
1 Esophagus, Upper **2** Esophagus, Middle **3** Esophagus, Lower **4** Esophagogastric Junction **5** Esophagus **6** Stomach **7** Stomach, Pylorus **8** Small Intestine **9** Duodenum **A** Jejunum **B** Ileum **C** Ileocecal Valve **E** Large Intestine **F** Large Intestine, Right **G** Large Intestine, Left **H** Cecum **K** Ascending Colon **L** Transverse Colon **M** Descending Colon **N** Sigmoid Colon **P** Rectum	**Ø** Open **3** Percutaneous **4** Percutaneous Endoscopic	**C** Extraluminal Device **D** Intraluminal Device **Z** No Device	**Z** No Qualifier
1 Esophagus, Upper **2** Esophagus, Middle **3** Esophagus, Lower **4** Esophagogastric Junction **5** Esophagus **6** Stomach **7** Stomach, Pylorus **8** Small Intestine **9** Duodenum **A** Jejunum **B** Ileum **C** Ileocecal Valve **E** Large Intestine **F** Large Intestine, Right **G** Large Intestine, Left **H** Cecum **K** Ascending Colon **L** Transverse Colon **M** Descending Colon **N** Sigmoid Colon **P** Rectum **Q** Anus	**7** Via Natural or Artificial Opening **8** Via Natural or Artificial Opening Endoscopic	**D** Intraluminal Device **Z** No Device	**Z** No Qualifier
Q Anus	**Ø** Open **3** Percutaneous **4** Percutaneous Endoscopic **X** External	**C** Extraluminal Device **D** Intraluminal Device **Z** No Device	**Z** No Qualifier

Ø Medical and Surgical
D Gastrointestinal System
W Revision Correcting, to the extent possible, a portion of a malfunctioning device or the position of a displaced device

Body Part Character 4	Approach Character 5	Device Character 6	Qualifier Character 7
Ø Upper Intestinal Tract **D** Lower Intestinal Tract	**Ø** Open **3** Percutaneous **4** Percutaneous Endoscopic **7** Via Natural or Artificial Opening **8** Via Natural or Artificial Opening Endoscopic **X** External	**Ø** Drainage Device **2** Monitoring Device **3** Infusion Device **7** Autologous Tissue Substitute **C** Extraluminal Device **D** Intraluminal Device **J** Synthetic Substitute **K** Nonautologous Tissue Substitute **U** Feeding Device	**Z** No Qualifier
5 Esophagus	**7** Via Natural or Artificial Opening **8** Via Natural or Artificial Opening Endoscopic **X** External	**B** Airway	**Z** No Qualifier

ØDW Continued on next page

Ø Medical and Surgical
D Gastrointestinal System
W Revision — Correcting, to the extent possible, a portion of a malfunctioning device or the position of a displaced device

ØDW Continued

Body Part Character 4	Approach Character 5	Device Character 6	Qualifier Character 7
6 Stomach	Ø Open 3 Percutaneous 4 Percutaneous Endoscopic	Ø Drainage Device 2 Monitoring Device 3 Infusion Device 7 Autologous Tissue Substitute C Extraluminal Device D Intraluminal Device J Synthetic Substitute K Nonautologous Tissue Substitute M Stimulator Lead U Feeding Device	Z No Qualifier
6 Stomach	7 Via Natural or Artificial Opening 8 Via Natural or Artificial Opening Endoscopic X External	Ø Drainage Device 2 Monitoring Device 3 Infusion Device 7 Autologous Tissue Substitute C Extraluminal Device D Intraluminal Device J Synthetic Substitute K Nonautologous Tissue Substitute U Feeding Device	Z No Qualifier
8 Small Intestine E Large Intestine	Ø Open 4 Percutaneous Endoscopic 7 Via Natural or Artificial Opening 8 Via Natural or Artificial Opening Endoscopic	7 Autologous Tissue Substitute J Synthetic Substitute K Nonautologous Tissue Substitute	Z No Qualifier
Q Anus	Ø Open 3 Percutaneous 4 Percutaneous Endoscopic 7 Via Natural or Artificial Opening 8 Via Natural or Artificial Opening Endoscopic	L Artificial Sphincter	Z No Qualifier
R Anal Sphincter	Ø Open 3 Percutaneous 4 Percutaneous Endoscopic	M Stimulator Lead	Z No Qualifier
U Omentum V Mesentery W Peritoneum	Ø Open 3 Percutaneous 4 Percutaneous Endoscopic	Ø Drainage Device 7 Autologous Tissue Substitute J Synthetic Substitute K Nonautologous Tissue Substitute	Z No Qualifier

Ø Medical and Surgical
D Gastrointestinal System
X Transfer — Moving, without taking out, all or a portion of a body part to another location to take over the function of all or a portion of a body part

Body Part Character 4	Approach Character 5	Device Character 6	Qualifier Character 7
6 Stomach 8 Small Intestine E Large Intestine	Ø Open 4 Percutaneous Endoscopic	Z No Device	5 Esophagus

Ø Medical and Surgical
D Gastrointestinal System
Y Transplantation — Putting in or on all or a portion of a living body part taken from another individual or animal to physically take the place and/or function of all or a portion of a similar body part

Body Part Character 4	Approach Character 5	Device Character 6	Qualifier Character 7
5 Esophagus 6 Stomach 8 Small Intestine E Large Intestine	Ø Open	Z No Device	Ø Allogeneic 1 Syngeneic 2 Zooplastic

Hepatobiliary System and Pancreas ØF1–ØFY

Ø Medical and Surgical
F Hepatobiliary System and Pancreas
1 Bypass   Altering the route of passage of the contents of a tubular body part

Body Part Character 4	Approach Character 5	Device Character 6	Qualifier Character 7
4 Gallbladder 5 Hepatic Duct, Right 6 Hepatic Duct, Left 8 Cystic Duct 9 Common Bile Duct	Ø Open 4 Percutaneous Endoscopic	D Intraluminal Device Z No Device	3 Duodenum 4 Stomach 5 Hepatic Duct, Right 6 Hepatic Duct, Left 7 Hepatic Duct, Caudate 8 Cystic Duct 9 Common Bile Duct B Small Intestine
D Pancreatic Duct F Pancreatic Duct, Accessory G Pancreas	Ø Open 4 Percutaneous Endoscopic	D Intraluminal Device Z No Device	3 Duodenum B Small Intestine C Large Intestine

Ø Medical and Surgical
F Hepatobiliary System and Pancreas
2 Change   Taking out or off a device from a body part and putting back an identical or similar device in or on the same body part without cutting or puncturing the skin or a mucous membrane

Body Part Character 4	Approach Character 5	Device Character 6	Qualifier Character 7
Ø Liver 4 Gallbladder B Hepatobiliary Duct D Pancreatic Duct G Pancreas	X External	Ø Drainage Device Y Other Device	Z No Qualifier

Ø Medical and Surgical
F Hepatobiliary System and Pancreas
5 Destruction   Physical eradication of all or a portion of a body part by the direct use of energy, force, or a destructive agent

Body Part Character 4	Approach Character 5	Device Character 6	Qualifier Character 7
Ø Liver 1 Liver, Right Lobe 2 Liver, Left Lobe 4 Gallbladder G Pancreas	Ø Open 3 Percutaneous 4 Percutaneous Endoscopic	Z No Device	Z No Qualifier
5 Hepatic Duct, Right 6 Hepatic Duct, Left 8 Cystic Duct 9 Common Bile Duct C Ampulla of Vater D Pancreatic Duct F Pancreatic Duct, Accessory	Ø Open 3 Percutaneous 4 Percutaneous Endoscopic 7 Via Natural or Artificial Opening 8 Via Natural or Artificial Opening Endoscopic	Z No Device	Z No Qualifier

Ø Medical and Surgical
F Hepatobiliary System and Pancreas
7 Dilation   Expanding an orifice or the lumen of a tubular body part

Body Part Character 4	Approach Character 5	Device Character 6	Qualifier Character 7
5 Hepatic Duct, Right 6 Hepatic Duct, Left 8 Cystic Duct 9 Common Bile Duct C Ampulla of Vater D Pancreatic Duct F Pancreatic Duct, Accessory	Ø Open 3 Percutaneous 4 Percutaneous Endoscopic 7 Via Natural or Artificial Opening 8 Via Natural or Artificial Opening Endoscopic	D Intraluminal Device Z No Device	Z No Qualifier

 © 2011 Ingenix, Inc

Ø   Medical and Surgical
F   Hepatobiliary System and Pancreas
8   Division   Cutting into a body part without draining fluids and/or gases from the body part in order to separate or transect a body part

Body Part Character 4	Approach Character 5	Device Character 6	Qualifier Character 7
G Pancreas	**Ø** Open **3** Percutaneous **4** Percutaneous Endoscopic	**Z** No Device	**Z** No Qualifier

Ø   Medical and Surgical
F   Hepatobiliary System and Pancreas
9   Drainage   Taking or letting out fluids and/or gases from a body part

Body Part Character 4	Approach Character 5	Device Character 6	Qualifier Character 7
Ø Liver **1** Liver, Right Lobe **2** Liver, Left Lobe **4** Gallbladder **G** Pancreas	**Ø** Open **3** Percutaneous **4** Percutaneous Endoscopic	**Ø** Drainage Device	**Z** No Qualifier
Ø Liver **1** Liver, Right Lobe **2** Liver, Left Lobe **4** Gallbladder **G** Pancreas	**Ø** Open **3** Percutaneous **4** Percutaneous Endoscopic	**Z** No Device	**X** Diagnostic **Z** No Qualifier
5 Hepatic Duct, Right **6** Hepatic Duct, Left **8** Cystic Duct **9** Common Bile Duct **C** Ampulla of Vater **D** Pancreatic Duct **F** Pancreatic Duct, Accessory	**Ø** Open **3** Percutaneous **4** Percutaneous Endoscopic **7** Via Natural or Artificial Opening **8** Via Natural or Artificial Opening Endoscopic	**Ø** Drainage Device	**Z** No Qualifier
5 Hepatic Duct, Right **6** Hepatic Duct, Left **8** Cystic Duct **9** Common Bile Duct **C** Ampulla of Vater **D** Pancreatic Duct **F** Pancreatic Duct, Accessory	**Ø** Open **3** Percutaneous **4** Percutaneous Endoscopic **7** Via Natural or Artificial Opening **8** Via Natural or Artificial Opening Endoscopic	**Z** No Device	**X** Diagnostic **Z** No Qualifier

Ø   Medical and Surgical
F   Hepatobiliary System and Pancreas
B   Excision   Cutting out or off, without replacement, a portion of a body part

Body Part Character 4	Approach Character 5	Device Character 6	Qualifier Character 7
Ø Liver **1** Liver, Right Lobe **2** Liver, Left Lobe **4** Gallbladder **G** Pancreas	**Ø** Open **3** Percutaneous **4** Percutaneous Endoscopic	**Z** No Device	**X** Diagnostic **Z** No Qualifier
5 Hepatic Duct, Right **6** Hepatic Duct, Left **8** Cystic Duct **9** Common Bile Duct **C** Ampulla of Vater **D** Pancreatic Duct **F** Pancreatic Duct, Accessory	**Ø** Open **3** Percutaneous **4** Percutaneous Endoscopic **7** Via Natural or Artificial Opening **8** Via Natural or Artificial Opening Endoscopic	**Z** No Device	**X** Diagnostic **Z** No Qualifier

0   **Medical and Surgical**
F   **Hepatobiliary System and Pancreas**
C   **Extirpation**   Taking or cutting out solid matter from a body part

Body Part Character 4	Approach Character 5	Device Character 6	Qualifier Character 7
0 Liver **1** Liver, Right Lobe **2** Liver, Left Lobe **4** Gallbladder **G** Pancreas	**0** Open **3** Percutaneous **4** Percutaneous Endoscopic	**Z** No Device	**Z** No Qualifier
5 Hepatic Duct, Right **6** Hepatic Duct, Left **8** Cystic Duct **9** Common Bile Duct **C** Ampulla of Vater **D** Pancreatic Duct **F** Pancreatic Duct, Accessory	**0** Open **3** Percutaneous **4** Percutaneous Endoscopic **7** Via Natural or Artificial Opening **8** Via Natural or Artificial Opening Endoscopic	**Z** No Device	**Z** No Qualifier

0   **Medical and Surgical**
F   **Hepatobiliary System and Pancreas**
F   **Fragmentation**   Breaking solid matter in a body part into pieces

Body Part Character 4	Approach Character 5	Device Character 6	Qualifier Character 7
4 Gallbladder **5** Hepatic Duct, Right **6** Hepatic Duct, Left **8** Cystic Duct **9** Common Bile Duct **C** Ampulla of Vater **D** Pancreatic Duct **F** Pancreatic Duct, Accessory	**0** Open **3** Percutaneous **4** Percutaneous Endoscopic **7** Via Natural or Artificial Opening **8** Via Natural or Artificial Opening Endoscopic **X** External	**Z** No Device	**Z** No Qualifier

0   **Medical and Surgical**
F   **Hepatobiliary System and Pancreas**
H   **Insertion**   Putting in a nonbiological appliance that monitors, assists, performs, or prevents a physiological function but does not physically take the place of a body part

Body Part Character 4	Approach Character 5	Device Character 6	Qualifier Character 7
0 Liver **1** Liver, Right Lobe **2** Liver, Left Lobe **4** Gallbladder **G** Pancreas	**0** Open **3** Percutaneous **4** Percutaneous Endoscopic	**2** Monitoring Device **3** Infusion Device	**Z** No Qualifier
B Hepatobiliary Duct **D** Pancreatic Duct	**0** Open **3** Percutaneous **4** Percutaneous Endoscopic **7** Via Natural or Artificial Opening **8** Via Natural or Artificial Opening Endoscopic	**1** Radioactive Element **2** Monitoring Device **3** Infusion Device	**Z** No Qualifier

0   **Medical and Surgical**
F   **Hepatobiliary System and Pancreas**
J   **Inspection**   Visually and/or manually exploring a body part

Body Part Character 4	Approach Character 5	Device Character 6	Qualifier Character 7
0 Liver **4** Gallbladder **G** Pancreas	**0** Open **3** Percutaneous **4** Percutaneous Endoscopic **X** External	**Z** No Device	**Z** No Qualifier
B Hepatobiliary Duct **D** Pancreatic Duct	**0** Open **3** Percutaneous **4** Percutaneous Endoscopic **7** Via Natural or Artificial Opening **8** Via Natural or Artificial Opening Endoscopic	**Z** No Device	**Z** No Qualifier

Ø   Medical and Surgical
F   Hepatobiliary System and Pancreas
L   Occlusion   Completely closing an orifice or the lumen of a tubular body part

Body Part Character 4	Approach Character 5	Device Character 6	Qualifier Character 7
5 Hepatic Duct, Right 6 Hepatic Duct, Left 8 Cystic Duct 9 Common Bile Duct C Ampulla of Vater D Pancreatic Duct F Pancreatic Duct, Accessory	Ø Open 3 Percutaneous 4 Percutaneous Endoscopic	C Extraluminal Device D Intraluminal Device Z No Device	Z No Qualifier
5 Hepatic Duct, Right 6 Hepatic Duct, Left 8 Cystic Duct 9 Common Bile Duct C Ampulla of Vater D Pancreatic Duct F Pancreatic Duct, Accessory	7 Via Natural or Artificial Opening 8 Via Natural or Artificial Opening Endoscopic	D Intraluminal Device Z No Device	Z No Qualifier

Ø   Medical and Surgical
F   Hepatobiliary System and Pancreas
M   Reattachment   Putting back in or on all or a portion of a separated body part to its normal location or other suitable location

Body Part Character 4	Approach Character 5	Device Character 6	Qualifier Character 7
Ø Liver 1 Liver, Right Lobe 2 Liver, Left Lobe 4 Gallbladder 5 Hepatic Duct, Right 6 Hepatic Duct, Left 8 Cystic Duct 9 Common Bile Duct C Ampulla of Vater D Pancreatic Duct F Pancreatic Duct, Accessory G Pancreas	Ø Open 4 Percutaneous Endoscopic	Z No Device	Z No Qualifier

Ø   Medical and Surgical
F   Hepatobiliary System and Pancreas
N   Release   Freeing a body part from an abnormal physical constraint

Body Part Character 4	Approach Character 5	Device Character 6	Qualifier Character 7
Ø Liver 1 Liver, Right Lobe 2 Liver, Left Lobe 4 Gallbladder G Pancreas	Ø Open 3 Percutaneous 4 Percutaneous Endoscopic	Z No Device	Z No Qualifier
5 Hepatic Duct, Right 6 Hepatic Duct, Left 8 Cystic Duct 9 Common Bile Duct C Ampulla of Vater D Pancreatic Duct F Pancreatic Duct, Accessory	Ø Open 3 Percutaneous 4 Percutaneous Endoscopic 7 Via Natural or Artificial Opening 8 Via Natural or Artificial Opening Endoscopic	Z No Device	Z No Qualifier

Ø   Medical and Surgical
F   Hepatobiliary System and Pancreas
P   Removal   Taking out or off a device from a body part

Body Part Character 4	Approach Character 5	Device Character 6	Qualifier Character 7
Ø Liver	**Ø** Open **3** Percutaneous **4** Percutaneous Endoscopic **X** External	**Ø** Drainage Device **2** Monitoring Device **3** Infusion Device	**Z** No Qualifier
4 Gallbladder **G** Pancreas	**Ø** Open **3** Percutaneous **4** Percutaneous Endoscopic **X** External	**Ø** Drainage Device **2** Monitoring Device **3** Infusion Device **D** Intraluminal Device	**Z** No Qualifier
B Hepatobiliary Duct **D** Pancreatic Duct	**Ø** Open **3** Percutaneous **4** Percutaneous Endoscopic **7** Via Natural or Artificial Opening **8** Via Natural or Artificial Opening Endoscopic	**Ø** Drainage Device **1** Radioactive Element **2** Monitoring Device **3** Infusion Device **7** Autologous Tissue Substitute **C** Extraluminal Device **D** Intraluminal Device **J** Synthetic Substitute **K** Nonautologous Tissue Substitute	**Z** No Qualifier
B Hepatobiliary Duct **D** Pancreatic Duct	**X** External	**Ø** Drainage Device **1** Radioactive Element **2** Monitoring Device **3** Infusion Device **D** Intraluminal Device	**Z** No Qualifier

Ø   Medical and Surgical
F   Hepatobiliary System and Pancreas
Q   Repair   Restoring, to the extent possible, a body part to its normal anatomic structure and function

Body Part Character 4	Approach Character 5	Device Character 6	Qualifier Character 7
Ø Liver **1** Liver, Right Lobe **2** Liver, Left Lobe **4** Gallbladder **G** Pancreas	**Ø** Open **3** Percutaneous **4** Percutaneous Endoscopic	**Z** No Device	**Z** No Qualifier
5 Hepatic Duct, Right **6** Hepatic Duct, Left **8** Cystic Duct **9** Common Bile Duct **C** Ampulla of Vater **D** Pancreatic Duct **F** Pancreatic Duct, Accessory	**Ø** Open **3** Percutaneous **4** Percutaneous Endoscopic **7** Via Natural or Artificial Opening **8** Via Natural or Artificial Opening Endoscopic	**Z** No Device	**Z** No Qualifier

Ø   Medical and Surgical
F   Hepatobiliary System and Pancreas
R   Replacement   Putting in or on biological or synthetic material that physically takes the place and/or function of all or a portion of a body part

Body Part Character 4	Approach Character 5	Device Character 6	Qualifier Character 7
5 Hepatic Duct, Right **6** Hepatic Duct, Left **8** Cystic Duct **9** Common Bile Duct **C** Ampulla of Vater **D** Pancreatic Duct **F** Pancreatic Duct, Accessory	**Ø** Open **4** Percutaneous Endoscopic	**7** Autologous Tissue Substitute **J** Synthetic Substitute **K** Nonautologous Tissue Substitute	**Z** No Qualifier

     Revised Text in **BLUE**   © 2011 Ingenix, Inc

0 Medical and Surgical
F Hepatobiliary System and Pancreas
S Reposition   Moving to its normal location or other suitable location all or a portion of a body part

Body Part Character 4	Approach Character 5	Device Character 6	Qualifier Character 7
0 Liver 4 Gallbladder 5 Hepatic Duct, Right 6 Hepatic Duct, Left 8 Cystic Duct 9 Common Bile Duct C Ampulla of Vater D Pancreatic Duct F Pancreatic Duct, Accessory G Pancreas	0 Open 4 Percutaneous Endoscopic	Z No Device	Z No Qualifier

0 Medical and Surgical
F Hepatobiliary System and Pancreas
T Resection   Cutting out or off, without replacement, all of a body part

Body Part Character 4	Approach Character 5	Device Character 6	Qualifier Character 7
0 Liver 1 Liver, Right Lobe 2 Liver, Left Lobe 4 Gallbladder G Pancreas	0 Open 4 Percutaneous Endoscopic	Z No Device	Z No Qualifier
5 Hepatic Duct, Right 6 Hepatic Duct, Left 8 Cystic Duct 9 Common Bile Duct C Ampulla of Vater D Pancreatic Duct F Pancreatic Duct, Accessory	0 Open 4 Percutaneous Endoscopic 7 Via Natural or Artificial Opening 8 Via Natural or Artificial Opening Endoscopic	Z No Device	Z No Qualifier

0 Medical and Surgical
F Hepatobiliary System and Pancreas
U Supplement   Putting in or on biological or synthetic material that physically reinforces and/or augments the function of a portion of a body part

Body Part Character 4	Approach Character 5	Device Character 6	Qualifier Character 7
5 Hepatic Duct, Right 6 Hepatic Duct, Left 8 Cystic Duct 9 Common Bile Duct C Ampulla of Vater D Pancreatic Duct F Pancreatic Duct, Accessory	0 Open 3 Percutaneous 4 Percutaneous Endoscopic	7 Autologous Tissue Substitute J Synthetic Substitute K Nonautologous Tissue Substitute	Z No Qualifier

0 Medical and Surgical
F Hepatobiliary System and Pancreas
V Restriction   Partially closing an orifice or the lumen of a tubular body part

Body Part Character 4	Approach Character 5	Device Character 6	Qualifier Character 7
5 Hepatic Duct, Right 6 Hepatic Duct, Left 8 Cystic Duct 9 Common Bile Duct C Ampulla of Vater D Pancreatic Duct F Pancreatic Duct, Accessory	0 Open 3 Percutaneous 4 Percutaneous Endoscopic	C Extraluminal Device D Intraluminal Device Z No Device	Z No Qualifier
5 Hepatic Duct, Right 6 Hepatic Duct, Left 8 Cystic Duct 9 Common Bile Duct C Ampulla of Vater D Pancreatic Duct F Pancreatic Duct, Accessory	7 Via Natural or Artificial Opening 8 Via Natural or Artificial Opening Endoscopic	D Intraluminal Device Z No Device	Z No Qualifier

Ø   Medical and Surgical
F   Hepatobiliary System and Pancreas
W   Revision   Correcting, to the extent possible, a portion of a malfunctioning device or the position of a displaced device

Body Part Character 4	Approach Character 5	Device Character 6	Qualifier Character 7
Ø Liver	Ø Open 3 Percutaneous 4 Percutaneous Endoscopic X External	Ø Drainage Device 2 Monitoring Device 3 Infusion Device	Z No Qualifier
4 Gallbladder G Pancreas	Ø Open 3 Percutaneous 4 Percutaneous Endoscopic X External	Ø Drainage Device 2 Monitoring Device 3 Infusion Device D Intraluminal Device	Z No Qualifier
B Hepatobiliary Duct D Pancreatic Duct	Ø Open 3 Percutaneous 4 Percutaneous Endoscopic 7 Via Natural or Artificial Opening 8 Via Natural or Artificial Opening Endoscopic X External	Ø Drainage Device 2 Monitoring Device 3 Infusion Device 7 Autologous Tissue Substitute C Extraluminal Device D Intraluminal Device J Synthetic Substitute K Nonautologous Tissue Substitute	Z No Qualifier

Ø   Medical and Surgical
F   Hepatobiliary System and Pancreas
Y   Transplantation   Putting in or on all or a portion of a living body part taken from another individual or animal to physically take the place and/or function of all or a portion of a similar body part

Body Part Character 4	Approach Character 5	Device Character 6	Qualifier Character 7
Ø Liver G Pancreas	Ø Open	Z No Device	Ø Allogeneic 1 Syngeneic 2 Zooplastic

         Revised Text in **BLUE**

Endocrine System 0G2–0GW

0 Medical and Surgical
G Endocrine System
2 Change   Taking out or off a device from a body part and putting back an identical or similar device in or on the same body part without cutting or puncturing the skin or a mucous membrane

Body Part Character 4	Approach Character 5	Device Character 6	Qualifier Character 7
0 Pituitary Gland 1 Pineal Body 5 Adrenal Gland K Thyroid Gland R Parathyroid Gland S Endocrine Gland	X External	0 Drainage Device Y Other Device	Z No Qualifier

0 Medical and Surgical
G Endocrine System
5 Destruction   Physical eradication of all or a portion of a body part by the direct use of energy, force, or a destructive agent

Body Part Character 4	Approach Character 5	Device Character 6	Qualifier Character 7
0 Pituitary Gland 1 Pineal Body 2 Adrenal Gland, Left 3 Adrenal Gland, Right 4 Adrenal Glands, Bilateral 6 Carotid Body, Left 7 Carotid Body, Right 8 Carotid Bodies, Bilateral 9 Para-aortic Body B Coccygeal Glomus C Glomus Jugulare D Aortic Body F Paraganglion Extremity G Thyroid Gland Lobe, Left H Thyroid Gland Lobe, Right K Thyroid Gland L Superior Parathyroid Gland, Right M Superior Parathyroid Gland, Left N Inferior Parathyroid Gland, Right P Inferior Parathyroid Gland, Left Q Parathyroid Glands, Multiple R Parathyroid Gland	0 Open 3 Percutaneous 4 Percutaneous Endoscopic	Z No Device	Z No Qualifier

0 Medical and Surgical
G Endocrine System
8 Division   Cutting into a body part without draining fluids and/or gases from the body part in order to separate or transect a body part

Body Part Character 4	Approach Character 5	Device Character 6	Qualifier Character 7
0 Pituitary Gland J Thyroid Gland Isthmus	0 Open 3 Percutaneous 4 Percutaneous Endoscopic	Z No Device	Z No Qualifier

0   **Medical and Surgical**
G   **Endocrine System**
9   **Drainage**   Taking or letting out fluids and/or gases from a body part

Body Part Character 4	Approach Character 5	Device Character 6	Qualifier Character 7
0 Pituitary Gland **1** Pineal Body **2** Adrenal Gland, Left **3** Adrenal Gland, Right **4** Adrenal Glands, Bilateral **6** Carotid Body, Left **7** Carotid Body, Right **8** Carotid Bodies, Bilateral **9** Para-aortic Body **B** Coccygeal Glomus **C** Glomus Jugulare **D** Aortic Body **F** Paraganglion Extremity **G** Thyroid Gland Lobe, Left **H** Thyroid Gland Lobe, Right **K** Thyroid Gland **L** Superior Parathyroid Gland, Right **M** Superior Parathyroid Gland, Left **N** Inferior Parathyroid Gland, Right **P** Inferior Parathyroid Gland, Left **Q** Parathyroid Glands, Multiple **R** Parathyroid Gland	**0** Open **3** Percutaneous **4** Percutaneous Endoscopic	**0** Drainage Device	**Z** No Qualifier
0 Pituitary Gland **1** Pineal Body **2** Adrenal Gland, Left **3** Adrenal Gland, Right **4** Adrenal Glands, Bilateral **6** Carotid Body, Left **7** Carotid Body, Right **8** Carotid Bodies, Bilateral **9** Para-aortic Body **B** Coccygeal Glomus **C** Glomus Jugulare **D** Aortic Body **F** Paraganglion Extremity **G** Thyroid Gland Lobe, Left **H** Thyroid Gland Lobe, Right **K** Thyroid Gland **L** Superior Parathyroid Gland, Right **M** Superior Parathyroid Gland, Left **N** Inferior Parathyroid Gland, Right **P** Inferior Parathyroid Gland, Left **Q** Parathyroid Glands, Multiple **R** Parathyroid Gland	**0** Open **3** Percutaneous **4** Percutaneous Endoscopic	**Z** No Device	**X** Diagnostic **Z** No Qualifier

0   **Medical and Surgical**
G   **Endocrine System**
B   **Excision**   Cutting out or off, without replacement, a portion of a body part

Body Part Character 4	Approach Character 5	Device Character 6	Qualifier Character 7
0 Pituitary Gland **1** Pineal Body **2** Adrenal Gland, Left **3** Adrenal Gland, Right **4** Adrenal Glands, Bilateral **6** Carotid Body, Left **7** Carotid Body, Right **8** Carotid Bodies, Bilateral **9** Para-aortic Body **B** Coccygeal Glomus **C** Glomus Jugulare **D** Aortic Body **F** Paraganglion Extremity **G** Thyroid Gland Lobe, Left **H** Thyroid Gland Lobe, Right **L** Superior Parathyroid Gland, Right **M** Superior Parathyroid Gland, Left **N** Inferior Parathyroid Gland, Right **P** Inferior Parathyroid Gland, Left **Q** Parathyroid Glands, Multiple **R** Parathyroid Gland	**0** Open **3** Percutaneous **4** Percutaneous Endoscopic	**Z** No Device	**X** Diagnostic **Z** No Qualifier

0 **Medical and Surgical**
G **Endocrine System**
C **Extirpation**   Taking or cutting out solid matter from a body part

Body Part Character 4	Approach Character 5	Device Character 6	Qualifier Character 7
0 Pituitary Gland **1** Pineal Body **2** Adrenal Gland, Left **3** Adrenal Gland, Right **4** Adrenal Glands, Bilateral **6** Carotid Body, Left **7** Carotid Body, Right **8** Carotid Bodies, Bilateral **9** Para-aortic Body **B** Coccygeal Glomus **C** Glomus Jugulare **D** Aortic Body **F** Paraganglion Extremity **G** Thyroid Gland Lobe, Left **H** Thyroid Gland Lobe, Right **K** Thyroid Gland **L** Superior Parathyroid Gland, Right **M** Superior Parathyroid Gland, Left **N** Inferior Parathyroid Gland, Right **P** Inferior Parathyroid Gland, Left **Q** Parathyroid Glands, Multiple **R** Parathyroid Gland	**0** Open **3** Percutaneous **4** Percutaneous Endoscopic	**Z** No Device	**Z** No Qualifier

0 **Medical and Surgical**
G **Endocrine System**
H **Insertion**   Putting in a nonbiological appliance that monitors, assists, performs, or prevents a physiological function but does not physically take the place of a body part

Body Part Character 4	Approach Character 5	Device Character 6	Qualifier Character 7
S Endocrine Gland	**0** Open **3** Percutaneous **4** Percutaneous Endoscopic	**2** Monitoring Device **3** Infusion Device	**Z** No Qualifier

0 **Medical and Surgical**
G **Endocrine System**
J **Inspection**   Visually and/or manually exploring a body part

Body Part Character 4	Approach Character 5	Device Character 6	Qualifier Character 7
0 Pituitary Gland **1** Pineal Body **5** Adrenal Gland **K** Thyroid Gland **R** Parathyroid Gland **S** Endocrine Gland	**0** Open **3** Percutaneous **4** Percutaneous Endoscopic	**Z** No Device	**Z** No Qualifier

0 **Medical and Surgical**
G **Endocrine System**
M **Reattachment**   Putting back in or on all or a portion of a separated body part to its normal location or other suitable location

Body Part Character 4	Approach Character 5	Device Character 6	Qualifier Character 7
2 Adrenal Gland, Left **3** Adrenal Gland, Right **G** Thyroid Gland Lobe, Left **H** Thyroid Gland Lobe, Right **L** Superior Parathyroid Gland, Right **M** Superior Parathyroid Gland, Left **N** Inferior Parathyroid Gland, Right **P** Inferior Parathyroid Gland, Left **Q** Parathyroid Glands, Multiple **R** Parathyroid Gland	**0** Open **4** Percutaneous Endoscopic	**Z** No Device	**Z** No Qualifier

Ø   **Medical and Surgical**
G   **Endocrine System**
N   **Release**   Freeing a body part from an abnormal physical constraint

Body Part Character 4	Approach Character 5	Device Character 6	Qualifier Character 7
Ø Pituitary Gland 1 Pineal Body 2 Adrenal Gland, Left 3 Adrenal Gland, Right 4 Adrenal Glands, Bilateral 6 Carotid Body, Left 7 Carotid Body, Right 8 Carotid Bodies, Bilateral 9 Para-aortic Body B Coccygeal Glomus C Glomus Jugulare D Aortic Body F Paraganglion Extremity G Thyroid Gland Lobe, Left H Thyroid Gland Lobe, Right K Thyroid Gland L Superior Parathyroid Gland, Right M Superior Parathyroid Gland, Left N Inferior Parathyroid Gland, Right P Inferior Parathyroid Gland, Left Q Parathyroid Glands, Multiple R Parathyroid Gland	Ø Open 3 Percutaneous 4 Percutaneous Endoscopic	Z No Device	Z No Qualifier

Ø   **Medical and Surgical**
G   **Endocrine System**
P   **Removal**   Taking out or off a device from a body part

Body Part Character 4	Approach Character 5	Device Character 6	Qualifier Character 7
Ø Pituitary Gland 1 Pineal Body 5 Adrenal Gland K Thyroid Gland R Parathyroid Gland	Ø Open 3 Percutaneous 4 Percutaneous Endoscopic X External	Ø Drainage Device	Z No Qualifier
S Endocrine Gland	Ø Open 3 Percutaneous 4 Percutaneous Endoscopic X External	Ø Drainage Device 2 Monitoring Device 3 Infusion Device	Z No Qualifier

Ø   **Medical and Surgical**
G   **Endocrine System**
Q   **Repair**   Restoring, to the extent possible, a body part to its normal anatomic structure and function

Body Part Character 4	Approach Character 5	Device Character 6	Qualifier Character 7
Ø Pituitary Gland 1 Pineal Body 2 Adrenal Gland, Left 3 Adrenal Gland, Right 4 Adrenal Glands, Bilateral 6 Carotid Body, Left 7 Carotid Body, Right 8 Carotid Bodies, Bilateral 9 Para-aortic Body B Coccygeal Glomus C Glomus Jugulare D Aortic Body F Paraganglion Extremity G Thyroid Gland Lobe, Left H Thyroid Gland Lobe, Right J Thyroid Gland Isthmus K Thyroid Gland L Superior Parathyroid Gland, Right M Superior Parathyroid Gland, Left N Inferior Parathyroid Gland, Right P Inferior Parathyroid Gland, Left Q Parathyroid Glands, Multiple R Parathyroid Gland	Ø Open 3 Percutaneous 4 Percutaneous Endoscopic	Z No Device	Z No Qualifier

0   **Medical and Surgical**
G   **Endocrine System**
S   **Reposition**   Moving to its normal location or other suitable location all or a portion of a body part

Body Part Character 4	Approach Character 5	Device Character 6	Qualifier Character 7
2 Adrenal Gland, Left **3** Adrenal Gland, Right **G** Thyroid Gland Lobe, Left **H** Thyroid Gland Lobe, Right **L** Superior Parathyroid Gland, Right **M** Superior Parathyroid Gland, Left **N** Inferior Parathyroid Gland, Right **P** Inferior Parathyroid Gland, Left **Q** Parathyroid Glands, Multiple **R** Parathyroid Gland	**0** Open **4** Percutaneous Endoscopic	**Z** No Device	**Z** No Qualifier

0   **Medical and Surgical**
G   **Endocrine System**
T   **Resection**   Cutting out or off, without replacement, all of a body part

Body Part Character 4	Approach Character 5	Device Character 6	Qualifier Character 7
0 Pituitary Gland **1** Pineal Body **2** Adrenal Gland, Left **3** Adrenal Gland, Right **4** Adrenal Glands, Bilateral **6** Carotid Body, Left **7** Carotid Body, Right **8** Carotid Bodies, Bilateral **9** Para-aortic Body **B** Coccygeal Glomus **C** Glomus Jugulare **D** Aortic Body **F** Paraganglion Extremity **G** Thyroid Gland Lobe, Left **H** Thyroid Gland Lobe, Right **K** Thyroid Gland **L** Superior Parathyroid Gland, Right **M** Superior Parathyroid Gland, Left **N** Inferior Parathyroid Gland, Right **P** Inferior Parathyroid Gland, Left **Q** Parathyroid Glands, Multiple **R** Parathyroid Gland	**0** Open **4** Percutaneous Endoscopic	**Z** No Device	**Z** No Qualifier

0   **Medical and Surgical**
G   **Endocrine System**
W   **Revision**   Correcting, to the extent possible, a portion of a malfunctioning device or the position of a displaced device

Body Part Character 4	Approach Character 5	Device Character 6	Qualifier Character 7
0 Pituitary Gland **1** Pineal Body **5** Adrenal Gland **K** Thyroid Gland **R** Parathyroid Gland	**0** Open **3** Percutaneous **4** Percutaneous Endoscopic **X** External	**0** Drainage Device	**Z** No Qualifier
S Endocrine Gland	**0** Open **3** Percutaneous **4** Percutaneous Endoscopic **X** External	**0** Drainage Device **2** Monitoring Device **3** Infusion Device	**Z** No Qualifier

Skin and Breast ØHØ–ØHX

Ø   **Medical and Surgical**
H   **Skin and Breast**
Ø   **Alteration**   Modifying the anatomic structure of a body part without affecting the function of the body part

Body Part Character 4	Approach Character 5	Device Character 6	Qualifier Character 7
T Breast, Right **U** Breast, Left **V** Breast, Bilateral	**Ø** Open **3** Percutaneous **X** External	**7** Autologous Tissue Substitute **J** Synthetic Substitute **K** Nonautologous Tissue Substitute **Z** No Device	**Z** No Qualifier

Ø   **Medical and Surgical**
H   **Skin and Breast**
2   **Change**   Taking out or off a device from a body part and putting back an identical or similar device in or on the same body part without cutting or puncturing the skin or a mucous membrane

Body Part Character 4	Approach Character 5	Device Character 6	Qualifier Character 7
P Skin **T** Breast, Right **U** Breast, Left	**X** External	**Ø** Drainage Device **Y** Other Device	**Z** No Qualifier

Ø   **Medical and Surgical**
H   **Skin and Breast**
5   **Destruction**   Physical eradication of all or a portion of a body part by the direct use of energy, force, or a destructive agent

Body Part Character 4	Approach Character 5	Device Character 6	Qualifier Character 7
Ø Skin, Scalp **1** Skin, Face **2** Skin, Right Ear **3** Skin, Left Ear **4** Skin, Neck **5** Skin, Chest **6** Skin, Back **7** Skin, Abdomen **8** Skin, Buttock **9** Skin, Perineum **A** Skin, Genitalia **B** Skin, Right Upper Arm **C** Skin, Left Upper Arm **D** Skin, Right Lower Arm **E** Skin, Left Lower Arm **F** Skin, Right Hand **G** Skin, Left Hand **H** Skin, Right Upper Leg **J** Skin, Left Upper Leg **K** Skin, Right Lower Leg **L** Skin, Left Lower Leg **M** Skin, Right Foot **N** Skin, Left Foot	**X** External	**Z** No Device	**D** Multiple **Z** No Qualifier
Q Finger Nail **R** Toe Nail	**X** External	**Z** No Device	**Z** No Qualifier
T Breast, Right **U** Breast, Left **V** Breast, Bilateral **W** Nipple, Right **X** Nipple, Left	**Ø** Open **3** Percutaneous **7** Via Natural or Artificial Opening **8** Via Natural or Artificial Opening Endoscopic **X** External	**Z** No Device	**Z** No Qualifier

0　**Medical and Surgical**
H　**Skin and Breast**
8　**Division**　　　　Cutting into a body part without draining fluids and/or gases from the body part in order to separate or transect a body part

Body Part Character 4	Approach Character 5	Device Character 6	Qualifier Character 7
0 Skin, Scalp **1** Skin, Face **2** Skin, Right Ear **3** Skin, Left Ear **4** Skin, Neck **5** Skin, Chest **6** Skin, Back **7** Skin, Abdomen **8** Skin, Buttock **9** Skin, Perineum **A** Skin, Genitalia **B** Skin, Right Upper Arm **C** Skin, Left Upper Arm **D** Skin, Right Lower Arm **E** Skin, Left Lower Arm **F** Skin, Right Hand **G** Skin, Left Hand **H** Skin, Right Upper Leg **J** Skin, Left Upper Leg **K** Skin, Right Lower Leg **L** Skin, Left Lower Leg **M** Skin, Right Foot **N** Skin, Left Foot	**X** External	**Z** No Device	**Z** No Qualifier

0　**Medical and Surgical**
H　**Skin and Breast**
9　**Drainage**　　　　Taking or letting out fluids and/or gases from a body part

Body Part Character 4	Approach Character 5	Device Character 6	Qualifier Character 7
0 Skin, Scalp **1** Skin, Face **2** Skin, Right Ear **3** Skin, Left Ear **4** Skin, Neck **5** Skin, Chest **6** Skin, Back **7** Skin, Abdomen **8** Skin, Buttock **9** Skin, Perineum **A** Skin, Genitalia **B** Skin, Right Upper Arm **C** Skin, Left Upper Arm **D** Skin, Right Lower Arm **E** Skin, Left Lower Arm **F** Skin, Right Hand **G** Skin, Left Hand **H** Skin, Right Upper Leg **J** Skin, Left Upper Leg **K** Skin, Right Lower Leg **L** Skin, Left Lower Leg **M** Skin, Right Foot **N** Skin, Left Foot **Q** Finger Nail **R** Toe Nail	**X** External	**0** Drainage Device	**Z** No Qualifier

0H9 Continued on next page

Ø Medical and Surgical
H Skin and Breast
9 Drainage   Taking or letting out fluids and/or gases from a body part

ØH9 Continued

Body Part Character 4	Approach Character 5	Device Character 6	Qualifier Character 7
Ø Skin, Scalp **1** Skin, Face **2** Skin, Right Ear **3** Skin, Left Ear **4** Skin, Neck **5** Skin, Chest **6** Skin, Back **7** Skin, Abdomen **8** Skin, Buttock **9** Skin, Perineum **A** Skin, Genitalia **B** Skin, Right Upper Arm **C** Skin, Left Upper Arm **D** Skin, Right Lower Arm **E** Skin, Left Lower Arm **F** Skin, Right Hand **G** Skin, Left Hand **H** Skin, Right Upper Leg **J** Skin, Left Upper Leg **K** Skin, Right Lower Leg **L** Skin, Left Lower Leg **M** Skin, Right Foot **N** Skin, Left Foot **Q** Finger Nail **R** Toe Nail	**X** External	**Z** No Device	**X** Diagnostic **Z** No Qualifier
T Breast, Right **U** Breast, Left **V** Breast, Bilateral **W** Nipple, Right **X** Nipple, Left	**Ø** Open **3** Percutaneous **7** Via Natural or Artificial Opening **8** Via Natural or Artificial Opening Endoscopic **X** External	**Ø** Drainage Device	**Z** No Qualifier
T Breast, Right **U** Breast, Left **V** Breast, Bilateral **W** Nipple, Right **X** Nipple, Left	**Ø** Open **3** Percutaneous **7** Via Natural or Artificial Opening **8** Via Natural or Artificial Opening Endoscopic **X** External	**Z** No Device	**X** Diagnostic **Z** No Qualifier

Ø Medical and Surgical
H Skin and Breast
B Excision   Cutting out or off, without replacement, a portion of a body part

Body Part Character 4	Approach Character 5	Device Character 6	Qualifier Character 7
Ø Skin, Scalp **1** Skin, Face **2** Skin, Right Ear **3** Skin, Left Ear **4** Skin, Neck **5** Skin, Chest **6** Skin, Back **7** Skin, Abdomen **8** Skin, Buttock **9** Skin, Perineum **A** Skin, Genitalia **B** Skin, Right Upper Arm **C** Skin, Left Upper Arm **D** Skin, Right Lower Arm **E** Skin, Left Lower Arm **F** Skin, Right Hand **G** Skin, Left Hand **H** Skin, Right Upper Leg **J** Skin, Left Upper Leg **K** Skin, Right Lower Leg **L** Skin, Left Lower Leg **M** Skin, Right Foot **N** Skin, Left Foot **Q** Finger Nail **R** Toe Nail	**X** External	**Z** No Device	**X** Diagnostic **Z** No Qualifier
T Breast, Right **U** Breast, Left **V** Breast, Bilateral **W** Nipple, Right **X** Nipple, Left **Y** Supernumerary Breast	**Ø** Open **3** Percutaneous **7** Via Natural or Artificial Opening **8** Via Natural or Artificial Opening Endoscopic **X** External	**Z** No Device	**X** Diagnostic **Z** No Qualifier

0   **Medical and Surgical**
H   **Skin and Breast**
C   **Extirpation**   Taking or cutting out solid matter from a body part

Body Part Character 4	Approach Character 5	Device Character 6	Qualifier Character 7
0 Skin, Scalp **1** Skin, Face **2** Skin, Right Ear **3** Skin, Left Ear **4** Skin, Neck **5** Skin, Chest **6** Skin, Back **7** Skin, Abdomen **8** Skin, Buttock **9** Skin, Perineum **A** Skin, Genitalia **B** Skin, Right Upper Arm **C** Skin, Left Upper Arm **D** Skin, Right Lower Arm **E** Skin, Left Lower Arm **F** Skin, Right Hand **G** Skin, Left Hand **H** Skin, Right Upper Leg **J** Skin, Left Upper Leg **K** Skin, Right Lower Leg **L** Skin, Left Lower Leg **M** Skin, Right Foot **N** Skin, Left Foot **Q** Finger Nail **R** Toe Nail	**X** External	**Z** No Device	**Z** No Qualifier
T Breast, Right **U** Breast, Left **V** Breast, Bilateral **W** Nipple, Right **X** Nipple, Left	**0** Open **3** Percutaneous **7** Via Natural or Artificial Opening **8** Via Natural or Artificial Opening Endoscopic **X** External	**Z** No Device	**Z** No Qualifier

0   **Medical and Surgical**
H   **Skin and Breast**
D   **Extraction**   Pulling or stripping out or off all or a portion of a body part by the use of force

Body Part Character 4	Approach Character 5	Device Character 6	Qualifier Character 7
0 Skin, Scalp **1** Skin, Face **2** Skin, Right Ear **3** Skin, Left Ear **4** Skin, Neck **5** Skin, Chest **6** Skin, Back **7** Skin, Abdomen **8** Skin, Buttock **9** Skin, Perineum **A** Skin, Genitalia **B** Skin, Right Upper Arm **C** Skin, Left Upper Arm **D** Skin, Right Lower Arm **E** Skin, Left Lower Arm **F** Skin, Right Hand **G** Skin, Left Hand **H** Skin, Right Upper Leg **J** Skin, Left Upper Leg **K** Skin, Right Lower Leg **L** Skin, Left Lower Leg **M** Skin, Right Foot **N** Skin, Left Foot **Q** Finger Nail **R** Toe Nail **S** Hair	**X** External	**Z** No Device	**Z** No Qualifier

Skin and Breast

Ø Medical and Surgical
H Skin and Breast
H Insertion   Putting in a nonbiological appliance that monitors, assists, performs, or prevents a physiological function but does not physically take the place of a body part

Body Part Character 4	Approach Character 5	Device Character 6	Qualifier Character 7
T Breast, Right U Breast, Left V Breast, Bilateral W Nipple, Right X Nipple, Left	Ø Open 3 Percutaneous 7 Via Natural or Artificial Opening 8 Via Natural or Artificial Opening Endoscopic	1 Radioactive Element N Tissue Expander	Z No Qualifier
T Breast, Right U Breast, Left V Breast, Bilateral W Nipple, Right X Nipple, Left	X External	1 Radioactive Element	Z No Qualifier

Ø Medical and Surgical
H Skin and Breast
J Inspection   Visually and/or manually exploring a body part

Body Part Character 4	Approach Character 5	Device Character 6	Qualifier Character 7
P Skin Q Finger Nail R Toe Nail	X External	Z No Device	Z No Qualifier
T Breast, Right U Breast, Left	Ø Open 3 Percutaneous 7 Via Natural or Artificial Opening 8 Via Natural or Artificial Opening Endoscopic X External	Z No Device	Z No Qualifier

Ø Medical and Surgical
H Skin and Breast
M Reattachment   Putting back in or on all or a portion of a separated body part to its normal location or other suitable location

Body Part Character 4	Approach Character 5	Device Character 6	Qualifier Character 7
Ø Skin, Scalp 1 Skin, Face 2 Skin, Right Ear 3 Skin, Left Ear 4 Skin, Neck 5 Skin, Chest 6 Skin, Back 7 Skin, Abdomen 8 Skin, Buttock 9 Skin, Perineum A Skin, Genitalia B Skin, Right Upper Arm C Skin, Left Upper Arm D Skin, Right Lower Arm E Skin, Left Lower Arm F Skin, Right Hand G Skin, Left Hand H Skin, Right Upper Leg J Skin, Left Upper Leg K Skin, Right Lower Leg L Skin, Left Lower Leg M Skin, Right Foot N Skin, Left Foot T Breast, Right U Breast, Left V Breast, Bilateral W Nipple, Right X Nipple, Left	X External	Z No Device	Z No Qualifier

Ø Medical and Surgical
H Skin and Breast
N Release — Freeing a body part from an abnormal physical constraint

Body Part Character 4	Approach Character 5	Device Character 6	Qualifier Character 7
Ø Skin, Scalp 1 Skin, Face 2 Skin, Right Ear 3 Skin, Left Ear 4 Skin, Neck 5 Skin, Chest 6 Skin, Back 7 Skin, Abdomen 8 Skin, Buttock 9 Skin, Perineum A Skin, Genitalia B Skin, Right Upper Arm C Skin, Left Upper Arm D Skin, Right Lower Arm E Skin, Left Lower Arm F Skin, Right Hand G Skin, Left Hand H Skin, Right Upper Leg J Skin, Left Upper Leg K Skin, Right Lower Leg L Skin, Left Lower Leg M Skin, Right Foot N Skin, Left Foot Q Finger Nail R Toe Nail	X External	Z No Device	Z No Qualifier
T Breast, Right U Breast, Left V Breast, Bilateral W Nipple, Right X Nipple, Left	Ø Open 3 Percutaneous 7 Via Natural or Artificial Opening 8 Via Natural or Artificial Opening Endoscopic X External	Z No Device	Z No Qualifier

Ø Medical and Surgical
H Skin and Breast
P Removal — Taking out or off a device from a body part

Body Part Character 4	Approach Character 5	Device Character 6	Qualifier Character 7
P Skin Q Finger Nail R Toe Nail	X External	Ø Drainage Device 7 Autologous Tissue Substitute J Synthetic Substitute K Nonautologous Tissue Substitute	Z No Qualifier
S Hair	X External	7 Autologous Tissue Substitute J Synthetic Substitute K Nonautologous Tissue Substitute	Z No Qualifier
T Breast, Right U Breast, Left	Ø Open 3 Percutaneous 7 Via Natural or Artificial Opening 8 Via Natural or Artificial Opening Endoscopic	Ø Drainage Device 1 Radioactive Element 7 Autologous Tissue Substitute J Synthetic Substitute K Nonautologous Tissue Substitute N Tissue Expander	Z No Qualifier
T Breast, Right U Breast, Left	X External	Ø Drainage Device 1 Radioactive Element 7 Autologous Tissue Substitute J Synthetic Substitute K Nonautologous Tissue Substitute	Z No Qualifier

Ø Medical and Surgical
H Skin and Breast
Q Repair   Restoring, to the extent possible, a body part to its normal anatomic structure and function

Body Part Character 4	Approach Character 5	Device Character 6	Qualifier Character 7
Ø Skin, Scalp 1 Skin, Face 2 Skin, Right Ear 3 Skin, Left Ear 4 Skin, Neck 5 Skin, Chest 6 Skin, Back 7 Skin, Abdomen 8 Skin, Buttock 9 Skin, Perineum A Skin, Genitalia B Skin, Right Upper Arm C Skin, Left Upper Arm D Skin, Right Lower Arm E Skin, Left Lower Arm F Skin, Right Hand G Skin, Left Hand H Skin, Right Upper Leg J Skin, Left Upper Leg K Skin, Right Lower Leg L Skin, Left Lower Leg M Skin, Right Foot N Skin, Left Foot Q Finger Nail R Toe Nail	X External	Z No Device	Z No Qualifier
T Breast, Right U Breast, Left V Breast, Bilateral W Nipple, Right X Nipple, Left Y Supernumerary Breast	Ø Open 3 Percutaneous 7 Via Natural or Artificial Opening 8 Via Natural or Artificial Opening Endoscopic X External	Z No Device	Z No Qualifier

Ø Medical and Surgical
H Skin and Breast
R Replacement   Putting in or on biological or synthetic material that physically takes the place and/or function of all or a portion of a body part

Body Part Character 4	Approach Character 5	Device Character 6	Qualifier Character 7
Ø Skin, Scalp 1 Skin, Face 2 Skin, Right Ear 3 Skin, Left Ear 4 Skin, Neck 5 Skin, Chest 6 Skin, Back 7 Skin, Abdomen 8 Skin, Buttock 9 Skin, Perineum A Skin, Genitalia B Skin, Right Upper Arm C Skin, Left Upper Arm D Skin, Right Lower Arm E Skin, Left Lower Arm F Skin, Right Hand G Skin, Left Hand H Skin, Right Upper Leg J Skin, Left Upper Leg K Skin, Right Lower Leg L Skin, Left Lower Leg M Skin, Right Foot N Skin, Left Foot	X External	7 Autologous Tissue Substitute K Nonautologous Tissue Substitute	3 Full Thickness 4 Partial Thickness

ØHR Continued on next page

Ø　Medical and Surgical
H　Skin and Breast
R　Replacement　　Putting in or on biological or synthetic material that physically takes the place and/or function of all or a portion of a body part

Body Part Character 4	Approach Character 5	Device Character 6	Qualifier Character 7
Ø Skin, Scalp **1** Skin, Face **2** Skin, Right Ear **3** Skin, Left Ear **4** Skin, Neck **5** Skin, Chest **6** Skin, Back **7** Skin, Abdomen **8** Skin, Buttock **9** Skin, Perineum **A** Skin, Genitalia **B** Skin, Right Upper Arm **C** Skin, Left Upper Arm **D** Skin, Right Lower Arm **E** Skin, Left Lower Arm **F** Skin, Right Hand **G** Skin, Left Hand **H** Skin, Right Upper Leg **J** Skin, Left Upper Leg **K** Skin, Right Lower Leg **L** Skin, Left Lower Leg **M** Skin, Right Foot **N** Skin, Left Foot	**X** External	**J** Synthetic Substitute	**3** Full Thickness **4** Partial Thickness **Z** No Qualifier
Q Finger Nail **R** Toe Nail **S** Hair	**X** External	**7** Autologous Tissue Substitute **J** Synthetic Substitute **K** Nonautologous Tissue Substitute	**Z** No Qualifier
T Breast, Right **U** Breast, Left **V** Breast, Bilateral	**Ø** Open	**7** Autologous Tissue Substitute	**5** Latissimus Dorsi Myocutaneous Flap **6** Transverse Rectus Abdominis Myocutaneous Flap **7** Deep Inferior Epigastric Artery Perforator Flap **8** Superficial Inferior Epigastric Artery Flap **9** Gluteal Artery Perforator Flap **Z** No Qualifier
T Breast, Right **U** Breast, Left **V** Breast, Bilateral	**Ø** Open	**J** Synthetic Substitute **K** Nonautologous Tissue Substitute	**Z** No Qualifier
T Breast, Right **U** Breast, Left **V** Breast, Bilateral	**3** Percutaneous **X** External	**7** Autologous Tissue Substitute **J** Synthetic Substitute **K** Nonautologous Tissue Substitute	**Z** No Qualifier
W Nipple, Right **X** Nipple, Left	**Ø** Open **3** Percutaneous **X** External	**7** Autologous Tissue Substitute **J** Synthetic Substitute **K** Nonautologous Tissue Substitute	**Z** No Qualifier

Ø　Medical and Surgical
H　Skin and Breast
S　Reposition　　Moving to its normal location or other suitable location all or a portion of a body part

Body Part Character 4	Approach Character 5	Device Character 6	Qualifier Character 7
S Hair **W** Nipple, Right **X** Nipple, Left	**X** External	**Z** No Device	**Z** No Qualifier
T Breast, Right **U** Breast, Left **V** Breast, Bilateral	**Ø** Open	**Z** No Device	**Z** No Qualifier

Skin and Breast

ØHT–ØHX

Ø   Medical and Surgical
H   Skin and Breast
T   Resection   Cutting out or off, without replacement, all of a body part

Body Part Character 4	Approach Character 5	Device Character 6	Qualifier Character 7
Q Finger Nail R Toe Nail W Nipple, Right X Nipple, Left	X External	Z No Device	Z No Qualifier
T Breast, Right U Breast, Left V Breast, Bilateral Y Supernumerary Breast	Ø Open	Z No Device	Z No Qualifier

Ø   Medical and Surgical
H   Skin and Breast
U   Supplement   Putting in or on biological or synthetic material that physically reinforces and/or augments the function of a portion of a body part

Body Part Character 4	Approach Character 5	Device Character 6	Qualifier Character 7
T Breast, Right U Breast, Left V Breast, Bilateral W Nipple, Right X Nipple, Left	Ø Open 3 Percutaneous 7 Via Natural or Artificial Opening 8 Via Natural or Artificial Opening Endoscopic X External	7 Autologous Tissue Substitute J Synthetic Substitute K Nonautologous Tissue Substitute	Z No Qualifier

Ø   Medical and Surgical
H   Skin and Breast
W   Revision   Correcting, to the extent possible, a portion of a malfunctioning device or the position of a displaced device

Body Part Character 4	Approach Character 5	Device Character 6	Qualifier Character 7
P Skin Q Finger Nail R Toe Nail T Breast, Right U Breast, Left	X External	Ø Drainage Device 7 Autologous Tissue Substitute J Synthetic Substitute K Nonautologous Tissue Substitute	Z No Qualifier
S Hair	X External	7 Autologous Tissue Substitute J Synthetic Substitute K Nonautologous Tissue Substitute	Z No Qualifier
T Breast, Right U Breast, Left	Ø Open 3 Percutaneous 7 Via Natural or Artificial Opening 8 Via Natural or Artificial Opening Endoscopic	Ø Drainage Device 7 Autologous Tissue Substitute J Synthetic Substitute K Nonautologous Tissue Substitute N Tissue Expander	Z No Qualifier

Ø   Medical and Surgical
H   Skin and Breast
X   Transfer   Moving, without taking out, all or a portion of a body part to another location to take over the function of all or a portion of a body part

Body Part Character 4	Approach Character 5	Device Character 6	Qualifier Character 7
Ø Skin, Scalp 1 Skin, Face 2 Skin, Right Ear 3 Skin, Left Ear 4 Skin, Neck 5 Skin, Chest 6 Skin, Back 7 Skin, Abdomen 8 Skin, Buttock 9 Skin, Perineum A Skin, Genitalia B Skin, Right Upper Arm C Skin, Left Upper Arm D Skin, Right Lower Arm E Skin, Left Lower Arm F Skin, Right Hand G Skin, Left Hand H Skin, Right Upper Leg J Skin, Left Upper Leg K Skin, Right Lower Leg L Skin, Left Lower Leg M Skin, Right Foot N Skin, Left Foot	X External	Z No Device	Z No Qualifier

Revised Text in **BLUE**   © 2011 Ingenix, Inc

Subcutaneous Tissue and Fascia ØJØ–ØJX

Ø   **Medical and Surgical**
J   **Subcutaneous Tissue and Fascia**
Ø   **Alteration**   Modifying the anatomic structure of a body part without affecting the function of the body part

Body Part Character 4	Approach Character 5	Device Character 6	Qualifier Character 7
1 Subcutaneous Tissue and Fascia, Face **4** Subcutaneous Tissue and Fascia, Anterior Neck **5** Subcutaneous Tissue and Fascia, Posterior Neck **6** Subcutaneous Tissue and Fascia, Chest **7** Subcutaneous Tissue and Fascia, Back **8** Subcutaneous Tissue and Fascia, Abdomen **9** Subcutaneous Tissue and Fascia, Buttock **D** Subcutaneous Tissue and Fascia, Right Upper Arm **F** Subcutaneous Tissue and Fascia, Left Upper Arm **G** Subcutaneous Tissue and Fascia, Right Lower Arm **H** Subcutaneous Tissue and Fascia, Left Lower Arm **L** Subcutaneous Tissue and Fascia, Right Upper Leg **M** Subcutaneous Tissue and Fascia, Left Upper Leg **N** Subcutaneous Tissue and Fascia, Right Lower Leg **P** Subcutaneous Tissue and Fascia, Left Lower Leg	**Ø** Open **3** Percutaneous	**Z** No Device	**Z** No Qualifier

Ø   **Medical and Surgical**
J   **Subcutaneous Tissue and Fascia**
2   **Change**   Taking out or off a device from a body part and putting back an identical or similar device in or on the same body part without cutting or puncturing the skin or a mucous membrane

Body Part Character 4	Approach Character 5	Device Character 6	Qualifier Character 7
S Subcutaneous Tissue and Fascia, Head and Neck **T** Subcutaneous Tissue and Fascia, Trunk **V** Subcutaneous Tissue and Fascia, Upper Extremity **W** Subcutaneous Tissue and Fascia, Lower Extremity	**X** External	**Ø** Drainage Device **Y** Other Device	**Z** No Qualifier

Ø   **Medical and Surgical**
J   **Subcutaneous Tissue and Fascia**
5   **Destruction**   Physical eradication of all or a portion of a body part by the direct use of energy, force, or a destructive agent

Body Part Character 4	Approach Character 5	Device Character 6	Qualifier Character 7
Ø Subcutaneous Tissue and Fascia, Scalp **1** Subcutaneous Tissue and Fascia, Face **4** Subcutaneous Tissue and Fascia, Anterior Neck **5** Subcutaneous Tissue and Fascia, Posterior Neck **6** Subcutaneous Tissue and Fascia, Chest **7** Subcutaneous Tissue and Fascia, Back **8** Subcutaneous Tissue and Fascia, Abdomen **9** Subcutaneous Tissue and Fascia, Buttock **B** Subcutaneous Tissue and Fascia, Perineum **C** Subcutaneous Tissue and Fascia, Pelvic Region **D** Subcutaneous Tissue and Fascia, Right Upper Arm **F** Subcutaneous Tissue and Fascia, Left Upper Arm **G** Subcutaneous Tissue and Fascia, Right Lower Arm **H** Subcutaneous Tissue and Fascia, Left Lower Arm **J** Subcutaneous Tissue and Fascia, Right Hand **K** Subcutaneous Tissue and Fascia, Left Hand **L** Subcutaneous Tissue and Fascia, Right Upper Leg **M** Subcutaneous Tissue and Fascia, Left Upper Leg **N** Subcutaneous Tissue and Fascia, Right Lower Leg **P** Subcutaneous Tissue and Fascia, Left Lower Leg **Q** Subcutaneous Tissue and Fascia, Right Foot **R** Subcutaneous Tissue and Fascia, Left Foot	**Ø** Open **3** Percutaneous	**Z** No Device	**Z** No Qualifier

0   **Medical and Surgical**
J   **Subcutaneous Tissue and Fascia**
8   **Division**   Cutting into a body part without draining fluids and/or gases from the body part in order to separate or transect a body part

Body Part Character 4	Approach Character 5	Device Character 6	Qualifier Character 7
0 Subcutaneous Tissue and Fascia, Scalp 1 Subcutaneous Tissue and Fascia, Face 4 Subcutaneous Tissue and Fascia, Anterior Neck 5 Subcutaneous Tissue and Fascia, Posterior Neck 6 Subcutaneous Tissue and Fascia, Chest 7 Subcutaneous Tissue and Fascia, Back 8 Subcutaneous Tissue and Fascia, Abdomen 9 Subcutaneous Tissue and Fascia, Buttock B Subcutaneous Tissue and Fascia, Perineum C Subcutaneous Tissue and Fascia, Pelvic Region D Subcutaneous Tissue and Fascia, Right Upper Arm F Subcutaneous Tissue and Fascia, Left Upper Arm G Subcutaneous Tissue and Fascia, Right Lower Arm H Subcutaneous Tissue and Fascia, Left Lower Arm J Subcutaneous Tissue and Fascia, Right Hand K Subcutaneous Tissue and Fascia, Left Hand L Subcutaneous Tissue and Fascia, Right Upper Leg M Subcutaneous Tissue and Fascia, Left Upper Leg N Subcutaneous Tissue and Fascia, Right Lower Leg P Subcutaneous Tissue and Fascia, Left Lower Leg Q Subcutaneous Tissue and Fascia, Right Foot R Subcutaneous Tissue and Fascia, Left Foot S Subcutaneous Tissue and Fascia, Head and Neck T Subcutaneous Tissue and Fascia, Trunk V Subcutaneous Tissue and Fascia, Upper Extremity W Subcutaneous Tissue and Fascia, Lower Extremity	0 Open 3 Percutaneous	Z No Device	Z No Qualifier

0   **Medical and Surgical**
J   **Subcutaneous Tissue and Fascia**
9   **Drainage**   Taking or letting out fluids and/or gases from a body part

Body Part Character 4	Approach Character 5	Device Character 6	Qualifier Character 7
0 Subcutaneous Tissue and Fascia, Scalp 1 Subcutaneous Tissue and Fascia, Face 4 Subcutaneous Tissue and Fascia, Anterior Neck 5 Subcutaneous Tissue and Fascia, Posterior Neck 6 Subcutaneous Tissue and Fascia, Chest 7 Subcutaneous Tissue and Fascia, Back 8 Subcutaneous Tissue and Fascia, Abdomen 9 Subcutaneous Tissue and Fascia, Buttock B Subcutaneous Tissue and Fascia, Perineum C Subcutaneous Tissue and Fascia, Pelvic Region D Subcutaneous Tissue and Fascia, Right Upper Arm F Subcutaneous Tissue and Fascia, Left Upper Arm G Subcutaneous Tissue and Fascia, Right Lower Arm H Subcutaneous Tissue and Fascia, Left Lower Arm J Subcutaneous Tissue and Fascia, Right Hand K Subcutaneous Tissue and Fascia, Left Hand L Subcutaneous Tissue and Fascia, Right Upper Leg M Subcutaneous Tissue and Fascia, Left Upper Leg N Subcutaneous Tissue and Fascia, Right Lower Leg P Subcutaneous Tissue and Fascia, Left Lower Leg Q Subcutaneous Tissue and Fascia, Right Foot R Subcutaneous Tissue and Fascia, Left Foot	0 Open 3 Percutaneous	0 Drainage Device	Z No Qualifier

0J9 Continued on next page

    Revised Text in **BLUE**

ICD-10-PCS (2011 Draft)

Ø Medical and Surgical　　　　　　　　　　　　　　　　　　　　　　　*ØJ9 Continued*
J Subcutaneous Tissue and Fascia
9 Drainage　　　Taking or letting out fluids and/or gases from a body part

Body Part Character 4	Approach Character 5	Device Character 6	Qualifier Character 7
Ø Subcutaneous Tissue and Fascia, Scalp 1 Subcutaneous Tissue and Fascia, Face 4 Subcutaneous Tissue and Fascia, Anterior Neck 5 Subcutaneous Tissue and Fascia, Posterior Neck 6 Subcutaneous Tissue and Fascia, Chest 7 Subcutaneous Tissue and Fascia, Back 8 Subcutaneous Tissue and Fascia, Abdomen 9 Subcutaneous Tissue and Fascia, Buttock B Subcutaneous Tissue and Fascia, Perineum C Subcutaneous Tissue and Fascia, Pelvic Region D Subcutaneous Tissue and Fascia, Right Upper Arm F Subcutaneous Tissue and Fascia, Left Upper Arm G Subcutaneous Tissue and Fascia, Right Lower Arm H Subcutaneous Tissue and Fascia, Left Lower Arm J Subcutaneous Tissue and Fascia, Right Hand K Subcutaneous Tissue and Fascia, Left Hand L Subcutaneous Tissue and Fascia, Right Upper Leg M Subcutaneous Tissue and Fascia, Left Upper Leg N Subcutaneous Tissue and Fascia, Right Lower Leg P Subcutaneous Tissue and Fascia, Left Lower Leg Q Subcutaneous Tissue and Fascia, Right Foot R Subcutaneous Tissue and Fascia, Left Foot	Ø Open 3 Percutaneous	Z No Device	X Diagnostic Z No Qualifier

Ø Medical and Surgical
J Subcutaneous Tissue and Fascia
B Excision　　　Cutting out or off, without replacement, a portion of a body part

Body Part Character 4	Approach Character 5	Device Character 6	Qualifier Character 7
Ø Subcutaneous Tissue and Fascia, Scalp 1 Subcutaneous Tissue and Fascia, Face 4 Subcutaneous Tissue and Fascia, Anterior Neck 5 Subcutaneous Tissue and Fascia, Posterior Neck 6 Subcutaneous Tissue and Fascia, Chest 7 Subcutaneous Tissue and Fascia, Back 8 Subcutaneous Tissue and Fascia, Abdomen 9 Subcutaneous Tissue and Fascia, Buttock B Subcutaneous Tissue and Fascia, Perineum C Subcutaneous Tissue and Fascia, Pelvic Region D Subcutaneous Tissue and Fascia, Right Upper Arm F Subcutaneous Tissue and Fascia, Left Upper Arm G Subcutaneous Tissue and Fascia, Right Lower Arm H Subcutaneous Tissue and Fascia, Left Lower Arm J Subcutaneous Tissue and Fascia, Right Hand K Subcutaneous Tissue and Fascia, Left Hand L Subcutaneous Tissue and Fascia, Right Upper Leg M Subcutaneous Tissue and Fascia, Left Upper Leg N Subcutaneous Tissue and Fascia, Right Lower Leg P Subcutaneous Tissue and Fascia, Left Lower Leg Q Subcutaneous Tissue and Fascia, Right Foot R Subcutaneous Tissue and Fascia, Left Foot	Ø Open 3 Percutaneous	Z No Device	X Diagnostic Z No Qualifier

Ø   **Medical and Surgical**
J   **Subcutaneous Tissue and Fascia**
C   **Extirpation**   Taking or cutting out solid matter from a body part

Body Part Character 4	Approach Character 5	Device Character 6	Qualifier Character 7
Ø Subcutaneous Tissue and Fascia, Scalp **1** Subcutaneous Tissue and Fascia, Face **4** Subcutaneous Tissue and Fascia, Anterior Neck **5** Subcutaneous Tissue and Fascia, Posterior Neck **6** Subcutaneous Tissue and Fascia, Chest **7** Subcutaneous Tissue and Fascia, Back **8** Subcutaneous Tissue and Fascia, Abdomen **9** Subcutaneous Tissue and Fascia, Buttock **B** Subcutaneous Tissue and Fascia, Perineum **C** Subcutaneous Tissue and Fascia, Pelvic Region **D** Subcutaneous Tissue and Fascia, Right Upper Arm **F** Subcutaneous Tissue and Fascia, Left Upper Arm **G** Subcutaneous Tissue and Fascia, Right Lower Arm **H** Subcutaneous Tissue and Fascia, Left Lower Arm **J** Subcutaneous Tissue and Fascia, Right Hand **K** Subcutaneous Tissue and Fascia, Left Hand **L** Subcutaneous Tissue and Fascia, Right Upper Leg **M** Subcutaneous Tissue and Fascia, Left Upper Leg **N** Subcutaneous Tissue and Fascia, Right Lower Leg **P** Subcutaneous Tissue and Fascia, Left Lower Leg **Q** Subcutaneous Tissue and Fascia, Right Foot **R** Subcutaneous Tissue and Fascia, Left Foot	**Ø** Open **3** Percutaneous	**Z** No Device	**Z** No Qualifier

Ø   **Medical and Surgical**
J   **Subcutaneous Tissue and Fascia**
D   **Extraction**   Pulling or stripping out or off all or a portion of a body part by the use of force

Body Part Character 4	Approach Character 5	Device Character 6	Qualifier Character 7
Ø Subcutaneous Tissue and Fascia, Scalp **1** Subcutaneous Tissue and Fascia, Face **4** Subcutaneous Tissue and Fascia, Anterior Neck **5** Subcutaneous Tissue and Fascia, Posterior Neck **6** Subcutaneous Tissue and Fascia, Chest **7** Subcutaneous Tissue and Fascia, Back **8** Subcutaneous Tissue and Fascia, Abdomen **9** Subcutaneous Tissue and Fascia, Buttock **B** Subcutaneous Tissue and Fascia, Perineum **C** Subcutaneous Tissue and Fascia, Pelvic Region **D** Subcutaneous Tissue and Fascia, Right Upper Arm **F** Subcutaneous Tissue and Fascia, Left Upper Arm **G** Subcutaneous Tissue and Fascia, Right Lower Arm **H** Subcutaneous Tissue and Fascia, Left Lower Arm **J** Subcutaneous Tissue and Fascia, Right Hand **K** Subcutaneous Tissue and Fascia, Left Hand **L** Subcutaneous Tissue and Fascia, Right Upper Leg **M** Subcutaneous Tissue and Fascia, Left Upper Leg **N** Subcutaneous Tissue and Fascia, Right Lower Leg **P** Subcutaneous Tissue and Fascia, Left Lower Leg **Q** Subcutaneous Tissue and Fascia, Right Foot **R** Subcutaneous Tissue and Fascia, Left Foot	**Ø** Open **3** Percutaneous	**Z** No Device	**Z** No Qualifier

Ø **Medical and Surgical**
J **Subcutaneous Tissue and Fascia**
H **Insertion**   Putting in a nonbiological appliance that monitors, assists, performs, or prevents a physiological function but does not physically take the place of a body part

Body Part Character 4	Approach Character 5	Device Character 6	Qualifier Character 7
Ø Subcutaneous Tissue and Fascia, Scalp 1 Subcutaneous Tissue and Fascia, Face 4 Subcutaneous Tissue and Fascia, Anterior Neck 5 Subcutaneous Tissue and Fascia, Posterior Neck 9 Subcutaneous Tissue and Fascia, Buttock B Subcutaneous Tissue and Fascia, Perineum C Subcutaneous Tissue and Fascia, Pelvic Region J Subcutaneous Tissue and Fascia, Right Hand K Subcutaneous Tissue and Fascia, Left Hand Q Subcutaneous Tissue and Fascia, Right Foot R Subcutaneous Tissue and Fascia, Left Foot	Ø Open 3 Percutaneous	N Tissue Expander	Z No Qualifier
6 Subcutaneous Tissue and Fascia, Chest 7 Subcutaneous Tissue and Fascia, Back 8 Subcutaneous Tissue and Fascia, Abdomen	Ø Open 3 Percutaneous	M Stimulator Generator	6 Single Array 7 Dual Array 8 Single Array Rechargeable 9 Dual Array Rechargeable Z No Qualifier
6 Subcutaneous Tissue and Fascia, Chest 8 Subcutaneous Tissue and Fascia, Abdomen	Ø Open 3 Percutaneous	2 Monitoring Device	D Hemodynamic Z No Qualifier
6 Subcutaneous Tissue and Fascia, Chest 8 Subcutaneous Tissue and Fascia, Abdomen	Ø Open 3 Percutaneous	P Cardiac Rhythm Related Device	Ø Pacemaker, Single Chamber 1 Pacemaker, Single Chamber Rate Responsive 2 Pacemaker, Dual Chamber 3 Cardiac Resynchronization Pacemaker Pulse Generator 4 Defibrillator Generator 5 Cardiac Resynchronization Defibrillator Pulse Generator A Contractility Modulation Device Y Other Cardiac Rhythm Related Device Z No Qualifier
6 Subcutaneous Tissue and Fascia, Chest 8 Subcutaneous Tissue and Fascia, Abdomen D Subcutaneous Tissue and Fascia, Right Upper Arm F Subcutaneous Tissue and Fascia, Left Upper Arm G Subcutaneous Tissue and Fascia, Right Lower Arm H Subcutaneous Tissue and Fascia, Left Lower Arm L Subcutaneous Tissue and Fascia, Right Upper Leg M Subcutaneous Tissue and Fascia, Left Upper Leg N Subcutaneous Tissue and Fascia, Right Lower Leg P Subcutaneous Tissue and Fascia, Left Lower Leg	Ø Open 3 Percutaneous	H Contraceptive Device N Tissue Expander V Infusion Pump W Reservoir X Vascular Access Device	Z No Qualifier
7 Subcutaneous Tissue and Fascia, Back	Ø Open 3 Percutaneous	N Tissue Expander V Infusion Pump	Z No Qualifier
S Subcutaneous Tissue and Fascia, Head and Neck V Subcutaneous Tissue and Fascia, Upper Extremity W Subcutaneous Tissue and Fascia, Lower Extremity	Ø Open 3 Percutaneous	1 Radioactive Element 3 Infusion Device	Z No Qualifier
T Subcutaneous Tissue and Fascia, Trunk	Ø Open 3 Percutaneous	1 Radioactive Element 3 Infusion Device V Infusion Pump	Z No Qualifier

Ø **Medical and Surgical**
J **Subcutaneous Tissue and Fascia**
J **Inspection**   Visually and/or manually exploring a body part

Body Part Character 4	Approach Character 5	Device Character 6	Qualifier Character 7
S Subcutaneous Tissue and Fascia, Head and Neck T Subcutaneous Tissue and Fascia, Trunk V Subcutaneous Tissue and Fascia, Upper Extremity W Subcutaneous Tissue and Fascia, Lower Extremity	Ø Open 3 Percutaneous X External	Z No Device	Z No Qualifier

Ø   **Medical and Surgical**
J   **Subcutaneous Tissue and Fascia**
N   **Release**   Freeing a body part from an abnormal physical constraint

Body Part Character 4	Approach Character 5	Device Character 6	Qualifier Character 7
Ø Subcutaneous Tissue and Fascia, Scalp **1** Subcutaneous Tissue and Fascia, Face **4** Subcutaneous Tissue and Fascia, Anterior Neck **5** Subcutaneous Tissue and Fascia, Posterior Neck **6** Subcutaneous Tissue and Fascia, Chest **7** Subcutaneous Tissue and Fascia, Back **8** Subcutaneous Tissue and Fascia, Abdomen **9** Subcutaneous Tissue and Fascia, Buttock **B** Subcutaneous Tissue and Fascia, Perineum **C** Subcutaneous Tissue and Fascia, Pelvic Region **D** Subcutaneous Tissue and Fascia, Right Upper Arm **F** Subcutaneous Tissue and Fascia, Left Upper Arm **G** Subcutaneous Tissue and Fascia, Right Lower Arm **H** Subcutaneous Tissue and Fascia, Left Lower Arm **J** Subcutaneous Tissue and Fascia, Right Hand **K** Subcutaneous Tissue and Fascia, Left Hand **L** Subcutaneous Tissue and Fascia, Right Upper Leg **M** Subcutaneous Tissue and Fascia, Left Upper Leg **N** Subcutaneous Tissue and Fascia, Right Lower Leg **P** Subcutaneous Tissue and Fascia, Left Lower Leg **Q** Subcutaneous Tissue and Fascia, Right Foot **R** Subcutaneous Tissue and Fascia, Left Foot	**Ø** Open **3** Percutaneous **X** External	**Z** No Device	**Z** No Qualifier

Ø   **Medical and Surgical**
J   **Subcutaneous Tissue and Fascia**
P   **Removal**   Taking out or off a device from a body part

Body Part Character 4	Approach Character 5	Device Character 6	Qualifier Character 7
S Subcutaneous Tissue and Fascia, Head and Neck	**Ø** Open **3** Percutaneous	**Ø** Drainage Device **1** Radioactive Element **3** Infusion Device **7** Autologous Tissue Substitute **J** Synthetic Substitute **K** Nonautologous Tissue Substitute **N** Tissue Expander	**Z** No Qualifier
S Subcutaneous Tissue and Fascia, Head and Neck	**X** External	**Ø** Drainage Device **1** Radioactive Element **3** Infusion Device	**Z** No Qualifier
T Subcutaneous Tissue and Fascia, Trunk	**Ø** Open **3** Percutaneous	**Ø** Drainage Device **1** Radioactive Element **2** Monitoring Device **3** Infusion Device **7** Autologous Tissue Substitute **H** Contraceptive Device **J** Synthetic Substitute **K** Nonautologous Tissue Substitute **M** Stimulator Generator **N** Tissue Expander **P** Cardiac Rhythm Related Device **V** Infusion Pump **W** Reservoir **X** Vascular Access Device	**Z** No Qualifier
T Subcutaneous Tissue and Fascia, Trunk	**X** External	**Ø** Drainage Device **1** Radioactive Element **2** Monitoring Device **3** Infusion Device **H** Contraceptive Device **V** Infusion Pump **X** Vascular Access Device	**Z** No Qualifier

ØJP Continued on next page

     Revised Text in **BLUE**

Ø   **Medical and Surgical**   *ØJP Continued*
J   **Subcutaneous Tissue and Fascia**
P   **Removal**   Taking out or off a device from a body part

Body Part Character 4	Approach Character 5	Device Character 6	Qualifier Character 7
V Subcutaneous Tissue and Fascia, Upper Extremity **W** Subcutaneous Tissue and Fascia, Lower Extremity	**Ø** Open **3** Percutaneous	**Ø** Drainage Device **1** Radioactive Element **3** Infusion Device **7** Autologous Tissue Substitute **H** Contraceptive Device **J** Synthetic Substitute **K** Nonautologous Tissue Substitute **N** Tissue Expander **V** Infusion Pump **W** Reservoir **X** Vascular Access Device	**Z** No Qualifier
V Subcutaneous Tissue and Fascia, Upper Extremity **W** Subcutaneous Tissue and Fascia, Lower Extremity	**X** External	**Ø** Drainage Device **1** Radioactive Element **3** Infusion Device **H** Contraceptive Device **V** Infusion Pump **X** Vascular Access Device	**Z** No Qualifier

Ø   **Medical and Surgical**
J   **Subcutaneous Tissue and Fascia**
Q   **Repair**   Restoring, to the extent possible, a body part to its normal anatomic structure and function

Body Part Character 4	Approach Character 5	Device Character 6	Qualifier Character 7
Ø Subcutaneous Tissue and Fascia, Scalp **1** Subcutaneous Tissue and Fascia, Face **4** Subcutaneous Tissue and Fascia, Anterior Neck **5** Subcutaneous Tissue and Fascia, Posterior Neck **6** Subcutaneous Tissue and Fascia, Chest **7** Subcutaneous Tissue and Fascia, Back **8** Subcutaneous Tissue and Fascia, Abdomen **9** Subcutaneous Tissue and Fascia, Buttock **B** Subcutaneous Tissue and Fascia, Perineum **C** Subcutaneous Tissue and Fascia, Pelvic Region **D** Subcutaneous Tissue and Fascia, Right Upper Arm **F** Subcutaneous Tissue and Fascia, Left Upper Arm **G** Subcutaneous Tissue and Fascia, Right Lower Arm **H** Subcutaneous Tissue and Fascia, Left Lower Arm **J** Subcutaneous Tissue and Fascia, Right Hand **K** Subcutaneous Tissue and Fascia, Left Hand **L** Subcutaneous Tissue and Fascia, Right Upper Leg **M** Subcutaneous Tissue and Fascia, Left Upper Leg **N** Subcutaneous Tissue and Fascia, Right Lower Leg **P** Subcutaneous Tissue and Fascia, Left Lower Leg **Q** Subcutaneous Tissue and Fascia, Right Foot **R** Subcutaneous Tissue and Fascia, Left Foot	**Ø** Open **3** Percutaneous	**Z** No Device	**Z** No Qualifier

Ø   **Medical and Surgical**
J   **Subcutaneous Tissue and Fascia**
R   **Replacement**   Putting in or on biological or synthetic material that physically takes the place and/or function of all or a portion of a body part

Body Part Character 4	Approach Character 5	Device Character 6	Qualifier Character 7
Ø Subcutaneous Tissue and Fascia, Scalp **1** Subcutaneous Tissue and Fascia, Face **4** Subcutaneous Tissue and Fascia, Anterior Neck **5** Subcutaneous Tissue and Fascia, Posterior Neck **6** Subcutaneous Tissue and Fascia, Chest **7** Subcutaneous Tissue and Fascia, Back **8** Subcutaneous Tissue and Fascia, Abdomen **9** Subcutaneous Tissue and Fascia, Buttock **B** Subcutaneous Tissue and Fascia, Perineum **C** Subcutaneous Tissue and Fascia, Pelvic Region **D** Subcutaneous Tissue and Fascia, Right Upper Arm **F** Subcutaneous Tissue and Fascia, Left Upper Arm **G** Subcutaneous Tissue and Fascia, Right Lower Arm **H** Subcutaneous Tissue and Fascia, Left Lower Arm **J** Subcutaneous Tissue and Fascia, Right Hand **K** Subcutaneous Tissue and Fascia, Left Hand **L** Subcutaneous Tissue and Fascia, Right Upper Leg **M** Subcutaneous Tissue and Fascia, Left Upper Leg **N** Subcutaneous Tissue and Fascia, Right Lower Leg **P** Subcutaneous Tissue and Fascia, Left Lower Leg **Q** Subcutaneous Tissue and Fascia, Right Foot **R** Subcutaneous Tissue and Fascia, Left Foot	**Ø** Open **3** Percutaneous	**7** Autologous Tissue Substitute **J** Synthetic Substitute **K** Nonautologous Tissue Substitute	**Z** No Qualifier

Ø Medical and Surgical
J Subcutaneous Tissue and Fascia
U Supplement: Putting in or on biological or synthetic material that physically reinforces and/or augments the function of a portion of a body part

Body Part Character 4	Approach Character 5	Device Character 6	Qualifier Character 7
Ø Subcutaneous Tissue and Fascia, Scalp **1** Subcutaneous Tissue and Fascia, Face **4** Subcutaneous Tissue and Fascia, Anterior Neck **5** Subcutaneous Tissue and Fascia, Posterior Neck **6** Subcutaneous Tissue and Fascia, Chest **7** Subcutaneous Tissue and Fascia, Back **8** Subcutaneous Tissue and Fascia, Abdomen **9** Subcutaneous Tissue and Fascia, Buttock **B** Subcutaneous Tissue and Fascia, Perineum **C** Subcutaneous Tissue and Fascia, Pelvic Region **D** Subcutaneous Tissue and Fascia, Right Upper Arm **F** Subcutaneous Tissue and Fascia, Left Upper Arm **G** Subcutaneous Tissue and Fascia, Right Lower Arm **H** Subcutaneous Tissue and Fascia, Left Lower Arm **J** Subcutaneous Tissue and Fascia, Right Hand **K** Subcutaneous Tissue and Fascia, Left Hand **L** Subcutaneous Tissue and Fascia, Right Upper Leg **M** Subcutaneous Tissue and Fascia, Left Upper Leg **N** Subcutaneous Tissue and Fascia, Right Lower Leg **P** Subcutaneous Tissue and Fascia, Left Lower Leg **Q** Subcutaneous Tissue and Fascia, Right Foot **R** Subcutaneous Tissue and Fascia, Left Foot	**Ø** Open **3** Percutaneous	**7** Autologous Tissue Substitute **J** Synthetic Substitute **K** Nonautologous Tissue Substitute	**Z** No Qualifier

Subcutaneous Tissue and Fascia

ØJW–ØJX

Ø   Medical and Surgical
J   Subcutaneous Tissue and Fascia
W   Revision   Correcting, to the extent possible, a portion of a malfunctioning device or the position of a displaced device

Body Part Character 4	Approach Character 5	Device Character 6	Qualifier Character 7
S Subcutaneous Tissue and Fascia, Head and Neck	Ø Open 3 Percutaneous X External	Ø Drainage Device 3 Infusion Device 7 Autologous Tissue Substitute J Synthetic Substitute K Nonautologous Tissue Substitute N Tissue Expander	Z No Qualifier
T Subcutaneous Tissue and Fascia, Trunk	Ø Open 3 Percutaneous X External	Ø Drainage Device 2 Monitoring Device 3 Infusion Device 7 Autologous Tissue Substitute H Contraceptive Device J Synthetic Substitute K Nonautologous Tissue Substitute M Stimulator Generator N Tissue Expander P Cardiac Rhythm Related Device V Infusion Pump W Reservoir X Vascular Access Device	Z No Qualifier

V Subcutaneous Tissue and Fascia, Upper
   Extremity
W Subcutaneous Tissue and Fascia, Lower
    Extremity
	Ø Open
	3 Percutaneous
	X External
		Ø Drainage Device
		3 Infusion Device
		7 Autologous Tissue Substitute
		H Contraceptive Device
		J Synthetic Substitute
		K Nonautologous Tissue
		   Substitute
		N Tissue Expander
		V Infusion Pump
		W Reservoir
		X Vascular Access Device
			Z No Qualifier

Ø   Medical and Surgical
J   Subcutaneous Tissue and Fascia
X   Transfer   Moving, without taking out, all or a portion of a body part to another location to take over the function of all or a portion of a body part

Body Part Character 4	Approach Character 5	Device Character 6	Qualifier Character 7

Ø Subcutaneous Tissue and Fascia, Scalp
1 Subcutaneous Tissue and Fascia, Face
4 Subcutaneous Tissue and Fascia, Anterior Neck
5 Subcutaneous Tissue and Fascia, Posterior Neck
6 Subcutaneous Tissue and Fascia, Chest
7 Subcutaneous Tissue and Fascia, Back
8 Subcutaneous Tissue and Fascia, Abdomen
9 Subcutaneous Tissue and Fascia, Buttock
B Subcutaneous Tissue and Fascia, Perineum
C Subcutaneous Tissue and Fascia, Pelvic Region
D Subcutaneous Tissue and Fascia, Right Upper
   Arm
F Subcutaneous Tissue and Fascia, Left Upper
   Arm
G Subcutaneous Tissue and Fascia, Right Lower
   Arm
H Subcutaneous Tissue and Fascia, Left Lower
   Arm
J Subcutaneous Tissue and Fascia, Right Hand
K Subcutaneous Tissue and Fascia, Left Hand
L Subcutaneous Tissue and Fascia, Right Upper
   Leg
M Subcutaneous Tissue and Fascia, Left Upper Leg
N Subcutaneous Tissue and Fascia, Right Lower
   Leg
P Subcutaneous Tissue and Fascia, Left Lower Leg
Q Subcutaneous Tissue and Fascia, Right Foot
R Subcutaneous Tissue and Fascia, Left Foot
	Ø Open
	3 Percutaneous
		Z No Device	B Skin and Subcutaneous Tissue
			C Skin, Subcutaneous Tissue and
			   Fascia
			Z No Qualifier

            Revised Text in **BLUE**

Muscles 0K2–0KX

0 Medical and Surgical
K Muscles
2 Change   Taking out or off a device from a body part and putting back an identical or similar device in or on the same body part without cutting or puncturing the skin or a mucous membrane

Body Part Character 4	Approach Character 5	Device Character 6	Qualifier Character 7
X Upper Muscle **Y** Lower Muscle	**X** External	**0** Drainage Device **Y** Other Device	**Z** No Qualifier

0 Medical and Surgical
K Muscles
5 Destruction   Physical eradication of all or a portion of a body part by the direct use of energy, force, or a destructive agent

Body Part Character 4	Approach Character 5	Device Character 6	Qualifier Character 7
0 Head Muscle **1** Facial Muscle **2** Neck Muscle, Right **3** Neck Muscle, Left **4** Tongue, Palate, Pharynx Muscle **5** Shoulder Muscle, Right **6** Shoulder Muscle, Left **7** Upper Arm Muscle, Right **8** Upper Arm Muscle, Left **9** Lower Arm and Wrist Muscle, Right **B** Lower Arm and Wrist Muscle, Left **C** Hand Muscle, Right **D** Hand Muscle, Left **F** Trunk Muscle, Right **G** Trunk Muscle, Left **H** Thorax Muscle, Right **J** Thorax Muscle, Left **K** Abdomen Muscle, Right **L** Abdomen Muscle, Left **M** Perineum Muscle **N** Hip Muscle, Right **P** Hip Muscle, Left **Q** Upper Leg Muscle, Right **R** Upper Leg Muscle, Left **S** Lower Leg Muscle, Right **T** Lower Leg Muscle, Left **V** Foot Muscle, Right **W** Foot Muscle, Left	**0** Open **3** Percutaneous **4** Percutaneous Endoscopic	**Z** No Device	**Z** No Qualifier

Ø Medical and Surgical
K Muscles
8 Division   Cutting into a body part without draining fluids and/or gases from the body part in order to separate or transect a body part

Body Part Character 4	Approach Character 5	Device Character 6	Qualifier Character 7
Ø Head Muscle 1 Facial Muscle 2 Neck Muscle, Right 3 Neck Muscle, Left 4 Tongue, Palate, Pharynx Muscle 5 Shoulder Muscle, Right 6 Shoulder Muscle, Left 7 Upper Arm Muscle, Right 8 Upper Arm Muscle, Left 9 Lower Arm and Wrist Muscle, Right B Lower Arm and Wrist Muscle, Left C Hand Muscle, Right D Hand Muscle, Left F Trunk Muscle, Right G Trunk Muscle, Left H Thorax Muscle, Right J Thorax Muscle, Left K Abdomen Muscle, Right L Abdomen Muscle, Left M Perineum Muscle N Hip Muscle, Right P Hip Muscle, Left Q Upper Leg Muscle, Right R Upper Leg Muscle, Left S Lower Leg Muscle, Right T Lower Leg Muscle, Left V Foot Muscle, Right W Foot Muscle, Left	Ø Open 3 Percutaneous 4 Percutaneous Endoscopic	Z No Device	Z No Qualifier

Ø Medical and Surgical
K Muscles
9 Drainage   Taking or letting out fluids and/or gases from a body part

Body Part Character 4	Approach Character 5	Device Character 6	Qualifier Character 7
Ø Head Muscle 1 Facial Muscle 2 Neck Muscle, Right 3 Neck Muscle, Left 4 Tongue, Palate, Pharynx Muscle 5 Shoulder Muscle, Right 6 Shoulder Muscle, Left 7 Upper Arm Muscle, Right 8 Upper Arm Muscle, Left 9 Lower Arm and Wrist Muscle, Right B Lower Arm and Wrist Muscle, Left C Hand Muscle, Right D Hand Muscle, Left F Trunk Muscle, Right G Trunk Muscle, Left H Thorax Muscle, Right J Thorax Muscle, Left K Abdomen Muscle, Right L Abdomen Muscle, Left M Perineum Muscle N Hip Muscle, Right P Hip Muscle, Left Q Upper Leg Muscle, Right R Upper Leg Muscle, Left S Lower Leg Muscle, Right T Lower Leg Muscle, Left V Foot Muscle, Right W Foot Muscle, Left	Ø Open 3 Percutaneous 4 Percutaneous Endoscopic	Ø Drainage Device	Z No Qualifier

ØK9 Continued on next page

0   **Medical and Surgical**   *0K9 Continued*
K   **Muscles**
9   **Drainage**   Taking or letting out fluids and/or gases from a body part

Body Part Character 4	Approach Character 5	Device Character 6	Qualifier Character 7
0 Head Muscle **1** Facial Muscle **2** Neck Muscle, Right **3** Neck Muscle, Left **4** Tongue, Palate, Pharynx Muscle **5** Shoulder Muscle, Right **6** Shoulder Muscle, Left **7** Upper Arm Muscle, Right **8** Upper Arm Muscle, Left **9** Lower Arm and Wrist Muscle, Right **B** Lower Arm and Wrist Muscle, Left **C** Hand Muscle, Right **D** Hand Muscle, Left **F** Trunk Muscle, Right **G** Trunk Muscle, Left **H** Thorax Muscle, Right **J** Thorax Muscle, Left **K** Abdomen Muscle, Right **L** Abdomen Muscle, Left **M** Perineum Muscle **N** Hip Muscle, Right **P** Hip Muscle, Left **Q** Upper Leg Muscle, Right **R** Upper Leg Muscle, Left **S** Lower Leg Muscle, Right **T** Lower Leg Muscle, Left **V** Foot Muscle, Right **W** Foot Muscle, Left	**0** Open **3** Percutaneous **4** Percutaneous Endoscopic	**Z** No Device	**X** Diagnostic **Z** No Qualifier

0   **Medical and Surgical**
K   **Muscles**
B   **Excision**   Cutting out or off, without replacement, a portion of a body part

Body Part Character 4	Approach Character 5	Device Character 6	Qualifier Character 7
0 Head Muscle **1** Facial Muscle **2** Neck Muscle, Right **3** Neck Muscle, Left **4** Tongue, Palate, Pharynx Muscle **5** Shoulder Muscle, Right **6** Shoulder Muscle, Left **7** Upper Arm Muscle, Right **8** Upper Arm Muscle, Left **9** Lower Arm and Wrist Muscle, Right **B** Lower Arm and Wrist Muscle, Left **C** Hand Muscle, Right **D** Hand Muscle, Left **F** Trunk Muscle, Right **G** Trunk Muscle, Left **H** Thorax Muscle, Right **J** Thorax Muscle, Left **K** Abdomen Muscle, Right **L** Abdomen Muscle, Left **M** Perineum Muscle **N** Hip Muscle, Right **P** Hip Muscle, Left **Q** Upper Leg Muscle, Right **R** Upper Leg Muscle, Left **S** Lower Leg Muscle, Right **T** Lower Leg Muscle, Left **V** Foot Muscle, Right **W** Foot Muscle, Left	**0** Open **3** Percutaneous **4** Percutaneous Endoscopic	**Z** No Device	**X** Diagnostic **Z** No Qualifier

Ø Medical and Surgical
K Muscles
C Extirpation   Taking or cutting out solid matter from a body part

Body Part Character 4	Approach Character 5	Device Character 6	Qualifier Character 7
Ø Head Muscle **1** Facial Muscle **2** Neck Muscle, Right **3** Neck Muscle, Left **4** Tongue, Palate, Pharynx Muscle **5** Shoulder Muscle, Right **6** Shoulder Muscle, Left **7** Upper Arm Muscle, Right **8** Upper Arm Muscle, Left **9** Lower Arm and Wrist Muscle, Right **B** Lower Arm and Wrist Muscle, Left **C** Hand Muscle, Right **D** Hand Muscle, Left **F** Trunk Muscle, Right **G** Trunk Muscle, Left **H** Thorax Muscle, Right **J** Thorax Muscle, Left **K** Abdomen Muscle, Right **L** Abdomen Muscle, Left **M** Perineum Muscle **N** Hip Muscle, Right **P** Hip Muscle, Left **Q** Upper Leg Muscle, Right **R** Upper Leg Muscle, Left **S** Lower Leg Muscle, Right **T** Lower Leg Muscle, Left **V** Foot Muscle, Right **W** Foot Muscle, Left	**Ø** Open **3** Percutaneous **4** Percutaneous Endoscopic	**Z** No Device	**Z** No Qualifier

Ø Medical and Surgical
K Muscles
H Insertion   Putting in a nonbiological appliance that monitors, assists, performs, or prevents a physiological function but does not physically take the place of a body part

Body Part Character 4	Approach Character 5	Device Character 6	Qualifier Character 7
X Upper Muscle **Y** Lower Muscle	**Ø** Open **3** Percutaneous **4** Percutaneous Endoscopic	**M** Stimulator Lead	**Z** No Qualifier

Ø Medical and Surgical
K Muscles
J Inspection   Visually and/or manually exploring a body part

Body Part Character 4	Approach Character 5	Device Character 6	Qualifier Character 7
X Upper Muscle **Y** Lower Muscle	**Ø** Open **3** Percutaneous **4** Percutaneous Endoscopic **X** External	**Z** No Device	**Z** No Qualifier

Revised Text in **BLUE**   © 2011 Ingenix, Inc

Ø Medical and Surgical
K Muscles
M Reattachment   Putting back in or on all or a portion of a separated body part to its normal location or other suitable location

Body Part Character 4	Approach Character 5	Device Character 6	Qualifier Character 7
Ø Head Muscle **1** Facial Muscle **2** Neck Muscle, Right **3** Neck Muscle, Left **4** Tongue, Palate, Pharynx Muscle **5** Shoulder Muscle, Right **6** Shoulder Muscle, Left **7** Upper Arm Muscle, Right **8** Upper Arm Muscle, Left **9** Lower Arm and Wrist Muscle, Right **B** Lower Arm and Wrist Muscle, Left **C** Hand Muscle, Right **D** Hand Muscle, Left **F** Trunk Muscle, Right **G** Trunk Muscle, Left **H** Thorax Muscle, Right **J** Thorax Muscle, Left **K** Abdomen Muscle, Right **L** Abdomen Muscle, Left **M** Perineum Muscle **N** Hip Muscle, Right **P** Hip Muscle, Left **Q** Upper Leg Muscle, Right **R** Upper Leg Muscle, Left **S** Lower Leg Muscle, Right **T** Lower Leg Muscle, Left **V** Foot Muscle, Right **W** Foot Muscle, Left	**Ø** Open **4** Percutaneous Endoscopic	**Z** No Device	**Z** No Qualifier

Ø Medical and Surgical
K Muscles
N Release   Freeing a body part from an abnormal physical constraint

Body Part Character 4	Approach Character 5	Device Character 6	Qualifier Character 7
Ø Head Muscle **1** Facial Muscle **2** Neck Muscle, Right **3** Neck Muscle, Left **4** Tongue, Palate, Pharynx Muscle **5** Shoulder Muscle, Right **6** Shoulder Muscle, Left **7** Upper Arm Muscle, Right **8** Upper Arm Muscle, Left **9** Lower Arm and Wrist Muscle, Right **B** Lower Arm and Wrist Muscle, Left **C** Hand Muscle, Right **D** Hand Muscle, Left **F** Trunk Muscle, Right **G** Trunk Muscle, Left **H** Thorax Muscle, Right **J** Thorax Muscle, Left **K** Abdomen Muscle, Right **L** Abdomen Muscle, Left **M** Perineum Muscle **N** Hip Muscle, Right **P** Hip Muscle, Left **Q** Upper Leg Muscle, Right **R** Upper Leg Muscle, Left **S** Lower Leg Muscle, Right **T** Lower Leg Muscle, Left **V** Foot Muscle, Right **W** Foot Muscle, Left	**Ø** Open **3** Percutaneous **4** Percutaneous Endoscopic **X** External	**Z** No Device	**Z** No Qualifier

Ø   Medical and Surgical
K   Muscles
P   Removal   Taking out or off a device from a body part

Body Part Character 4	Approach Character 5	Device Character 6	Qualifier Character 7
X Upper Muscle Y Lower Muscle	Ø Open 3 Percutaneous 4 Percutaneous Endoscopic	Ø Drainage Device 7 Autologous Tissue Substitute J Synthetic Substitute K Nonautologous Tissue Substitute M Stimulator Lead	Z No Qualifier
X Upper Muscle Y Lower Muscle	X External	Ø Drainage Device M Stimulator Lead	Z No Qualifier

Ø   Medical and Surgical
K   Muscles
Q   Repair   Restoring, to the extent possible, a body part to its normal anatomic structure and function

Body Part Character 4	Approach Character 5	Device Character 6	Qualifier Character 7
Ø Head Muscle 1 Facial Muscle 2 Neck Muscle, Right 3 Neck Muscle, Left 4 Tongue, Palate, Pharynx Muscle 5 Shoulder Muscle, Right 6 Shoulder Muscle, Left 7 Upper Arm Muscle, Right 8 Upper Arm Muscle, Left 9 Lower Arm and Wrist Muscle, Right B Lower Arm and Wrist Muscle, Left C Hand Muscle, Right D Hand Muscle, Left F Trunk Muscle, Right G Trunk Muscle, Left H Thorax Muscle, Right J Thorax Muscle, Left K Abdomen Muscle, Right L Abdomen Muscle, Left M Perineum Muscle N Hip Muscle, Right P Hip Muscle, Left Q Upper Leg Muscle, Right R Upper Leg Muscle, Left S Lower Leg Muscle, Right T Lower Leg Muscle, Left V Foot Muscle, Right W Foot Muscle, Left	Ø Open 3 Percutaneous 4 Percutaneous Endoscopic	Z No Device	Z No Qualifier

0 **Medical and Surgical**
K **Muscles**
S **Reposition**　　Moving to its normal location or other suitable location all or a portion of a body part

Body Part Character 4	Approach Character 5	Device Character 6	Qualifier Character 7
0 Head Muscle	**0** Open	**Z** No Device	**Z** No Qualifier
1 Facial Muscle	**4** Percutaneous Endoscopic		
2 Neck Muscle, Right			
3 Neck Muscle, Left			
4 Tongue, Palate, Pharynx Muscle			
5 Shoulder Muscle, Right			
6 Shoulder Muscle, Left			
7 Upper Arm Muscle, Right			
8 Upper Arm Muscle, Left			
9 Lower Arm and Wrist Muscle, Right			
B Lower Arm and Wrist Muscle, Left			
C Hand Muscle, Right			
D Hand Muscle, Left			
F Trunk Muscle, Right			
G Trunk Muscle, Left			
H Thorax Muscle, Right			
J Thorax Muscle, Left			
K Abdomen Muscle, Right			
L Abdomen Muscle, Left			
M Perineum Muscle			
N Hip Muscle, Right			
P Hip Muscle, Left			
Q Upper Leg Muscle, Right			
R Upper Leg Muscle, Left			
S Lower Leg Muscle, Right			
T Lower Leg Muscle, Left			
V Foot Muscle, Right			
W Foot Muscle, Left			

0 **Medical and Surgical**
K **Muscles**
T **Resection**　　Cutting out or off, without replacement, all of a body part

Body Part Character 4	Approach Character 5	Device Character 6	Qualifier Character 7
0 Head Muscle	**0** Open	**Z** No Device	**Z** No Qualifier
1 Facial Muscle	**4** Percutaneous Endoscopic		
2 Neck Muscle, Right			
3 Neck Muscle, Left			
4 Tongue, Palate, Pharynx Muscle			
5 Shoulder Muscle, Right			
6 Shoulder Muscle, Left			
7 Upper Arm Muscle, Right			
8 Upper Arm Muscle, Left			
9 Lower Arm and Wrist Muscle, Right			
B Lower Arm and Wrist Muscle, Left			
C Hand Muscle, Right			
D Hand Muscle, Left			
F Trunk Muscle, Right			
G Trunk Muscle, Left			
H Thorax Muscle, Right			
J Thorax Muscle, Left			
K Abdomen Muscle, Right			
L Abdomen Muscle, Left			
M Perineum Muscle			
N Hip Muscle, Right			
P Hip Muscle, Left			
Q Upper Leg Muscle, Right			
R Upper Leg Muscle, Left			
S Lower Leg Muscle, Right			
T Lower Leg Muscle, Left			
V Foot Muscle, Right			
W Foot Muscle, Left			

Ø   Medical and Surgical
K   Muscles
U   Supplement   Putting in or on biological or synthetic material that physically reinforces and/or augments the function of a portion of a body part

Body Part Character 4	Approach Character 5	Device Character 6	Qualifier Character 7
Ø Head Muscle 1 Facial Muscle 2 Neck Muscle, Right 3 Neck Muscle, Left 4 Tongue, Palate, Pharynx Muscle 5 Shoulder Muscle, Right 6 Shoulder Muscle, Left 7 Upper Arm Muscle, Right 8 Upper Arm Muscle, Left 9 Lower Arm and Wrist Muscle, Right B Lower Arm and Wrist Muscle, Left C Hand Muscle, Right D Hand Muscle, Left F Trunk Muscle, Right G Trunk Muscle, Left H Thorax Muscle, Right J Thorax Muscle, Left K Abdomen Muscle, Right L Abdomen Muscle, Left M Perineum Muscle N Hip Muscle, Right P Hip Muscle, Left Q Upper Leg Muscle, Right R Upper Leg Muscle, Left S Lower Leg Muscle, Right T Lower Leg Muscle, Left V Foot Muscle, Right W Foot Muscle, Left	Ø Open 4 Percutaneous Endoscopic	7 Autologous Tissue Substitute J Synthetic Substitute K Nonautologous Tissue Substitute	Z No Qualifier

Ø   Medical and Surgical
K   Muscles
W   Revision   Correcting, to the extent possible, a portion of a malfunctioning device or the position of a displaced device

Body Part Character 4	Approach Character 5	Device Character 6	Qualifier Character 7
X Upper Muscle Y Lower Muscle	Ø Open 3 Percutaneous 4 Percutaneous Endoscopic X External	Ø Drainage Device 7 Autologous Tissue Substitute J Synthetic Substitute K Nonautologous Tissue Substitute M Stimulator Lead	Z No Qualifier

Ø   Medical and Surgical
K   Muscles
X   Transfer   Moving, without taking out, all or a portion of a body part to another location to take over the function of all or a portion of a body part

Body Part Character 4	Approach Character 5	Device Character 6	Qualifier Character 7
Ø Head Muscle **1** Facial Muscle **2** Neck Muscle, Right **3** Neck Muscle, Left **4** Tongue, Palate, Pharynx Muscle **5** Shoulder Muscle, Right **6** Shoulder Muscle, Left **7** Upper Arm Muscle, Right **8** Upper Arm Muscle, Left **9** Lower Arm and Wrist Muscle, Right **B** Lower Arm and Wrist Muscle, Left **C** Hand Muscle, Right **D** Hand Muscle, Left **F** Trunk Muscle, Right **G** Trunk Muscle, Left **H** Thorax Muscle, Right **J** Thorax Muscle, Left **M** Perineum Muscle **N** Hip Muscle, Right **P** Hip Muscle, Left **Q** Upper Leg Muscle, Right **R** Upper Leg Muscle, Left **S** Lower Leg Muscle, Right **T** Lower Leg Muscle, Left **V** Foot Muscle, Right **W** Foot Muscle, Left	**Ø** Open **4** Percutaneous Endoscopic	**Z** No Device	**Ø** Skin **1** Subcutaneous Tissue **2** Skin and Subcutaneous Tissue **Z** No Qualifier
K Abdomen Muscle, Right **L** Abdomen Muscle, Left	**Ø** Open **4** Percutaneous Endoscopic	**Z** No Device	**Ø** Skin **1** Subcutaneous Tissue **2** Skin and Subcutaneous Tissue **6** Transverse Rectus Abdominis Myocutaneous Flap **Z** No Qualifier

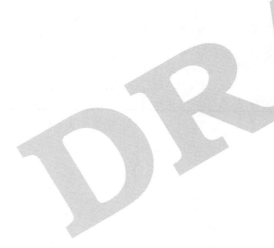

Tendons ØL2–ØLX

Ø Medical and Surgical
L Tendons
2 Change   Taking out or off a device from a body part and putting back an identical or similar device in or on the same body part without cutting or puncturing the skin or a mucous membrane

Body Part Character 4	Approach Character 5	Device Character 6	Qualifier Character 7
X Upper Tendon Y Lower Tendon	X External	Ø Drainage Device Y Other Device	Z No Qualifier

Ø Medical and Surgical
L Tendons
5 Destruction   Physical eradication of all or a portion of a body part by the direct use of energy, force, or a destructive agent

Body Part Character 4	Approach Character 5	Device Character 6	Qualifier Character 7
Ø Head and Neck Tendon 1 Shoulder Tendon, Right 2 Shoulder Tendon, Left 3 Upper Arm Tendon, Right 4 Upper Arm Tendon, Left 5 Lower Arm and Wrist Tendon, Right 6 Lower Arm and Wrist Tendon, Left 7 Hand Tendon, Right 8 Hand Tendon, Left 9 Trunk Tendon, Right B Trunk Tendon, Left C Thorax Tendon, Right D Thorax Tendon, Left F Abdomen Tendon, Right G Abdomen Tendon, Left H Perineum Tendon J Hip Tendon, Right K Hip Tendon, Left L Upper Leg Tendon, Right M Upper Leg Tendon, Left N Lower Leg Tendon, Right P Lower Leg Tendon, Left Q Knee Tendon, Right R Knee Tendon, Left S Ankle Tendon, Right T Ankle Tendon, Left V Foot Tendon, Right W Foot Tendon, Left	Ø Open 3 Percutaneous 4 Percutaneous Endoscopic	Z No Device	Z No Qualifier

   Revised Text in **BLUE**   © 2011 Ingenix, Inc

0   **Medical and Surgical**
L   **Tendons**
8   **Division**   Cutting into a body part without draining fluids and/or gases from the body part in order to separate or transect a body part

Body Part Character 4	Approach Character 5	Device Character 6	Qualifier Character 7
0 Head and Neck Tendon 1 Shoulder Tendon, Right 2 Shoulder Tendon, Left 3 Upper Arm Tendon, Right 4 Upper Arm Tendon, Left 5 Lower Arm and Wrist Tendon, Right 6 Lower Arm and Wrist Tendon, Left 7 Hand Tendon, Right 8 Hand Tendon, Left 9 Trunk Tendon, Right B Trunk Tendon, Left C Thorax Tendon, Right D Thorax Tendon, Left F Abdomen Tendon, Right G Abdomen Tendon, Left H Perineum Tendon J Hip Tendon, Right K Hip Tendon, Left L Upper Leg Tendon, Right M Upper Leg Tendon, Left N Lower Leg Tendon, Right P Lower Leg Tendon, Left Q Knee Tendon, Right R Knee Tendon, Left S Ankle Tendon, Right T Ankle Tendon, Left V Foot Tendon, Right W Foot Tendon, Left	0 Open 3 Percutaneous 4 Percutaneous Endoscopic	Z No Device	Z No Qualifier

0   **Medical and Surgical**
L   **Tendons**
9   **Drainage**   Taking or letting out fluids and/or gases from a body part

Body Part Character 4	Approach Character 5	Device Character 6	Qualifier Character 7
0 Head and Neck Tendon 1 Shoulder Tendon, Right 2 Shoulder Tendon, Left 3 Upper Arm Tendon, Right 4 Upper Arm Tendon, Left 5 Lower Arm and Wrist Tendon, Right 6 Lower Arm and Wrist Tendon, Left 7 Hand Tendon, Right 8 Hand Tendon, Left 9 Trunk Tendon, Right B Trunk Tendon, Left C Thorax Tendon, Right D Thorax Tendon, Left F Abdomen Tendon, Right G Abdomen Tendon, Left H Perineum Tendon J Hip Tendon, Right K Hip Tendon, Left L Upper Leg Tendon, Right M Upper Leg Tendon, Left N Lower Leg Tendon, Right P Lower Leg Tendon, Left Q Knee Tendon, Right R Knee Tendon, Left S Ankle Tendon, Right T Ankle Tendon, Left V Foot Tendon, Right W Foot Tendon, Left	0 Open 3 Percutaneous 4 Percutaneous Endoscopic	0 Drainage Device	Z No Qualifier

0L9 Continued on next page

0   **Medical and Surgical**   *0L9 Continued*
L   **Tendons**
9   **Drainage**   Taking or letting out fluids and/or gases from a body part

Body Part Character 4	Approach Character 5	Device Character 6	Qualifier Character 7
0 Head and Neck Tendon **1** Shoulder Tendon, Right **2** Shoulder Tendon, Left **3** Upper Arm Tendon, Right **4** Upper Arm Tendon, Left **5** Lower Arm and Wrist Tendon, Right **6** Lower Arm and Wrist Tendon, Left **7** Hand Tendon, Right **8** Hand Tendon, Left **9** Trunk Tendon, Right **B** Trunk Tendon, Left **C** Thorax Tendon, Right **D** Thorax Tendon, Left **F** Abdomen Tendon, Right **G** Abdomen Tendon, Left **H** Perineum Tendon **J** Hip Tendon, Right **K** Hip Tendon, Left **L** Upper Leg Tendon, Right **M** Upper Leg Tendon, Left **N** Lower Leg Tendon, Right **P** Lower Leg Tendon, Left **Q** Knee Tendon, Right **R** Knee Tendon, Left **S** Ankle Tendon, Right **T** Ankle Tendon, Left **V** Foot Tendon, Right **W** Foot Tendon, Left	**0** Open **3** Percutaneous **4** Percutaneous Endoscopic	**Z** No Device	**X** Diagnostic **Z** No Qualifier

0   **Medical and Surgical**
L   **Tendons**
B   **Excision**   Cutting out or off, without replacement, a portion of a body part

Body Part Character 4	Approach Character 5	Device Character 6	Qualifier Character 7
0 Head and Neck Tendon **1** Shoulder Tendon, Right **2** Shoulder Tendon, Left **3** Upper Arm Tendon, Right **4** Upper Arm Tendon, Left **5** Lower Arm and Wrist Tendon, Right **6** Lower Arm and Wrist Tendon, Left **7** Hand Tendon, Right **8** Hand Tendon, Left **9** Trunk Tendon, Right **B** Trunk Tendon, Left **C** Thorax Tendon, Right **D** Thorax Tendon, Left **F** Abdomen Tendon, Right **G** Abdomen Tendon, Left **H** Perineum Tendon **J** Hip Tendon, Right **K** Hip Tendon, Left **L** Upper Leg Tendon, Right **M** Upper Leg Tendon, Left **N** Lower Leg Tendon, Right **P** Lower Leg Tendon, Left **Q** Knee Tendon, Right **R** Knee Tendon, Left **S** Ankle Tendon, Right **T** Ankle Tendon, Left **V** Foot Tendon, Right **W** Foot Tendon, Left	**0** Open **3** Percutaneous **4** Percutaneous Endoscopic	**Z** No Device	**X** Diagnostic **Z** No Qualifier

      Revised Text in **BLUE**

Ø   **Medical and Surgical**
L   **Tendons**
C   **Extirpation**   Taking or cutting out solid matter from a body part

Body Part Character 4	Approach Character 5	Device Character 6	Qualifier Character 7
Ø Head and Neck Tendon 1 Shoulder Tendon, Right 2 Shoulder Tendon, Left 3 Upper Arm Tendon, Right 4 Upper Arm Tendon, Left 5 Lower Arm and Wrist Tendon, Right 6 Lower Arm and Wrist Tendon, Left 7 Hand Tendon, Right 8 Hand Tendon, Left 9 Trunk Tendon, Right B Trunk Tendon, Left C Thorax Tendon, Right D Thorax Tendon, Left F Abdomen Tendon, Right G Abdomen Tendon, Left H Perineum Tendon J Hip Tendon, Right K Hip Tendon, Left L Upper Leg Tendon, Right M Upper Leg Tendon, Left N Lower Leg Tendon, Right P Lower Leg Tendon, Left Q Knee Tendon, Right R Knee Tendon, Left S Ankle Tendon, Right T Ankle Tendon, Left V Foot Tendon, Right W Foot Tendon, Left	Ø Open 3 Percutaneous 4 Percutaneous Endoscopic	Z No Device	Z No Qualifier

Ø   **Medical and Surgical**
L   **Tendons**
J   **Inspection**   Visually and/or manually exploring a body part

Body Part Character 4	Approach Character 5	Device Character 6	Qualifier Character 7
X Upper Tendon Y Lower Tendon	Ø Open 3 Percutaneous 4 Percutaneous Endoscopic X External	Z No Device	Z No Qualifier

Ø   **Medical and Surgical**
L   **Tendons**
M   **Reattachment**   Putting back in or on all or a portion of a separated body part to its normal location or other suitable location

Body Part Character 4	Approach Character 5	Device Character 6	Qualifier Character 7
Ø Head and Neck Tendon 1 Shoulder Tendon, Right 2 Shoulder Tendon, Left 3 Upper Arm Tendon, Right 4 Upper Arm Tendon, Left 5 Lower Arm and Wrist Tendon, Right 6 Lower Arm and Wrist Tendon, Left 7 Hand Tendon, Right 8 Hand Tendon, Left 9 Trunk Tendon, Right B Trunk Tendon, Left C Thorax Tendon, Right D Thorax Tendon, Left F Abdomen Tendon, Right G Abdomen Tendon, Left H Perineum Tendon J Hip Tendon, Right K Hip Tendon, Left L Upper Leg Tendon, Right M Upper Leg Tendon, Left N Lower Leg Tendon, Right P Lower Leg Tendon, Left Q Knee Tendon, Right R Knee Tendon, Left S Ankle Tendon, Right T Ankle Tendon, Left V Foot Tendon, Right W Foot Tendon, Left	Ø Open 4 Percutaneous Endoscopic	Z No Device	Z No Qualifier

Ø   **Medical and Surgical**
L   **Tendons**
N   **Release**   Freeing a body part from an abnormal physical constraint

Body Part Character 4	Approach Character 5	Device Character 6	Qualifier Character 7
Ø Head and Neck Tendon **1** Shoulder Tendon, Right **2** Shoulder Tendon, Left **3** Upper Arm Tendon, Right **4** Upper Arm Tendon, Left **5** Lower Arm and Wrist Tendon, Right **6** Lower Arm and Wrist Tendon, Left **7** Hand Tendon, Right **8** Hand Tendon, Left **9** Trunk Tendon, Right **B** Trunk Tendon, Left **C** Thorax Tendon, Right **D** Thorax Tendon, Left **F** Abdomen Tendon, Right **G** Abdomen Tendon, Left **H** Perineum Tendon **J** Hip Tendon, Right **K** Hip Tendon, Left **L** Upper Leg Tendon, Right **M** Upper Leg Tendon, Left **N** Lower Leg Tendon, Right **P** Lower Leg Tendon, Left **Q** Knee Tendon, Right **R** Knee Tendon, Left **S** Ankle Tendon, Right **T** Ankle Tendon, Left **V** Foot Tendon, Right **W** Foot Tendon, Left	**Ø** Open **3** Percutaneous **4** Percutaneous Endoscopic **X** External	**Z** No Device	**Z** No Qualifier

Ø   **Medical and Surgical**
L   **Tendons**
P   **Removal**   Taking out or off a device from a body part

Body Part Character 4	Approach Character 5	Device Character 6	Qualifier Character 7
X Upper Tendon **Y** Lower Tendon	**Ø** Open **3** Percutaneous **4** Percutaneous Endoscopic	**Ø** Drainage Device **7** Autologous Tissue Substitute **J** Synthetic Substitute **K** Nonautologous Tissue Substitute	**Z** No Qualifier
X Upper Tendon **Y** Lower Tendon	**X** External	**Ø** Drainage Device	**Z** No Qualifier

Revised Text in **BLUE**

Ø　Medical and Surgical
L　Tendons
Q　Repair　　　　　Restoring, to the extent possible, a body part to its normal anatomic structure and function

Body Part Character 4	Approach Character 5	Device Character 6	Qualifier Character 7
Ø　Head and Neck Tendon 1　Shoulder Tendon, Right 2　Shoulder Tendon, Left 3　Upper Arm Tendon, Right 4　Upper Arm Tendon, Left 5　Lower Arm and Wrist Tendon, Right 6　Lower Arm and Wrist Tendon, Left 7　Hand Tendon, Right 8　Hand Tendon, Left 9　Trunk Tendon, Right B　Trunk Tendon, Left C　Thorax Tendon, Right D　Thorax Tendon, Left F　Abdomen Tendon, Right G　Abdomen Tendon, Left H　Perineum Tendon J　Hip Tendon, Right K　Hip Tendon, Left L　Upper Leg Tendon, Right M　Upper Leg Tendon, Left N　Lower Leg Tendon, Right P　Lower Leg Tendon, Left Q　Knee Tendon, Right R　Knee Tendon, Left S　Ankle Tendon, Right T　Ankle Tendon, Left V　Foot Tendon, Right W　Foot Tendon, Left	Ø　Open 3　Percutaneous 4　Percutaneous Endoscopic	Z　No Device	Z　No Qualifier

Ø　Medical and Surgical
L　Tendons
R　Replacement　　　　　Putting in or on biological or synthetic material that physically takes the place and/or function of all or a portion of a body part

Body Part Character 4	Approach Character 5	Device Character 6	Qualifier Character 7
Ø　Head and Neck Tendon 1　Shoulder Tendon, Right 2　Shoulder Tendon, Left 3　Upper Arm Tendon, Right 4　Upper Arm Tendon, Left 5　Lower Arm and Wrist Tendon, Right 6　Lower Arm and Wrist Tendon, Left 7　Hand Tendon, Right 8　Hand Tendon, Left 9　Trunk Tendon, Right B　Trunk Tendon, Left C　Thorax Tendon, Right D　Thorax Tendon, Left F　Abdomen Tendon, Right G　Abdomen Tendon, Left H　Perineum Tendon J　Hip Tendon, Right K　Hip Tendon, Left L　Upper Leg Tendon, Right M　Upper Leg Tendon, Left N　Lower Leg Tendon, Right P　Lower Leg Tendon, Left Q　Knee Tendon, Right R　Knee Tendon, Left S　Ankle Tendon, Right T　Ankle Tendon, Left V　Foot Tendon, Right W　Foot Tendon, Left	Ø　Open 4　Percutaneous Endoscopic	7　Autologous Tissue Substitute J　Synthetic Substitute K　Nonautologous Tissue Substitute	Z　No Qualifier

Ø   Medical and Surgical
L   Tendons
S   Reposition   Moving to its normal location or other suitable location all or a portion of a body part

Body Part Character 4	Approach Character 5	Device Character 6	Qualifier Character 7
Ø Head and Neck Tendon 1 Shoulder Tendon, Right 2 Shoulder Tendon, Left 3 Upper Arm Tendon, Right 4 Upper Arm Tendon, Left 5 Lower Arm and Wrist Tendon, Right 6 Lower Arm and Wrist Tendon, Left 7 Hand Tendon, Right 8 Hand Tendon, Left 9 Trunk Tendon, Right B Trunk Tendon, Left C Thorax Tendon, Right D Thorax Tendon, Left F Abdomen Tendon, Right G Abdomen Tendon, Left H Perineum Tendon J Hip Tendon, Right K Hip Tendon, Left L Upper Leg Tendon, Right M Upper Leg Tendon, Left N Lower Leg Tendon, Right P Lower Leg Tendon, Left Q Knee Tendon, Right R Knee Tendon, Left S Ankle Tendon, Right T Ankle Tendon, Left V Foot Tendon, Right W Foot Tendon, Left	Ø Open 4 Percutaneous Endoscopic	Z No Device	Z No Qualifier

Ø   Medical and Surgical
L   Tendons
T   Resection   Cutting out or off, without replacement, all of a body part

Body Part Character 4	Approach Character 5	Device Character 6	Qualifier Character 7
Ø Head and Neck Tendon 1 Shoulder Tendon, Right 2 Shoulder Tendon, Left 3 Upper Arm Tendon, Right 4 Upper Arm Tendon, Left 5 Lower Arm and Wrist Tendon, Right 6 Lower Arm and Wrist Tendon, Left 7 Hand Tendon, Right 8 Hand Tendon, Left 9 Trunk Tendon, Right B Trunk Tendon, Left C Thorax Tendon, Right D Thorax Tendon, Left F Abdomen Tendon, Right G Abdomen Tendon, Left H Perineum Tendon J Hip Tendon, Right K Hip Tendon, Left L Upper Leg Tendon, Right M Upper Leg Tendon, Left N Lower Leg Tendon, Right P Lower Leg Tendon, Left Q Knee Tendon, Right R Knee Tendon, Left S Ankle Tendon, Right T Ankle Tendon, Left V Foot Tendon, Right W Foot Tendon, Left	Ø Open 4 Percutaneous Endoscopic	Z No Device	Z No Qualifier

Ø   **Medical and Surgical**
L   **Tendons**
U   **Supplement**   Putting in or on biological or synthetic material that physically reinforces and/or augments the function of a portion of a body part

Body Part Character 4	Approach Character 5	Device Character 6	Qualifier Character 7
Ø Head and Neck Tendon 1 Shoulder Tendon, Right 2 Shoulder Tendon, Left 3 Upper Arm Tendon, Right 4 Upper Arm Tendon, Left 5 Lower Arm and Wrist Tendon, Right 6 Lower Arm and Wrist Tendon, Left 7 Hand Tendon, Right 8 Hand Tendon, Left 9 Trunk Tendon, Right B Trunk Tendon, Left C Thorax Tendon, Right D Thorax Tendon, Left F Abdomen Tendon, Right G Abdomen Tendon, Left H Perineum Tendon J Hip Tendon, Right K Hip Tendon, Left L Upper Leg Tendon, Right M Upper Leg Tendon, Left N Lower Leg Tendon, Right P Lower Leg Tendon, Left Q Knee Tendon, Right R Knee Tendon, Left S Ankle Tendon, Right T Ankle Tendon, Left V Foot Tendon, Right W Foot Tendon, Left	Ø Open 4 Percutaneous Endoscopic	7 Autologous Tissue Substitute J Synthetic Substitute K Nonautologous Tissue Substitute	Z No Qualifier

Ø   **Medical and Surgical**
L   **Tendons**
W   **Revision**   Correcting, to the extent possible, a portion of a malfunctioning device or the position of a displaced device

Body Part Character 4	Approach Character 5	Device Character 6	Qualifier Character 7
X Upper Tendon Y Lower Tendon	Ø Open 3 Percutaneous 4 Percutaneous Endoscopic X External	Ø Drainage Device 7 Autologous Tissue Substitute J Synthetic Substitute K Nonautologous Tissue Substitute	Z No Qualifier

Ø   **Medical and Surgical**
L   **Tendons**
X   **Transfer**   Moving, without taking out, all or a portion of a body part to another location to take over the function of all or a portion of a body part

Body Part Character 4	Approach Character 5	Device Character 6	Qualifier Character 7
Ø Head and Neck Tendon 1 Shoulder Tendon, Right 2 Shoulder Tendon, Left 3 Upper Arm Tendon, Right 4 Upper Arm Tendon, Left 5 Lower Arm and Wrist Tendon, Right 6 Lower Arm and Wrist Tendon, Left 7 Hand Tendon, Right 8 Hand Tendon, Left 9 Trunk Tendon, Right B Trunk Tendon, Left C Thorax Tendon, Right D Thorax Tendon, Left F Abdomen Tendon, Right G Abdomen Tendon, Left H Perineum Tendon J Hip Tendon, Right K Hip Tendon, Left L Upper Leg Tendon, Right M Upper Leg Tendon, Left N Lower Leg Tendon, Right P Lower Leg Tendon, Left Q Knee Tendon, Right R Knee Tendon, Left S Ankle Tendon, Right T Ankle Tendon, Left V Foot Tendon, Right W Foot Tendon, Left	Ø Open 4 Percutaneous Endoscopic	Z No Device	Z No Qualifier

Bursae and Ligaments ØM2–ØMX

Ø   **Medical and Surgical**
M   **Bursae and Ligaments**
2   **Change**   Taking out or off a device from a body part and putting back an identical or similar device in or on the same body part without cutting or puncturing the skin or a mucous membrane

Body Part Character 4	Approach Character 5	Device Character 6	Qualifier Character 7
X Upper Bursa and Ligament **Y** Lower Bursa and Ligament	**X** External	**Ø** Drainage Device **Y** Other Device	**Z** No Qualifier

Ø   **Medical and Surgical**
M   **Bursae and Ligaments**
5   **Destruction**   Physical eradication of all or a portion of a body part by the direct use of energy, force, or a destructive agent

Body Part Character 4	Approach Character 5	Device Character 6	Qualifier Character 7
Ø Head and Neck Bursa and Ligament **1** Shoulder Bursa and Ligament, Right **2** Shoulder Bursa and Ligament, Left **3** Elbow Bursa and Ligament, Right **4** Elbow Bursa and Ligament, Left **5** Wrist Bursa and Ligament, Right **6** Wrist Bursa and Ligament, Left **7** Hand Bursa and Ligament, Right **8** Hand Bursa and Ligament, Left **9** Upper Extremity Bursa and Ligament, Right **B** Upper Extremity Bursa and Ligament, Left **C** Trunk Bursa and Ligament, Right **D** Trunk Bursa and Ligament, Left **F** Thorax Bursa and Ligament, Right **G** Thorax Bursa and Ligament, Left **H** Abdomen Bursa and Ligament, Right **J** Abdomen Bursa and Ligament, Left **K** Perineum Bursa and Ligament **L** Hip Bursa and Ligament, Right **M** Hip Bursa and Ligament, Left **N** Knee Bursa and Ligament, Right **P** Knee Bursa and Ligament, Left **Q** Ankle Bursa and Ligament, Right **R** Ankle Bursa and Ligament, Left **S** Foot Bursa and Ligament, Right **T** Foot Bursa and Ligament, Left **V** Lower Extremity Bursa and Ligament, Right **W** Lower Extremity Bursa and Ligament, Left	**Ø** Open **3** Percutaneous **4** Percutaneous Endoscopic	**Z** No Device	**Z** No Qualifier

     Revised Text in **BLUE**

Ø **Medical and Surgical**
M **Bursae and Ligaments**
8 **Division**   Cutting into a body part without draining fluids and/or gases from the body part in order to separate or transect a body part

Body Part Character 4	Approach Character 5	Device Character 6	Qualifier Character 7
Ø Head and Neck Bursa and Ligament	Ø Open	Z No Device	Z No Qualifier
1 Shoulder Bursa and Ligament, Right	3 Percutaneous		
2 Shoulder Bursa and Ligament, Left	4 Percutaneous Endoscopic		
3 Elbow Bursa and Ligament, Right			
4 Elbow Bursa and Ligament, Left			
5 Wrist Bursa and Ligament, Right			
6 Wrist Bursa and Ligament, Left			
7 Hand Bursa and Ligament, Right			
8 Hand Bursa and Ligament, Left			
9 Upper Extremity Bursa and Ligament, Right			
B Upper Extremity Bursa and Ligament, Left			
C Trunk Bursa and Ligament, Right			
D Trunk Bursa and Ligament, Left			
F Thorax Bursa and Ligament, Right			
G Thorax Bursa and Ligament, Left			
H Abdomen Bursa and Ligament, Right			
J Abdomen Bursa and Ligament, Left			
K Perineum Bursa and Ligament			
L Hip Bursa and Ligament, Right			
M Hip Bursa and Ligament, Left			
N Knee Bursa and Ligament, Right			
P Knee Bursa and Ligament, Left			
Q Ankle Bursa and Ligament, Right			
R Ankle Bursa and Ligament, Left			
S Foot Bursa and Ligament, Right			
T Foot Bursa and Ligament, Left			
V Lower Extremity Bursa and Ligament, Right			
W Lower Extremity Bursa and Ligament, Left			

Ø **Medical and Surgical**
M **Bursae and Ligaments**
9 **Drainage**   Taking or letting out fluids and/or gases from a body part

Body Part Character 4	Approach Character 5	Device Character 6	Qualifier Character 7
Ø Head and Neck Bursa and Ligament	Ø Open	Ø Drainage Device	Z No Qualifier
1 Shoulder Bursa and Ligament, Right	3 Percutaneous		
2 Shoulder Bursa and Ligament, Left	4 Percutaneous Endoscopic		
3 Elbow Bursa and Ligament, Right			
4 Elbow Bursa and Ligament, Left			
5 Wrist Bursa and Ligament, Right			
6 Wrist Bursa and Ligament, Left			
7 Hand Bursa and Ligament, Right			
8 Hand Bursa and Ligament, Left			
9 Upper Extremity Bursa and Ligament, Right			
B Upper Extremity Bursa and Ligament, Left			
C Trunk Bursa and Ligament, Right			
D Trunk Bursa and Ligament, Left			
F Thorax Bursa and Ligament, Right			
G Thorax Bursa and Ligament, Left			
H Abdomen Bursa and Ligament, Right			
J Abdomen Bursa and Ligament, Left			
K Perineum Bursa and Ligament			
L Hip Bursa and Ligament, Right			
M Hip Bursa and Ligament, Left			
N Knee Bursa and Ligament, Right			
P Knee Bursa and Ligament, Left			
Q Ankle Bursa and Ligament, Right			
R Ankle Bursa and Ligament, Left			
S Foot Bursa and Ligament, Right			
T Foot Bursa and Ligament, Left			
V Lower Extremity Bursa and Ligament, Right			
W Lower Extremity Bursa and Ligament, Left			

ØM9 Continued on next page

Ø   Medical and Surgical
M   Bursae and Ligaments
9   Drainage   Taking or letting out fluids and/or gases from a body part

ØM9 Continued

Body Part Character 4	Approach Character 5	Device Character 6	Qualifier Character 7
Ø Head and Neck Bursa and Ligament 1 Shoulder Bursa and Ligament, Right 2 Shoulder Bursa and Ligament, Left 3 Elbow Bursa and Ligament, Right 4 Elbow Bursa and Ligament, Left 5 Wrist Bursa and Ligament, Right 6 Wrist Bursa and Ligament, Left 7 Hand Bursa and Ligament, Right 8 Hand Bursa and Ligament, Left 9 Upper Extremity Bursa and Ligament, Right B Upper Extremity Bursa and Ligament, Left C Trunk Bursa and Ligament, Right D Trunk Bursa and Ligament, Left F Thorax Bursa and Ligament, Right G Thorax Bursa and Ligament, Left H Abdomen Bursa and Ligament, Right J Abdomen Bursa and Ligament, Left K Perineum Bursa and Ligament L Hip Bursa and Ligament, Right M Hip Bursa and Ligament, Left N Knee Bursa and Ligament, Right P Knee Bursa and Ligament, Left Q Ankle Bursa and Ligament, Right R Ankle Bursa and Ligament, Left S Foot Bursa and Ligament, Right T Foot Bursa and Ligament, Left V Lower Extremity Bursa and Ligament, Right W Lower Extremity Bursa and Ligament, Left	Ø Open 3 Percutaneous 4 Percutaneous Endoscopic	Z No Device	X Diagnostic Z No Qualifier

Ø   Medical and Surgical
M   Bursae and Ligaments
B   Excision   Cutting out or off, without replacement, a portion of a body part

Body Part Character 4	Approach Character 5	Device Character 6	Qualifier Character 7
Ø Head and Neck Bursa and Ligament 1 Shoulder Bursa and Ligament, Right 2 Shoulder Bursa and Ligament, Left 3 Elbow Bursa and Ligament, Right 4 Elbow Bursa and Ligament, Left 5 Wrist Bursa and Ligament, Right 6 Wrist Bursa and Ligament, Left 7 Hand Bursa and Ligament, Right 8 Hand Bursa and Ligament, Left 9 Upper Extremity Bursa and Ligament, Right B Upper Extremity Bursa and Ligament, Left C Trunk Bursa and Ligament, Right D Trunk Bursa and Ligament, Left F Thorax Bursa and Ligament, Right G Thorax Bursa and Ligament, Left H Abdomen Bursa and Ligament, Right J Abdomen Bursa and Ligament, Left K Perineum Bursa and Ligament L Hip Bursa and Ligament, Right M Hip Bursa and Ligament, Left N Knee Bursa and Ligament, Right P Knee Bursa and Ligament, Left Q Ankle Bursa and Ligament, Right R Ankle Bursa and Ligament, Left S Foot Bursa and Ligament, Right T Foot Bursa and Ligament, Left V Lower Extremity Bursa and Ligament, Right W Lower Extremity Bursa and Ligament, Left	Ø Open 3 Percutaneous 4 Percutaneous Endoscopic	Z No Device	X Diagnostic Z No Qualifier

     Revised Text in **BLUE**

Ø Medical and Surgical
M Bursae and Ligaments
C Extirpation   Taking or cutting out solid matter from a body part

Body Part Character 4	Approach Character 5	Device Character 6	Qualifier Character 7
Ø Head and Neck Bursa and Ligament 1 Shoulder Bursa and Ligament, Right 2 Shoulder Bursa and Ligament, Left 3 Elbow Bursa and Ligament, Right 4 Elbow Bursa and Ligament, Left 5 Wrist Bursa and Ligament, Right 6 Wrist Bursa and Ligament, Left 7 Hand Bursa and Ligament, Right 8 Hand Bursa and Ligament, Left 9 Upper Extremity Bursa and Ligament, Right B Upper Extremity Bursa and Ligament, Left C Trunk Bursa and Ligament, Right D Trunk Bursa and Ligament, Left F Thorax Bursa and Ligament, Right G Thorax Bursa and Ligament, Left H Abdomen Bursa and Ligament, Right J Abdomen Bursa and Ligament, Left K Perineum Bursa and Ligament L Hip Bursa and Ligament, Right M Hip Bursa and Ligament, Left N Knee Bursa and Ligament, Right P Knee Bursa and Ligament, Left Q Ankle Bursa and Ligament, Right R Ankle Bursa and Ligament, Left S Foot Bursa and Ligament, Right T Foot Bursa and Ligament, Left V Lower Extremity Bursa and Ligament, Right W Lower Extremity Bursa and Ligament, Left	Ø Open 3 Percutaneous 4 Percutaneous Endoscopic	Z No Device	Z No Qualifier

Ø Medical and Surgical
M Bursae and Ligaments
D Extraction   Pulling or stripping out or off all or a portion of a body part by the use of force

Body Part Character 4	Approach Character 5	Device Character 6	Qualifier Character 7
Ø Head and Neck Bursa and Ligament 1 Shoulder Bursa and Ligament, Right 2 Shoulder Bursa and Ligament, Left 3 Elbow Bursa and Ligament, Right 4 Elbow Bursa and Ligament, Left 5 Wrist Bursa and Ligament, Right 6 Wrist Bursa and Ligament, Left 7 Hand Bursa and Ligament, Right 8 Hand Bursa and Ligament, Left 9 Upper Extremity Bursa and Ligament, Right B Upper Extremity Bursa and Ligament, Left C Trunk Bursa and Ligament, Right D Trunk Bursa and Ligament, Left F Thorax Bursa and Ligament, Right G Thorax Bursa and Ligament, Left H Abdomen Bursa and Ligament, Right J Abdomen Bursa and Ligament, Left K Perineum Bursa and Ligament L Hip Bursa and Ligament, Right M Hip Bursa and Ligament, Left N Knee Bursa and Ligament, Right P Knee Bursa and Ligament, Left Q Ankle Bursa and Ligament, Right R Ankle Bursa and Ligament, Left S Foot Bursa and Ligament, Right T Foot Bursa and Ligament, Left V Lower Extremity Bursa and Ligament, Right W Lower Extremity Bursa and Ligament, Left	Ø Open 3 Percutaneous 4 Percutaneous Endoscopic	Z No Device	Z No Qualifier

Ø   **Medical and Surgical**
M   **Bursae and Ligaments**
J   **Inspection**   Visually and/or manually exploring a body part

Body Part Character 4	Approach Character 5	Device Character 6	Qualifier Character 7
X Upper Bursa and Ligament **Y** Lower Bursa and Ligament	**Ø** Open **3** Percutaneous **4** Percutaneous Endoscopic **X** External	**Z** No Device	**Z** No Qualifier

Ø   **Medical and Surgical**
M   **Bursae and Ligaments**
M   **Reattachment**   Putting back in or on all or a portion of a separated body part to its normal location or other suitable location

Body Part Character 4	Approach Character 5	Device Character 6	Qualifier Character 7
Ø Head and Neck Bursa and Ligament **1** Shoulder Bursa and Ligament, Rightv **2** Shoulder Bursa and Ligament, Left **3** Elbow Bursa and Ligament, Right **4** Elbow Bursa and Ligament, Left **5** Wrist Bursa and Ligament, Right **6** Wrist Bursa and Ligament, Left **7** Hand Bursa and Ligament, Right **8** Hand Bursa and Ligament, Left **9** Upper Extremity Bursa and Ligament, Right **B** Upper Extremity Bursa and Ligament, Left **C** Trunk Bursa and Ligament, Right **D** Trunk Bursa and Ligament, Left **F** Thorax Bursa and Ligament, Right **G** Thorax Bursa and Ligament, Left **H** Abdomen Bursa and Ligament, Right **J** Abdomen Bursa and Ligament, Left **K** Perineum Bursa and Ligament **L** Hip Bursa and Ligament, Right **M** Hip Bursa and Ligament, Left **N** Knee Bursa and Ligament, Right **P** Knee Bursa and Ligament, Left **Q** Ankle Bursa and Ligament, Right **R** Ankle Bursa and Ligament, Left **S** Foot Bursa and Ligament, Right **T** Foot Bursa and Ligament, Left **V** Lower Extremity Bursa and Ligament, Right **W** Lower Extremity Bursa and Ligament, Left	**Ø** Open **4** Percutaneous Endoscopic	**Z** No Device	**Z** No Qualifier

Ø Medical and Surgical
M Bursae and Ligaments
N Release   Freeing a body part from an abnormal physical constraint

Body Part Character 4	Approach Character 5	Device Character 6	Qualifier Character 7

Ø Head and Neck Bursa and Ligament
1 Shoulder Bursa and Ligament, Right
2 Shoulder Bursa and Ligament, Left
3 Elbow Bursa and Ligament, Right
4 Elbow Bursa and Ligament, Left
5 Wrist Bursa and Ligament, Right
6 Wrist Bursa and Ligament, Left
7 Hand Bursa and Ligament, Right
8 Hand Bursa and Ligament, Left
9 Upper Extremity Bursa and
   Ligament, Right
B Upper Extremity Bursa and
   Ligament, Left
C Trunk Bursa and Ligament, Right
D Trunk Bursa and Ligament, Left
F Thorax Bursa and Ligament, Right
G Thorax Bursa and Ligament, Left
H Abdomen Bursa and Ligament,
   Right
J Abdomen Bursa and Ligament, Left
K Perineum Bursa and Ligament
L Hip Bursa and Ligament, Right
M Hip Bursa and Ligament, Left
N Knee Bursa and Ligament, Right
P Knee Bursa and Ligament, Left
Q Ankle Bursa and Ligament, Right
R Ankle Bursa and Ligament, Left
S Foot Bursa and Ligament, Right
T Foot Bursa and Ligament, Left
V Lower Extremity Bursa and
   Ligament, Right
W Lower Extremity Bursa and
   Ligament, Left
	Ø Open
	3 Percutaneous
	4 Percutaneous Endoscopic
	X External
		Z No Device	Z No Qualifier

Ø Medical and Surgical
M Bursae and Ligaments
P Removal   Taking out or off a device from a body part

Body Part Character 4	Approach Character 5	Device Character 6	Qualifier Character 7
X Upper Bursa and Ligament Y Lower Bursa and Ligament	Ø Open 3 Percutaneous 4 Percutaneous Endoscopic	Ø Drainage Device 7 Autologous Tissue Substitute J Synthetic Substitute K Nonautologous Tissue Substitute	Z No Qualifier
X Upper Bursa and Ligament Y Lower Bursa and Ligament	X External	Ø Drainage Device	Z No Qualifier

Bursae and Ligaments

Ø Medical and Surgical
M Bursae and Ligaments
Q Repair   Restoring, to the extent possible, a body part to its normal anatomic structure and function

Body Part Character 4	Approach Character 5	Device Character 6	Qualifier Character 7
Ø Head and Neck Bursa and Ligament **1** Shoulder Bursa and Ligament, Right **2** Shoulder Bursa and Ligament, Left **3** Elbow Bursa and Ligament, Right **4** Elbow Bursa and Ligament, Left **5** Wrist Bursa and Ligament, Right **6** Wrist Bursa and Ligament, Left **7** Hand Bursa and Ligament, Right **8** Hand Bursa and Ligament, Left **9** Upper Extremity Bursa and Ligament, Right **B** Upper Extremity Bursa and Ligament, Left **C** Trunk Bursa and Ligament, Right **D** Trunk Bursa and Ligament, Left **F** Thorax Bursa and Ligament, Right **G** Thorax Bursa and Ligament, Left **H** Abdomen Bursa and Ligament, Right **J** Abdomen Bursa and Ligament, Left **K** Perineum Bursa and Ligament **L** Hip Bursa and Ligament, Right **M** Hip Bursa and Ligament, Left **N** Knee Bursa and Ligament, Right **P** Knee Bursa and Ligament, Left **Q** Ankle Bursa and Ligament, Right **R** Ankle Bursa and Ligament, Left **S** Foot Bursa and Ligament, Right **T** Foot Bursa and Ligament, Left **V** Lower Extremity Bursa and Ligament, Right **W** Lower Extremity Bursa and Ligament, Left	**Ø** Open **3** Percutaneous **4** Percutaneous Endoscopic	**Z** No Device	**Z** No Qualifier

Ø Medical and Surgical
M Bursae and Ligaments
S Reposition   Moving to its normal location or other suitable location all or a portion of a body part

Body Part Character 4	Approach Character 5	Device Character 6	Qualifier Character 7
Ø Head and Neck Bursa and Ligament **1** Shoulder Bursa and Ligament, Right **2** Shoulder Bursa and Ligament, Left **3** Elbow Bursa and Ligament, Right **4** Elbow Bursa and Ligament, Left **5** Wrist Bursa and Ligament, Right **6** Wrist Bursa and Ligament, Left **7** Hand Bursa and Ligament, Right **8** Hand Bursa and Ligament, Left **9** Upper Extremity Bursa and Ligament, Right **B** Upper Extremity Bursa and Ligament, Left **C** Trunk Bursa and Ligament, Right **D** Trunk Bursa and Ligament, Left **F** Thorax Bursa and Ligament, Right **G** Thorax Bursa and Ligament, Left **H** Abdomen Bursa and Ligament, Right **J** Abdomen Bursa and Ligament, Left **K** Perineum Bursa and Ligament **L** Hip Bursa and Ligament, Right **M** Hip Bursa and Ligament, Left **N** Knee Bursa and Ligament, Right **P** Knee Bursa and Ligament, Left **Q** Ankle Bursa and Ligament, Right **R** Ankle Bursa and Ligament, Left **S** Foot Bursa and Ligament, Right **T** Foot Bursa and Ligament, Left **V** Lower Extremity Bursa and Ligament, Right **W** Lower Extremity Bursa and Ligament, Left	**Ø** Open **4** Percutaneous Endoscopic	**Z** No Device	**Z** No Qualifier

        Revised Text in **BLUE**   © 2011 Ingenix, Inc

Ø　Medical and Surgical
M　Bursae and Ligaments
T　Resection　　Cutting out or off, without replacement, all of a body part

Body Part Character 4	Approach Character 5	Device Character 6	Qualifier Character 7
Ø　Head and Neck Bursa and Ligament 1　Shoulder Bursa and Ligament, Right 2　Shoulder Bursa and Ligament, Left 3　Elbow Bursa and Ligament, Right 4　Elbow Bursa and Ligament, Left 5　Wrist Bursa and Ligament, Right 6　Wrist Bursa and Ligament, Left 7　Hand Bursa and Ligament, Right 8　Hand Bursa and Ligament, Left 9　Upper Extremity Bursa and Ligament, Right B　Upper Extremity Bursa and Ligament, Left C　Trunk Bursa and Ligament, Right D　Trunk Bursa and Ligament, Left F　Thorax Bursa and Ligament, Right G　Thorax Bursa and Ligament, Left H　Abdomen Bursa and Ligament, Right J　Abdomen Bursa and Ligament, Left K　Perineum Bursa and Ligament L　Hip Bursa and Ligament, Right M　Hip Bursa and Ligament, Left N　Knee Bursa and Ligament, Right P　Knee Bursa and Ligament, Left Q　Ankle Bursa and Ligament, Right R　Ankle Bursa and Ligament, Left S　Foot Bursa and Ligament, Right T　Foot Bursa and Ligament, Left V　Lower Extremity Bursa and Ligament, Right W　Lower Extremity Bursa and Ligament, Left	Ø　Open 4　Percutaneous Endoscopic	Z　No Device	Z　No Qualifier

Ø　Medical and Surgical
M　Bursae and Ligaments
U　Supplement　　Putting in or on biological or synthetic material that physically reinforces and/or augments the function of a portion of a body part

Body Part Character 4	Approach Character 5	Device Character 6	Qualifier Character 7
Ø　Head and Neck Bursa and Ligament 1　Shoulder Bursa and Ligament, Right 2　Shoulder Bursa and Ligament, Left 3　Elbow Bursa and Ligament, Right 4　Elbow Bursa and Ligament, Left 5　Wrist Bursa and Ligament, Right 6　Wrist Bursa and Ligament, Left 7　Hand Bursa and Ligament, Right 8　Hand Bursa and Ligament, Left 9　Upper Extremity Bursa and Ligament, Right B　Upper Extremity Bursa and Ligament, Left C　Trunk Bursa and Ligament, Right D　Trunk Bursa and Ligament, Left F　Thorax Bursa and Ligament, Right G　Thorax Bursa and Ligament, Left H　Abdomen Bursa and Ligament, Right J　Abdomen Bursa and Ligament, Left K　Perineum Bursa and Ligament L　Hip Bursa and Ligament, Right M　Hip Bursa and Ligament, Left N　Knee Bursa and Ligament, Right P　Knee Bursa and Ligament, Left Q　Ankle Bursa and Ligament, Right R　Ankle Bursa and Ligament, Left S　Foot Bursa and Ligament, Right T　Foot Bursa and Ligament, Left V　Lower Extremity Bursa and Ligament, Right W　Lower Extremity Bursa and Ligament, Left	Ø　Open 4　Percutaneous Endoscopic	7　Autologous Tissue Substitute J　Synthetic Substitute K　Nonautologous Tissue Substitute	Z　No Qualifier

Ø   **Medical and Surgical**
M   **Bursae and Ligaments**
W   **Revision**   Correcting, to the extent possible, a portion of a malfunctioning device or the position of a displaced device

Body Part Character 4	Approach Character 5	Device Character 6	Qualifier Character 7
X Upper Bursa and Ligament **Y** Lower Bursa and Ligament	**Ø** Open **3** Percutaneous **4** Percutaneous Endoscopic **X** External	**Ø** Drainage Device **7** Autologous Tissue Substitute **J** Synthetic Substitute **K** Nonautologous Tissue Substitute	**Z** No Qualifier

Ø   **Medical and Surgical**
M   **Bursae and Ligaments**
X   **Transfer**   Moving, without taking out, all or a portion of a body part to another location to take over the function of all or a portion of a body part

Body Part Character 4	Approach Character 5	Device Character 6	Qualifier Character 7
Ø Head and Neck Bursa and Ligament **1** Shoulder Bursa and Ligament, Right **2** Shoulder Bursa and Ligament, Left **3** Elbow Bursa and Ligament, Right **4** Elbow Bursa and Ligament, Left **5** Wrist Bursa and Ligament, Right **6** Wrist Bursa and Ligament, Left **7** Hand Bursa and Ligament, Right **8** Hand Bursa and Ligament, Left **9** Upper Extremity Bursa and Ligament, Right **B** Upper Extremity Bursa and Ligament, Left **C** Trunk Bursa and Ligament, Right **D** Trunk Bursa and Ligament, Left **F** Thorax Bursa and Ligament, Right **G** Thorax Bursa and Ligament, Left **H** Abdomen Bursa and Ligament, Right **J** Abdomen Bursa and Ligament, Left **K** Perineum Bursa and Ligament **L** Hip Bursa and Ligament, Right **M** Hip Bursa and Ligament, Left **N** Knee Bursa and Ligament, Right **P** Knee Bursa and Ligament, Left **Q** Ankle Bursa and Ligament, Right **R** Ankle Bursa and Ligament, Left **S** Foot Bursa and Ligament, Right **T** Foot Bursa and Ligament, Left **V** Lower Extremity Bursa and Ligament, Right **W** Lower Extremity Bursa and Ligament, Left	**Ø** Open **4** Percutaneous Endoscopic	**Z** No Device	**Z** No Qualifier

      Revised Text in **BLUE**

Head and Facial Bones ØN2–ØNW

Ø   **Medical and Surgical**
N   **Head and Facial Bones**
2   **Change**   Taking out or off a device from a body part and putting back an identical or similar device in or on the same body part without cutting or puncturing the skin or a mucous membrane

Body Part Character 4	Approach Character 5	Device Character 6	Qualifier Character 7
Ø Skull B Nasal Bone W Facial Bone	X External	Ø Drainage Device Y Other Device	Z No Qualifier

Ø   **Medical and Surgical**
N   **Head and Facial Bones**
5   **Destruction**   Physical eradication of all or a portion of a body part by the direct use of energy, force, or a destructive agent

Body Part Character 4	Approach Character 5	Device Character 6	Qualifier Character 7
Ø Skull 1 Frontal Bone, Right 2 Frontal Bone, Left 3 Parietal Bone, Right 4 Parietal Bone, Left 5 Temporal Bone, Right 6 Temporal Bone, Left 7 Occipital Bone, Right 8 Occipital Bone, Left B Nasal Bone C Sphenoid Bone, Right D Sphenoid Bone, Left F Ethmoid Bone, Right G Ethmoid Bone, Left H Lacrimal Bone, Right J Lacrimal Bone, Left K Palatine Bone, Right L Palatine Bone, Left M Zygomatic Bone, Right N Zygomatic Bone, Left P Orbit, Right Q Orbit, Left R Maxilla, Right S Maxilla, Left T Mandible, Right V Mandible, Left X Hyoid Bone	Ø Open 3 Percutaneous 4 Percutaneous Endoscopic	Z No Device	Z No Qualifier

Ø **Medical and Surgical**
N **Head and Facial Bones**
8 **Division**   Cutting into a body part without draining fluids and/or gases from the body part in order to separate or transect a body part

Body Part Character 4	Approach Character 5	Device Character 6	Qualifier Character 7
Ø Skull 1 Frontal Bone, Right 2 Frontal Bone, Left 3 Parietal Bone, Right 4 Parietal Bone, Left 5 Temporal Bone, Right 6 Temporal Bone, Left 7 Occipital Bone, Right 8 Occipital Bone, Left B Nasal Bone C Sphenoid Bone, Right D Sphenoid Bone, Left F Ethmoid Bone, Right G Ethmoid Bone, Left H Lacrimal Bone, Right J Lacrimal Bone, Left K Palatine Bone, Right L Palatine Bone, Left M Zygomatic Bone, Right N Zygomatic Bone, Left P Orbit, Right Q Orbit, Left R Maxilla, Right S Maxilla, Left T Mandible, Right V Mandible, Left X Hyoid Bone	Ø Open 3 Percutaneous 4 Percutaneous Endoscopic	Z No Device	Z No Qualifier

Ø **Medical and Surgical**
N **Head and Facial Bones**
9 **Drainage**   Taking or letting out fluids and/or gases from a body part

Body Part Character 4	Approach Character 5	Device Character 6	Qualifier Character 7
Ø Skull 1 Frontal Bone, Right 2 Frontal Bone, Left 3 Parietal Bone, Right 4 Parietal Bone, Left 5 Temporal Bone, Right 6 Temporal Bone, Left 7 Occipital Bone, Right 8 Occipital Bone, Left B Nasal Bone C Sphenoid Bone, Right D Sphenoid Bone, Left F Ethmoid Bone, Right G Ethmoid Bone, Left H Lacrimal Bone, Right J Lacrimal Bone, Left K Palatine Bone, Right L Palatine Bone, Left M Zygomatic Bone, Right N Zygomatic Bone, Left P Orbit, Right Q Orbit, Left R Maxilla, Right S Maxilla, Left T Mandible, Right V Mandible, Left X Hyoid Bone	Ø Open 3 Percutaneous 4 Percutaneous Endoscopic	Ø Drainage Device	Z No Qualifier

ØN9 Continued on next page

Revised Text in **BLUE**   © 2011 Ingenix, Inc

Ø   Medical and Surgical
N   Head and Facial Bones
9   Drainage   Taking or letting out fluids and/or gases from a body part

ØN9 Continued

Body Part Character 4	Approach Character 5	Device Character 6	Qualifier Character 7
Ø Skull	Ø Open	Z No Device	X Diagnostic
1 Frontal Bone, Right	3 Percutaneous		Z No Qualifier
2 Frontal Bone, Left	4 Percutaneous Endoscopic		
3 Parietal Bone, Right			
4 Parietal Bone, Left			
5 Temporal Bone, Right			
6 Temporal Bone, Left			
7 Occipital Bone, Right			
8 Occipital Bone, Left			
B Nasal Bone			
C Sphenoid Bone, Right			
D Sphenoid Bone, Left			
F Ethmoid Bone, Right			
G Ethmoid Bone, Left			
H Lacrimal Bone, Right			
J Lacrimal Bone, Left			
K Palatine Bone, Right			
L Palatine Bone, Left			
M Zygomatic Bone, Right			
N Zygomatic Bone, Left			
P Orbit, Right			
Q Orbit, Left			
R Maxilla, Right			
S Maxilla, Left			
T Mandible, Right			
V Mandible, Left			
X Hyoid Bone			

Ø   Medical and Surgical
N   Head and Facial Bones
B   Excision   Cutting out or off, without replacement, a portion of a body part

Body Part Character 4	Approach Character 5	Device Character 6	Qualifier Character 7
Ø Skull	Ø Open	Z No Device	X Diagnostic
1 Frontal Bone, Right	3 Percutaneous		Z No Qualifier
2 Frontal Bone, Left	4 Percutaneous Endoscopic		
3 Parietal Bone, Right			
4 Parietal Bone, Left			
5 Temporal Bone, Right			
6 Temporal Bone, Left			
7 Occipital Bone, Right			
8 Occipital Bone, Left			
B Nasal Bone			
C Sphenoid Bone, Right			
D Sphenoid Bone, Left			
F Ethmoid Bone, Right			
G Ethmoid Bone, Left			
H Lacrimal Bone, Right			
J Lacrimal Bone, Left			
K Palatine Bone, Right			
L Palatine Bone, Left			
M Zygomatic Bone, Right			
N Zygomatic Bone, Left			
P Orbit, Right			
Q Orbit, Left			
R Maxilla, Right			
S Maxilla, Left			
T Mandible, Right			
V Mandible, Left			
X Hyoid Bone			

Ø   **Medical and Surgical**
N   **Head and Facial Bones**
C   **Extirpation**   Taking or cutting out solid matter from a body part

Body Part Character 4	Approach Character 5	Device Character 6	Qualifier Character 7
1 Frontal Bone, Right **2** Frontal Bone, Left **3** Parietal Bone, Right **4** Parietal Bone, Left **5** Temporal Bone, Right **6** Temporal Bone, Left **7** Occipital Bone, Right **8** Occipital Bone, Left **B** Nasal Bone **C** Sphenoid Bone, Right **D** Sphenoid Bone, Left **F** Ethmoid Bone, Right **G** Ethmoid Bone, Left **H** Lacrimal Bone, Right **J** Lacrimal Bone, Left **K** Palatine Bone, Right **L** Palatine Bone, Left **M** Zygomatic Bone, Right **N** Zygomatic Bone, Left **P** Orbit, Right **Q** Orbit, Left **R** Maxilla, Right **S** Maxilla, Left **T** Mandible, Right **V** Mandible, Left **X** Hyoid Bone	**Ø** Open **3** Percutaneous **4** Percutaneous Endoscopic	**Z** No Device	**Z** No Qualifier

Ø   **Medical and Surgical**
N   **Head and Facial Bones**
H   **Insertion**   Putting in a nonbiological appliance that monitors, assists, performs, or prevents a physiological function but does not physically take the place of a body part

Body Part Character 4	Approach Character 5	Device Character 6	Qualifier Character 7
Ø Skull	**Ø** Open	**4** Internal Fixation Device **5** External Fixation Device **M** Bone Growth Stimulator **N** **Neurostimulator Generator**	**Z** No Qualifier
Ø Skull	**3** Percutaneous **4** Percutaneous Endoscopic	**4** Internal Fixation Device **5** External Fixation Device **M** Bone Growth Stimulator	**Z** No Qualifier
1 Frontal Bone, Right **2** Frontal Bone, Left **3** Parietal Bone, Right **4** Parietal Bone, Left **7** Occipital Bone, Right **8** Occipital Bone, Left **C** Sphenoid Bone, Right **D** Sphenoid Bone, Left **F** Ethmoid Bone, Right **G** Ethmoid Bone, Left **H** Lacrimal Bone, Right **J** Lacrimal Bone, Left **K** Palatine Bone, Right **L** Palatine Bone, Left **M** Zygomatic Bone, Right **N** Zygomatic Bone, Left **P** Orbit, Right **Q** Orbit, Left **X** Hyoid Bone	**Ø** Open **3** Percutaneous **4** Percutaneous Endoscopic	**4** Internal Fixation Device	**Z** No Qualifier
5 Temporal Bone, Right **6** Temporal Bone, Left	**Ø** Open **3** Percutaneous **4** Percutaneous Endoscopic	**4** Internal Fixation Device **S** Hearing Device	**Z** No Qualifier
B Nasal Bone	**Ø** Open **3** Percutaneous **4** Percutaneous Endoscopic	**4** Internal Fixation Device **M** Bone Growth Stimulator	**Z** No Qualifier
R Maxilla, Right **S** Maxilla, Left **T** Mandible, Right **V** Mandible, Left	**Ø** Open **3** Percutaneous **4** Percutaneous Endoscopic	**4** Internal Fixation Device **5** External Fixation Device	**Z** No Qualifier
W Facial Bone	**Ø** Open **3** Percutaneous **4** Percutaneous Endoscopic	**M** Bone Growth Stimulator	**Z** No Qualifier

Ø　**Medical and Surgical**
N　**Head and Facial Bones**
J　**Inspection**　　Visually and/or manually exploring a body part

Body Part Character 4	Approach Character 5	Device Character 6	Qualifier Character 7
Ø Skull B Nasal Bone W Facial Bone	Ø Open 3 Percutaneous 4 Percutaneous Endoscopic X External	Z No Device	Z No Qualifier

Ø　**Medical and Surgical**
N　**Head and Facial Bones**
N　**Release**　　Freeing a body part from an abnormal physical constraint

Body Part Character 4	Approach Character 5	Device Character 6	Qualifier Character 7
1 Frontal Bone, Right 2 Frontal Bone, Left 3 Parietal Bone, Right 4 Parietal Bone, Left 5 Temporal Bone, Right 6 Temporal Bone, Left 7 Occipital Bone, Right 8 Occipital Bone, Left B Nasal Bone C Sphenoid Bone, Right D Sphenoid Bone, Left F Ethmoid Bone, Right G Ethmoid Bone, Left H Lacrimal Bone, Right J Lacrimal Bone, Left K Palatine Bone, Right L Palatine Bone, Left M Zygomatic Bone, Right N Zygomatic Bone, Left P Orbit, Right Q Orbit, Left R Maxilla, Right S Maxilla, Left T Mandible, Right V Mandible, Left X Hyoid Bone	Ø Open 3 Percutaneous 4 Percutaneous Endoscopic	Z No Device	Z No Qualifier

Ø　**Medical and Surgical**
N　**Head and Facial Bones**
P　**Removal**　　Taking out or off a device from a body part

Body Part Character 4	Approach Character 5	Device Character 6	Qualifier Character 7
Ø Skull	Ø Open	Ø Drainage Device 4 Internal Fixation Device 5 External Fixation Device 7 Autologous Tissue Substitute J Synthetic Substitute K Nonautologous Tissue Substitute M Bone Growth Stimulator **N Neurostimulator Generator** S Hearing Device	Z No Qualifier
Ø Skull	3 Percutaneous 4 Percutaneous Endoscopic	Ø Drainage Device 4 Internal Fixation Device 5 External Fixation Device 7 Autologous Tissue Substitute J Synthetic Substitute K Nonautologous Tissue Substitute M Bone Growth Stimulator S Hearing Device	Z No Qualifier
Ø Skull	X External	Ø Drainage Device 4 Internal Fixation Device 5 External Fixation Device M Bone Growth Stimulator S Hearing Device	Z No Qualifier
B Nasal Bone W Facial Bone	Ø Open 3 Percutaneous 4 Percutaneous Endoscopic	Ø Drainage Device 4 Internal Fixation Device 7 Autologous Tissue Substitute J Synthetic Substitute K Nonautologous Tissue Substitute M Bone Growth Stimulator	Z No Qualifier

ØNP Continued on next page

ØNP Continued

Ø   **Medical and Surgical**
N   **Head and Facial Bones**
P   **Removal**   Taking out or off a device from a body part

Body Part Character 4	Approach Character 5	Device Character 6	Qualifier Character 7
B Nasal Bone **W** Facial Bone	**X** External	**Ø** Drainage Device **4** Internal Fixation Device **M** Bone Growth Stimulator	**Z** No Qualifier

Ø   **Medical and Surgical**
N   **Head and Facial Bones**
Q   **Repair**   Restoring, to the extent possible, a body part to its normal anatomic structure and function

Body Part Character 4	Approach Character 5	Device Character 6	Qualifier Character 7
Ø Skull **1** Frontal Bone, Right **2** Frontal Bone, Left **3** Parietal Bone, Right **4** Parietal Bone, Left **5** Temporal Bone, Right **6** Temporal Bone, Left **7** Occipital Bone, Right **8** Occipital Bone, Left **B** Nasal Bone **C** Sphenoid Bone, Right **D** Sphenoid Bone, Left **F** Ethmoid Bone, Right **G** Ethmoid Bone, Left **H** Lacrimal Bone, Right **J** Lacrimal Bone, Left **K** Palatine Bone, Right **L** Palatine Bone, Left **M** Zygomatic Bone, Right **N** Zygomatic Bone, Left **P** Orbit, Right **Q** Orbit, Left **R** Maxilla, Right **S** Maxilla, Left **T** Mandible, Right **V** Mandible, Left **X** Hyoid Bone	**Ø** Open **3** Percutaneous **4** Percutaneous Endoscopic **X** External	**Z** No Device	**Z** No Qualifier

Ø   **Medical and Surgical**
N   **Head and Facial Bones**
R   **Replacement**   Putting in or on biological or synthetic material that physically takes the place and/or function of all or a portion of a body part

Body Part Character 4	Approach Character 5	Device Character 6	Qualifier Character 7
Ø Skull **1** Frontal Bone, Right **2** Frontal Bone, Left **3** Parietal Bone, Right **4** Parietal Bone, Left **5** Temporal Bone, Right **6** Temporal Bone, Left **7** Occipital Bone, Right **8** Occipital Bone, Left **B** Nasal Bone **C** Sphenoid Bone, Right **D** Sphenoid Bone, Left **F** Ethmoid Bone, Right **G** Ethmoid Bone, Left **H** Lacrimal Bone, Right **J** Lacrimal Bone, Left **K** Palatine Bone, Right **L** Palatine Bone, Left **M** Zygomatic Bone, Right **N** Zygomatic Bone, Left **P** Orbit, Right **Q** Orbit, Left **R** Maxilla, Right **S** Maxilla, Left **T** Mandible, Right **V** Mandible, Left **X** Hyoid Bone	**Ø** Open **3** Percutaneous **4** Percutaneous Endoscopic	**7** Autologous Tissue Substitute **J** Synthetic Substitute **K** Nonautologous Tissue Substitute	**Z** No Qualifier

         Revised Text in **BLUE**

Ø   **Medical and Surgical**
N   **Head and Facial Bones**
S   **Reposition**   Moving to its normal location or other suitable location all or a portion of a body part

Body Part Character 4	Approach Character 5	Device Character 6	Qualifier Character 7
Ø Skull **1** Frontal Bone, Right **2** Frontal Bone, Left **3** Parietal Bone, Right **4** Parietal Bone, Left **5** Temporal Bone, Right **6** Temporal Bone, Left **7** Occipital Bone, Right **8** Occipital Bone, Left **B** Nasal Bone **C** Sphenoid Bone, Right **D** Sphenoid Bone, Left **F** Ethmoid Bone, Right **G** Ethmoid Bone, Left **H** Lacrimal Bone, Right **J** Lacrimal Bone, Left **K** Palatine Bone, Right **L** Palatine Bone, Left **M** Zygomatic Bone, Right **N** Zygomatic Bone, Left **P** Orbit, Right **Q** Orbit, Left **R** Maxilla, Right **S** Maxilla, Left **T** Mandible, Right **V** Mandible, Left **X** Hyoid Bone	**X** External	**Z** No Device	**Z** No Qualifier
Ø Skull **R** Maxilla, Right **S** Maxilla, Left **T** Mandible, Right **V** Mandible, Left	**Ø** Open **3** Percutaneous **4** Percutaneous Endoscopic	**4** Internal Fixation Device **5** External Fixation Device **Z** No Device	**Z** No Qualifier
1 Frontal Bone, Right **2** Frontal Bone, Left **3** Parietal Bone, Right **4** Parietal Bone, Left **5** Temporal Bone, Right **6** Temporal Bone, Left **7** Occipital Bone, Right **8** Occipital Bone, Left **B** Nasal Bone **C** Sphenoid Bone, Right **D** Sphenoid Bone, Left **F** Ethmoid Bone, Right **G** Ethmoid Bone, Left **H** Lacrimal Bone, Right **J** Lacrimal Bone, Left **K** Palatine Bone, Right **L** Palatine Bone, Left **M** Zygomatic Bone, Right **N** Zygomatic Bone, Left **P** Orbit, Right **Q** Orbit, Left **X** Hyoid Bone	**Ø** Open **3** Percutaneous **4** Percutaneous Endoscopic	**4** Internal Fixation Device **Z** No Device	**Z** No Qualifier

Ø   **Medical and Surgical**
N   **Head and Facial Bones**
T   **Resection**   Cutting out or off, without replacement, all of a body part

Body Part Character 4	Approach Character 5	Device Character 6	Qualifier Character 7
1 Frontal Bone, Right 2 Frontal Bone, Left 3 Parietal Bone, Right 4 Parietal Bone, Left 5 Temporal Bone, Right 6 Temporal Bone, Left 7 Occipital Bone, Right 8 Occipital Bone, Left B Nasal Bone C Sphenoid Bone, Right D Sphenoid Bone, Left F Ethmoid Bone, Right G Ethmoid Bone, Left H Lacrimal Bone, Right J Lacrimal Bone, Left K Palatine Bone, Right L Palatine Bone, Left M Zygomatic Bone, Right N Zygomatic Bone, Left P Orbit, Right Q Orbit, Left R Maxilla, Right S Maxilla, Left T Mandible, Right V Mandible, Left X Hyoid Bone	Ø Open	Z No Device	Z No Qualifier

Ø   **Medical and Surgical**
N   **Head and Facial Bones**
U   **Supplement**   Putting in or on biological or synthetic material that physically reinforces and/or augments the function of a portion of a body part

Body Part Character 4	Approach Character 5	Device Character 6	Qualifier Character 7
Ø Skull 1 Frontal Bone, Right 2 Frontal Bone, Left 3 Parietal Bone, Right 4 Parietal Bone, Left 5 Temporal Bone, Right 6 Temporal Bone, Left 7 Occipital Bone, Right 8 Occipital Bone, Left B Nasal Bone C Sphenoid Bone, Right D Sphenoid Bone, Left F Ethmoid Bone, Right G Ethmoid Bone, Left H Lacrimal Bone, Right J Lacrimal Bone, Left K Palatine Bone, Right L Palatine Bone, Left M Zygomatic Bone, Right N Zygomatic Bone, Left P Orbit, Right Q Orbit, Left R Maxilla, Right S Maxilla, Left T Mandible, Right V Mandible, Left X Hyoid Bone	Ø Open 3 Percutaneous 4 Percutaneous Endoscopic	7 Autologous Tissue Substitute J Synthetic Substitute K Nonautologous Tissue Substitute	Z No Qualifier

Revised Text in **BLUE**

Ø   Medical and Surgical
N   Head and Facial Bones
W   Revision   Correcting, to the extent possible, a portion of a malfunctioning device or the position of a displaced device

Body Part Character 4	Approach Character 5	Device Character 6	Qualifier Character 7
Ø Skull	Ø Open	Ø Drainage Device 4 Internal Fixation Device 5 External Fixation Device 7 Autologous Tissue Substitute J Synthetic Substitute K Nonautologous Tissue Substitute M Bone Growth Stimulator N **Neurostimulator Generator** S Hearing Device	Z No Qualifier
Ø Skull	3 Percutaneous 4 Percutaneous Endoscopic X External	Ø Drainage Device 4 Internal Fixation Device 5 External Fixation Device 7 Autologous Tissue Substitute J Synthetic Substitute K Nonautologous Tissue Substitute M Bone Growth Stimulator S Hearing Device	Z No Qualifier
B Nasal Bone W Facial Bone	Ø Open 3 Percutaneous 4 Percutaneous Endoscopic X External	Ø Drainage Device 4 Internal Fixation Device 7 Autologous Tissue Substitute J Synthetic Substitute K Nonautologous Tissue Substitute M Bone Growth Stimulator	Z No Qualifier

Upper Bones ØP2–ØPW

Ø   **Medical and Surgical**
P   **Upper Bones**
2   **Change**   Taking out or off a device from a body part and putting back an identical or similar device in or on the same body part without cutting or puncturing the skin or a mucous membrane

Body Part Character 4	Approach Character 5	Device Character 6	Qualifier Character 7
Y Upper Bone	**X** External	**Ø** Drainage Device **Y** Other Device	**Z** No Qualifier

Ø   **Medical and Surgical**
P   **Upper Bones**
5   **Destruction**   Physical eradication of all or a portion of a body part by the direct use of energy, force, or a destructive agent

Body Part Character 4	Approach Character 5	Device Character 6	Qualifier Character 7
Ø Sternum **1** Rib, Right **2** Rib, Left **3** Cervical Vertebra **4** Thoracic Vertebra **5** Scapula, Right **6** Scapula, Left **7** Glenoid Cavity, Right **8** Glenoid Cavity, Left **9** Clavicle, Right **B** Clavicle, Left **C** Humeral Head, Right **D** Humeral Head, Left **F** Humeral Shaft, Right **G** Humeral Shaft, Left **H** Radius, Right **J** Radius, Left **K** Ulna, Right **L** Ulna, Left **M** Carpal, Right **N** Carpal, Left **P** Metacarpal, Right **Q** Metacarpal, Left **R** Thumb Phalanx, Right **S** Thumb Phalanx, Left **T** Finger Phalanx, Right **V** Finger Phalanx, Left	**Ø** Open **3** Percutaneous **4** Percutaneous Endoscopic	**Z** No Device	**Z** No Qualifier

Ø   **Medical and Surgical**
P   **Upper Bones**
8   **Division**   Cutting into a body part without draining fluids and/or gases from the body part in order to separate or transect a body part

Body Part Character 4	Approach Character 5	Device Character 6	Qualifier Character 7
Ø Sternum **1** Rib, Right **2** Rib, Left **3** Cervical Vertebra **4** Thoracic Vertebra **5** Scapula, Right **6** Scapula, Left **7** Glenoid Cavity, Right **8** Glenoid Cavity, Left **9** Clavicle, Right **B** Clavicle, Left **C** Humeral Head, Right **D** Humeral Head, Left **F** Humeral Shaft, Right **G** Humeral Shaft, Left **H** Radius, Right **J** Radius, Left **K** Ulna, Right **L** Ulna, Left **M** Carpal, Right **N** Carpal, Left **P** Metacarpal, Right **Q** Metacarpal, Left **R** Thumb Phalanx, Right **S** Thumb Phalanx, Left **T** Finger Phalanx, Right **V** Finger Phalanx, Left	**Ø** Open **3** Percutaneous **4** Percutaneous Endoscopic	**Z** No Device	**Z** No Qualifier

0   **Medical and Surgical**
P   **Upper Bones**
9   **Drainage**   Taking or letting out fluids and/or gases from a body part

Body Part Character 4	Approach Character 5	Device Character 6	Qualifier Character 7
0 Sternum **1** Rib, Right **2** Rib, Left **3** Cervical Vertebra **4** Thoracic Vertebra **5** Scapula, Right **6** Scapula, Left **7** Glenoid Cavity, Right **8** Glenoid Cavity, Left **9** Clavicle, Right **B** Clavicle, Left **C** Humeral Head, Right **D** Humeral Head, Left **F** Humeral Shaft, Right **G** Humeral Shaft, Left **H** Radius, Right **J** Radius, Left **K** Ulna, Right **L** Ulna, Left **M** Carpal, Right **N** Carpal, Left **P** Metacarpal, Right **Q** Metacarpal, Left **R** Thumb Phalanx, Right **S** Thumb Phalanx, Left **T** Finger Phalanx, Right **V** Finger Phalanx, Left	**0** Open **3** Percutaneous **4** Percutaneous Endoscopic	**0** Drainage Device	**Z** No Qualifier
0 Sternum **1** Rib, Right **2** Rib, Left **3** Cervical Vertebra **4** Thoracic Vertebra **5** Scapula, Right **6** Scapula, Left **7** Glenoid Cavity, Right **8** Glenoid Cavity, Left **9** Clavicle, Right **B** Clavicle, Left **C** Humeral Head, Right **D** Humeral Head, Left **F** Humeral Shaft, Right **G** Humeral Shaft, Left **H** Radius, Right **J** Radius, Left **K** Ulna, Right **L** Ulna, Left **M** Carpal, Right **N** Carpal, Left **P** Metacarpal, Right **Q** Metacarpal, Left **R** Thumb Phalanx, Right **S** Thumb Phalanx, Left **T** Finger Phalanx, Right **V** Finger Phalanx, Left	**0** Open **3** Percutaneous **4** Percutaneous Endoscopic	**Z** No Device	**X** Diagnostic **Z** No Qualifier

Ø   **Medical and Surgical**
P   **Upper Bones**
B   **Excision**   Cutting out or off, without replacement, a portion of a body part

Body Part Character 4	Approach Character 5	Device Character 6	Qualifier Character 7
Ø Sternum 1 Rib, Right 2 Rib, Left 3 Cervical Vertebra 4 Thoracic Vertebra 5 Scapula, Right 6 Scapula, Left 7 Glenoid Cavity, Right 8 Glenoid Cavity, Left 9 Clavicle, Right B Clavicle, Left C Humeral Head, Right D Humeral Head, Left F Humeral Shaft, Right G Humeral Shaft, Left H Radius, Right J Radius, Left K Ulna, Right L Ulna, Left M Carpal, Right N Carpal, Left P Metacarpal, Right Q Metacarpal, Left R Thumb Phalanx, Right S Thumb Phalanx, Left T Finger Phalanx, Right V Finger Phalanx, Left	Ø Open 3 Percutaneous 4 Percutaneous Endoscopic	Z No Device	X Diagnostic Z No Qualifier

Ø   **Medical and Surgical**
P   **Upper Bones**
C   **Extirpation**   Taking or cutting out solid matter from a body part

Body Part Character 4	Approach Character 5	Device Character 6	Qualifier Character 7
Ø Sternum 1 Rib, Right 2 Rib, Left 3 Cervical Vertebra 4 Thoracic Vertebra 5 Scapula, Right 6 Scapula, Left 7 Glenoid Cavity, Right 8 Glenoid Cavity, Left 9 Clavicle, Right B Clavicle, Left C Humeral Head, Right D Humeral Head, Left F Humeral Shaft, Right G Humeral Shaft, Left H Radius, Right J Radius, Left K Ulna, Right L Ulna, Left M Carpal, Right N Carpal, Left P Metacarpal, Right Q Metacarpal, Left R Thumb Phalanx, Right S Thumb Phalanx, Left T Finger Phalanx, Right V Finger Phalanx, Left	Ø Open 3 Percutaneous 4 Percutaneous Endoscopic	Z No Device	Z No Qualifier

Ø   **Medical and Surgical**
P   **Upper Bones**
H   **Insertion**   Putting in a nonbiological appliance that monitors, assists, performs, or prevents a physiological function but does not physically take the place of a body part

Body Part Character 4	Approach Character 5	Device Character 6	Qualifier Character 7
Ø Sternum	Ø Open 3 Percutaneous 4 Percutaneous Endoscopic	4 Internal Fixation Device	8 **Rigid Plate** Z No Qualifier
1 Rib, Right 2 Rib, Left 3 Cervical Vertebra 4 Thoracic Vertebra 5 Scapula, Right 6 Scapula, Left 7 Glenoid Cavity, Right 8 Glenoid Cavity, Left 9 Clavicle, Right B Clavicle, Left	Ø Open 3 Percutaneous 4 Percutaneous Endoscopic	4 Internal Fixation Device	Z No Qualifier
C Humeral Head, Right D Humeral Head, Left F Humeral Shaft, Right G Humeral Shaft, Left H Radius, Right J Radius, Left K Ulna, Right L Ulna, Left	Ø Open 3 Percutaneous 4 Percutaneous Endoscopic	4 Internal Fixation Device 6 Intramedullary Fixation Device	Z No Qualifier
C Humeral Head, Right D Humeral Head, Left F Humeral Shaft, Right G Humeral Shaft, Left H Radius, Right J Radius, Left K Ulna, Right L Ulna, Left	Ø Open 3 Percutaneous 4 Percutaneous Endoscopic	5 External Fixation Device	3 Monoplanar 4 Ring 5 Hybrid 9 Limb Lengthening Device Z No Qualifier
M Carpal, Right N Carpal, Left P Metacarpal, Right Q Metacarpal, Left R Thumb Phalanx, Right S Thumb Phalanx, Left T Finger Phalanx, Right V Finger Phalanx, Left	Ø Open 3 Percutaneous 4 Percutaneous Endoscopic	4 Internal Fixation Device 5 External Fixation Device	Z No Qualifier

Ø   **Medical and Surgical**
P   **Upper Bones**
J   **Inspection**   Visually and/or manually exploring a body part

Body Part Character 4	Approach Character 5	Device Character 6	Qualifier Character 7
Y Upper Bone	Ø Open 3 Percutaneous 4 Percutaneous Endoscopic X External	Z No Device	Z No Qualifier

Ø   **Medical and Surgical**
P   **Upper Bones**
N   **Release**   Freeing a body part from an abnormal physical constraint

Body Part Character 4	Approach Character 5	Device Character 6	Qualifier Character 7
Ø Sternum **1** Rib, Right **2** Rib, Left **3** Cervical Vertebra **4** Thoracic Vertebra **5** Scapula, Right **6** Scapula, Left **7** Glenoid Cavity, Right **8** Glenoid Cavity, Left **9** Clavicle, Right **B** Clavicle, Left **C** Humeral Head, Right **D** Humeral Head, Left **F** Humeral Shaft, Right **G** Humeral Shaft, Left **H** Radius, Right **J** Radius, Left **K** Ulna, Right **L** Ulna, Left **M** Carpal, Right **N** Carpal, Left **P** Metacarpal, Right **Q** Metacarpal, Left **R** Thumb Phalanx, Right **S** Thumb Phalanx, Left **T** Finger Phalanx, Right **V** Finger Phalanx, Left	**Ø** Open **3** Percutaneous **4** Percutaneous Endoscopic	**Z** No Device	**Z** No Qualifier

Ø   **Medical and Surgical**
P   **Upper Bones**
P   **Removal**   Taking out or off a device from a body part

Body Part Character 4	Approach Character 5	Device Character 6	Qualifier Character 7
Ø Sternum **1** Rib, Right **2** Rib, Left **3** Cervical Vertebra **4** Thoracic Vertebra **5** Scapula, Right **6** Scapula, Left **7** Glenoid Cavity, Right **8** Glenoid Cavity, Left **9** Clavicle, Right **B** Clavicle, Left	**Ø** Open **3** Percutaneous **4** Percutaneous Endoscopic	**4** Internal Fixation Device **7** Autologous Tissue Substitute **J** Synthetic Substitute **K** Nonautologous Tissue Substitute	**Z** No Qualifier
Ø Sternum **1** Rib, Right **2** Rib, Left **3** Cervical Vertebra **4** Thoracic Vertebra **5** Scapula, Right **6** Scapula, Left **7** Glenoid Cavity, Right **8** Glenoid Cavity, Left **9** Clavicle, Right **B** Clavicle, Left	**X** External	**4** Internal Fixation Device	**Z** No Qualifier
C Humeral Head, Right **D** Humeral Head, Left **F** Humeral Shaft, Right **G** Humeral Shaft, Left **H** Radius, Right **J** Radius, Left **K** Ulna, Right **L** Ulna, Left	**Ø** Open **3** Percutaneous **4** Percutaneous Endoscopic	**4** Internal Fixation Device **5** External Fixation Device **6** Intramedullary Fixation Device **7** Autologous Tissue Substitute **J** Synthetic Substitute **K** Nonautologous Tissue Substitute	**Z** No Qualifier

ØPP Continued on next page

Ø   **Medical and Surgical**   *ØPP Continued*
P   **Upper Bones**
P   **Removal**   Taking out or off a device from a body part

Body Part Character 4	Approach Character 5	Device Character 6	Qualifier Character 7
C Humeral Head, Right **D** Humeral Head, Left **F** Humeral Shaft, Right **G** Humeral Shaft, Left **H** Radius, Right **J** Radius, Left **K** Ulna, Right **L** Ulna, Left **M** Carpal, Right **N** Carpal, Left **P** Metacarpal, Right **Q** Metacarpal, Left **R** Thumb Phalanx, Right **S** Thumb Phalanx, Left **T** Finger Phalanx, Right **V** Finger Phalanx, Left	**X** External	**4** Internal Fixation Device **5** External Fixation Device	**Z** No Qualifier
M Carpal, Right **N** Carpal, Left **P** Metacarpal, Right **Q** Metacarpal, Left **R** Thumb Phalanx, Right **S** Thumb Phalanx, Left **T** Finger Phalanx, Right **V** Finger Phalanx, Left	**Ø** Open **3** Percutaneous **4** Percutaneous Endoscopic	**4** Internal Fixation Device **5** External Fixation Device **7** Autologous Tissue Substitute **J** Synthetic Substitute **K** Nonautologous Tissue Substitute	**Z** No Qualifier
Y Upper Bone	**Ø** Open **3** Percutaneous **4** Percutaneous Endoscopic **X** External	**Ø** Drainage Device **M** Bone Growth Stimulator	**Z** No Qualifier

Ø   **Medical and Surgical**
P   **Upper Bones**
Q   **Repair**   Restoring, to the extent possible, a body part to its normal anatomic structure and function

Body Part Character 4	Approach Character 5	Device Character 6	Qualifier Character 7
Ø Sternum **1** Rib, Right **2** Rib, Left **3** Cervical Vertebra **4** Thoracic Vertebra **5** Scapula, Right **6** Scapula, Left **7** Glenoid Cavity, Right **8** Glenoid Cavity, Left **9** Clavicle, Right **B** Clavicle, Left **C** Humeral Head, Right **D** Humeral Head, Left **F** Humeral Shaft, Right **G** Humeral Shaft, Left **H** Radius, Right **J** Radius, Left **K** Ulna, Right **L** Ulna, Left **M** Carpal, Right **N** Carpal, Left **P** Metacarpal, Right **Q** Metacarpal, Left **R** Thumb Phalanx, Right **S** Thumb Phalanx, Left **T** Finger Phalanx, Right **V** Finger Phalanx, Left	**Ø** Open **3** Percutaneous **4** Percutaneous Endoscopic **X** External	**Z** No Device	**Z** No Qualifier

Upper Bones

ØPR–ØPS

Ø   Medical and Surgical
P   Upper Bones
R   Replacement   Putting in or on biological or synthetic material that physically takes the place and/or function of all or a portion of a body part

Body Part Character 4	Approach Character 5	Device Character 6	Qualifier Character 7
Ø Sternum 1 Rib, Right 2 Rib, Left 3 Cervical Vertebra 4 Thoracic Vertebra 5 Scapula, Right 6 Scapula, Left 7 Glenoid Cavity, Right 8 Glenoid Cavity, Left 9 Clavicle, Right B Clavicle, Left C Humeral Head, Right D Humeral Head, Left F Humeral Shaft, Right G Humeral Shaft, Left H Radius, Right J Radius, Left K Ulna, Right L Ulna, Left M Carpal, Right N Carpal, Left P Metacarpal, Right Q Metacarpal, Left R Thumb Phalanx, Right S Thumb Phalanx, Left T Finger Phalanx, Right V Finger Phalanx, Left	Ø Open 3 Percutaneous 4 Percutaneous Endoscopic	7 Autologous Tissue Substitute J Synthetic Substitute K Nonautologous Tissue Substitute	Z No Qualifier

Ø   Medical and Surgical
P   Upper Bones
S   Reposition   Moving to its normal location or other suitable location all or a portion of a body part

Body Part Character 4	Approach Character 5	Device Character 6	Qualifier Character 7
Ø Sternum	Ø Open 3 Percutaneous 4 Percutaneous Endoscopic	4 Internal Fixation Device	8 **Rigid Plate** Z No Qualifier
Ø Sternum	Ø Open 3 Percutaneous 4 Percutaneous Endoscopic	Z No Device	Z No Qualifier
1 Rib, Right 2 Rib, Left 3 Cervical Vertebra 4 Thoracic Vertebra 5 Scapula, Right 6 Scapula, Left 7 Glenoid Cavity, Right 8 Glenoid Cavity, Left 9 Clavicle, Right B Clavicle, Left	Ø Open 3 Percutaneous 4 Percutaneous Endoscopic	4 Internal Fixation Device Z No Device	Z No Qualifier
Ø Sternum 1 Rib, Right 2 Rib, Left 3 Cervical Vertebra 4 Thoracic Vertebra 5 Scapula, Right 6 Scapula, Left 7 Glenoid Cavity, Right 8 Glenoid Cavity, Left 9 Clavicle, Right B Clavicle, Left	X External	Z No Device	Z No Qualifier
C Humeral Head, Right D Humeral Head, Left F Humeral Shaft, Right G Humeral Shaft, Left H Radius, Right J Radius, Left K Ulna, Right L Ulna, Left	Ø Open 3 Percutaneous 4 Percutaneous Endoscopic	4 Internal Fixation Device 6 Intramedullary Fixation Device Z No Device	Z No Qualifier

ØPS Continued on next page

© 2011 Ingenix, Inc

0   **Medical and Surgical**   *0PS Continued*
P   **Upper Bones**
S   **Reposition**   Moving to its normal location or other suitable location all or a portion of a body part

Body Part Character 4	Approach Character 5	Device Character 6	Qualifier Character 7
C Humeral Head, Right **D** Humeral Head, Left **F** Humeral Shaft, Right **G** Humeral Shaft, Left **H** Radius, Right **J** Radius, Left **K** Ulna, Right **L** Ulna, Left	**0** Open **3** Percutaneous **4** Percutaneous Endoscopic	**5** External Fixation Device	**3** Monoplanar **4** Ring **5** Hybrid **Z** No Qualifier
C Humeral Head, Right **D** Humeral Head, Left **F** Humeral Shaft, Right **G** Humeral Shaft, Left **H** Radius, Right **J** Radius, Left **K** Ulna, Right **L** Ulna, Left	**X** External	**Z** No Device	**Z** No Qualifier
M Carpal, Right **N** Carpal, Left **P** Metacarpal, Right **Q** Metacarpal, Left **R** Thumb Phalanx, Right **S** Thumb Phalanx, Left **T** Finger Phalanx, Right **V** Finger Phalanx, Left	**0** Open **3** Percutaneous **4** Percutaneous Endoscopic	**4** Internal Fixation Device **Z** No Device	**Z** No Qualifier
M Carpal, Right **N** Carpal, Left **P** Metacarpal, Right **Q** Metacarpal, Left **R** Thumb Phalanx, Right **S** Thumb Phalanx, Left **T** Finger Phalanx, Right **V** Finger Phalanx, Left	**0** Open **3** Percutaneous **4** Percutaneous Endoscopic	**5** External Fixation Device	**3** Monoplanar **4** Ring **5** Hybrid **Z** No Qualifier

0   **Medical and Surgical**
P   **Upper Bones**
T   **Resection**   Cutting out or off, without replacement, all of a body part

Body Part Character 4	Approach Character 5	Device Character 6	Qualifier Character 7
0 Sternum **1** Rib, Right **2** Rib, Left **5** Scapula, Right **6** Scapula, Left **7** Glenoid Cavity, Right **8** Glenoid Cavity, Left **9** Clavicle, Right **B** Clavicle, Left **C** Humeral Head, Right **D** Humeral Head, Left **F** Humeral Shaft, Right **G** Humeral Shaft, Left **H** Radius, Right **J** Radius, Left **K** Ulna, Right **L** Ulna, Left **M** Carpal, Right **N** Carpal, Left **P** Metacarpal, Right **Q** Metacarpal, Left **R** Thumb Phalanx, Right **S** Thumb Phalanx, Left **T** Finger Phalanx, Right **V** Finger Phalanx, Left	**0** Open	**Z** No Device	**Z** No Qualifier

Ø   Medical and Surgical
P   Upper Bones
U   Supplement   Putting in or on biological or synthetic material that physically reinforces and/or augments the function of a portion of a body part

Body Part Character 4	Approach Character 5	Device Character 6	Qualifier Character 7
Ø Sternum **1** Rib, Right **2** Rib, Left **3** Cervical Vertebra **4** Thoracic Vertebra **5** Scapula, Right **6** Scapula, Left **7** Glenoid Cavity, Right **8** Glenoid Cavity, Left **9** Clavicle, Right **B** Clavicle, Left **C** Humeral Head, Right **D** Humeral Head, Left **F** Humeral Shaft, Right **G** Humeral Shaft, Left **H** Radius, Right **J** Radius, Left **K** Ulna, Right **L** Ulna, Left **M** Carpal, Right **N** Carpal, Left **P** Metacarpal, Right **Q** Metacarpal, Left **R** Thumb Phalanx, Right **S** Thumb Phalanx, Left **T** Finger Phalanx, Right **V** Finger Phalanx, Left	**Ø** Open **3** Percutaneous **4** Percutaneous Endoscopic	**7** Autologous Tissue Substitute **J** Synthetic Substitute **K** Nonautologous Tissue Substitute	**Z** No Qualifier

Ø   Medical and Surgical
P   Upper Bones
W   Revision   Correcting, to the extent possible, a portion of a malfunctioning device or the position of a displaced device

Body Part Character 4	Approach Character 5	Device Character 6	Qualifier Character 7
Ø Sternum **1** Rib, Right **2** Rib, Left **3** Cervical Vertebra **4** Thoracic Vertebra **5** Scapula, Right **6** Scapula, Left **7** Glenoid Cavity, Right **8** Glenoid Cavity, Left **9** Clavicle, Right **B** Clavicle, Left	**Ø** Open **3** Percutaneous **4** Percutaneous Endoscopic **X** External	**4** Internal Fixation Device **7** Autologous Tissue Substitute **J** Synthetic Substitute **K** Nonautologous Tissue Substitute	**Z** No Qualifier
C Humeral Head, Right **D** Humeral Head, Left **F** Humeral Shaft, Right **G** Humeral Shaft, Left **H** Radius, Right **J** Radius, Left **K** Ulna, Right **L** Ulna, Left	**Ø** Open **3** Percutaneous **4** Percutaneous Endoscopic **X** External	**4** Internal Fixation Device **5** External Fixation Device **6** Intramedullary Fixation Device **7** Autologous Tissue Substitute **J** Synthetic Substitute **K** Nonautologous Tissue Substitute	**Z** No Qualifier
M Carpal, Right **N** Carpal, Left **P** Metacarpal, Right **Q** Metacarpal, Left **R** Thumb Phalanx, Right **S** Thumb Phalanx, Left **T** Finger Phalanx, Right **V** Finger Phalanx, Left	**Ø** Open **3** Percutaneous **4** Percutaneous Endoscopic **X** External	**4** Internal Fixation Device **5** External Fixation Device **7** Autologous Tissue Substitute **J** Synthetic Substitute **K** Nonautologous Tissue Substitute	**Z** No Qualifier
Y Upper Bone	**Ø** Open **3** Percutaneous **4** Percutaneous Endoscopic **X** External	**Ø** Drainage Device **M** Bone Growth Stimulator	**Z** No Qualifier

Lower Bones 0Q2–0QW

0　Medical and Surgical
Q　Lower Bones
2　Change　　Taking out or off a device from a body part and putting back an identical or similar device in or on the same body part without cutting or puncturing the skin or a mucous membrane

Body Part Character 4	Approach Character 5	Device Character 6	Qualifier Character 7
Y　Lower Bone	X　External	0　Drainage Device Y　Other Device	Z　No Qualifier

0　Medical and Surgical
Q　Lower Bones
5　Destruction　　Physical eradication of all or a portion of a body part by the direct use of energy, force, or a destructive agent

Body Part Character 4	Approach Character 5	Device Character 6	Qualifier Character 7
0　Lumbar Vertebra 1　Sacrum 2　Pelvic Bone, Right 3　Pelvic Bone, Left 4　Acetabulum, Right 5　Acetabulum, Left 6　Upper Femur, Right 7　Upper Femur, Left 8　Femoral Shaft, Right 9　Femoral Shaft, Left B　Lower Femur, Right C　Lower Femur, Left D　Patella, Right F　Patella, Left G　Tibia, Right H　Tibia, Left J　Fibula, Right K　Fibula, Left L　Tarsal, Right M　Tarsal, Left N　Metatarsal, Right P　Metatarsal, Left Q　Toe Phalanx, Right R　Toe Phalanx, Left S　Coccyx	0　Open 3　Percutaneous 4　Percutaneous Endoscopic	Z　No Device	Z　No Qualifier

0　Medical and Surgical
Q　Lower Bones
8　Division　　Cutting into a body part without draining fluids and/or gases from the body part in order to separate or transect a body part

Body Part Character 4	Approach Character 5	Device Character 6	Qualifier Character 7
0　Lumbar Vertebra 1　Sacrum 2　Pelvic Bone, Right 3　Pelvic Bone, Left 4　Acetabulum, Right 5　Acetabulum, Left 6　Upper Femur, Right 7　Upper Femur, Left 8　Femoral Shaft, Right 9　Femoral Shaft, Left B　Lower Femur, Right C　Lower Femur, Left D　Patella, Right F　Patella, Left G　Tibia, Right H　Tibia, Left J　Fibula, Right K　Fibula, Left L　Tarsal, Right M　Tarsal, Left N　Metatarsal, Right P　Metatarsal, Left Q　Toe Phalanx, Right R　Toe Phalanx, Left S　Coccyx	0　Open 3　Percutaneous 4　Percutaneous Endoscopic	Z　No Device	Z　No Qualifier

Ø   Medical and Surgical
Q   Lower Bones
9   Drainage   Taking or letting out fluids and/or gases from a body part

Body Part Character 4	Approach Character 5	Device Character 6	Qualifier Character 7
Ø Lumbar Vertebra 1 Sacrum 2 Pelvic Bone, Right 3 Pelvic Bone, Left 4 Acetabulum, Right 5 Acetabulum, Left 6 Upper Femur, Right 7 Upper Femur, Left 8 Femoral Shaft, Right 9 Femoral Shaft, Left B Lower Femur, Right C Lower Femur, Left D Patella, Right F Patella, Left G Tibia, Right H Tibia, Left J Fibula, Right K Fibula, Left L Tarsal, Right M Tarsal, Left N Metatarsal, Right P Metatarsal, Left Q Toe Phalanx, Right R Toe Phalanx, Left S Coccyx	Ø Open 3 Percutaneous 4 Percutaneous Endoscopic	Ø Drainage Device	Z No Qualifier
Ø Lumbar Vertebra 1 Sacrum 2 Pelvic Bone, Right 3 Pelvic Bone, Left 4 Acetabulum, Right 5 Acetabulum, Left 6 Upper Femur, Right 7 Upper Femur, Left 8 Femoral Shaft, Right 9 Femoral Shaft, Left B Lower Femur, Right C Lower Femur, Left D Patella, Right F Patella, Left G Tibia, Right H Tibia, Left J Fibula, Right K Fibula, Left L Tarsal, Right M Tarsal, Left N Metatarsal, Right P Metatarsal, Left Q Toe Phalanx, Right R Toe Phalanx, Left S Coccyx	Ø Open 3 Percutaneous 4 Percutaneous Endoscopic	Z No Device	X Diagnostic Z No Qualifier

Revised Text in **BLUE**

0　Medical and Surgical
Q　Lower Bones
B　Excision　　　Cutting out or off, without replacement, a portion of a body part

Body Part Character 4	Approach Character 5	Device Character 6	Qualifier Character 7
0　Lumbar Vertebra 1　Sacrum 2　Pelvic Bone, Right 3　Pelvic Bone, Left 4　Acetabulum, Right 5　Acetabulum, Left 6　Upper Femur, Right 7　Upper Femur, Left 8　Femoral Shaft, Right 9　Femoral Shaft, Left B　Lower Femur, Right C　Lower Femur, Left D　Patella, Right F　Patella, Left G　Tibia, Right H　Tibia, Left J　Fibula, Right K　Fibula, Left L　Tarsal, Right M　Tarsal, Left N　Metatarsal, Right P　Metatarsal, Left Q　Toe Phalanx, Right R　Toe Phalanx, Left S　Coccyx	0　Open 3　Percutaneous 4　Percutaneous Endoscopic	Z　No Device	X　Diagnostic Z　No Qualifier

0　Medical and Surgical
Q　Lower Bones
C　Extirpation　　　Taking or cutting out solid matter from a body part

Body Part Character 4	Approach Character 5	Device Character 6	Qualifier Character 7
0　Lumbar Vertebra 1　Sacrum 2　Pelvic Bone, Right 3　Pelvic Bone, Left 4　Acetabulum, Right 5　Acetabulum, Left 6　Upper Femur, Right 7　Upper Femur, Left 8　Femoral Shaft, Right 9　Femoral Shaft, Left B　Lower Femur, Right C　Lower Femur, Left D　Patella, Right F　Patella, Left G　Tibia, Right H　Tibia, Left J　Fibula, Right K　Fibula, Left L　Tarsal, Right M　Tarsal, Left N　Metatarsal, Right P　Metatarsal, Left Q　Toe Phalanx, Right R　Toe Phalanx, Left S　Coccyx	0　Open 3　Percutaneous 4　Percutaneous Endoscopic	Z　No Device	Z　No Qualifier

0   Medical and Surgical
Q   Lower Bones
H   Insertion   Putting in a nonbiological appliance that monitors, assists, performs, or prevents a physiological function but does not physically take the place of a body part

Body Part Character 4	Approach Character 5	Device Character 6	Qualifier Character 7
0 Lumbar Vertebra 1 Sacrum 2 Pelvic Bone, Right 3 Pelvic Bone, Left 4 Acetabulum, Right 5 Acetabulum, Left D Patella, Right F Patella, Left L Tarsal, Right M Tarsal, Left N Metatarsal, Right P Metatarsal, Left Q Toe Phalanx, Right R Toe Phalanx, Left S Coccyx	0 Open 3 Percutaneous 4 Percutaneous Endoscopic	4 Internal Fixation Device 5 External Fixation Device	Z No Qualifier
6 Upper Femur, Right 7 Upper Femur, Left 8 Femoral Shaft, Right 9 Femoral Shaft, Left B Lower Femur, Right C Lower Femur, Left G Tibia, Right H Tibia, Left J Fibula, Right K Fibula, Left	0 Open 3 Percutaneous 4 Percutaneous Endoscopic	4 Internal Fixation Device 6 Intramedullary Fixation Device	Z No Qualifier
6 Upper Femur, Right 7 Upper Femur, Left 8 Femoral Shaft, Right 9 Femoral Shaft, Left B Lower Femur, Right C Lower Femur, Left G Tibia, Right H Tibia, Left J Fibula, Right K Fibula, Left	0 Open 3 Percutaneous 4 Percutaneous Endoscopic	5 External Fixation Device	3 Monoplanar 4 Ring 5 Hybrid 9 Limb Lengthening Device Z No Qualifier
Y Lower Bone	0 Open 3 Percutaneous 4 Percutaneous Endoscopic	M Bone Growth Stimulator	Z No Qualifier

0   Medical and Surgical
Q   Lower Bones
J   Inspection   Visually and/or manually exploring a body part

Body Part Character 4	Approach Character 5	Device Character 6	Qualifier Character 7
Y Lower Bone	0 Open 3 Percutaneous 4 Percutaneous Endoscopic X External	Z No Device	Z No Qualifier

Revised Text in **BLUE**

Ø Medical and Surgical
Q Lower Bones
N Release　　　Freeing a body part from an abnormal physical constraint

Body Part Character 4	Approach Character 5	Device Character 6	Qualifier Character 7
Ø Lumbar Vertebra 1 Sacrum 2 Pelvic Bone, Right 3 Pelvic Bone, Left 4 Acetabulum, Right 5 Acetabulum, Left 6 Upper Femur, Right 7 Upper Femur, Left 8 Femoral Shaft, Right 9 Femoral Shaft, Left B Lower Femur, Right C Lower Femur, Left D Patella, Right F Patella, Left G Tibia, Right H Tibia, Left J Fibula, Right K Fibula, Left L Tarsal, Right M Tarsal, Left N Metatarsal, Right P Metatarsal, Left Q Toe Phalanx, Right R Toe Phalanx, Left S Coccyx	Ø Open 3 Percutaneous 4 Percutaneous Endoscopic	Z No Device	Z No Qualifier

Ø Medical and Surgical
Q Lower Bones
P Removal　　　Taking out or off a device from a body part

Body Part Character 4	Approach Character 5	Device Character 6	Qualifier Character 7
Ø Lumbar Vertebra 1 Sacrum 4 Acetabulum, Right 5 Acetabulum, Left S Coccyx	Ø Open 3 Percutaneous 4 Percutaneous Endoscopic	4 Internal Fixation Device 7 Autologous Tissue Substitute J Synthetic Substitute K Nonautologous Tissue Substitute	Z No Qualifier
Ø Lumbar Vertebra 1 Sacrum 4 Acetabulum, Right 5 Acetabulum, Left S Coccyx	X External	4 Internal Fixation Device	Z No Qualifier
2 Pelvic Bone, Right 3 Pelvic Bone, Left 6 Upper Femur, Right 7 Upper Femur, Left 8 Femoral Shaft, Right 9 Femoral Shaft, Left B Lower Femur, Right C Lower Femur, Left D Patella, Right F Patella, Left G Tibia, Right H Tibia, Left J Fibula, Right K Fibula, Left L Tarsal, Right M Tarsal, Left N Metatarsal, Right P Metatarsal, Left Q Toe Phalanx, Right R Toe Phalanx, Left	X External	4 Internal Fixation Device 5 External Fixation Device	Z No Qualifier

ØQP Continued on next page

ØQP Continued

Ø **Medical and Surgical**
Q **Lower Bones**
P **Removal**   Taking out or off a device from a body part

Body Part Character 4	Approach Character 5	Device Character 6	Qualifier Character 7
2 Pelvic Bone, Right **3** Pelvic Bone, Left **D** Patella, Right **F** Patella, Left **L** Tarsal, Right **M** Tarsal, Left **N** Metatarsal, Right **P** Metatarsal, Left **Q** Toe Phalanx, Right **R** Toe Phalanx, Left	**Ø** Open **3** Percutaneous **4** Percutaneous Endoscopic	**4** Internal Fixation Device **5** External Fixation Device **7** Autologous Tissue Substitute **J** Synthetic Substitute **K** Nonautologous Tissue Substitute	**Z** No Qualifier
6 Upper Femur, Right **7** Upper Femur, Left **8** Femoral Shaft, Right **9** Femoral Shaft, Left **B** Lower Femur, Right **C** Lower Femur, Left **G** Tibia, Right **H** Tibia, Left **J** Fibula, Right **K** Fibula, Left	**Ø** Open **3** Percutaneous **4** Percutaneous Endoscopic	**4** Internal Fixation Device **5** External Fixation Device **6** Intramedullary Fixation Device **7** Autologous Tissue Substitute **J** Synthetic Substitute **K** Nonautologous Tissue Substitute	**Z** No Qualifier
Y Lower Bone	**Ø** Open **3** Percutaneous **4** Percutaneous Endoscopic **X** External	**Ø** Drainage Device **M** Bone Growth Stimulator	**Z** No Qualifier

Ø **Medical and Surgical**
Q **Lower Bones**
Q **Repair**   Restoring, to the extent possible, a body part to its normal anatomic structure and function

Body Part Character 4	Approach Character 5	Device Character 6	Qualifier Character 7
Ø Lumbar Vertebra **1** Sacrum **2** Pelvic Bone, Right **3** Pelvic Bone, Left **4** Acetabulum, Right **5** Acetabulum, Left **6** Upper Femur, Right **7** Upper Femur, Left **8** Femoral Shaft, Right **9** Femoral Shaft, Left **B** Lower Femur, Right **C** Lower Femur, Left **D** Patella, Right **F** Patella, Left **G** Tibia, Right **H** Tibia, Left **J** Fibula, Right **K** Fibula, Left **L** Tarsal, Right **M** Tarsal, Left **N** Metatarsal, Right **P** Metatarsal, Left **Q** Toe Phalanx, Right **R** Toe Phalanx, Left **S** Coccyx	**Ø** Open **3** Percutaneous **4** Percutaneous Endoscopic **X** External	**Z** No Device	**Z** No Qualifier

ØQP–ØQQ

Lower Bones

0 Medical and Surgical
Q Lower Bones
R Replacement   Putting in or on biological or synthetic material that physically takes the place and/or function of all or a portion of a body part

Body Part Character 4	Approach Character 5	Device Character 6	Qualifier Character 7
0 Lumbar Vertebra 1 Sacrum 2 Pelvic Bone, Right 3 Pelvic Bone, Left 4 Acetabulum, Right 5 Acetabulum, Left 6 Upper Femur, Right 7 Upper Femur, Left 8 Femoral Shaft, Right 9 Femoral Shaft, Left B Lower Femur, Right C Lower Femur, Left D Patella, Right F Patella, Left G Tibia, Right H Tibia, Left J Fibula, Right K Fibula, Left L Tarsal, Right M Tarsal, Left N Metatarsal, Right P Metatarsal, Left Q Toe Phalanx, Right R Toe Phalanx, Left S Coccyx	0 Open 3 Percutaneous 4 Percutaneous Endoscopic	7 Autologous Tissue Substitute J Synthetic Substitute K Nonautologous Tissue Substitute	Z No Qualifier

0 Medical and Surgical
Q Lower Bones
S Reposition   Moving to its normal location or other suitable location all or a portion of a body part

Body Part Character 4	Approach Character 5	Device Character 6	Qualifier Character 7
0 Lumbar Vertebra 1 Sacrum 2 Pelvic Bone, Right 3 Pelvic Bone, Left 4 Acetabulum, Right 5 Acetabulum, Left 6 Upper Femur, Right 7 Upper Femur, Left 8 Femoral Shaft, Right 9 Femoral Shaft, Left B Lower Femur, Right C Lower Femur, Left D Patella, Right F Patella, Left G Tibia, Right H Tibia, Left J Fibula, Right K Fibula, Left L Tarsal, Right M Tarsal, Left N Metatarsal, Right P Metatarsal, Left Q Toe Phalanx, Right R Toe Phalanx, Left S Coccyx	X External	Z No Device	Z No Qualifier
0 Lumbar Vertebra 1 Sacrum 2 Pelvic Bone, Right 3 Pelvic Bone, Left 4 Acetabulum, Right 5 Acetabulum, Left D Patella, Right F Patella, Left L Tarsal, Right M Tarsal, Left N Metatarsal, Right P Metatarsal, Left Q Toe Phalanx, Right R Toe Phalanx, Left S Coccyx	0 Open 3 Percutaneous 4 Percutaneous Endoscopic	4 Internal Fixation Device Z No Device	Z No Qualifier

0QS Continued on next page

Lower Bones

ØQS–ØQT

Ø   **Medical and Surgical**   *ØQS Continued*
Q   **Lower Bones**
S   **Reposition**   Moving to its normal location or other suitable location all or a portion of a body part

Body Part Character 4	Approach Character 5	Device Character 6	Qualifier Character 7
2 Pelvic Bone, Right 3 Pelvic Bone, Left 6 Upper Femur, Right 7 Upper Femur, Left 8 Femoral Shaft, Right 9 Femoral Shaft, Left B Lower Femur, Right C Lower Femur, Left D Patella, Right F Patella, Left G Tibia, Right H Tibia, Left J Fibula, Right K Fibula, Left L Tarsal, Right M Tarsal, Left N Metatarsal, Right P Metatarsal, Left Q Toe Phalanx, Right R Toe Phalanx, Left	Ø Open 3 Percutaneous 4 Percutaneous Endoscopic	5 External Fixation Device	3 Monoplanar 4 Ring 5 Hybrid Z No Qualifier
6 Upper Femur, Right 7 Upper Femur, Left 8 Femoral Shaft, Right 9 Femoral Shaft, Left B Lower Femur, Right C Lower Femur, Left G Tibia, Right H Tibia, Left J Fibula, Right K Fibula, Left	Ø Open 3 Percutaneous 4 Percutaneous Endoscopic	4 Internal Fixation Device 6 Intramedullary Fixation Device Z No Device	Z No Qualifier

Ø   **Medical and Surgical**
Q   **Lower Bones**
T   **Resection**   Cutting out or off, without replacement, all of a body part

Body Part Character 4	Approach Character 5	Device Character 6	Qualifier Character 7
2 Pelvic Bone, Right 3 Pelvic Bone, Left 4 Acetabulum, Right 5 Acetabulum, Left 6 Upper Femur, Right 7 Upper Femur, Left 8 Femoral Shaft, Right 9 Femoral Shaft, Left B Lower Femur, Right C Lower Femur, Left D Patella, Right F Patella, Left G Tibia, Right H Tibia, Left J Fibula, Right K Fibula, Left L Tarsal, Right M Tarsal, Left N Metatarsal, Right P Metatarsal, Left Q Toe Phalanx, Right R Toe Phalanx, Left S Coccyx	Ø Open	Z No Device	Z No Qualifier

Ø　Medical and Surgical
Q　Lower Bones
U　Supplement　　Putting in or on biological or synthetic material that physically reinforces and/or augments the function of a portion of a body part

Body Part Character 4	Approach Character 5	Device Character 6	Qualifier Character 7
Ø Lumbar Vertebra 1 Sacrum 2 Pelvic Bone, Right 3 Pelvic Bone, Left 4 Acetabulum, Right 5 Acetabulum, Left 6 Upper Femur, Right 7 Upper Femur, Left 8 Femoral Shaft, Right 9 Femoral Shaft, Left B Lower Femur, Right C Lower Femur, Left D Patella, Right F Patella, Left G Tibia, Right H Tibia, Left J Fibula, Right K Fibula, Left L Tarsal, Right M Tarsal, Left N Metatarsal, Right P Metatarsal, Left Q Toe Phalanx, Right R Toe Phalanx, Left S Coccyx	Ø Open 3 Percutaneous 4 Percutaneous Endoscopic	7 Autologous Tissue Substitute J Synthetic Substitute K Nonautologous Tissue Substitute	Z No Qualifier

Ø　Medical and Surgical
Q　Lower Bones
W　Revision　　Correcting, to the extent possible, a portion of a malfunctioning device or the position of a displaced device

Body Part Character 4	Approach Character 5	Device Character 6	Qualifier Character 7
Ø Lumbar Vertebra 1 Sacrum 4 Acetabulum, Right 5 Acetabulum, Left S Coccyx	Ø Open 3 Percutaneous 4 Percutaneous Endoscopic X External	4 Internal Fixation Device 7 Autologous Tissue Substitute J Synthetic Substitute K Nonautologous Tissue Substitute	Z No Qualifier
2 Pelvic Bone, Right 3 Pelvic Bone, Left D Patella, Right F Patella, Left L Tarsal, Right M Tarsal, Left N Metatarsal, Right P Metatarsal, Left Q Toe Phalanx, Right R Toe Phalanx, Left	Ø Open 3 Percutaneous 4 Percutaneous Endoscopic X External	4 Internal Fixation Device 5 External Fixation Device 7 Autologous Tissue Substitute J Synthetic Substitute K Nonautologous Tissue Substitute	Z No Qualifier
6 Upper Femur, Right 7 Upper Femur, Left 8 Femoral Shaft, Right 9 Femoral Shaft, Left B Lower Femur, Right C Lower Femur, Left G Tibia, Right H Tibia, Left J Fibula, Right K Fibula, Left	Ø Open 3 Percutaneous 4 Percutaneous Endoscopic X External	4 Internal Fixation Device 5 External Fixation Device 6 Intramedullary Fixation Device 7 Autologous Tissue Substitute J Synthetic Substitute K Nonautologous Tissue Substitute	Z No Qualifier
Y Lower Bone	Ø Open 3 Percutaneous 4 Percutaneous Endoscopic X External	Ø Drainage Device M Bone Growth Stimulator	Z No Qualifier

Upper Joints ØR2–ØRW

Ø   Medical and Surgical
R   Upper Joints
2   Change   Taking out or off a device from a body part and putting back an identical or similar device in or on the same body part without cutting or puncturing the skin or a mucous membrane

Body Part Character 4	Approach Character 5	Device Character 6	Qualifier Character 7
Y Upper Joint	X External	Ø Drainage Device Y Other Device	Z No Qualifier

Ø   Medical and Surgical
R   Upper Joints
5   Destruction   Physical eradication of all or a portion of a body part by the direct use of energy, force, or a destructive agent

Body Part Character 4	Approach Character 5	Device Character 6	Qualifier Character 7
Ø Occipital-cervical Joint 1 Cervical Vertebral Joint 3 Cervical Vertebral Disc 4 Cervicothoracic Vertebral Joint 5 Cervicothoracic Vertebral Disc 6 Thoracic Vertebral Joint 9 Thoracic Vertebral Disc A Thoracolumbar Vertebral Joint B Thoracolumbar Vertebral Disc C Temporomandibular Joint, Right D Temporomandibular Joint, Left E Sternoclavicular Joint, Right F Sternoclavicular Joint, Left G Acromioclavicular Joint, Right H Acromioclavicular Joint, Left J Shoulder Joint, Right K Shoulder Joint, Left L Elbow Joint, Right M Elbow Joint, Left N Wrist Joint, Right P Wrist Joint, Left Q Carpal Joint, Right R Carpal Joint, Left S Metacarpocarpal Joint, Right T Metacarpocarpal Joint, Left U Metacarpophalangeal Joint, Right V Metacarpophalangeal Joint, Left W Finger Phalangeal Joint, Right X Finger Phalangeal Joint, Left	Ø Open 3 Percutaneous 4 Percutaneous Endoscopic	Z No Device	Z No Qualifier

0   **Medical and Surgical**
R   **Upper Joints**
9   **Drainage**   Taking or letting out fluids and/or gases from a body part

Body Part Character 4	Approach Character 5	Device Character 6	Qualifier Character 7
0 Occipital-cervical Joint **1** Cervical Vertebral Joint **3** Cervical Vertebral Disc **4** Cervicothoracic Vertebral Joint **5** Cervicothoracic Vertebral Disc **6** Thoracic Vertebral Joint **9** Thoracic Vertebral Disc **A** Thoracolumbar Vertebral Joint **B** Thoracolumbar Vertebral Disc **C** Temporomandibular Joint, Right **D** Temporomandibular Joint, Left **E** Sternoclavicular Joint, Right **F** Sternoclavicular Joint, Left **G** Acromioclavicular Joint, Right **H** Acromioclavicular Joint, Left **J** Shoulder Joint, Right **K** Shoulder Joint, Left **L** Elbow Joint, Right **M** Elbow Joint, Left **N** Wrist Joint, Right **P** Wrist Joint, Left **Q** Carpal Joint, Right **R** Carpal Joint, Left **S** Metacarpocarpal Joint, Right **T** Metacarpocarpal Joint, Left **U** Metacarpophalangeal Joint, Right **V** Metacarpophalangeal Joint, Left **W** Finger Phalangeal Joint, Right **X** Finger Phalangeal Joint, Left	**0** Open **3** Percutaneous **4** Percutaneous Endoscopic	**0** Drainage Device	**Z** No Qualifier
0 Occipital-cervical Joint **1** Cervical Vertebral Joint **3** Cervical Vertebral Disc **4** Cervicothoracic Vertebral Joint **5** Cervicothoracic Vertebral Disc **6** Thoracic Vertebral Joint **9** Thoracic Vertebral Disc **A** Thoracolumbar Vertebral Joint **B** Thoracolumbar Vertebral Disc **C** Temporomandibular Joint, Right **D** Temporomandibular Joint, Left **E** Sternoclavicular Joint, Right **F** Sternoclavicular Joint, Left **G** Acromioclavicular Joint, Right **H** Acromioclavicular Joint, Left **J** Shoulder Joint, Right **K** Shoulder Joint, Left **L** Elbow Joint, Right **M** Elbow Joint, Left **N** Wrist Joint, Right **P** Wrist Joint, Left **Q** Carpal Joint, Right **R** Carpal Joint, Left **S** Metacarpocarpal Joint, Right **T** Metacarpocarpal Joint, Left **U** Metacarpophalangeal Joint, Right **V** Metacarpophalangeal Joint, Left **W** Finger Phalangeal Joint, Right **X** Finger Phalangeal Joint, Left	**0** Open **3** Percutaneous **4** Percutaneous Endoscopic	**Z** No Device	**X** Diagnostic **Z** No Qualifier

       Revised Text in **BLUE**

Ø   **Medical and Surgical**
R   **Upper Joints**
B   **Excision**   Cutting out or off, without replacement, a portion of a body part

Body Part Character 4	Approach Character 5	Device Character 6	Qualifier Character 7
Ø Occipital-cervical Joint 1 Cervical Vertebral Joint 3 Cervical Vertebral Disc 4 Cervicothoracic Vertebral Joint 5 Cervicothoracic Vertebral Disc 6 Thoracic Vertebral Joint 9 Thoracic Vertebral Disc A Thoracolumbar Vertebral Joint B Thoracolumbar Vertebral Disc C Temporomandibular Joint, Right D Temporomandibular Joint, Left E Sternoclavicular Joint, Right F Sternoclavicular Joint, Left G Acromioclavicular Joint, Right H Acromioclavicular Joint, Left J Shoulder Joint, Right K Shoulder Joint, Left L Elbow Joint, Right M Elbow Joint, Left N Wrist Joint, Right P Wrist Joint, Left Q Carpal Joint, Right R Carpal Joint, Left S Metacarpocarpal Joint, Right T Metacarpocarpal Joint, Left U Metacarpophalangeal Joint, Right V Metacarpophalangeal Joint, Left W Finger Phalangeal Joint, Right X Finger Phalangeal Joint, Left	Ø Open 3 Percutaneous 4 Percutaneous Endoscopic	Z No Device	X Diagnostic Z No Qualifier

Ø   **Medical and Surgical**
R   **Upper Joints**
C   **Extirpation**   Taking or cutting out solid matter from a body part

Body Part Character 4	Approach Character 5	Device Character 6	Qualifier Character 7
Ø Occipital-cervical Joint 1 Cervical Vertebral Joint 3 Cervical Vertebral Disc 4 Cervicothoracic Vertebral Joint 5 Cervicothoracic Vertebral Disc 6 Thoracic Vertebral Joint 9 Thoracic Vertebral Disc A Thoracolumbar Vertebral Joint B Thoracolumbar Vertebral Disc C Temporomandibular Joint, Right D Temporomandibular Joint, Left E Sternoclavicular Joint, Right F Sternoclavicular Joint, Left G Acromioclavicular Joint, Right H Acromioclavicular Joint, Left J Shoulder Joint, Right K Shoulder Joint, Left L Elbow Joint, Right M Elbow Joint, Left N Wrist Joint, Right P Wrist Joint, Left Q Carpal Joint, Right R Carpal Joint, Left S Metacarpocarpal Joint, Right T Metacarpocarpal Joint, Left U Metacarpophalangeal Joint, Right V Metacarpophalangeal Joint, Left W Finger Phalangeal Joint, Right X Finger Phalangeal Joint, Left	Ø Open 3 Percutaneous 4 Percutaneous Endoscopic	Z No Device	Z No Qualifier

Ø   Medical and Surgical
R   Upper Joints
G   Fusion   Joining together portions of an articular body part rendering the articular body part immobile

Body Part Character 4	Approach Character 5	Device Character 6	Qualifier Character 7
Ø Occipital-cervical Joint **1** Cervical Vertebral Joint **2** Cervical Vertebral Joints, 2 or more **4** Cervicothoracic Vertebral Joint **6** Thoracic Vertebral Joint **7** Thoracic Vertebral Joints, 2 to 7 **8** Thoracic Vertebral Joints, 8 or more **A** Thoracolumbar Vertebral Joint	**Ø** Open **3** Percutaneous **4** Percutaneous Endoscopic	**3** Interbody Internal Fixation Device **4** Internal Fixation Device **7** Autologous Tissue Substitute **J** Synthetic Substitute **K** Nonautologous Tissue Substitute **Z** No Device	**Ø** Anterior Approach, Anterior Column **1** Posterior Approach, Posterior Column **J** Posterior Approach, Anterior Column
C Temporomandibular Joint, Right **D** Temporomandibular Joint, Left **E** Sternoclavicular Joint, Right **F** Sternoclavicular Joint, Left **G** Acromioclavicular Joint, Right **H** Acromioclavicular Joint, Left **J** Shoulder Joint, Right **K** Shoulder Joint, Left	**Ø** Open **3** Percutaneous **4** Percutaneous Endoscopic	**4** Internal Fixation Device **7** Autologous Tissue Substitute **J** Synthetic Substitute **K** Nonautologous Tissue Substitute **Z** No Device	**Z** No Qualifier
L Elbow Joint, Right **M** Elbow Joint, Left **N** Wrist Joint, Right **P** Wrist Joint, Left **Q** Carpal Joint, Right **R** Carpal Joint, Left **S** Metacarpocarpal Joint, Right **T** Metacarpocarpal Joint, Left **U** Metacarpophalangeal Joint, Right **V** Metacarpophalangeal Joint, Left **W** Finger Phalangeal Joint, Right **X** Finger Phalangeal Joint, Left	**Ø** Open **3** Percutaneous **4** Percutaneous Endoscopic	**4** Internal Fixation Device **5** External Fixation Device **7** Autologous Tissue Substitute **J** Synthetic Substitute **K** Nonautologous Tissue Substitute **Z** No Device	**Z** No Qualifier

Ø   Medical and Surgical
R   Upper Joints
H   Insertion   Putting in a nonbiological appliance that monitors, assists, performs, or prevents a physiological function but does not physically take the place of a body part

Body Part Character 4	Approach Character 5	Device Character 6	Qualifier Character 7
Ø Occipital-cervical Joint **1** Cervical Vertebral Joint **4** Cervicothoracic Vertebral Joint **6** Thoracic Vertebral Joint **A** Thoracolumbar Vertebral Joint	**Ø** Open **3** Percutaneous **4** Percutaneous Endoscopic	**3** Infusion Device **8** Spacer	**Z** No Qualifier
Ø Occipital-cervical Joint **1** Cervical Vertebral Joint **4** Cervicothoracic Vertebral Joint **6** Thoracic Vertebral Joint **A** Thoracolumbar Vertebral Joint	**Ø** Open **3** Percutaneous **4** Percutaneous Endoscopic	**4** Internal Fixation Device	**2** Interspinous Process **3** Pedicle-based Dynamic Stabilization **Z** No Qualifier
3 Cervical Vertebral Disc **5** Cervicothoracic Vertebral Disc **9** Thoracic Vertebral Disc **B** Thoracolumbar Vertebral Disc	**Ø** Open **3** Percutaneous **4** Percutaneous Endoscopic	**3** Infusion Device	**Z** No Qualifier
C Temporomandibular Joint, Right **D** Temporomandibular Joint, Left **E** Sternoclavicular Joint, Right **F** Sternoclavicular Joint, Left **G** Acromioclavicular Joint, Right **H** Acromioclavicular Joint, Left **J** Shoulder Joint, Right **K** Shoulder Joint, Left	**Ø** Open **3** Percutaneous **4** Percutaneous Endoscopic	**3** Infusion Device **4** Internal Fixation Device **8** Spacer	**Z** No Qualifier
L Elbow Joint, Right **M** Elbow Joint, Left **N** Wrist Joint, Right **P** Wrist Joint, Left **Q** Carpal Joint, Right **R** Carpal Joint, Left **S** Metacarpocarpal Joint, Right **T** Metacarpocarpal Joint, Left **U** Metacarpophalangeal Joint, Right **V** Metacarpophalangeal Joint, Left **W** Finger Phalangeal Joint, Right **X** Finger Phalangeal Joint, Left	**Ø** Open **3** Percutaneous **4** Percutaneous Endoscopic	**3** Infusion Device **4** Internal Fixation Device **5** External Fixation Device **8** Spacer	**Z** No Qualifier

Ø   Medical and Surgical
R   Upper Joints
J   Inspection   Visually and/or manually exploring a body part

Body Part Character 4	Approach Character 5	Device Character 6	Qualifier Character 7
Ø Occipital-cervical Joint 1 Cervical Vertebral Joint 3 Cervical Vertebral Disc 4 Cervicothoracic Vertebral Joint 5 Cervicothoracic Vertebral Disc 6 Thoracic Vertebral Joint 9 Thoracic Vertebral Disc A Thoracolumbar Vertebral Joint B Thoracolumbar Vertebral Disc C Temporomandibular Joint, Right D Temporomandibular Joint, Left E Sternoclavicular Joint, Right F Sternoclavicular Joint, Left G Acromioclavicular Joint, Right H Acromioclavicular Joint, Left J Shoulder Joint, Right K Shoulder Joint, Left L Elbow Joint, Right M Elbow Joint, Left N Wrist Joint, Right P Wrist Joint, Left Q Carpal Joint, Right R Carpal Joint, Left S Metacarpocarpal Joint, Right T Metacarpocarpal Joint, Left U Metacarpophalangeal Joint, Right V Metacarpophalangeal Joint, Left W Finger Phalangeal Joint, Right X Finger Phalangeal Joint, Left	Ø Open 3 Percutaneous 4 Percutaneous Endoscopic X External	Z No Device	Z No Qualifier

Ø   Medical and Surgical
R   Upper Joints
N   Release   Freeing a body part from an abnormal physical constraint

Body Part Character 4	Approach Character 5	Device Character 6	Qualifier Character 7
Ø Occipital-cervical Joint 1 Cervical Vertebral Joint 3 Cervical Vertebral Disc 4 Cervicothoracic Vertebral Joint 5 Cervicothoracic Vertebral Disc 6 Thoracic Vertebral Joint 9 Thoracic Vertebral Disc A Thoracolumbar Vertebral Joint B Thoracolumbar Vertebral Disc C Temporomandibular Joint, Right D Temporomandibular Joint, Left E Sternoclavicular Joint, Right F Sternoclavicular Joint, Left G Acromioclavicular Joint, Right H Acromioclavicular Joint, Left J Shoulder Joint, Right K Shoulder Joint, Left L Elbow Joint, Right M Elbow Joint, Left N Wrist Joint, Right P Wrist Joint, Left Q Carpal Joint, Right R Carpal Joint, Left S Metacarpocarpal Joint, Right T Metacarpocarpal Joint, Left U Metacarpophalangeal Joint, Right V Metacarpophalangeal Joint, Left W Finger Phalangeal Joint, Right X Finger Phalangeal Joint, Left	Ø Open 3 Percutaneous 4 Percutaneous Endoscopic X External	Z No Device	Z No Qualifier

Revised Text in **BLUE**

Ø Medical and Surgical
R Upper Joints
P Removal Taking out or off a device from a body part

Body Part Character 4	Approach Character 5	Device Character 6	Qualifier Character 7
Ø Occipital-cervical Joint 1 Cervical Vertebral Joint 4 Cervicothoracic Vertebral Joint 6 Thoracic Vertebral Joint A Thoracolumbar Vertebral Joint C Temporomandibular Joint, Right D Temporomandibular Joint, Left E Sternoclavicular Joint, Right F Sternoclavicular Joint, Left G Acromioclavicular Joint, Right H Acromioclavicular Joint, Left J Shoulder Joint, Right K Shoulder Joint, Left	Ø Open 3 Percutaneous 4 Percutaneous Endoscopic	Ø Drainage Device 3 Infusion Device 4 Internal Fixation Device 7 Autologous Tissue Substitute 8 Spacer J Synthetic Substitute K Nonautologous Tissue Substitute	Z No Qualifier
Ø Occipital-cervical Joint 1 Cervical Vertebral Joint 4 Cervicothoracic Vertebral Joint 6 Thoracic Vertebral Joint A Thoracolumbar Vertebral Joint C Temporomandibular Joint, Right D Temporomandibular Joint, Left E Sternoclavicular Joint, Right F Sternoclavicular Joint, Left G Acromioclavicular Joint, Right H Acromioclavicular Joint, Left J Shoulder Joint, Right K Shoulder Joint, Left	X External	Ø Drainage Device 3 Infusion Device 4 Internal Fixation Device	Z No Qualifier
3 Cervical Vertebral Disc 5 Cervicothoracic Vertebral Disc 9 Thoracic Vertebral Disc B Thoracolumbar Vertebral Disc	Ø Open 3 Percutaneous 4 Percutaneous Endoscopic	Ø Drainage Device 3 Infusion Device 7 Autologous Tissue Substitute J Synthetic Substitute K Nonautologous Tissue Substitute	Z No Qualifier
3 Cervical Vertebral Disc 5 Cervicothoracic Vertebral Disc 9 Thoracic Vertebral Disc B Thoracolumbar Vertebral Disc	X External	Ø Drainage Device 3 Infusion Device	Z No Qualifier
L Elbow Joint, Right M Elbow Joint, Left N Wrist Joint, Right P Wrist Joint, Left Q Carpal Joint, Right R Carpal Joint, Left S Metacarpocarpal Joint, Right T Metacarpocarpal Joint, Left U Metacarpophalangeal Joint, Right V Metacarpophalangeal Joint, Left W Finger Phalangeal Joint, Right X Finger Phalangeal Joint, Left	Ø Open 3 Percutaneous 4 Percutaneous Endoscopic	Ø Drainage Device 3 Infusion Device 4 Internal Fixation Device 5 External Fixation Device 7 Autologous Tissue Substitute 8 Spacer J Synthetic Substitute K Nonautologous Tissue Substitute	Z No Qualifier
L Elbow Joint, Right M Elbow Joint, Left N Wrist Joint, Right P Wrist Joint, Left Q Carpal Joint, Right R Carpal Joint, Left S Metacarpocarpal Joint, Right T Metacarpocarpal Joint, Left U Metacarpophalangeal Joint, Right V Metacarpophalangeal Joint, Left W Finger Phalangeal Joint, Right X Finger Phalangeal Joint, Left	X External	Ø Drainage Device 3 Infusion Device 4 Internal Fixation Device 5 External Fixation Device	Z No Qualifier

Ø Medical and Surgical
R Upper Joints
Q Repair   Restoring, to the extent possible, a body part to its normal anatomic structure and function

Body Part Character 4	Approach Character 5	Device Character 6	Qualifier Character 7
Ø Occipital-cervical Joint 1 Cervical Vertebral Joint 3 Cervical Vertebral Disc 4 Cervicothoracic Vertebral Joint 5 Cervicothoracic Vertebral Disc 6 Thoracic Vertebral Joint 9 Thoracic Vertebral Disc A Thoracolumbar Vertebral Joint B Thoracolumbar Vertebral Disc C Temporomandibular Joint, Right D Temporomandibular Joint, Left E Sternoclavicular Joint, Right F Sternoclavicular Joint, Left G Acromioclavicular Joint, Right H Acromioclavicular Joint, Left J Shoulder Joint, Right K Shoulder Joint, Left L Elbow Joint, Right M Elbow Joint, Left N Wrist Joint, Right P Wrist Joint, Left Q Carpal Joint, Right R Carpal Joint, Left S Metacarpocarpal Joint, Right T Metacarpocarpal Joint, Left U Metacarpophalangeal Joint, Right V Metacarpophalangeal Joint, Left W Finger Phalangeal Joint, Right X Finger Phalangeal Joint, Left	Ø Open 3 Percutaneous 4 Percutaneous Endoscopic X External	Z No Device	Z No Qualifier

Ø Medical and Surgical
R Upper Joints
R Replacement   Putting in or on biological or synthetic material that physically takes the place and/or function of all or a portion of a body part

Body Part Character 4	Approach Character 5	Device Character 6	Qualifier Character 7
Ø Occipital-cervical Joint 1 Cervical Vertebral Joint 4 Cervicothoracic Vertebral Joint 6 Thoracic Vertebral Joint A Thoracolumbar Vertebral Joint	Ø Open	7 Autologous Tissue Substitute K Nonautologous Tissue Substitute	Z No Qualifier
Ø Occipital-cervical Joint 1 Cervical Vertebral Joint 4 Cervicothoracic Vertebral Joint 6 Thoracic Vertebral Joint A Thoracolumbar Vertebral Joint	Ø Open	J Synthetic Substitute	4 Facet Z No Qualifier
3 Cervical Vertebral Disc 5 Cervicothoracic Vertebral Disc 9 Thoracic Vertebral Disc B Thoracolumbar Vertebral Disc C Temporomandibular Joint, Right D Temporomandibular Joint, Left E Sternoclavicular Joint, Right F Sternoclavicular Joint, Left G Acromioclavicular Joint, Right H Acromioclavicular Joint, Left J Shoulder Joint, Right K Shoulder Joint, Left L Elbow Joint, Right M Elbow Joint, Left N Wrist Joint, Right P Wrist Joint, Left Q Carpal Joint, Right R Carpal Joint, Left S Metacarpocarpal Joint, Right T Metacarpocarpal Joint, Left U Metacarpophalangeal Joint, Right V Metacarpophalangeal Joint, Left W Finger Phalangeal Joint, Right X Finger Phalangeal Joint, Left	Ø Open	7 Autologous Tissue Substitute J Synthetic Substitute K Nonautologous Tissue Substitute	Z No Qualifier
J Shoulder Joint, Right K Shoulder Joint, Left	Ø Open	7 Autologous Tissue Substitute K Nonautologous Tissue Substitute	Z No Qualifier

ØRR Continued on next page

Revised Text in **BLUE**
© 2011 Ingenix, Inc

Ø　Medical and Surgical
R　Upper Joints
R　Replacement　Putting in or on biological or synthetic material that physically takes the place and/or function of all or a portion of a body part

ØRR Continued

Body Part Character 4	Approach Character 5	Device Character 6	Qualifier Character 7
J Shoulder Joint, Right **K** Shoulder Joint, Left	**Ø** Open	**J** Synthetic Substitute	**5** Reverse Ball and Socket **6** Humeral Surface **7** Glenoid Surface **Z** No Qualifier

Ø　Medical and Surgical
R　Upper Joints
S　Reposition　Moving to its normal location or other suitable location all or a portion of a body part

Body Part Character 4	Approach Character 5	Device Character 6	Qualifier Character 7
Ø Occipital-cervical Joint **1** Cervical Vertebral Joint **4** Cervicothoracic Vertebral Joint **6** Thoracic Vertebral Joint **A** Thoracolumbar Vertebral Joint **C** Temporomandibular Joint, Right **D** Temporomandibular Joint, Left **E** Sternoclavicular Joint, Right **F** Sternoclavicular Joint, Left **G** Acromioclavicular Joint, Right **H** Acromioclavicular Joint, Left **J** Shoulder Joint, Right **K** Shoulder Joint, Left	**Ø** Open **3** Percutaneous **4** Percutaneous Endoscopic **X** External	**4** Internal Fixation Device **Z** No Device	**Z** No Qualifier
L Elbow Joint, Right **M** Elbow Joint, Left **N** Wrist Joint, Right **P** Wrist Joint, Left **Q** Carpal Joint, Right **R** Carpal Joint, Left **S** Metacarpocarpal Joint, Right **T** Metacarpocarpal Joint, Left **U** Metacarpophalangeal Joint, Right **V** Metacarpophalangeal Joint, Left **W** Finger Phalangeal Joint, Right **X** Finger Phalangeal Joint, Left	**Ø** Open **3** Percutaneous **4** Percutaneous Endoscopic **X** External	**4** Internal Fixation Device **5** External Fixation Device **Z** No Device	**Z** No Qualifier

Ø　Medical and Surgical
R　Upper Joints
T　Resection　Cutting out or off, without replacement, all of a body part

Body Part Character 4	Approach Character 5	Device Character 6	Qualifier Character 7
3 Cervical Vertebral Disc **4** Cervicothoracic Vertebral Joint **5** Cervicothoracic Vertebral Disc **9** Thoracic Vertebral Disc **B** Thoracolumbar Vertebral Disc **C** Temporomandibular Joint, Right **D** Temporomandibular Joint, Left **E** Sternoclavicular Joint, Right **F** Sternoclavicular Joint, Left **G** Acromioclavicular Joint, Right **H** Acromioclavicular Joint, Left **J** Shoulder Joint, Right **K** Shoulder Joint, Left **L** Elbow Joint, Right **M** Elbow Joint, Left **N** Wrist Joint, Right **P** Wrist Joint, Left **Q** Carpal Joint, Right **R** Carpal Joint, Left **S** Metacarpocarpal Joint, Right **T** Metacarpocarpal Joint, Left **U** Metacarpophalangeal Joint, Right **V** Metacarpophalangeal Joint, Left **W** Finger Phalangeal Joint, Right **X** Finger Phalangeal Joint, Left	**Ø** Open	**Z** No Device	**Z** No Qualifier

Ø   **Medical and Surgical**
R   **Upper Joints**
U   **Supplement**   Putting in or on biological or synthetic material that physically reinforces and/or augments the function of a portion of a body part

Body Part Character 4	Approach Character 5	Device Character 6	Qualifier Character 7
Ø Occipital-cervical Joint **1** Cervical Vertebral Joint **4** Cervicothoracic Vertebral Joint **6** Thoracic Vertebral Joint **A** Thoracolumbar Vertebral Joint	**Ø** Open	**7** Autologous Tissue Substitute **K** Nonautologous Tissue Substitute	**Z** No Qualifier
Ø Occipital-cervical Joint **1** Cervical Vertebral Joint **4** Cervicothoracic Vertebral Joint **6** Thoracic Vertebral Joint **A** Thoracolumbar Vertebral Joint	**Ø** Open	**J** Synthetic Substitute	**4** Facet **Z** No Qualifier
Ø Occipital-cervical Joint **1** Cervical Vertebral Joint **4** Cervicothoracic Vertebral Joint **6** Thoracic Vertebral Joint **A** Thoracolumbar Vertebral Joint	**3** Percutaneous **4** Percutaneous Endoscopic	**7** Autologous Tissue Substitute **J** Synthetic Substitute **K** Nonautologous Tissue Substitute	**Z** No Qualifier
3 Cervical Vertebral Disc **5** Cervicothoracic Vertebral Disc **9** Thoracic Vertebral Disc **B** Thoracolumbar Vertebral Disc **C** Temporomandibular Joint, Right **D** Temporomandibular Joint, Left **E** Sternoclavicular Joint, Right **F** Sternoclavicular Joint, Left **G** Acromioclavicular Joint, Right **H** Acromioclavicular Joint, Left **J** Shoulder Joint, Right **K** Shoulder Joint, Left **L** Elbow Joint, Right **M** Elbow Joint, Left **N** Wrist Joint, Right **P** Wrist Joint, Left **Q** Carpal Joint, Right **R** Carpal Joint, Left **S** Metacarpocarpal Joint, Right **T** Metacarpocarpal Joint, Left **U** Metacarpophalangeal Joint, Right **V** Metacarpophalangeal Joint, Left **W** Finger Phalangeal Joint, Right **X** Finger Phalangeal Joint, Left	**Ø** Open **3** Percutaneous **4** Percutaneous Endoscopic	**7** Autologous Tissue Substitute **J** Synthetic Substitute **K** Nonautologous Tissue Substitute	**Z** No Qualifier

Ø　Medical and Surgical
R　Upper Joints
W　Revision　　Correcting, to the extent possible, a portion of a malfunctioning device or the position of a displaced device

Body Part Character 4	Approach Character 5	Device Character 6	Qualifier Character 7
Ø Occipital-cervical Joint 1 Cervical Vertebral Joint 4 Cervicothoracic Vertebral Joint 6 Thoracic Vertebral Joint A Thoracolumbar Vertebral Joint C Temporomandibular Joint, Right D Temporomandibular Joint, Left E Sternoclavicular Joint, Right F Sternoclavicular Joint, Left G Acromioclavicular Joint, Right H Acromioclavicular Joint, Left J Shoulder Joint, Right K Shoulder Joint, Left	Ø Open 3 Percutaneous 4 Percutaneous Endoscopic X External	Ø Drainage Device 3 Infusion Device 4 Internal Fixation Device 7 Autologous Tissue Substitute 8 Spacer J Synthetic Substitute K Nonautologous Tissue Substitute	Z No Qualifier
3 Cervical Vertebral Disc 5 Cervicothoracic Vertebral Disc 9 Thoracic Vertebral Disc B Thoracolumbar Vertebral Disc	Ø Open 3 Percutaneous 4 Percutaneous Endoscopic X External	Ø Drainage Device 3 Infusion Device 7 Autologous Tissue Substitute J Synthetic Substitute K Nonautologous Tissue Substitute	Z No Qualifier
L Elbow Joint, Right M Elbow Joint, Left N Wrist Joint, Right P Wrist Joint, Left Q Carpal Joint, Right R Carpal Joint, Left S Metacarpocarpal Joint, Right T Metacarpocarpal Joint, Left U Metacarpophalangeal Joint, Right V Metacarpophalangeal Joint, Left W Finger Phalangeal Joint, Right X Finger Phalangeal Joint, Left	Ø Open 3 Percutaneous 4 Percutaneous Endoscopic X External	Ø Drainage Device 3 Infusion Device 4 Internal Fixation Device 5 External Fixation Device 7 Autologous Tissue Substitute 8 Spacer J Synthetic Substitute K Nonautologous Tissue Substitute	Z No Qualifier

Lower Joints ØS2–ØSW

Ø   Medical and Surgical
S   Lower Joints
2   Change   Taking out or off a device from a body part and putting back an identical or similar device in or on the same body part without cutting or puncturing the skin or a mucous membrane

Body Part Character 4	Approach Character 5	Device Character 6	Qualifier Character 7
Y Lower Joint	X External	Ø Drainage Device Y Other Device	Z No Qualifier

Ø   Medical and Surgical
S   Lower Joints
5   Destruction   Physical eradication of all or a portion of a body part by the direct use of energy, force, or a destructive agent

Body Part Character 4	Approach Character 5	Device Character 6	Qualifier Character 7
Ø Lumbar Vertebral Joint 2 Lumbar Vertebral Disc 3 Lumbosacral Joint 4 Lumbosacral Disc 5 Sacrococcygeal Joint 6 Coccygeal Joint 7 Sacroiliac Joint, Right 8 Sacroiliac Joint, Left 9 Hip Joint, Right B Hip Joint, Left C Knee Joint, Right D Knee Joint, Left F Ankle Joint, Right G Ankle Joint, Left H Tarsal Joint, Right J Tarsal Joint, Left K Metatarsal-Tarsal Joint, Right L Metatarsal-Tarsal Joint, Left M Metatarsal-Phalangeal Joint, Right N Metatarsal-Phalangeal Joint, Left P Toe Phalangeal Joint, Right Q Toe Phalangeal Joint, Left	Ø Open 3 Percutaneous 4 Percutaneous Endoscopic	Z No Device	Z No Qualifier

Ø   Medical and Surgical
S   Lower Joints
9   Drainage   Taking or letting out fluids and/or gases from a body part

Body Part Character 4	Approach Character 5	Device Character 6	Qualifier Character 7
Ø Lumbar Vertebral Joint 2 Lumbar Vertebral Disc 3 Lumbosacral Joint 4 Lumbosacral Disc 5 Sacrococcygeal Joint 6 Coccygeal Joint 7 Sacroiliac Joint, Right 8 Sacroiliac Joint, Left 9 Hip Joint, Right B Hip Joint, Left C Knee Joint, Right D Knee Joint, Left F Ankle Joint, Right G Ankle Joint, Left H Tarsal Joint, Right J Tarsal Joint, Left K Metatarsal-Tarsal Joint, Right L Metatarsal-Tarsal Joint, Left M Metatarsal-Phalangeal Joint, Right N Metatarsal-Phalangeal Joint, Left P Toe Phalangeal Joint, Right Q Toe Phalangeal Joint, Left	Ø Open 3 Percutaneous 4 Percutaneous Endoscopic	Ø Drainage Device	Z No Qualifier

ØS9 Continued on next page

                Revised Text in **BLUE**

Ø   Medical and Surgical
S   Lower Joints
9   Drainage   Taking or letting out fluids and/or gases from a body part

ØS9 Continued

Body Part Character 4	Approach Character 5	Device Character 6	Qualifier Character 7
Ø Lumbar Vertebral Joint 2 Lumbar Vertebral Disc 3 Lumbosacral Joint 4 Lumbosacral Disc 5 Sacrococcygeal Joint 6 Coccygeal Joint 7 Sacroiliac Joint, Right 8 Sacroiliac Joint, Left 9 Hip Joint, Right B Hip Joint, Left C Knee Joint, Right D Knee Joint, Left F Ankle Joint, Right G Ankle Joint, Left H Tarsal Joint, Right J Tarsal Joint, Left K Metatarsal-Tarsal Joint, Right L Metatarsal-Tarsal Joint, Left M Metatarsal-Phalangeal Joint, Right N Metatarsal-Phalangeal Joint, Left P Toe Phalangeal Joint, Right Q Toe Phalangeal Joint, Left	Ø Open 3 Percutaneous 4 Percutaneous Endoscopic	Z No Device	X Diagnostic Z No Qualifier

Ø   Medical and Surgical
S   Lower Joints
B   Excision   Cutting out or off, without replacement, a portion of a body part

Body Part Character 4	Approach Character 5	Device Character 6	Qualifier Character 7
Ø Lumbar Vertebral Joint 2 Lumbar Vertebral Disc 3 Lumbosacral Joint 4 Lumbosacral Disc 5 Sacrococcygeal Joint 6 Coccygeal Joint 7 Sacroiliac Joint, Right 8 Sacroiliac Joint, Left 9 Hip Joint, Right B Hip Joint, Left C Knee Joint, Right D Knee Joint, Left F Ankle Joint, Right G Ankle Joint, Left H Tarsal Joint, Right J Tarsal Joint, Left K Metatarsal-Tarsal Joint, Right L Metatarsal-Tarsal Joint, Left M Metatarsal-Phalangeal Joint, Right N Metatarsal-Phalangeal Joint, Left P Toe Phalangeal Joint, Right Q Toe Phalangeal Joint, Left	Ø Open 3 Percutaneous 4 Percutaneous Endoscopic	Z No Device	X Diagnostic Z No Qualifier

Ø Medical and Surgical
S Lower Joints
C Extirpation Taking or cutting out solid matter from a body part

Body Part Character 4	Approach Character 5	Device Character 6	Qualifier Character 7
Ø Lumbar Vertebral Joint **2** Lumbar Vertebral Disc **3** Lumbosacral Joint **4** Lumbosacral Disc **5** Sacrococcygeal Joint **6** Coccygeal Joint **7** Sacroiliac Joint, Right **8** Sacroiliac Joint, Left **9** Hip Joint, Right **B** Hip Joint, Left **C** Knee Joint, Right **D** Knee Joint, Left **F** Ankle Joint, Right **G** Ankle Joint, Left **H** Tarsal Joint, Right **J** Tarsal Joint, Left **K** Metatarsal-Tarsal Joint, Right **L** Metatarsal-Tarsal Joint, Left **M** Metatarsal-Phalangeal Joint, Right **N** Metatarsal-Phalangeal Joint, Left **P** Toe Phalangeal Joint, Right **Q** Toe Phalangeal Joint, Left	**Ø** Open **3** Percutaneous **4** Percutaneous Endoscopic	**Z** No Device	**Z** No Qualifier

Ø Medical and Surgical
S Lower Joints
G Fusion Joining together portions of an articular body part rendering the articular body part immobile

Body Part Character 4	Approach Character 5	Device Character 6	Qualifier Character 7
Ø Lumbar Vertebral Joint **1** Lumbar Vertebral Joints, **2** or more **3** Lumbosacral Joint	**Ø** Open **3** Percutaneous **4** Percutaneous Endoscopic	**3** Interbody Internal Fixation Device **4** Internal Fixation Device **7** Autologous Tissue Substitute **J** Synthetic Substitute **K** Nonautologous Tissue Substitute **Z** No Device	**Ø** Anterior Approach, Anterior Column **1** Posterior Approach, Posterior Column **J** Posterior Approach, Anterior Column
5 Sacrococcygeal Joint **6** Coccygeal Joint **7** Sacroiliac Joint, Right **8** Sacroiliac Joint, Left	**Ø** Open **3** Percutaneous **4** Percutaneous Endoscopic	**4** Internal Fixation Device **7** Autologous Tissue Substitute **J** Synthetic Substitute **K** Nonautologous Tissue Substitute **Z** No Device	**Z** No Qualifier
9 Hip Joint, Right **B** Hip Joint, Left **C** Knee Joint, Right **D** Knee Joint, Left **F** Ankle Joint, Right **G** Ankle Joint, Left **H** Tarsal Joint, Right **J** Tarsal Joint, Left **K** Metatarsal-Tarsal Joint, Right **L** Metatarsal-Tarsal Joint, Left **M** Metatarsal-Phalangeal Joint, Right **N** Metatarsal-Phalangeal Joint, Left **P** Toe Phalangeal Joint, Right **Q** Toe Phalangeal Joint, Left	**Ø** Open **3** Percutaneous **4** Percutaneous Endoscopic	**4** Internal Fixation Device **5** External Fixation Device **7** Autologous Tissue Substitute **J** Synthetic Substitute **K** Nonautologous Tissue Substitute **Z** No Device	**Z** No Qualifier

Ø　**Medical and Surgical**
S　**Lower Joints**
H　**Insertion**　　Putting in a nonbiological appliance that monitors, assists, performs, or prevents a physiological function but does not physically take the place of a body part

Body Part Character 4	Approach Character 5	Device Character 6	Qualifier Character 7
Ø Lumbar Vertebral Joint **2** Lumbar Vertebral Disc **3** Lumbosacral Joint **4** Lumbosacral Disc	**Ø** Open **3** Percutaneous **4** Percutaneous Endoscopic	**3** Infusion Device **8** Spacer	**Z** No Qualifier
Ø Lumbar Vertebral Joint **3** Lumbosacral Joint	**Ø** Open **3** Percutaneous **4** Percutaneous Endoscopic	**4** Internal Fixation Device	**2** Interspinous Process **3** Pedicle-based Dynamic 　 Stabilization **Z** No Qualifier
5 Sacrococcygeal Joint **6** Coccygeal Joint **7** Sacroiliac Joint, Right **8** Sacroiliac Joint, Left	**Ø** Open **3** Percutaneous **4** Percutaneous Endoscopic	**3** Infusion Device **4** Internal Fixation Device **8** Spacer	**Z** No Qualifier
9 Hip Joint, Right **B** Hip Joint, Left **C** Knee Joint, Right **D** Knee Joint, Left **F** Ankle Joint, Right **G** Ankle Joint, Left **H** Tarsal Joint, Right **J** Tarsal Joint, Left **K** Metatarsal-Tarsal Joint, Right **L** Metatarsal-Tarsal Joint, Left **M** Metatarsal-Phalangeal Joint, Right **N** Metatarsal-Phalangeal Joint, Left **P** Toe Phalangeal Joint, Right **Q** Toe Phalangeal Joint, Left	**Ø** Open **3** Percutaneous **4** Percutaneous Endoscopic	**3** Infusion Device **4** Internal Fixation Device **5** External Fixation Device **8** Spacer	**Z** No Qualifier

Ø　**Medical and Surgical**
S　**Lower Joints**
J　**Inspection**　　Visually and/or manually exploring a body part

Body Part Character 4	Approach Character 5	Device Character 6	Qualifier Character 7
Ø Lumbar Vertebral Joint **2** Lumbar Vertebral Disc **3** Lumbosacral Joint **4** Lumbosacral Disc **5** Sacrococcygeal Joint **6** Coccygeal Joint **7** Sacroiliac Joint, Right **8** Sacroiliac Joint, Left **9** Hip Joint, Right **B** Hip Joint, Left **C** Knee Joint, Right **D** Knee Joint, Left **F** Ankle Joint, Right **G** Ankle Joint, Left **H** Tarsal Joint, Right **J** Tarsal Joint, Left **K** Metatarsal-Tarsal Joint, Right **L** Metatarsal-Tarsal Joint, Left **M** Metatarsal-Phalangeal Joint, Right **N** Metatarsal-Phalangeal Joint, Left **P** Toe Phalangeal Joint, Right **Q** Toe Phalangeal Joint, Left	**Ø** Open **3** Percutaneous **4** Percutaneous Endoscopic **X** External	**Z** No Device	**Z** No Qualifier

Lower Joints

Ø Medical and Surgical
S Lower Joints
N Release   Freeing a body part from an abnormal physical constraint

Body Part Character 4	Approach Character 5	Device Character 6	Qualifier Character 7
Ø Lumbar Vertebral Joint 2 Lumbar Vertebral Disc 3 Lumbosacral Joint 4 Lumbosacral Disc 5 Sacrococcygeal Joint 6 Coccygeal Joint 7 Sacroiliac Joint, Right 8 Sacroiliac Joint, Left 9 Hip Joint, Right B Hip Joint, Left C Knee Joint, Right D Knee Joint, Left F Ankle Joint, Right G Ankle Joint, Left H Tarsal Joint, Right J Tarsal Joint, Left K Metatarsal-Tarsal Joint, Right L Metatarsal-Tarsal Joint, Left M Metatarsal-Phalangeal Joint, Right N Metatarsal-Phalangeal Joint, Left P Toe Phalangeal Joint, Right Q Toe Phalangeal Joint, Left	Ø Open 3 Percutaneous 4 Percutaneous Endoscopic X External	Z No Device	Z No Qualifier

Ø Medical and Surgical
S Lower Joints
P Removal   Taking out or off a device from a body part

Body Part Character 4	Approach Character 5	Device Character 6	Qualifier Character 7
Ø Lumbar Vertebral Joint 3 Lumbosacral Joint 5 Sacrococcygeal Joint 6 Coccygeal Joint 7 Sacroiliac Joint, Right 8 Sacroiliac Joint, Left	Ø Open 3 Percutaneous 4 Percutaneous Endoscopic	Ø Drainage Device 3 Infusion Device 4 Internal Fixation Device 7 Autologous Tissue Substitute 8 Spacer J Synthetic Substitute K Nonautologous Tissue Substitute	Z No Qualifier
Ø Lumbar Vertebral Joint 3 Lumbosacral Joint 5 Sacrococcygeal Joint 6 Coccygeal Joint 7 Sacroiliac Joint, Right 8 Sacroiliac Joint, Left	X External	Ø Drainage Device 3 Infusion Device 4 Internal Fixation Device	Z No Qualifier
2 Lumbar Vertebral Disc 4 Lumbosacral Disc	Ø Open 3 Percutaneous 4 Percutaneous Endoscopic	Ø Drainage Device 3 Infusion Device 7 Autologous Tissue Substitute J Synthetic Substitute K Nonautologous Tissue Substitute	Z No Qualifier
2 Lumbar Vertebral Disc 4 Lumbosacral Disc	X External	Ø Drainage Device 3 Infusion Device	Z No Qualifier
9 Hip Joint, Right B Hip Joint, Left	Ø Open	Ø Drainage Device 3 Infusion Device 4 Internal Fixation Device 5 External Fixation Device 7 Autologous Tissue Substitute 8 Spacer 9 Liner B Resurfacing Device J Synthetic Substitute K Nonautologous Tissue Substitute	Z No Qualifier

ØSP Continued on next page

    Revised Text in **BLUE**   © 2011 Ingenix, Inc

Ø Medical and Surgical
S Lower Joints
P Removal   Taking out or off a device from a body part

Body Part Character 4	Approach Character 5	Device Character 6	Qualifier Character 7
9 Hip Joint, Right **B** Hip Joint, Left **C** Knee Joint, Right **D** Knee Joint, Left	**3** Percutaneous **4** Percutaneous Endoscopic	**Ø** Drainage Device **3** Infusion Device **4** Internal Fixation Device **5** External Fixation Device **7** Autologous Tissue Substitute **8** Spacer **J** Synthetic Substitute **K** Nonautologous Tissue Substitute	**Z** No Qualifier
9 Hip Joint, Right **B** Hip Joint, Left **C** Knee Joint, Right **D** Knee Joint, Left **F** Ankle Joint, Right **G** Ankle Joint, Left **H** Tarsal Joint, Right **J** Tarsal Joint, Left **K** Metatarsal-Tarsal Joint, Right **L** Metatarsal-Tarsal Joint, Left **M** Metatarsal-Phalangeal Joint, Right **N** Metatarsal-Phalangeal Joint, Left **P** Toe Phalangeal Joint, Right **Q** Toe Phalangeal Joint, Left	**X** External	**Ø** Drainage Device **3** Infusion Device **4** Internal Fixation Device **5** External Fixation Device	**Z** No Qualifier
C Knee Joint, Right **D** Knee Joint, Left	**Ø** Open	**Ø** Drainage Device **3** Infusion Device **4** Internal Fixation Device **5** External Fixation Device **7** Autologous Tissue Substitute **8** Spacer **9** Liner **J** Synthetic Substitute **K** Nonautologous Tissue Substitute	**Z** No Qualifier
F Ankle Joint, Right **G** Ankle Joint, Left **H** Tarsal Joint, Right **J** Tarsal Joint, Left **K** Metatarsal-Tarsal Joint, Right **L** Metatarsal-Tarsal Joint, Left **M** Metatarsal-Phalangeal Joint, Right **N** Metatarsal-Phalangeal Joint, Left **P** Toe Phalangeal Joint, Right **Q** Toe Phalangeal Joint, Left	**Ø** Open **3** Percutaneous **4** Percutaneous Endoscopic	**Ø** Drainage Device **3** Infusion Device **4** Internal Fixation Device **5** External Fixation Device **7** Autologous Tissue Substitute **8** Spacer **J** Synthetic Substitute **K** Nonautologous Tissue Substitute	**Z** No Qualifier

Ø Medical and Surgical
S Lower Joints
Q Repair   Restoring, to the extent possible, a body part to its normal anatomic structure and function

Body Part Character 4	Approach Character 5	Device Character 6	Qualifier Character 7
Ø Lumbar Vertebral Joint **2** Lumbar Vertebral Disc **3** Lumbosacral Joint **4** Lumbosacral Disc **5** Sacrococcygeal Joint **6** Coccygeal Joint **7** Sacroiliac Joint, Right **8** Sacroiliac Joint, Left **9** Hip Joint, Right **B** Hip Joint, Left **C** Knee Joint, Right **D** Knee Joint, Left **F** Ankle Joint, Right **G** Ankle Joint, Left **H** Tarsal Joint, Right **J** Tarsal Joint, Left **K** Metatarsal-Tarsal Joint, Right **L** Metatarsal-Tarsal Joint, Left **M** Metatarsal-Phalangeal Joint, Right **N** Metatarsal-Phalangeal Joint, Left **P** Toe Phalangeal Joint, Right **Q** Toe Phalangeal Joint, Left	**Ø** Open **3** Percutaneous **4** Percutaneous Endoscopic **X** External	**Z** No Device	**Z** No Qualifier

Lower Joints

ØSR–ØSS

Ø   Medical and Surgical
S   Lower Joints
R   Replacement   Putting in or on biological or synthetic material that physically takes the place and/or function of all or a portion of a body part

Body Part Character 4	Approach Character 5	Device Character 6	Qualifier Character 7
Ø Lumbar Vertebral Joint **3** Lumbosacral Joint	**Ø** Open	**J** Synthetic Substitute	**4** Facet **Z** No Qualifier
Ø Lumbar Vertebral Joint **3** Lumbosacral Joint **9** Hip Joint, Right **A** Hip Joint, Acetabular Surface, Right **B** Hip Joint, Left **E** Hip Joint, Acetabular Surface, Left **R** Hip Joint, Femoral Surface, Right **S** Hip Joint, Femoral Surface, Left	**Ø** Open	**7** Autologous Tissue Substitute **K** Nonautologous Tissue Substitute	**Z** No Qualifier
2 Lumbar Vertebral Disc **4** Lumbosacral Disc **5** Sacrococcygeal Joint **6** Coccygeal Joint **7** Sacroiliac Joint, Right **8** Sacroiliac Joint, Left **C** Knee Joint, Right **D** Knee Joint, Left **F** Ankle Joint, Right **G** Ankle Joint, Left **H** Tarsal Joint, Right **J** Tarsal Joint, Left **K** Metatarsal-Tarsal Joint, Right **L** Metatarsal-Tarsal Joint, Left **M** Metatarsal-Phalangeal Joint, Right **N** Metatarsal-Phalangeal Joint, Left **P** Toe Phalangeal Joint, Right **Q** Toe Phalangeal Joint, Left **T** Knee Joint, Femoral Surface, Right **U** Knee Joint, Femoral Surface, Left **V** Knee Joint, Tibial Surface, Right **W** Knee Joint, Tibial Surface, Left	**Ø** Open	**7** Autologous Tissue Substitute **J** Synthetic Substitute **K** Nonautologous Tissue Substitute	**Z** No Qualifier
9 Hip Joint, Right **B** Hip Joint, Left	**Ø** Open	**J** Synthetic Substitute	**5** Metal on Polyethylene **6** Metal on Metal **7** Ceramic on Ceramic **8** Ceramic on Polyethylene **Z** No Qualifier
A Hip Joint, Acetabular Surface, Right **E** Hip Joint, Acetabular Surface, Left	**Ø** Open	**J** Synthetic Substitute	**F** Metal **G** Ceramic **H** Polyethylene **Z** No Qualifier
R Hip Joint, Femoral Surface, Right **S** Hip Joint, Femoral Surface, Left	**Ø** Open	**J** Synthetic Substitute	**F** Metal **G** Ceramic **Z** No Qualifier

Ø   Medical and Surgical
S   Lower Joints
S   Reposition   Moving to its normal location or other suitable location all or a portion of a body part

Body Part Character 4	Approach Character 5	Device Character 6	Qualifier Character 7
Ø Lumbar Vertebral Joint **3** Lumbosacral Joint **5** Sacrococcygeal Joint **6** Coccygeal Joint **7** Sacroiliac Joint, Right **8** Sacroiliac Joint, Left	**Ø** Open **3** Percutaneous **4** Percutaneous Endoscopic **X** External	**4** Internal Fixation Device **Z** No Device	**Z** No Qualifier
9 Hip Joint, Right **B** Hip Joint, Left **C** Knee Joint, Right **D** Knee Joint, Left **F** Ankle Joint, Right **G** Ankle Joint, Left **H** Tarsal Joint, Right **J** Tarsal Joint, Left **K** Metatarsal-Tarsal Joint, Right **L** Metatarsal-Tarsal Joint, Left **M** Metatarsal-Phalangeal Joint, Right **N** Metatarsal-Phalangeal Joint, Left **P** Toe Phalangeal Joint, Right **Q** Toe Phalangeal Joint, Left	**Ø** Open **3** Percutaneous **4** Percutaneous Endoscopic **X** External	**4** Internal Fixation Device **5** External Fixation Device **Z** No Device	**Z** No Qualifier

Ø Medical and Surgical
S Lower Joints
T Resection Cutting out or off, without replacement, all of a body part

Body Part Character 4	Approach Character 5	Device Character 6	Qualifier Character 7
2 Lumbar Vertebral Disc 4 Lumbosacral Disc 5 Sacrococcygeal Joint 6 Coccygeal Joint 7 Sacroiliac Joint, Right 8 Sacroiliac Joint, Left 9 Hip Joint, Right B Hip Joint, Left C Knee Joint, Right D Knee Joint, Left F Ankle Joint, Right G Ankle Joint, Left H Tarsal Joint, Right J Tarsal Joint, Left K Metatarsal-Tarsal Joint, Right L Metatarsal-Tarsal Joint, Left M Metatarsal-Phalangeal Joint, Right N Metatarsal-Phalangeal Joint, Left P Toe Phalangeal Joint, Right Q Toe Phalangeal Joint, Left	Ø Open	Z No Device	Z No Qualifier

Ø Medical and Surgical
S Lower Joints
U Supplement Putting in or on biological or synthetic material that physically reinforces and/or augments the function of a portion of a body part

Body Part Character 4	Approach Character 5	Device Character 6	Qualifier Character 7
Ø Lumbar Vertebral Joint 3 Lumbosacral Joint	Ø Open	7 Autologous Tissue Substitute K Nonautologous Tissue Substitute	Z No Qualifier
Ø Lumbar Vertebral Joint 3 Lumbosacral Joint	Ø Open	J Synthetic Substitute	4 Facet Z No Qualifier
Ø Lumbar Vertebral Joint 3 Lumbosacral Joint 9 Hip Joint, Right B Hip Joint, Left	3 Percutaneous 4 Percutaneous Endoscopic	7 Autologous Tissue Substitute J Synthetic Substitute K Nonautologous Tissue Substitute	Z No Qualifier
2 Lumbar Vertebral Disc 4 Lumbosacral Disc 5 Sacrococcygeal Joint 6 Coccygeal Joint 7 Sacroiliac Joint, Right 8 Sacroiliac Joint, Left C Knee Joint, Right D Knee Joint, Left F Ankle Joint, Right G Ankle Joint, Left H Tarsal Joint, Right J Tarsal Joint, Left K Metatarsal-Tarsal Joint, Right L Metatarsal-Tarsal Joint, Left M Metatarsal-Phalangeal Joint, Right N Metatarsal-Phalangeal Joint, Left P Toe Phalangeal Joint, Right Q Toe Phalangeal Joint, Left	Ø Open 3 Percutaneous 4 Percutaneous Endoscopic	7 Autologous Tissue Substitute J Synthetic Substitute K Nonautologous Tissue Substitute	Z No Qualifier
9 Hip Joint, Right B Hip Joint, Left	Ø Open	7 Autologous Tissue Substitute 9 Liner B Resurfacing Device J Synthetic Substitute K Nonautologous Tissue Substitute	Z No Qualifier
A Hip Joint, Acetabular Surface, Right E Hip Joint, Acetabular Surface, Left R Hip Joint, Femoral Surface, Right S Hip Joint, Femoral Surface, Left	Ø Open	9 Liner B Resurfacing Device	Z No Qualifier
C Knee Joint, Right D Knee Joint, Left	Ø Open	9 Liner	C Patellar Surface Z No Qualifier
T Knee Joint, Femoral Surface, Right U Knee Joint, Femoral Surface, Left V Knee Joint, Tibial Surface, Right W Knee Joint, Tibial Surface, Left	Ø Open	9 Liner	Z No Qualifier

Ø   **Medical and Surgical**
S   **Lower Joints**
W   **Revision**   Correcting, to the extent possible, a portion of a malfunctioning device or the position of a displaced device

Body Part Character 4	Approach Character 5	Device Character 6	Qualifier Character 7
Ø Lumbar Vertebral Joint 3 Lumbosacral Joint 5 Sacrococcygeal Joint 6 Coccygeal Joint 7 Sacroiliac Joint, Right 8 Sacroiliac Joint, Left	Ø Open 3 Percutaneous 4 Percutaneous Endoscopic X External	Ø Drainage Device 3 Infusion Device 4 Internal Fixation Device 7 Autologous Tissue Substitute 8 Spacer J Synthetic Substitute K Nonautologous Tissue Substitute	Z No Qualifier
2 Lumbar Vertebral Disc 4 Lumbosacral Disc	Ø Open 3 Percutaneous 4 Percutaneous Endoscopic X External	Ø Drainage Device 3 Infusion Device 7 Autologous Tissue Substitute J Synthetic Substitute K Nonautologous Tissue Substitute	Z No Qualifier
9 Hip Joint, Right B Hip Joint, Left	Ø Open	Ø Drainage Device 3 Infusion Device 4 Internal Fixation Device 5 External Fixation Device 7 Autologous Tissue Substitute 8 Spacer 9 Liner B Resurfacing Device J Synthetic Substitute K Nonautologous Tissue Substitute	Z No Qualifier
9 Hip Joint, Right B Hip Joint, Left C Knee Joint, Right D Knee Joint, Left	3 Percutaneous 4 Percutaneous Endoscopic X External	Ø Drainage Device 3 Infusion Device 4 Internal Fixation Device 5 External Fixation Device 7 Autologous Tissue Substitute 8 Spacer J Synthetic Substitute K Nonautologous Tissue Substitute	Z No Qualifier
C Knee Joint, Right D Knee Joint, Left	Ø Open	Ø Drainage Device 3 Infusion Device 4 Internal Fixation Device 5 External Fixation Device 7 Autologous Tissue Substitute 8 Spacer 9 Liner J Synthetic Substitute K Nonautologous Tissue Substitute	Z No Qualifier
F Ankle Joint, Right G Ankle Joint, Left H Tarsal Joint, Right J Tarsal Joint, Left K Metatarsal-Tarsal Joint, Right L Metatarsal-Tarsal Joint, Left M Metatarsal-Phalangeal Joint, Right N Metatarsal-Phalangeal Joint, Left P Toe Phalangeal Joint, Right Q Toe Phalangeal Joint, Left	Ø Open 3 Percutaneous 4 Percutaneous Endoscopic X External	Ø Drainage Device 3 Infusion Device 4 Internal Fixation Device 5 External Fixation Device 7 Autologous Tissue Substitute 8 Spacer J Synthetic Substitute K Nonautologous Tissue Substitute	Z No Qualifier

Urinary System ØT1–ØTY

Ø   **Medical and Surgical**
T   **Urinary System**
1   **Bypass**   Altering the route of passage of the contents of a tubular body part

Body Part Character 4	Approach Character 5	Device Character 6	Qualifier Character 7
3 Kidney Pelvis, Right 4 Kidney Pelvis, Left	Ø Open 4 Percutaneous Endoscopic	7 Autologous Tissue Substitute J Synthetic Substitute K Nonautologous Tissue Substitute Z No Device	3 Kidney Pelvis, Right 4 Kidney Pelvis, Left 6 Ureter, Right 7 Ureter, Left 8 Colon 9 Colocutaneous A Ileum B Bladder C Ileocutaneous D Cutaneous
3 Kidney Pelvis, Right 4 Kidney Pelvis, Left 6 Ureter, Right 7 Ureter, Left 8 Ureters, Bilateral B Bladder	3 Percutaneous	J Synthetic Substitute	D Cutaneous
6 Ureter, Right 7 Ureter, Left 8 Ureters, Bilateral	Ø Open 4 Percutaneous Endoscopic	7 Autologous Tissue Substitute J Synthetic Substitute K Nonautologous Tissue Substitute Z No Device	6 Ureter, Right 7 Ureter, Left 8 Colon 9 Colocutaneous A Ileum B Bladder C Ileocutaneous D Cutaneous
B Bladder	Ø Open 4 Percutaneous Endoscopic	7 Autologous Tissue Substitute J Synthetic Substitute K Nonautologous Tissue Substitute Z No Device	9 Colocutaneous C Ileocutaneous D Cutaneous

Ø   **Medical and Surgical**
T   **Urinary System**
2   **Change**   Taking out or off a device from a body part and putting back an identical or similar device in or on the same body part without cutting or puncturing the skin or a mucous membrane

Body Part Character 4	Approach Character 5	Device Character 6	Qualifier Character 7
5 Kidney 9 Ureter B Bladder D Urethra	X External	Ø Drainage Device Y Other Device	Z No Qualifier

Ø   **Medical and Surgical**
T   **Urinary System**
5   **Destruction**   Physical eradication of all or a portion of a body part by the direct use of energy, force, or a destructive agent

Body Part Character 4	Approach Character 5	Device Character 6	Qualifier Character 7
Ø Kidney, Right 1 Kidney, Left 3 Kidney Pelvis, Right 4 Kidney Pelvis, Left 6 Ureter, Right 7 Ureter, Left B Bladder C Bladder Neck	Ø Open 3 Percutaneous 4 Percutaneous Endoscopic 7 Via Natural or Artificial Opening 8 Via Natural or Artificial Opening Endoscopic	Z No Device	Z No Qualifier
D Urethra	Ø Open 3 Percutaneous 4 Percutaneous Endoscopic 7 Via Natural or Artificial Opening 8 Via Natural or Artificial Opening Endoscopic X External	Z No Device	Z No Qualifier

Urinary System

ØT7–ØT9

Ø   Medical and Surgical
T   Urinary System
7   Dilation   Expanding an orifice or the lumen of a tubular body part

Body Part Character 4	Approach Character 5	Device Character 6	Qualifier Character 7
3 Kidney Pelvis, Right 4 Kidney Pelvis, Left 6 Ureter, Right 7 Ureter, Left 8 Ureters, Bilateral B Bladder C Bladder Neck D Urethra	Ø Open 3 Percutaneous 4 Percutaneous Endoscopic 7 Via Natural or Artificial Opening 8 Via Natural or Artificial Opening Endoscopic	D Intraluminal Device Z No Device	Z No Qualifier

Ø   Medical and Surgical
T   Urinary System
8   Division   Cutting into a body part without draining fluids and/or gases from the body part in order to separate or transect a body part

Body Part Character 4	Approach Character 5	Device Character 6	Qualifier Character 7
2 Kidneys, Bilateral C Bladder Neck	Ø Open 3 Percutaneous 4 Percutaneous Endoscopic	Z No Device	Z No Qualifier

Ø   Medical and Surgical
T   Urinary System
9   Drainage   Taking or letting out fluids and/or gases from a body part

Body Part Character 4	Approach Character 5	Device Character 6	Qualifier Character 7
Ø Kidney, Right 1 Kidney, Left 3 Kidney Pelvis, Right 4 Kidney Pelvis, Left 6 Ureter, Right 7 Ureter, Left 8 Ureters, Bilateral B Bladder C Bladder Neck	Ø Open 3 Percutaneous 4 Percutaneous Endoscopic 7 Via Natural or Artificial Opening 8 Via Natural or Artificial Opening Endoscopic	Ø Drainage Device	Z No Qualifier
Ø Kidney, Right 1 Kidney, Left 3 Kidney Pelvis, Right 4 Kidney Pelvis, Left 6 Ureter, Right 7 Ureter, Left 8 Ureters, Bilateral B Bladder C Bladder Neck	Ø Open 3 Percutaneous 4 Percutaneous Endoscopic 7 Via Natural or Artificial Opening 8 Via Natural or Artificial Opening Endoscopic	Z No Device	X Diagnostic Z No Qualifier
D Urethra	Ø Open 3 Percutaneous 4 Percutaneous Endoscopic 7 Via Natural or Artificial Opening 8 Via Natural or Artificial Opening Endoscopic X External	Ø Drainage Device	Z No Qualifier
D Urethra	Ø Open 3 Percutaneous 4 Percutaneous Endoscopic 7 Via Natural or Artificial Opening 8 Via Natural or Artificial Opening Endoscopic X External	Z No Device	X Diagnostic Z No Qualifier

0 Medical and Surgical
T Urinary System
B Excision　Cutting out or off, without replacement, a portion of a body part

Body Part Character 4	Approach Character 5	Device Character 6	Qualifier Character 7
0 Kidney, Right 1 Kidney, Left 3 Kidney Pelvis, Right 4 Kidney Pelvis, Left 6 Ureter, Right 7 Ureter, Left B Bladder C Bladder Neck	0 Open 3 Percutaneous 4 Percutaneous Endoscopic 7 Via Natural or Artificial Opening 8 Via Natural or Artificial Opening Endoscopic	Z No Device	X Diagnostic Z No Qualifier
D Urethra	0 Open 3 Percutaneous 4 Percutaneous Endoscopic 7 Via Natural or Artificial Opening 8 Via Natural or Artificial Opening Endoscopic X External	Z No Device	X Diagnostic Z No Qualifier

0 Medical and Surgical
T Urinary System
C Extirpation　Taking or cutting out solid matter from a body part

Body Part Character 4	Approach Character 5	Device Character 6	Qualifier Character 7
0 Kidney, Right 1 Kidney, Left 3 Kidney Pelvis, Right 4 Kidney Pelvis, Left 6 Ureter, Right 7 Ureter, Left B Bladder C Bladder Neck	0 Open 3 Percutaneous 4 Percutaneous Endoscopic 7 Via Natural or Artificial Opening 8 Via Natural or Artificial Opening Endoscopic	Z No Device	Z No Qualifier
D Urethra	0 Open 3 Percutaneous 4 Percutaneous Endoscopic 7 Via Natural or Artificial Opening 8 Via Natural or Artificial Opening Endoscopic X External	Z No Device	Z No Qualifier

0 Medical and Surgical
T Urinary System
D Extraction　Pulling or stripping out or off all or a portion of a body part by the use of force

Body Part Character 4	Approach Character 5	Device Character 6	Qualifier Character 7
0 Kidney, Right 1 Kidney, Left	0 Open 3 Percutaneous 4 Percutaneous Endoscopic	Z No Device	Z No Qualifier

0 Medical and Surgical
T Urinary System
F Fragmentation　Breaking solid matter in a body part into pieces

Body Part Character 4	Approach Character 5	Device Character 6	Qualifier Character 7
3 Kidney Pelvis, Right 4 Kidney Pelvis, Left 6 Ureter, Right 7 Ureter, Left B Bladder C Bladder Neck D Urethra	0 Open 3 Percutaneous 4 Percutaneous Endoscopic 7 Via Natural or Artificial Opening 8 Via Natural or Artificial Opening Endoscopic X External	Z No Device	Z No Qualifier

Ø   **Medical and Surgical**
T   **Urinary System**
H   **Insertion**   Putting in a nonbiological appliance that monitors, assists, performs, or prevents a physiological function but does not physically take the place of a body part

Body Part Character 4	Approach Character 5	Device Character 6	Qualifier Character 7
5 Kidney	**Ø** Open **3** Percutaneous **4** Percutaneous Endoscopic **7** Via Natural or Artificial Opening **8** Via Natural or Artificial Opening Endoscopic	**2** Monitoring Device **3** Infusion Device	**Z** No Qualifier
9 Ureter	**Ø** Open **3** Percutaneous **4** Percutaneous Endoscopic **7** Via Natural or Artificial Opening **8** Via Natural or Artificial Opening Endoscopic	**2** Monitoring Device **3** Infusion Device **M** Stimulator Lead	**Z** No Qualifier
B Bladder	**Ø** Open **3** Percutaneous **4** Percutaneous Endoscopic **7** Via Natural or Artificial Opening **8** Via Natural or Artificial Opening Endoscopic	**2** Monitoring Device **3** Infusion Device **L** Artificial Sphincter **M** Stimulator Lead	**Z** No Qualifier
C Bladder Neck	**Ø** Open **3** Percutaneous **4** Percutaneous Endoscopic **7** Via Natural or Artificial Opening **8** Via Natural or Artificial Opening Endoscopic	**L** Artificial Sphincter	**Z** No Qualifier
D Urethra	**Ø** Open **3** Percutaneous **4** Percutaneous Endoscopic **7** Via Natural or Artificial Opening **8** Via Natural or Artificial Opening Endoscopic **X** External	**2** Monitoring Device **3** Infusion Device **L** Artificial Sphincter	**Z** No Qualifier

Ø   **Medical and Surgical**
T   **Urinary System**
J   **Inspection**   Visually and/or manually exploring a body part

Body Part Character 4	Approach Character 5	Device Character 6	Qualifier Character 7
5 Kidney **9** Ureter **B** Bladder **D** Urethra	**Ø** Open **3** Percutaneous **4** Percutaneous Endoscopic **7** Via Natural or Artificial Opening **8** Via Natural or Artificial Opening Endoscopic **X** External	**Z** No Device	**Z** No Qualifier

Ø   **Medical and Surgical**
T   **Urinary System**
L   **Occlusion**   Completely closing an orifice or the lumen of a tubular body part

Body Part Character 4	Approach Character 5	Device Character 6	Qualifier Character 7
3 Kidney Pelvis, Right **4** Kidney Pelvis, Left **6** Ureter, Right **7** Ureter, Left **B** Bladder **C** Bladder Neck	**Ø** Open **3** Percutaneous **4** Percutaneous Endoscopic	**C** Extraluminal Device **D** Intraluminal Device **Z** No Device	**Z** No Qualifier
3 Kidney Pelvis, Right **4** Kidney Pelvis, Left **6** Ureter, Right **7** Ureter, Left **B** Bladder **C** Bladder Neck **D** Urethra	**7** Via Natural or Artificial Opening **8** Via Natural or Artificial Opening Endoscopic	**D** Intraluminal Device **Z** No Device	**Z** No Qualifier
D Urethra	**Ø** Open **3** Percutaneous **4** Percutaneous Endoscopic **X** External	**C** Extraluminal Device **D** Intraluminal Device **Z** No Device	**Z** No Qualifier

     Revised Text in **BLUE**

Ø Medical and Surgical
T Urinary System
M Reattachment Putting back in or on all or a portion of a separated body part to its normal location or other suitable location

Body Part Character 4	Approach Character 5	Device Character 6	Qualifier Character 7
Ø Kidney, Right 1 Kidney, Left 2 Kidneys, Bilateral 3 Kidney Pelvis, Right 4 Kidney Pelvis, Left 6 Ureter, Right 7 Ureter, Left 8 Ureters, Bilateral B Bladder C Bladder Neck D Urethra	Ø Open 4 Percutaneous Endoscopic	Z No Device	Z No Qualifier

Ø Medical and Surgical
T Urinary System
N Release Freeing a body part from an abnormal physical constraint

Body Part Character 4	Approach Character 5	Device Character 6	Qualifier Character 7
Ø Kidney, Right 1 Kidney, Left 3 Kidney Pelvis, Right 4 Kidney Pelvis, Left 6 Ureter, Right 7 Ureter, Left B Bladder C Bladder Neck	Ø Open 3 Percutaneous 4 Percutaneous Endoscopic 7 Via Natural or Artificial Opening 8 Via Natural or Artificial Opening Endoscopic	Z No Device	Z No Qualifier
D Urethra	Ø Open 3 Percutaneous 4 Percutaneous Endoscopic 7 Via Natural or Artificial Opening 8 Via Natural or Artificial Opening Endoscopic X External	Z No Device	Z No Qualifier

Ø Medical and Surgical
T Urinary System
P Removal Taking out or off a device from a body part

Body Part Character 4	Approach Character 5	Device Character 6	Qualifier Character 7
5 Kidney	Ø Open 3 Percutaneous 4 Percutaneous Endoscopic 7 Via Natural or Artificial Opening 8 Via Natural or Artificial Opening Endoscopic	Ø Drainage Device 2 Monitoring Device 3 Infusion Device 7 Autologous Tissue Substitute C Extraluminal Device D Intraluminal Device J Synthetic Substitute K Nonautologous Tissue Substitute	Z No Qualifier
5 Kidney	X External	Ø Drainage Device 2 Monitoring Device 3 Infusion Device D Intraluminal Device	Z No Qualifier
9 Ureter	Ø Open 3 Percutaneous 4 Percutaneous Endoscopic 7 Via Natural or Artificial Opening 8 Via Natural or Artificial Opening Endoscopic	Ø Drainage Device 2 Monitoring Device 3 Infusion Device 7 Autologous Tissue Substitute C Extraluminal Device D Intraluminal Device J Synthetic Substitute K Nonautologous Tissue Substitute M Stimulator Lead	Z No Qualifier
9 Ureter	X External	Ø Drainage Device 2 Monitoring Device 3 Infusion Device D Intraluminal Device M Stimulator Lead	Z No Qualifier

ØTP Continued on next page

Urinary System

0TP–0TR

0   **Medical and Surgical**   *0TP Continued*
T   **Urinary System**
P   **Removal**   Taking out or off a device from a body part

Body Part Character 4	Approach Character 5	Device Character 6	Qualifier Character 7
B Bladder	**0** Open **3** Percutaneous **4** Percutaneous Endoscopic **7** Via Natural or Artificial Opening **8** Via Natural or Artificial Opening Endoscopic	**0** Drainage Device **2** Monitoring Device **3** Infusion Device **7** Autologous Tissue Substitute **C** Extraluminal Device **D** Intraluminal Device **J** Synthetic Substitute **K** Nonautologous Tissue Substitute **L** Artificial Sphincter **M** Stimulator Lead	**Z** No Qualifier
B Bladder	**X** External	**0** Drainage Device **2** Monitoring Device **3** Infusion Device **D** Intraluminal Device **L** Artificial Sphincter **M** Stimulator Lead	**Z** No Qualifier
D Urethra	**0** Open **3** Percutaneous **4** Percutaneous Endoscopic **7** Via Natural or Artificial Opening **8** Via Natural or Artificial Opening Endoscopic	**0** Drainage Device **2** Monitoring Device **3** Infusion Device **7** Autologous Tissue Substitute **C** Extraluminal Device **D** Intraluminal Device **J** Synthetic Substitute **K** Nonautologous Tissue Substitute **L** Artificial Sphincter	**Z** No Qualifier
D Urethra	**X** External	**0** Drainage Device **2** Monitoring Device **3** Infusion Device **D** Intraluminal Device **L** Artificial Sphincter	**Z** No Qualifier

0   **Medical and Surgical**
T   **Urinary System**
Q   **Repair**   Restoring, to the extent possible, a body part to its normal anatomic structure and function

Body Part Character 4	Approach Character 5	Device Character 6	Qualifier Character 7
0 Kidney, Right **1** Kidney, Left **3** Kidney Pelvis, Right **4** Kidney Pelvis, Left **6** Ureter, Right **7** Ureter, Left **B** Bladder **C** Bladder Neck	**0** Open **3** Percutaneous **4** Percutaneous Endoscopic **7** Via Natural or Artificial Opening **8** Via Natural or Artificial Opening Endoscopic	**Z** No Device	**Z** No Qualifier
D Urethra	**0** Open **3** Percutaneous **4** Percutaneous Endoscopic **7** Via Natural or Artificial Opening **8** Via Natural or Artificial Opening Endoscopic **X** External	**Z** No Device	**Z** No Qualifier

0   **Medical and Surgical**
T   **Urinary System**
R   **Replacement**   Putting in or on biological or synthetic material that physically takes the place and/or function of all or a portion of a body part

Body Part Character 4	Approach Character 5	Device Character 6	Qualifier Character 7
3 Kidney Pelvis, Right **4** Kidney Pelvis, Left **6** Ureter, Right **7** Ureter, Left **B** Bladder **C** Bladder Neck	**0** Open **4** Percutaneous Endoscopic **7** Via Natural or Artificial Opening **8** Via Natural or Artificial Opening Endoscopic	**7** Autologous Tissue Substitute **J** Synthetic Substitute **K** Nonautologous Tissue Substitute	**Z** No Qualifier
D Urethra	**0** Open **4** Percutaneous Endoscopic **7** Via Natural or Artificial Opening **8** Via Natural or Artificial Opening Endoscopic **X** External	**7** Autologous Tissue Substitute **J** Synthetic Substitute **K** Nonautologous Tissue Substitute	**Z** No Qualifier

Ø   **Medical and Surgical**
T   **Urinary System**
S   **Reposition**   Moving to its normal location or other suitable location all or a portion of a body part

Body Part Character 4	Approach Character 5	Device Character 6	Qualifier Character 7
Ø Kidney, Right **1** Kidney, Left **2** Kidneys, Bilateral **3** Kidney Pelvis, Right **4** Kidney Pelvis, Left **6** Ureter, Right **7** Ureter, Left **8** Ureters, Bilateral **B** Bladder **C** Bladder Neck **D** Urethra	**Ø** Open **4** Percutaneous Endoscopic	**Z** No Device	**Z** No Qualifier

Ø   **Medical and Surgical**
T   **Urinary System**
T   **Resection**   Cutting out or off, without replacement, all of a body part

Body Part Character 4	Approach Character 5	Device Character 6	Qualifier Character 7
Ø Kidney, Right **1** Kidney, Left **2** Kidneys, Bilateral	**Ø** Open **4** Percutaneous Endoscopic	**Z** No Device	**Z** No Qualifier
3 Kidney Pelvis, Right **4** Kidney Pelvis, Left **6** Ureter, Right **7** Ureter, Left **B** Bladder **C** Bladder Neck **D** Urethra	**Ø** Open **4** Percutaneous Endoscopic **7** Via Natural or Artificial Opening **8** Via Natural or Artificial Opening Endoscopic	**Z** No Device	**Z** No Qualifier

Ø   **Medical and Surgical**
T   **Urinary System**
U   **Supplement**   Putting in or on biological or synthetic material that physically reinforces and/or augments the function of a portion of a body part

Body Part Character 4	Approach Character 5	Device Character 6	Qualifier Character 7
3 Kidney Pelvis, Right **4** Kidney Pelvis, Left **6** Ureter, Right **7** Ureter, Left **B** Bladder **C** Bladder Neck	**Ø** Open **4** Percutaneous Endoscopic **7** Via Natural or Artificial Opening **8** Via Natural or Artificial Opening Endoscopic	**7** Autologous Tissue Substitute **J** Synthetic Substitute **K** Nonautologous Tissue Substitute	**Z** No Qualifier
D Urethra	**Ø** Open **4** Percutaneous Endoscopic **7** Via Natural or Artificial Opening **8** Via Natural or Artificial Opening Endoscopic **X** External	**7** Autologous Tissue Substitute **J** Synthetic Substitute **K** Nonautologous Tissue Substitute	**Z** No Qualifier

Ø   **Medical and Surgical**
T   **Urinary System**
V   **Restriction**   Partially closing an orifice or the lumen of a tubular body part

Body Part Character 4	Approach Character 5	Device Character 6	Qualifier Character 7
3 Kidney Pelvis, Right **4** Kidney Pelvis, Left **6** Ureter, Right **7** Ureter, Left **B** Bladder **C** Bladder Neck **D** Urethra	**Ø** Open **3** Percutaneous **4** Percutaneous Endoscopic	**C** Extraluminal Device **D** Intraluminal Device **Z** No Device	**Z** No Qualifier
3 Kidney Pelvis, Right **4** Kidney Pelvis, Left **6** Ureter, Right **7** Ureter, Left **B** Bladder **C** Bladder Neck **D** Urethra	**7** Via Natural or Artificial Opening **8** Via Natural or Artificial Opening Endoscopic	**D** Intraluminal Device **Z** No Device	**Z** No Qualifier
D Urethra	**X** External	**Z** No Device	**Z** No Qualifier

Ø   Medical and Surgical
T   Urinary System
W   Revision   Correcting, to the extent possible, a portion of a malfunctioning device or the position of a displaced device

Body Part Character 4	Approach Character 5	Device Character 6	Qualifier Character 7
5 Kidney	Ø Open 3 Percutaneous 4 Percutaneous Endoscopic 7 Via Natural or Artificial Opening 8 Via Natural or Artificial Opening Endoscopic X External	Ø Drainage Device 2 Monitoring Device 3 Infusion Device 7 Autologous Tissue Substitute C Extraluminal Device D Intraluminal Device J Synthetic Substitute K Nonautologous Tissue Substitute	Z No Qualifier
9 Ureter	Ø Open 3 Percutaneous 4 Percutaneous Endoscopic 7 Via Natural or Artificial Opening 8 Via Natural or Artificial Opening Endoscopic X External	Ø Drainage Device 2 Monitoring Device 3 Infusion Device 7 Autologous Tissue Substitute C Extraluminal Device D Intraluminal Device J Synthetic Substitute K Nonautologous Tissue Substitute M Stimulator Lead	Z No Qualifier
B Bladder	Ø Open 3 Percutaneous 4 Percutaneous Endoscopic 7 Via Natural or Artificial Opening 8 Via Natural or Artificial Opening Endoscopic X External	Ø Drainage Device 2 Monitoring Device 3 Infusion Device 7 Autologous Tissue Substitute C Extraluminal Device D Intraluminal Device J Synthetic Substitute K Nonautologous Tissue Substitute L Artificial Sphincter M Stimulator Lead	Z No Qualifier
D Urethra	Ø Open 3 Percutaneous 4 Percutaneous Endoscopic 7 Via Natural or Artificial Opening 8 Via Natural or Artificial Opening Endoscopic X External	Ø Drainage Device 2 Monitoring Device 3 Infusion Device 7 Autologous Tissue Substitute C Extraluminal Device D Intraluminal Device J Synthetic Substitute K Nonautologous Tissue Substitute L Artificial Sphincter	Z No Qualifier

Ø   Medical and Surgical
T   Urinary System
Y   Transplantation   Putting in or on all or a portion of a living body part taken from another individual or animal to physically take the place and/or function of all or a portion of a similar body part

Body Part Character 4	Approach Character 5	Device Character 6	Qualifier Character 7
Ø Kidney, Right 1 Kidney, Left	Ø Open	Z No Device	Ø Allogeneic 1 Syngeneic 2 Zooplastic

       Revised Text in **BLUE**

Female Reproductive System 0U1–0UY

0   **Medical and Surgical**
U   **Female Reproductive System**
1   **Bypass**   Altering the route of passage of the contents of a tubular body part

Body Part Character 4	Approach Character 5	Device Character 6	Qualifier Character 7
5 Fallopian Tube, Right **6** Fallopian Tube, Left	**0** Open **4** Percutaneous Endoscopic	**7** Autologous Tissue Substitute **J** Synthetic Substitute **K** Nonautologous Tissue Substitute **Z** No Device	**5** Fallopian Tube, Right **6** Fallopian Tube, Left **9** Uterus

0   **Medical and Surgical**
U   **Female Reproductive System**
2   **Change**   Taking out or off a device from a body part and putting back an identical or similar device in or on the same body part without cutting or puncturing the skin or a mucous membrane

Body Part Character 4	Approach Character 5	Device Character 6	Qualifier Character 7
3 Ovary **8** Fallopian Tube **M** Vulva	**X** External	**0** Drainage Device **Y** Other Device	**Z** No Qualifier
D Uterus and Cervix	**X** External	**0** Drainage Device **H** Contraceptive Device **Y** Other Device	**Z** No Qualifier
H Vagina and Cul-de-sac	**X** External	**0** Drainage Device **G** Pessary **Y** Other Device	**Z** No Qualifier

0   **Medical and Surgical**
U   **Female Reproductive System**
5   **Destruction**   Physical eradication of all or a portion of a body part by the direct use of energy, force, or a destructive agent

Body Part Character 4	Approach Character 5	Device Character 6	Qualifier Character 7
0 Ovary, Right **1** Ovary, Left **2** Ovaries, Bilateral **4** Uterine Supporting Structure	**0** Open **3** Percutaneous **4** Percutaneous Endoscopic	**Z** No Device	**Z** No Qualifier
5 Fallopian Tube, Right **6** Fallopian Tube, Left **7** Fallopian Tubes, Bilateral **9** Uterus **B** Endometrium **C** Cervix **F** Cul-de-sac **K** Hymen	**0** Open **3** Percutaneous **4** Percutaneous Endoscopic **7** Via Natural or Artificial Opening **8** Via Natural or Artificial Opening Endoscopic	**Z** No Device	**Z** No Qualifier
G Vagina	**0** Open **3** Percutaneous **4** Percutaneous Endoscopic **7** Via Natural or Artificial Opening **8** Via Natural or Artificial Opening Endoscopic **X** External	**Z** No Device	**Z** No Qualifier
J Clitoris **L** Vestibular Gland **M** Vulva	**0** Open **X** External	**Z** No Device	**Z** No Qualifier

0   **Medical and Surgical**
U   **Female Reproductive System**
7   **Dilation**   Expanding an orifice or lumen of a tabular body part

Body Part Character 4	Approach Character 5	Device Character 6	Qualifier Character 7
5 Fallopian Tube, Right **6** Fallopian Tube, Left **7** Fallopian Tubes, Bilateral **9** Uterus **C** Cervix **G** Vagina **K** Hymen	**0** Open **3** Percutaneous **4** Percutaneous Endoscopic **7** Via Natural or Artificial Opening **8** Via Natural or Artificial Opening Endoscopic	**D** Intraluminal Device **Z** No Device	**Z** No Qualifier

0   **Medical and Surgical**
U   **Female Reproductive System**
8   **Division**   Cutting into a body part without draining fluids and/or gases from the body part in order to separate or transect a body part

Body Part Character 4	Approach Character 5	Device Character 6	Qualifier Character 7
0 Ovary, Right **1** Ovary, Left **2** Ovaries, Bilateral **4** Uterine Supporting Structure	**0** Open **3** Percutaneous **4** Percutaneous Endoscopic	**Z** No Device	**Z** No Qualifier
K Hymen	**7** Via Natural or Artificial Opening **8** Via Natural or Artificial Opening Endoscopic	**Z** No Device	**Z** No Qualifier

0   **Medical and Surgical**
U   **Female Reproductive System**
9   **Drainage**   Taking or letting out fluids and/or gases from a body part

Body Part Character 4	Approach Character 5	Device Character 6	Qualifier Character 7
0 Ovary, Right **1** Ovary, Left **2** Ovaries, Bilateral	**X** External	**Z** No Device	**Z** No Qualifier
0 Ovary, Right **1** Ovary, Left **2** Ovaries, Bilateral **4** Uterine Supporting Structure	**0** Open **3** Percutaneous **4** Percutaneous Endoscopic	**0** Drainage Device	**Z** No Qualifier
0 Ovary, Right **1** Ovary, Left **2** Ovaries, Bilateral **4** Uterine Supporting Structure	**0** Open **3** Percutaneous **4** Percutaneous Endoscopic	**Z** No Device	**X** Diagnostic **Z** No Qualifier
5 Fallopian Tube, Right **6** Fallopian Tube, Left **7** Fallopian Tubes, Bilateral **9** Uterus **C** Cervix **F** Cul-de-sac **K** Hymen	**0** Open **3** Percutaneous **4** Percutaneous Endoscopic **7** Via Natural or Artificial Opening **8** Via Natural or Artificial Opening Endoscopic	**0** Drainage Device	**Z** No Qualifier
5 Fallopian Tube, Right **6** Fallopian Tube, Left **7** Fallopian Tubes, Bilateral **9** Uterus **C** Cervix **F** Cul-de-sac **K** Hymen	**0** Open **3** Percutaneous **4** Percutaneous Endoscopic **7** Via Natural or Artificial Opening **8** Via Natural or Artificial Opening Endoscopic	**Z** No Device	**X** Diagnostic **Z** No Qualifier
G Vagina	**0** Open **3** Percutaneous **4** Percutaneous Endoscopic **7** Via Natural or Artificial Opening **8** Via Natural or Artificial Opening Endoscopic **X** External	**0** Drainage Device	**Z** No Qualifier
G Vagina	**0** Open **3** Percutaneous **4** Percutaneous Endoscopic **7** Via Natural or Artificial Opening **8** Via Natural or Artificial Opening Endoscopic **X** External	**Z** No Device	**X** Diagnostic **Z** No Qualifier
J Clitoris **L** Vestibular Gland **M** Vulva	**0** Open **X** External	**0** Drainage Device	**Z** No Qualifier
J Clitoris **L** Vestibular Gland **M** Vulva	**0** Open **X** External	**Z** No Device	**X** Diagnostic **Z** No Qualifier

Ø Medical and Surgical
U Female Reproductive System
B Excision   Cutting out or off, without replacement, a portion of a body part

Body Part Character 4	Approach Character 5	Device Character 6	Qualifier Character 7
Ø Ovary, Right 1 Ovary, Left 2 Ovaries, Bilateral 4 Uterine Supporting Structure 5 Fallopian Tube, Right 6 Fallopian Tube, Left 7 Fallopian Tubes, Bilateral 9 Uterus C Cervix F Cul-de-sac K Hymen	Ø Open 3 Percutaneous 4 Percutaneous Endoscopic 7 Via Natural or Artificial Opening 8 Via Natural or Artificial Opening Endoscopic	Z No Device	X Diagnostic Z No Qualifier
G Vagina	Ø Open 3 Percutaneous 4 Percutaneous Endoscopic 7 Via Natural or Artificial Opening 8 Via Natural or Artificial Opening Endoscopic X External	Z No Device	X Diagnostic Z No Qualifier
J Clitoris L Vestibular Gland M Vulva	Ø Open X External	Z No Device	X Diagnostic Z No Qualifier

Ø Medical and Surgical
U Female Reproductive System
C Extirpation   Taking or cutting out solid matter from a body part

Body Part Character 4	Approach Character 5	Device Character 6	Qualifier Character 7
Ø Ovary, Right 1 Ovary, Left 2 Ovaries, Bilateral 4 Uterine Supporting Structure	Ø Open 3 Percutaneous 4 Percutaneous Endoscopic	Z No Device	Z No Qualifier
5 Fallopian Tube, Right 6 Fallopian Tube, Left 7 Fallopian Tubes, Bilateral 9 Uterus B Endometrium C Cervix F Cul-de-sac K Hymen	Ø Open 3 Percutaneous 4 Percutaneous Endoscopic 7 Via Natural or Artificial Opening 8 Via Natural or Artificial Opening Endoscopic	Z No Device	Z No Qualifier
G Vagina	Ø Open 3 Percutaneous 4 Percutaneous Endoscopic 7 Via Natural or Artificial Opening 8 Via Natural or Artificial Opening Endoscopic X External	Z No Device	Z No Qualifier
J Clitoris L Vestibular Gland M Vulva	Ø Open X External	Z No Device	Z No Qualifier

Ø Medical and Surgical
U Female Reproductive System
D Extraction   Pulling or stripping out or off all or a portion of a body part by the use of force

Body Part Character 4	Approach Character 5	Device Character 6	Qualifier Character 7
B Endometrium	7 Via Natural or Artificial Opening 8 Via Natural or Artificial Opening Endoscopic	Z No Device	X Diagnostic Z No Qualifier
N Ova	Ø Open 3 Percutaneous 4 Percutaneous Endoscopic	Z No Device	Z No Qualifier

Ø   **Medical and Surgical**
U   **Female Reproductive System**
F   **Fragmentation**   Breaking solid matter in a body part into pieces

Body Part Character 4	Approach Character 5	Device Character 6	Qualifier Character 7
5 Fallopian Tube, Right 6 Fallopian Tube, Left 7 Fallopian Tubes, Bilateral 9 Uterus	Ø Open 3 Percutaneous 4 Percutaneous Endoscopic 7 Via Natural or Artificial Opening 8 Via Natural or Artificial Opening Endoscopic X External	Z No Device	Z No Qualifier

Ø   **Medical and Surgical**
U   **Female Reproductive System**
H   **Insertion**   Putting in a nonbiological appliance that monitors, assists, performs, or prevents a physiological function but does not physically take the place of a body part

Body Part Character 4	Approach Character 5	Device Character 6	Qualifier Character 7
3 Ovary	Ø Open 3 Percutaneous 4 Percutaneous Endoscopic	3 Infusion Device	Z No Qualifier
8 Fallopian Tube D Uterus and Cervix H Vagina and Cul-de-sac	Ø Open 3 Percutaneous 4 Percutaneous Endoscopic 7 Via Natural or Artificial Opening 8 Via Natural or Artificial Opening Endoscopic	3 Infusion Device	Z No Qualifier
9 Uterus C Cervix	7 Via Natural or Artificial Opening 8 Via Natural or Artificial Opening Endoscopic	H Contraceptive Device	Z No Qualifier
F Cul-de-sac	7 Via Natural or Artificial Opening 8 Via Natural or Artificial Opening Endoscopic	G Pessary	Z No Qualifier
G Vagina	Ø Open 3 Percutaneous 4 Percutaneous Endoscopic X External	1 Radioactive Element	Z No Qualifier
G Vagina	7 Via Natural or Artificial Opening 8 Via Natural or Artificial Opening Endoscopic	1 Radioactive Element G Pessary	Z No Qualifier

Ø   **Medical and Surgical**
U   **Female Reproductive System**
J   **Inspection**   Visually and/or manually exploring a body part

Body Part Character 4	Approach Character 5	Device Character 6	Qualifier Character 7
3 Ovary	Ø Open 3 Percutaneous 4 Percutaneous Endoscopic X External	Z No Device	Z No Qualifier
8 Fallopian Tube D Uterus and Cervix H Vagina and Cul-de-sac	Ø Open 3 Percutaneous 4 Percutaneous Endoscopic 7 Via Natural or Artificial Opening 8 Via Natural or Artificial Opening Endoscopic X External	Z No Device	Z No Qualifier
M Vulva	Ø Open X External	Z No Device	Z No Qualifier

0   Medical and Surgical
U   Female Reproductive System
L   Occlusion   Completely closing an orifice or the lumen of a tubular body part

Body Part Character 4	Approach Character 5	Device Character 6	Qualifier Character 7
5 Fallopian Tube, Right 6 Fallopian Tube, Left 7 Fallopian Tubes, Bilateral	0 Open 3 Percutaneous 4 Percutaneous Endoscopic	C Extraluminal Device D Intraluminal Device Z No Device	Z No Qualifier
5 Fallopian Tube, Right 6 Fallopian Tube, Left 7 Fallopian Tubes, Bilateral F Cul-de-sac G Vagina	7 Via Natural or Artificial Opening 8 Via Natural or Artificial Opening Endoscopic	D Intraluminal Device Z No Device	Z No Qualifier

0   Medical and Surgical
U   Female Reproductive System
M   Reattachment   Putting back in or on all or a portion of a separated body part to its normal location or other suitable location

Body Part Character 4	Approach Character 5	Device Character 6	Qualifier Character 7
0 Ovary, Right 1 Ovary, Left 2 Ovaries, Bilateral 4 Uterine Supporting Structure 5 Fallopian Tube, Right 6 Fallopian Tube, Left 7 Fallopian Tubes, Bilateral 9 Uterus C Cervix F Cul-de-sac G Vagina K Hymen	0 Open 4 Percutaneous Endoscopic	Z No Device	Z No Qualifier
J Clitoris M Vulva	X External	Z No Device	Z No Qualifier

0   Medical and Surgical
U   Female Reproductive System
N   Release   Freeing a body part from an abnormal physical constraint

Body Part Character 4	Approach Character 5	Device Character 6	Qualifier Character 7
0 Ovary, Right 1 Ovary, Left 2 Ovaries, Bilateral 4 Uterine Supporting Structure	0 Open 3 Percutaneous 4 Percutaneous Endoscopic	Z No Device	Z No Qualifier
5 Fallopian Tube, Right 6 Fallopian Tube, Left 7 Fallopian Tubes, Bilateral 9 Uterus C Cervix F Cul-de-sac K Hymen	0 Open 3 Percutaneous 4 Percutaneous Endoscopic 7 Via Natural or Artificial Opening 8 Via Natural or Artificial Opening Endoscopic	Z No Device	Z No Qualifier
G Vagina	0 Open 3 Percutaneous 4 Percutaneous Endoscopic 7 Via Natural or Artificial Opening 8 Via Natural or Artificial Opening Endoscopic X External	Z No Device	Z No Qualifier
J Clitoris L Vestibular Gland M Vulva	0 Open X External	Z No Device	Z No Qualifier

Female Reproductive System

ØUP–ØUQ

Ø   **Medical and Surgical**
U   **Female Reproductive System**
P   **Removal**   Taking out or off a device from a body part

Body Part Character 4	Approach Character 5	Device Character 6	Qualifier Character 7
3 Ovary	**Ø** Open **3** Percutaneous **4** Percutaneous Endoscopic **X** External	**Ø** Drainage Device **3** Infusion Device	**Z** No Qualifier
8 Fallopian Tube	**Ø** Open **3** Percutaneous **4** Percutaneous Endoscopic **7** Via Natural or Artificial Opening **8** Via Natural or Artificial Opening Endoscopic	**Ø** Drainage Device **3** Infusion Device **7** Autologous Tissue Substitute **C** Extraluminal Device **D** Intraluminal Device **J** Synthetic Substitute **K** Nonautologous Tissue Substitute	**Z** No Qualifier
8 Fallopian Tube	**X** External	**Ø** Drainage Device **3** Infusion Device **D** Intraluminal Device	**Z** No Qualifier
D Uterus and Cervix	**Ø** Open **3** Percutaneous **4** Percutaneous Endoscopic **7** Via Natural or Artificial Opening **8** Via Natural or Artificial Opening Endoscopic	**Ø** Drainage Device **3** Infusion Device **7** Autologous Tissue Substitute **C** Extraluminal Device **D** Intraluminal Device **H** Contraceptive Device **J** Synthetic Substitute **K** Nonautologous Tissue Substitute	**Z** No Qualifier
D Uterus and Cervix	**X** External	**Ø** Drainage Device **3** Infusion Device **D** Intraluminal Device **H** Contraceptive Device	**Z** No Qualifier
H Vagina and Cul-de-sac	**Ø** Open **3** Percutaneous **4** Percutaneous Endoscopic **7** Via Natural or Artificial Opening **8** Via Natural or Artificial Opening Endoscopic	**Ø** Drainage Device **3** Infusion Device **7** Autologous Tissue Substitute **D** Intraluminal Device **G** Pessary **J** Synthetic Substitute **K** Nonautologous Tissue Substitute	**Z** No Qualifier
H Vagina and Cul-de-sac	**X** External	**Ø** Drainage Device **1** Radioactive Element **3** Infusion Device **D** Intraluminal Device **G** Pessary	**Z** No Qualifier
M Vulva	**Ø** Open	**Ø** Drainage Device **7** Autologous Tissue Substitute **J** Synthetic Substitute **K** Nonautologous Tissue Substitute	**Z** No Qualifier
M Vulva	**X** External	**Ø** Drainage Device	**Z** No Qualifier

Ø   **Medical and Surgical**
U   **Female Reproductive System**
Q   **Repair**   Restoring, to the extent possible, a body part to its normal anatomic structure and function

Body Part Character 4	Approach Character 5	Device Character 6	Qualifier Character 7
Ø Ovary, Right **1** Ovary, Left **2** Ovaries, Bilateral **4** Uterine Supporting Structure	**Ø** Open **3** Percutaneous **4** Percutaneous Endoscopic	**Z** No Device	**Z** No Qualifier
5 Fallopian Tube, Right **6** Fallopian Tube, Left **7** Fallopian Tubes, Bilateral **9** Uterus **C** Cervix **F** Cul-de-sac **K** Hymen	**Ø** Open **3** Percutaneous **4** Percutaneous Endoscopic **7** Via Natural or Artificial Opening **8** Via Natural or Artificial Opening Endoscopic	**Z** No Device	**Z** No Qualifier
G Vagina	**Ø** Open **3** Percutaneous **4** Percutaneous Endoscopic **7** Via Natural or Artificial Opening **8** Via Natural or Artificial Opening Endoscopic **X** External	**Z** No Device	**Z** No Qualifier
J Clitoris **L** Vestibular Gland **M** Vulva	**Ø** Open **X** External	**Z** No Device	**Z** No Qualifier

       Revised Text in **BLUE**   © 2011 Ingenix, Inc

0 **Medical and Surgical**
U **Female Reproductive System**
S **Reposition**   Moving to its normal location or other suitable location all or a portion of a body part

Body Part Character 4	Approach Character 5	Device Character 6	Qualifier Character 7
0 Ovary, Right **1** Ovary, Left **2** Ovaries, Bilateral **4** Uterine Supporting Structure **5** Fallopian Tube, Right **6** Fallopian Tube, Left **7** Fallopian Tubes, Bilateral **C** Cervix **F** Cul-de-sac	**0** Open **4** Percutaneous Endoscopic	**Z** No Device	**Z** No Qualifier
9 Uterus **G** Vagina	**0** Open **4** Percutaneous Endoscopic **X** External	**Z** No Device	**Z** No Qualifier

0 **Medical and Surgical**
U **Female Reproductive System**
T **Resection**   Cutting out or off, without replacement, all of a body part

Body Part Character 4	Approach Character 5	Device Character 6	Qualifier Character 7
0 Ovary, Right **1** Ovary, Left **2** Ovaries, Bilateral **5** Fallopian Tube, Right **6** Fallopian Tube, Left **7** Fallopian Tubes, Bilateral **9** Uterus	**0** Open **4** Percutaneous Endoscopic **7** Via Natural or Artificial Opening **8** Via Natural or Artificial Opening Endoscopic **F** Via Natural or Artificial Opening With Percutaneous Endoscopic Assistance	**Z** No Device	**Z** No Qualifier
4 Uterine Supporting Structure **C** Cervix **F** Cul-de-sac **G** Vagina **K** Hymen	**0** Open **4** Percutaneous Endoscopic **7** Via Natural or Artificial Opening **8** Via Natural or Artificial Opening Endoscopic	**Z** No Device	**Z** No Qualifier
J Clitoris **L** Vestibular Gland **M** Vulva	**0** Open **X** External	**Z** No Device	**Z** No Qualifier

0 **Medical and Surgical**
U **Female Reproductive System**
U **Supplement**   Putting in or on biological or synthetic material that physically reinforces and/or augments the function of a portion of a body part

Body Part Character 4	Approach Character 5	Device Character 6	Qualifier Character 7
4 Uterine Supporting Structure	**0** Open **4** Percutaneous Endoscopic	**7** Autologous Tissue Substitute **J** Synthetic Substitute **K** Nonautologous Tissue Substitute	**Z** No Qualifier
5 Fallopian Tube, Right **6** Fallopian Tube, Left **7** Fallopian Tubes, Bilateral **F** Cul-de-sac **K** Hymen	**0** Open **4** Percutaneous Endoscopic **7** Via Natural or Artificial Opening **8** Via Natural or Artificial Opening Endoscopic	**7** Autologous Tissue Substitute **J** Synthetic Substitute **K** Nonautologous Tissue Substitute	**Z** No Qualifier
G Vagina	**0** Open **4** Percutaneous Endoscopic **7** Via Natural or Artificial Opening **8** Via Natural or Artificial Opening Endoscopic **X** External	**7** Autologous Tissue Substitute **J** Synthetic Substitute **K** Nonautologous Tissue Substitute	**Z** No Qualifier
J Clitoris **M** Vulva	**0** Open **X** External	**7** Autologous Tissue Substitute **J** Synthetic Substitute **K** Nonautologous Tissue Substitute	**Z** No Qualifier

Ø **Medical and Surgical**
U **Female Reproductive System**
V **Restriction**   Partially closing an orifice or the lumen of a tubular body part

Body Part Character 4	Approach Character 5	Device Character 6	Qualifier Character 7
C Cervix	**Ø** Open **3** Percutaneous **4** Percutaneous Endoscopic	**C** Extraluminal Device **D** Intraluminal Device **Z** No Device	**Z** No Qualifier
C Cervix	**7** Via Natural or Artificial Opening **8** Via Natural or Artificial Opening Endoscopic	**D** Intraluminal Device **Z** No Device	**Z** No Qualifier

Ø **Medical and Surgical**
U **Female Reproductive System**
W **Revision**   Correcting, to the extent possible, a portion of a malfunctioning device or the position of a displaced device

Body Part Character 4	Approach Character 5	Device Character 6	Qualifier Character 7
3 Ovary	**Ø** Open **3** Percutaneous **4** Percutaneous Endoscopic **X** External	**Ø** Drainage Device **3** Infusion Device	**Z** No Qualifier
8 Fallopian Tube	**Ø** Open **3** Percutaneous **4** Percutaneous Endoscopic **7** Via Natural or Artificial Opening **8** Via Natural or Artificial Opening Endoscopic **X** External	**Ø** Drainage Device **3** Infusion Device **7** Autologous Tissue Substitute **C** Extraluminal Device **D** Intraluminal Device **J** Synthetic Substitute **K** Nonautologous Tissue Substitute	**Z** No Qualifier
D Uterus and Cervix	**Ø** Open **3** Percutaneous **4** Percutaneous Endoscopic **7** Via Natural or Artificial Opening **8** Via Natural or Artificial Opening Endoscopic **X** External	**Ø** Drainage Device **3** Infusion Device **7** Autologous Tissue Substitute **C** Extraluminal Device **D** Intraluminal Device **H** Contraceptive Device **J** Synthetic Substitute **K** Nonautologous Tissue Substitute	**Z** No Qualifier
H Vagina and Cul-de-sac	**Ø** Open **3** Percutaneous **4** Percutaneous Endoscopic **7** Via Natural or Artificial Opening **8** Via Natural or Artificial Opening Endoscopic **X** External	**Ø** Drainage Device **3** Infusion Device **7** Autologous Tissue Substitute **D** Intraluminal Device **G** Pessary **J** Synthetic Substitute **K** Nonautologous Tissue Substitute	**Z** No Qualifier
M Vulva	**Ø** Open **X** External	**Ø** Drainage Device **7** Autologous Tissue Substitute **J** Synthetic Substitute **K** Nonautologous Tissue Substitute	**Z** No Qualifier

Ø **Medical and Surgical**
U **Female Reproductive System**
Y **Transplantation** Putting in or on all or a portion of a living body part taken from another individual or animal to physically take the place and/or function of all or a portion of a similar body part

Body Part Character 4	Approach Character 5	Device Character 6	Qualifier Character 7
Ø Ovary, Right **1** Ovary, Left	**Ø** Open	**Z** No Device	**Ø** **Allogeneic** **1** **Syngeneic** **2** **Zooplastic**

Revised Text in **BLUE**

Male Reproductive System ØV1–ØVW

Ø   **Medical and Surgical**
V   **Male Reproductive System**
1   **Bypass**   Altering the route of passage of the contents of a tubular body part

Body Part Character 4	Approach Character 5	Device Character 6	Qualifier Character 7
N Vas Deferens, Right P Vas Deferens, Left Q Vas Deferens, Bilateral	Ø Open 4 Percutaneous Endoscopic	7 Autologous Tissue Substitute J Synthetic Substitute K Nonautologous Tissue Substitute Z No Device	J Epididymis, Right K Epididymis, Left N Vas Deferens, Right P Vas Deferens, Left

Ø   **Medical and Surgical**
V   **Male Reproductive System**
2   **Change**   Taking out or off a device from a body part and putting back an identical or similar device in or on the same body part without cutting or puncturing the skin or a mucous membrane

Body Part Character 4	Approach Character 5	Device Character 6	Qualifier Character 7
4 Prostate and Seminal Vesicles 8 Scrotum and Tunica Vaginalis D Testis M Epididymis and Spermatic Cord R Vas Deferens S Penis	X External	Ø Drainage Device Y Other Device	Z No Qualifier

Ø   **Medical and Surgical**
V   **Male Reproductive System**
5   **Destruction**   Physical eradication of all or a portion of a body part by the direct use of energy, force, or a destructive agent

Body Part Character 4	Approach Character 5	Device Character 6	Qualifier Character 7
Ø Prostate	Ø Open 3 Percutaneous 4 Percutaneous Endoscopic 7 Via Natural or Artificial Opening 8 Via Natural or Artificial Opening Endoscopic	Z No Device	Z No Qualifier
1 Seminal Vesicle, Right 2 Seminal Vesicle, Left 3 Seminal Vesicles, Bilateral 6 Tunica Vaginalis, Right 7 Tunica Vaginalis, Left 9 Testis, Right B Testis, Left C Testes, Bilateral F Spermatic Cord, Right G Spermatic Cord, Left H Spermatic Cords, Bilateral J Epididymis, Right K Epididymis, Left L Epididymis, Bilateral N Vas Deferens, Right P Vas Deferens, Left Q Vas Deferens, Bilateral	Ø Open 3 Percutaneous 4 Percutaneous Endoscopic	Z No Device	Z No Qualifier
5 Scrotum S Penis T Prepuce	Ø Open 3 Percutaneous 4 Percutaneous Endoscopic X External	Z No Device	Z No Qualifier

Ø   **Medical and Surgical**
V   **Male Reproductive System**
7   **Dilation**   Expanding an orifice or the lumen of a tubular body part

Body Part Character 4	Approach Character 5	Device Character 6	Qualifier Character 7
N Vas Deferens, Right P Vas Deferens, Left Q Vas Deferens, Bilateral	Ø Open 3 Percutaneous 4 Percutaneous Endoscopic	D Intraluminal Device Z No Device	Z No Qualifier

Ø   **Medical and Surgical**
V   **Male Reproductive System**
9   **Drainage**   Taking or letting out fluids and/or gases from a body part

Body Part Character 4	Approach Character 5	Device Character 6	Qualifier Character 7
Ø Prostate	**Ø** Open **3** Percutaneous **4** Percutaneous Endoscopic **7** Via Natural or Artificial Opening **8** Via Natural or Artificial Opening Endoscopic	**Ø** Drainage Device	**Z** No Qualifier
Ø Prostate	**Ø** Open **3** Percutaneous **4** Percutaneous Endoscopic **7** Via Natural or Artificial Opening **8** Via Natural or Artificial Opening Endoscopic	**Z** No Device	**X** Diagnostic **Z** No Qualifier
1 Seminal Vesicle, Right **2** Seminal Vesicle, Left **3** Seminal Vesicles, Bilateral **6** Tunica Vaginalis, Right **7** Tunica Vaginalis, Left **9** Testis, Right **B** Testis, Left **C** Testes, Bilateral **F** Spermatic Cord, Right **G** Spermatic Cord, Left **H** Spermatic Cords, Bilateral **J** Epididymis, Right **K** Epididymis, Left **L** Epididymis, Bilateral **N** Vas Deferens, Right **P** Vas Deferens, Left **Q** Vas Deferens, Bilateral	**Ø** Open **3** Percutaneous **4** Percutaneous Endoscopic	**Ø** Drainage Device	**Z** No Qualifier
1 Seminal Vesicle, Right **2** Seminal Vesicle, Left **3** Seminal Vesicles, Bilateral **6** Tunica Vaginalis, Right **7** Tunica Vaginalis, Left **9** Testis, Right **B** Testis, Left **C** Testes, Bilateral **F** Spermatic Cord, Right **G** Spermatic Cord, Left **H** Spermatic Cords, Bilateral **J** Epididymis, Right **K** Epididymis, Left **L** Epididymis, Bilateral **N** Vas Deferens, Right **P** Vas Deferens, Left **Q** Vas Deferens, Bilateral	**Ø** Open **3** Percutaneous **4** Percutaneous Endoscopic	**Z** No Device	**X** Diagnostic **Z** No Qualifier
5 Scrotum **S** Penis **T** Prepuce	**Ø** Open **3** Percutaneous **4** Percutaneous Endoscopic **X** External	**Ø** Drainage Device	**Z** No Qualifier
5 Scrotum **S** Penis **T** Prepuce	**Ø** Open **3** Percutaneous **4** Percutaneous Endoscopic **X** External	**Z** No Device	**X** Diagnostic **Z** No Qualifier

         Revised Text in **BLUE**

Ø　**Medical and Surgical**
V　**Male Reproductive System**
B　**Excision**　　Cutting out or off, without replacement, a portion of a body part

Body Part Character 4	Approach Character 5	Device Character 6	Qualifier Character 7
Ø Prostate	Ø Open 3 Percutaneous 4 Percutaneous Endoscopic 7 Via Natural or Artificial Opening 8 Via Natural or Artificial Opening Endoscopic	Z No Device	X Diagnostic Z No Qualifier
1 Seminal Vesicle, Right 2 Seminal Vesicle, Left 3 Seminal Vesicles, Bilateral 6 Tunica Vaginalis, Right 7 Tunica Vaginalis, Left 9 Testis, Right B Testis, Left C Testes, Bilateral F Spermatic Cord, Right G Spermatic Cord, Left H Spermatic Cords, Bilateral J Epididymis, Right K Epididymis, Left L Epididymis, Bilateral N Vas Deferens, Right P Vas Deferens, Left Q Vas Deferens, Bilateral	Ø Open 3 Percutaneous 4 Percutaneous Endoscopic	Z No Device	X Diagnostic Z No Qualifier
5 Scrotum S Penis T Prepuce	Ø Open 3 Percutaneous 4 Percutaneous Endoscopic X External	Z No Device	X Diagnostic Z No Qualifier

Ø　**Medical and Surgical**
V　**Male Reproductive System**
C　**Extirpation**　　Taking or cutting out solid matter from a body part

Body Part Character 4	Approach Character 5	Device Character 6	Qualifier Character 7
Ø Prostate	Ø Open 3 Percutaneous 4 Percutaneous Endoscopic 7 Via Natural or Artificial Opening 8 Via Natural or Artificial Opening Endoscopic	Z No Device	Z No Qualifier
1 Seminal Vesicle, Right 2 Seminal Vesicle, Left 3 Seminal Vesicles, Bilateral 6 Tunica Vaginalis, Right 7 Tunica Vaginalis, Left 9 Testis, Right B Testis, Left C Testes, Bilateral F Spermatic Cord, Right G Spermatic Cord, Left H Spermatic Cords, Bilateral J Epididymis, Right K Epididymis, Left L Epididymis, Bilateral N Vas Deferens, Right P Vas Deferens, Left Q Vas Deferens, Bilateral	Ø Open 3 Percutaneous 4 Percutaneous Endoscopic	Z No Device	Z No Qualifier
5 Scrotum S Penis T Prepuce	Ø Open 3 Percutaneous 4 Percutaneous Endoscopic X External	Z No Device	Z No Qualifier

Ø   **Medical and Surgical**
V   **Male Reproductive System**
H   **Insertion**   Putting in a nonbiological appliance that monitors, assists, performs, or prevents a physiological function but does not physically take the place of a body part

Body Part Character 4	Approach Character 5	Device Character 6	Qualifier Character 7
Ø Prostate	Ø Open 3 Percutaneous 4 Percutaneous Endoscopic 7 Via Natural or Artificial Opening 8 Via Natural or Artificial Opening Endoscopic	1 Radioactive Element	Z No Qualifier
4 Prostate and Seminal Vesicles 8 Scrotum and Tunica Vaginalis D Testis M Epididymis and Spermatic Cord R Vas Deferens	Ø Open 3 Percutaneous 4 Percutaneous Endoscopic 7 Via Natural or Artificial Opening 8 Via Natural or Artificial Opening Endoscopic	3 Infusion Device	Z No Qualifier
S Penis	Ø Open 3 Percutaneous 4 Percutaneous Endoscopic X External	3 Infusion Device	Z No Qualifier

Ø   **Medical and Surgical**
V   **Male Reproductive System**
J   **Inspection**   Visually and/or manually exploring a body part

Body Part Character 4	Approach Character 5	Device Character 6	Qualifier Character 7
4 Prostate and Seminal Vesicles 8 Scrotum and Tunica Vaginalis D Testis M Epididymis and Spermatic Cord R Vas Deferens S Penis	Ø Open 3 Percutaneous 4 Percutaneous Endoscopic X External	Z No Device	Z No Qualifier

Ø   **Medical and Surgical**
V   **Male Reproductive System**
L   **Occlusion**   Completely closing an orifice or the lumen of a tubular body part

Body Part Character 4	Approach Character 5	Device Character 6	Qualifier Character 7
F Spermatic Cord, Right G Spermatic Cord, Left H Spermatic Cords, Bilateral N Vas Deferens, Right P Vas Deferens, Left Q Vas Deferens, Bilateral	Ø Open 3 Percutaneous 4 Percutaneous Endoscopic	C Extraluminal Device D Intraluminal Device Z No Device	Z No Qualifier

Ø   **Medical and Surgical**
V   **Male Reproductive System**
M   **Reattachment**   Putting back in or on all or a portion of a separated body part to its normal location or other suitable location

Body Part Character 4	Approach Character 5	Device Character 6	Qualifier Character 7
5 Scrotum S Penis	X External	Z No Device	Z No Qualifier
6 Tunica Vaginalis, Right 7 Tunica Vaginalis, Left 9 Testis, Right B Testis, Left C Testes, Bilateral F Spermatic Cord, Right G Spermatic Cord, Left H Spermatic Cords, Bilateral	Ø Open 4 Percutaneous Endoscopic	Z No Device	Z No Qualifier

Ø　Medical and Surgical
V　Male Reproductive System
N　Release　　　　Freeing a body part from an abnormal physical constraint

Body Part Character 4	Approach Character 5	Device Character 6	Qualifier Character 7
Ø　Prostate	Ø　Open 3　Percutaneous 4　Percutaneous Endoscopic 7　Via Natural or Artificial Opening 8　Via Natural or Artificial Opening Endoscopic	Z　No Device	Z　No Qualifier
1　Seminal Vesicle, Right 2　Seminal Vesicle, Left 3　Seminal Vesicles, Bilateral 6　Tunica Vaginalis, Right 7　Tunica Vaginalis, Left 9　Testis, Right B　Testis, Left C　Testes, Bilateral F　Spermatic Cord, Right G　Spermatic Cord, Left H　Spermatic Cords, Bilateral J　Epididymis, Right K　Epididymis, Left L　Epididymis, Bilateral N　Vas Deferens, Right P　Vas Deferens, Left Q　Vas Deferens, Bilateral	Ø　Open 3　Percutaneous 4　Percutaneous Endoscopic	Z　No Device	Z　No Qualifier
5　Scrotum S　Penis T　Prepuce	Ø　Open 3　Percutaneous 4　Percutaneous Endoscopic X　External	Z　No Device	Z　No Qualifier

Ø　Medical and Surgical
V　Male Reproductive System
P　Removal　　　　Taking out or off a device from a body part

Body Part Character 4	Approach Character 5	Device Character 6	Qualifier Character 7
4　Prostate and Seminal Vesicles	Ø　Open 3　Percutaneous 4　Percutaneous Endoscopic 7　Via Natural or Artificial Opening 8　Via Natural or Artificial Opening Endoscopic	Ø　Drainage Device 1　Radioactive Element 3　Infusion Device 7　Autologous Tissue Substitute J　Synthetic Substitute K　Nonautologous Tissue Substitute	Z　No Qualifier
4　Prostate and Seminal Vesicles	X　External	Ø　Drainage Device 1　Radioactive Element 3　Infusion Device	Z　No Qualifier
8　Scrotum and Tunica Vaginalis D　Testis M　Epididymis and Spermatic Cord S　Penis	X　External	Ø　Drainage Device 3　Infusion Device	Z　No Qualifier
8　Scrotum and Tunica Vaginalis D　Testis S　Penis	Ø　Open 3　Percutaneous 4　Percutaneous Endoscopic 7　Via Natural or Artificial Opening 8　Via Natural or Artificial Opening Endoscopic	Ø　Drainage Device 3　Infusion Device 7　Autologous Tissue Substitute J　Synthetic Substitute K　Nonautologous Tissue Substitute	Z　No Qualifier
M　Epididymis and Spermatic Cord	Ø　Open 3　Percutaneous 4　Percutaneous Endoscopic 7　Via Natural or Artificial Opening 8　Via Natural or Artificial Opening Endoscopic	Ø　Drainage Device 3　Infusion Device 7　Autologous Tissue Substitute C　Extraluminal Device J　Synthetic Substitute K　Nonautologous Tissue Substitute	Z　No Qualifier
R　Vas Deferens	Ø　Open 3　Percutaneous 4　Percutaneous Endoscopic 7　Via Natural or Artificial Opening 8　Via Natural or Artificial Opening Endoscopic	Ø　Drainage Device 3　Infusion Device 7　Autologous Tissue Substitute C　Extraluminal Device D　Intraluminal Device J　Synthetic Substitute K　Nonautologous Tissue Substitute	Z　No Qualifier
R　Vas Deferens	X　External	Ø　Drainage Device 3　Infusion Device D　Intraluminal Device	Z　No Qualifier

Male Reproductive System (side margin)

ØVQ–ØVS (side margin)

Ø Medical and Surgical
V Male Reproductive System
Q Repair   Restoring, to the extent possible, a body part to its normal anatomic structure and function

Body Part Character 4	Approach Character 5	Device Character 6	Qualifier Character 7
Ø Prostate	Ø Open 3 Percutaneous 4 Percutaneous Endoscopic 7 Via Natural or Artificial Opening 8 Via Natural or Artificial Opening Endoscopic	Z No Device	Z No Qualifier
1 Seminal Vesicle, Right 2 Seminal Vesicle, Left 3 Seminal Vesicles, Bilateral 6 Tunica Vaginalis, Right 7 Tunica Vaginalis, Left 9 Testis, Right B Testis, Left C Testes, Bilateral F Spermatic Cord, Right G Spermatic Cord, Left H Spermatic Cords, Bilateral J Epididymis, Right K Epididymis, Left L Epididymis, Bilateral N Vas Deferens, Right P Vas Deferens, Left Q Vas Deferens, Bilateral	Ø Open 3 Percutaneous 4 Percutaneous Endoscopic	Z No Device	Z No Qualifier
5 Scrotum S Penis T Prepuce	Ø Open 3 Percutaneous 4 Percutaneous Endoscopic X External	Z No Device	Z No Qualifier

Ø Medical and Surgical
V Male Reproductive System
R Replacement   Putting in or on biological or synthetic material that physically takes the place and/or function of all or a portion of a body part

Body Part Character 4	Approach Character 5	Device Character 6	Qualifier Character 7
9 Testis, Right B Testis, Left C Testes, Bilateral	Ø Open	J Synthetic Substitute	Z No Qualifier

Ø Medical and Surgical
V Male Reproductive System
S Reposition   Moving to its normal location or other suitable location all or a portion of a body part

Body Part Character 4	Approach Character 5	Device Character 6	Qualifier Character 7
9 Testis, Right B Testis, Left C Testes, Bilateral F Spermatic Cord, Right G Spermatic Cord, Left H Spermatic Cords, Bilateral	Ø Open 3 Percutaneous 4 Percutaneous Endoscopic	Z No Device	Z No Qualifier

0   **Medical and Surgical**
V   **Male Reproductive System**
T   **Resection**   Cutting out or off, without replacement, all of a body part

Body Part Character 4	Approach Character 5	Device Character 6	Qualifier Character 7
0 Prostate	**0** Open **4** Percutaneous Endoscopic **7** Via Natural or Artificial Opening **8** Via Natural or Artificial Opening Endoscopic	**Z** No Device	**Z** No Qualifier
1 Seminal Vesicle, Right **2** Seminal Vesicle, Left **3** Seminal Vesicles, Bilateral **6** Tunica Vaginalis, Right **7** Tunica Vaginalis, Left **9** Testis, Right **B** Testis, Left **C** Testes, Bilateral **F** Spermatic Cord, Right **G** Spermatic Cord, Left **H** Spermatic Cords, Bilateral **J** Epididymis, Right **K** Epididymis, Left **L** Epididymis, Bilateral **N** Vas Deferens, Right **P** Vas Deferens, Left **Q** Vas Deferens, Bilateral	**0** Open **4** Percutaneous Endoscopic	**Z** No Device	**Z** No Qualifier
5 Scrotum **S** Penis **T** Prepuce	**0** Open **4** Percutaneous Endoscopic **X** External	**Z** No Device	**Z** No Qualifier

0   **Medical and Surgical**
V   **Male Reproductive System**
U   **Supplement**   Putting in or on biological or synthetic material that physically reinforces and/or augments the function of a portion of a body part

Body Part Character 4	Approach Character 5	Device Character 6	Qualifier Character 7
1 Seminal Vesicle, Right **2** Seminal Vesicle, Left **3** Seminal Vesicles, Bilateral **6** Tunica Vaginalis, Right **7** Tunica Vaginalis, Left **F** Spermatic Cord, Right **G** Spermatic Cord, Left **H** Spermatic Cords, Bilateral **J** Epididymis, Right **K** Epididymis, Left **L** Epididymis, Bilateral **N** Vas Deferens, Right **P** Vas Deferens, Left **Q** Vas Deferens, Bilateral	**0** Open **4** Percutaneous Endoscopic	**7** Autologous Tissue Substitute **J** Synthetic Substitute **K** Nonautologous Tissue Substitute	**Z** No Qualifier
5 Scrotum **S** Penis **T** Prepuce	**0** Open **4** Percutaneous Endoscopic **X** External	**7** Autologous Tissue Substitute **J** Synthetic Substitute **K** Nonautologous Tissue Substitute	**Z** No Qualifier
9 Testis, Right **B** Testis, Left **C** Testes, Bilateral	**0** Open	**7** Autologous Tissue Substitute **J** Synthetic Substitute **K** Nonautologous Tissue Substitute	**Z** No Qualifier

Ø Medical and Surgical
V Male Reproductive System
W Revision   Correcting, to the extent possible, a portion of a malfunctioning device or the position of a displaced device

Body Part Character 4	Approach Character 5	Device Character 6	Qualifier Character 7
4 Prostate and Seminal Vesicles **8** Scrotum and Tunica Vaginalis **D** Testis **S** Penis	**Ø** Open **3** Percutaneous **4** Percutaneous Endoscopic **7** Via Natural or Artificial Opening **8** Via Natural or Artificial Opening Endoscopic **X** External	**Ø** Drainage Device **3** Infusion Device **7** Autologous Tissue Substitute **J** Synthetic Substitute **K** Nonautologous Tissue Substitute	**Z** No Qualifier
M Epididymis and Spermatic Cord	**Ø** Open **3** Percutaneous **4** Percutaneous Endoscopic **7** Via Natural or Artificial Opening **8** Via Natural or Artificial Opening Endoscopic **X** External	**Ø** Drainage Device **3** Infusion Device **7** Autologous Tissue Substitute **C** Extraluminal Device **J** Synthetic Substitute **K** Nonautologous Tissue Substitute	**Z** No Qualifier
R Vas Deferens	**Ø** Open **3** Percutaneous **4** Percutaneous Endoscopic **7** Via Natural or Artificial Opening **8** Via Natural or Artificial Opening Endoscopic **X** External	**Ø** Drainage Device **3** Infusion Device **7** Autologous Tissue Substitute **C** Extraluminal Device **D** Intraluminal Device **J** Synthetic Substitute **K** Nonautologous Tissue Substitute	**Z** No Qualifier

    Revised Text in **BLUE**

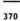

Anatomical Regions, General ØWØ-ØWW

Ø **Medical and Surgical**
W **Anatomical Regions, General**
Ø **Alteration**　　　　Modifying the anatomic structure of a body part without affecting the function of the body part

Body Part Character 4	Approach Character 5	Device Character 6	Qualifier Character 7
Ø Head **2** Face **4** Upper Jaw **5** Lower Jaw **6** Neck **8** Chest Wall **F** Abdominal Wall **K** Upper Back **L** Lower Back **M** Perineum, Male **N** Perineum, Female	**Ø** Open **3** Percutaneous **4** Percutaneous Endoscopic	**7** Autologous Tissue Substitute **J** Synthetic Substitute **K** Nonautologous Tissue Substitute **Z** No Device	**Z** No Qualifier

Ø **Medical and Surgical**
W **Anatomical Regions, General**
1 **Bypass**　　　　Altering the route of passage of the contents of a tubular body part

Body Part Character 4	Approach Character 5	Device Character 6	Qualifier Character 7
1 Cranial Cavity	**Ø** Open	**J** Synthetic Substitute	**9** Pleural Cavity, Right **B** Pleural Cavity, Left **G** Peritoneal Cavity **J** Pelvic Cavity
9 Pleural Cavity, Right **B** Pleural Cavity, Left **G** Peritoneal Cavity **J** Pelvic Cavity	**Ø** Open **4** Percutaneous Endoscopic	**J** Synthetic Substitute	**4** Cutaneous **9** Pleural Cavity, Right **B** Pleural Cavity, Left **G** Peritoneal Cavity **J** Pelvic Cavity **Y** Lower Vein
9 Pleural Cavity, Right **B** Pleural Cavity, Left **G** Peritoneal Cavity **J** Pelvic Cavity	**3** Percutaneous	**J** Synthetic Substitute	**4** Cutaneous

Ø **Medical and Surgical**
W **Anatomical Regions, General**
2 **Change**　　　　Taking out or off a device from a body part and putting back an identical or similar device in or on the same body part without cutting or puncturing the skin or a mucous membrane

Body Part Character 4	Approach Character 5	Device Character 6	Qualifier Character 7
Ø Head **1** Cranial Cavity **2** Face **4** Upper Jaw **5** Lower Jaw **6** Neck **8** Chest Wall **9** Pleural Cavity, Right **B** Pleural Cavity, Left **C** Mediastinum **D** Pericardial Cavity **F** Abdominal Wall **G** Peritoneal Cavity **H** Retroperitoneum **J** Pelvic Cavity **K** Upper Back **L** Lower Back **M** Perineum, Male **N** Perineum, Female	**X** External	**Ø** Drainage Device **Y** Other Device	**Z** No Qualifier

Ø   Medical and Surgical
W   Anatomical Regions, General
3   Control   Stopping, or attempting to stop, postprocedural bleeding

Body Part Character 4	Approach Character 5	Device Character 6	Qualifier Character 7
Ø Head **1** Cranial Cavity **2** Face **3** Oral Cavity and Throat **4** Upper Jaw **5** Lower Jaw **6** Neck **8** Chest Wall **9** Pleural Cavity, Right **B** Pleural Cavity, Left **C** Mediastinum **D** Pericardial Cavity **F** Abdominal Wall **G** Peritoneal Cavity **H** Retroperitoneum **J** Pelvic Cavity **K** Upper Back **L** Lower Back **M** Perineum, Male **N** Perineum, Female	**Ø** Open **3** Percutaneous **4** Percutaneous Endoscopic	**Z** No Device	**Z** No Qualifier
P Gastrointestinal Tract **Q** Respiratory Tract **R** Genitourinary Tract	**Ø** Open **3** Percutaneous **4** Percutaneous Endoscopic **7** Via Natural or Artificial Opening **8** Via Natural or Artificial Opening Endoscopic	**Z** No Device	**Z** No Qualifier

Ø   Medical and Surgical
W   Anatomical Regions, General
4   Creation   Making a new genital structure that does not take over the function of a body part

Body Part Character 4	Approach Character 5	Device Character 6	Qualifier Character 7
M Perineum, Male	**Ø** Open	**7** Autologous Tissue Substitute **J** Synthetic Substitute **K** Nonautologous Tissue Substitute **Z** No Device	**Ø** Vagina
N Perineum, Female	**Ø** Open	**7** Autologous Tissue Substitute **J** Synthetic Substitute **K** Nonautologous Tissue Substitute **Z** No Device	**1** Penis

Ø   Medical and Surgical
W   Anatomical Regions, General
8   Division   Cutting into a body part without draining fluids and/or gases from the body part in order to separate or transect a body part

Body Part Character 4	Approach Character 5	Device Character 6	Qualifier Character 7
N Perineum, Female	**X** External	**Z** No Device	**Z** No Qualifier

         Revised Text in **BLUE**   © 2011 Ingenix, Inc

0　Medical and Surgical
W　Anatomical Regions, General
9　Drainage　　　Taking or letting out fluids and/or gases from a body part

Body Part Character 4	Approach Character 5	Device Character 6	Qualifier Character 7
0 Head 1 Cranial Cavity 2 Face 3 Oral Cavity and Throat 4 Upper Jaw 5 Lower Jaw 6 Neck 8 Chest Wall 9 Pleural Cavity, Right B Pleural Cavity, Left C Mediastinum D Pericardial Cavity F Abdominal Wall G Peritoneal Cavity H Retroperitoneum J Pelvic Cavity K Upper Back L Lower Back M Perineum, Male N Perineum, Female	0 Open 3 Percutaneous 4 Percutaneous Endoscopic	0 Drainage Device	Z No Qualifier
0 Head 1 Cranial Cavity 2 Face 3 Oral Cavity and Throat 4 Upper Jaw 5 Lower Jaw 6 Neck 8 Chest Wall 9 Pleural Cavity, Right B Pleural Cavity, Left C Mediastinum D Pericardial Cavity F Abdominal Wall G Peritoneal Cavity H Retroperitoneum J Pelvic Cavity K Upper Back L Lower Back M Perineum, Male N Perineum, Female	0 Open 3 Percutaneous 4 Percutaneous Endoscopic	Z No Device	X Diagnostic Z No Qualifier

0　Medical and Surgical
W　Anatomical Regions, General
B　Excision　　　Cutting out or off, without replacement, a portion of a body part

Body Part Character 4	Approach Character 5	Device Character 6	Qualifier Character 7
0 Head 2 Face 4 Upper Jaw 5 Lower Jaw 8 Chest Wall K Upper Back L Lower Back M Perineum, Male N Perineum, Female	0 Open 3 Percutaneous 4 Percutaneous Endoscopic X External	Z No Device	X Diagnostic Z No Qualifier
6 Neck C Mediastinum F Abdominal Wall H Retroperitoneum	0 Open 3 Percutaneous 4 Percutaneous Endoscopic	Z No Device	X Diagnostic Z No Qualifier
6 Neck F Abdominal Wall	X External	Z No Device	2 Stoma X Diagnostic Z No Qualifier

Ø Medical and Surgical
W Anatomical Regions, General
C Extirpation   Taking or cutting out solid matter from a body part

Body Part Character 4	Approach Character 5	Device Character 6	Qualifier Character 7
1 Cranial Cavity 3 Oral Cavity and Throat 9 Pleural Cavity, Right B Pleural Cavity, Left C Mediastinum D Pericardial Cavity G Peritoneal Cavity J Pelvic Cavity	Ø Open 3 Percutaneous 4 Percutaneous Endoscopic X External	Z No Device	Z No Qualifier
P Gastrointestinal Tract Q Respiratory Tract R Genitourinary Tract	Ø Open 3 Percutaneous 4 Percutaneous Endoscopic 7 Via Natural or Artificial Opening 8 Via Natural or Artificial Opening Endoscopic X External	Z No Device	Z No Qualifier

Ø Medical and Surgical
W Anatomical Regions, General
F Fragmentation   Breaking solid matter in a body part into pieces

Body Part Character 4	Approach Character 5	Device Character 6	Qualifier Character 7
1 Cranial Cavity 3 Oral Cavity and Throat 9 Pleural Cavity, Right B Pleural Cavity, Left C Mediastinum D Pericardial Cavity G Peritoneal Cavity J Pelvic Cavity	Ø Open 3 Percutaneous 4 Percutaneous Endoscopic X External	Z No Device	Z No Qualifier
P Gastrointestinal Tract Q Respiratory Tract R Genitourinary Tract	Ø Open 3 Percutaneous 4 Percutaneous Endoscopic 7 Via Natural or Artificial Opening 8 Via Natural or Artificial Opening Endoscopic X External	Z No Device	Z No Qualifier

Ø Medical and Surgical
W Anatomical Regions, General
H Insertion   Putting in a nonbiological appliance that monitors, assists, performs, or prevents a physiological function but does not physically take the place of a body part

Body Part Character 4	Approach Character 5	Device Character 6	Qualifier Character 7
Ø Head 1 Cranial Cavity 2 Face 3 Oral Cavity and Throat 4 Upper Jaw 5 Lower Jaw 6 Neck 8 Chest Wall 9 Pleural Cavity, Right B Pleural Cavity, Left C Mediastinum D Pericardial Cavity F Abdominal Wall G Peritoneal Cavity H Retroperitoneum J Pelvic Cavity K Upper Back L Lower Back M Perineum, Male N Perineum, Female	Ø Open 3 Percutaneous 4 Percutaneous Endoscopic	1 Radioactive Element 3 Infusion Device Y Other Device	Z No Qualifier
P Gastrointestinal Tract Q Respiratory Tract R Genitourinary Tract	Ø Open 3 Percutaneous 4 Percutaneous Endoscopic 7 Via Natural or Artificial Opening 8 Via Natural or Artificial Opening Endoscopic	1 Radioactive Element 3 Infusion Device Y Other Device	Z No Qualifier

           Revised Text in **BLUE**   © 2Ø11 Ingenix, Inc

Ø Medical and Surgical
W Anatomical Regions, General
J Inspection   Visually and/or manually exploring a body part

Body Part Character 4	Approach Character 5	Device Character 6	Qualifier Character 7
Ø Head **2** Face **3** Oral Cavity and Throat **4** Upper Jaw **5** Lower Jaw **6** Neck **8** Chest Wall **F** Abdominal Wall **K** Upper Back **L** Lower Back **M** Perineum, Male **N** Perineum, Female	**Ø** Open **3** Percutaneous **4** Percutaneous Endoscopic **X** External	**Z** No Device	**Z** No Qualifier
1 Cranial Cavity **9** Pleural Cavity, Right **B** Pleural Cavity, Left **C** Mediastinum **D** Pericardial Cavity **G** Peritoneal Cavity **H** Retroperitoneum **J** Pelvic Cavity	**Ø** Open **3** Percutaneous **4** Percutaneous Endoscopic	**Z** No Device	**Z** No Qualifier
P Gastrointestinal Tract **Q** Respiratory Tract **R** Genitourinary Tract	**Ø** Open **3** Percutaneous **4** Percutaneous Endoscopic **7** Via Natural or Artificial Opening **8** Via Natural or Artificial Opening Endoscopic	**Z** No Device	**Z** No Qualifier

Ø Medical and Surgical
W Anatomical Regions, General
M Reattachment   Putting back in or on all or a portion of a separated body part to its normal location or other suitable location

Body Part Character 4	Approach Character 5	Device Character 6	Qualifier Character 7
2 Face **4** Upper Jaw **5** Lower Jaw **6** Neck **8** Chest Wall **F** Abdominal Wall **K** Upper Back **L** Lower Back **M** Perineum, Male **N** Perineum, Female	**Ø** Open	**Z** No Device	**Z** No Qualifier

Anatomical Regions, General

ØWP–ØWQ

Ø   Medical and Surgical
W   Anatomical Regions, General
P   Removal   Taking out or off a device from a body part

Body Part Character 4	Approach Character 5	Device Character 6	Qualifier Character 7
Ø Head 2 Face 4 Upper Jaw 5 Lower Jaw 6 Neck 8 Chest Wall C Mediastinum F Abdominal Wall K Upper Back L Lower Back M Perineum, Male N Perineum, Female	Ø Open 3 Percutaneous 4 Percutaneous Endoscopic X External	Ø Drainage Device 1 Radioactive Element 3 Infusion Device 7 Autologous Tissue Substitute J Synthetic Substitute K Nonautologous Tissue Substitute Y Other Device	Z No Qualifier
1 Cranial Cavity 9 Pleural Cavity, Right B Pleural Cavity, Left D Pericardial Cavity G Peritoneal Cavity H Retroperitoneum J Pelvic Cavity	X External	Ø Drainage Device 1 Radioactive Element 3 Infusion Device	Z No Qualifier
1 Cranial Cavity 9 Pleural Cavity, Right B Pleural Cavity, Left G Peritoneal Cavity J Pelvic Cavity	Ø Open 3 Percutaneous 4 Percutaneous Endoscopic	Ø Drainage Device 1 Radioactive Element 3 Infusion Device J Synthetic Substitute Y Other Device	Z No Qualifier
D Pericardial Cavity H Retroperitoneum	Ø Open 3 Percutaneous 4 Percutaneous Endoscopic	Ø Drainage Device 1 Radioactive Element 3 Infusion Device Y Other Device	Z No Qualifier
P Gastrointestinal Tract Q Respiratory Tract R Genitourinary Tract	Ø Open 3 Percutaneous 4 Percutaneous Endoscopic 7 Via Natural or Artificial Opening 8 Via Natural or Artificial Opening Endoscopic X External	1 Radioactive Element 3 Infusion Device Y Other Device	Z No Qualifier

Ø   Medical and Surgical
W   Anatomical Regions, General
Q   Repair   Restoring, to the extent possible, a body part to its normal anatomic structure and function

Body Part Character 4	Approach Character 5	Device Character 6	Qualifier Character 7
Ø Head 2 Face 4 Upper Jaw 5 Lower Jaw 8 Chest Wall K Upper Back L Lower Back M Perineum, Male N Perineum, Female	Ø Open 3 Percutaneous 4 Percutaneous Endoscopic X External	Z No Device	Z No Qualifier
6 Neck C Mediastinum F Abdominal Wall	Ø Open 3 Percutaneous 4 Percutaneous Endoscopic	Z No Device	Z No Qualifier
6 Neck F Abdominal Wall	X External	Z No Device	2 Stoma Z No Qualifier

0 **Medical and Surgical**
W **Anatomical Regions, General**
U **Supplement**   Putting in or on biological or synthetic material that physically reinforces and/or augments the function of a portion of a body part

Body Part Character 4	Approach Character 5	Device Character 6	Qualifier Character 7
0 Head 2 Face 4 Upper Jaw 5 Lower Jaw 6 Neck 8 Chest Wall C Mediastinum F Abdominal Wall K Upper Back L Lower Back M Perineum, Male N Perineum, Female	0 Open 4 Percutaneous Endoscopic	7 Autologous Tissue Substitute J Synthetic Substitute K Nonautologous Tissue Substitute	Z No Qualifier

0 **Medical and Surgical**
W **Anatomical Regions, General**
W **Revision**   Correcting, to the extent possible, a portion of a malfunctioning device or the position of a displaced device

Body Part Character 4	Approach Character 5	Device Character 6	Qualifier Character 7
0 Head 2 Face 4 Upper Jaw 5 Lower Jaw 6 Neck 8 Chest Wall C Mediastinum F Abdominal Wall K Upper Back L Lower Back M Perineum, Male N Perineum, Female	0 Open 3 Percutaneous 4 Percutaneous Endoscopic X External	0 Drainage Device 1 Radioactive Element 3 Infusion Device 7 Autologous Tissue Substitute J Synthetic Substitute K Nonautologous Tissue Substitute Y Other Device	Z No Qualifier
1 Cranial Cavity 9 Pleural Cavity, Right B Pleural Cavity, Left G Peritoneal Cavity J Pelvic Cavity	0 Open 3 Percutaneous 4 Percutaneous Endoscopic X External	0 Drainage Device 1 Radioactive Element 3 Infusion Device J Synthetic Substitute Y Other Device	Z No Qualifier
D Pericardial Cavity H Retroperitoneum	0 Open 3 Percutaneous 4 Percutaneous Endoscopic X External	0 Drainage Device 1 Radioactive Element 3 Infusion Device Y Other Device	Z No Qualifier
P Gastrointestinal Tract Q Respiratory Tract R Genitourinary Tract	0 Open 3 Percutaneous 4 Percutaneous Endoscopic 7 Via Natural or Artificial Opening 8 Via Natural or Artificial Opening Endoscopic X External	1 Radioactive Element 3 Infusion Device Y Other Device	Z No Qualifier

Anatomical Regions, Upper Extremities ØXØ–ØXX

Ø   **Medical and Surgical**
X   **Anatomical Regions, Upper Extremities**
Ø   **Alteration**   Modifying the anatomic structure of a body part without affecting the function of the body part

Body Part Character 4	Approach Character 5	Device Character 6	Qualifier Character 7
2 Shoulder Region, Right 3 Shoulder Region, Left 4 Axilla, Right 5 Axilla, Left 6 Upper Extremity, Right 7 Upper Extremity, Left 8 Upper Arm, Right 9 Upper Arm, Left B Elbow Region, Right C Elbow Region, Left D Lower Arm, Right F Lower Arm, Left G Wrist Region, Right H Wrist Region, Left	Ø Open 3 Percutaneous 4 Percutaneous Endoscopic	7 Autologous Tissue Substitute J Synthetic Substitute K Nonautologous Tissue Substitute Z No Device	Z No Qualifier

Ø   **Medical and Surgical**
X   **Anatomical Regions, Upper Extremities**
2   **Change**   Taking out or off a device from a body part and putting back an identical or similar device in or on the same body part without cutting or puncturing the skin or a mucous membrane

Body Part Character 4	Approach Character 5	Device Character 6	Qualifier Character 7
6 Upper Extremity, Right 7 Upper Extremity, Left	X External	Ø Drainage Device Y Other Device	Z No Qualifier

Ø   **Medical and Surgical**
X   **Anatomical Regions, Upper Extremities**
3   **Control**   Stopping, or attempting to stop, postprocedural bleeding

Body Part Character 4	Approach Character 5	Device Character 6	Qualifier Character 7
2 Shoulder Region, Right 3 Shoulder Region, Left 4 Axilla, Right 5 Axilla, Left 6 Upper Extremity, Right 7 Upper Extremity, Left 8 Upper Arm, Right 9 Upper Arm, Left B Elbow Region, Right C Elbow Region, Left D Lower Arm, Right F Lower Arm, Left G Wrist Region, Right H Wrist Region, Left J Hand, Right K Hand, Left	Ø Open 3 Percutaneous 4 Percutaneous Endoscopic	Z No Device	Z No Qualifier

0   **Medical and Surgical**
X   **Anatomical Regions, Upper Extremities**
6   **Detachment**   Cutting off all or a portion of the upper or lower extremities

Body Part Character 4	Approach Character 5	Device Character 6	Qualifier Character 7
0 Forequarter, Right 1 Forequarter, Left 2 Shoulder Region, Right 3 Shoulder Region, Left B Elbow Region, Right C Elbow Region, Left	0 Open	Z No Device	Z No Qualifier
8 Upper Arm, Right 9 Upper Arm, Left D Lower Arm, Right F Lower Arm, Left	0 Open	Z No Device	1 High 2 Mid 3 Low
J Hand, Right K Hand, Left	0 Open	Z No Device	0 Complete 4 Complete 1st Ray 5 Complete 2nd Ray 6 Complete 3rd Ray 7 Complete 4th Ray 8 Complete 5th Ray 9 Partial 1st Ray B Partial 2nd Ray C Partial 3rd Ray D Partial 4th Ray F Partial 5th Ray
L Thumb, Right M Thumb, Left N Index Finger, Right P Index Finger, Left Q Middle Finger, Right R Middle Finger, Left S Ring Finger, Right T Ring Finger, Left V Little Finger, Right W Little Finger, Left	0 Open	Z No Device	0 Complete 1 High 2 Mid 3 Low

0   **Medical and Surgical**
X   **Anatomical Regions, Upper Extremities**
9   **Drainage**   Taking or letting out fluids and/or gases from a body part

Body Part Character 4	Approach Character 5	Device Character 6	Qualifier Character 7
2 Shoulder Region, Right 3 Shoulder Region, Left 4 Axilla, Right 5 Axilla, Left 6 Upper Extremity, Right 7 Upper Extremity, Left 8 Upper Arm, Right 9 Upper Arm, Left B Elbow Region, Right C Elbow Region, Left D Lower Arm, Right F Lower Arm, Left G Wrist Region, Right H Wrist Region, Left J Hand, Right K Hand, Left	0 Open 3 Percutaneous 4 Percutaneous Endoscopic	0 Drainage Device	Z No Qualifier
2 Shoulder Region, Right 3 Shoulder Region, Left 4 Axilla, Right 5 Axilla, Left 6 Upper Extremity, Right 7 Upper Extremity, Left 8 Upper Arm, Right 9 Upper Arm, Left B Elbow Region, Right C Elbow Region, Left D Lower Arm, Right F Lower Arm, Left G Wrist Region, Right H Wrist Region, Left J Hand, Right K Hand, Left	0 Open 3 Percutaneous 4 Percutaneous Endoscopic	Z No Device	X Diagnostic Z No Qualifier

Anatomical Regions, Upper Extremities

ØXB–ØXJ

Ø   **Medical and Surgical**
X   **Anatomical Regions, Upper Extremities**
B   **Excision**   Cutting out or off, without replacement, a portion of a body part

Body Part Character 4	Approach Character 5	Device Character 6	Qualifier Character 7
2 Shoulder Region, Right 3 Shoulder Region, Left 4 Axilla, Right 5 Axilla, Left 6 Upper Extremity, Right 7 Upper Extremity, Left 8 Upper Arm, Right 9 Upper Arm, Left B Elbow Region, Right C Elbow Region, Left D Lower Arm, Right F Lower Arm, Left G Wrist Region, Right H Wrist Region, Left J Hand, Right K Hand, Left	Ø Open 3 Percutaneous 4 Percutaneous Endoscopic	Z No Device	X Diagnostic Z No Qualifier

Ø   **Medical and Surgical**
X   **Anatomical Regions, Upper Extremities**
H   **Insertion**   Putting in a nonbiological appliance that monitors, assists, performs, or prevents a physiological function but does not physically take the place of a body part

Body Part Character 4	Approach Character 5	Device Character 6	Qualifier Character 7
2 Shoulder Region, Right 3 Shoulder Region, Left 4 Axilla, Right 5 Axilla, Left 6 Upper Extremity, Right 7 Upper Extremity, Left 8 Upper Arm, Right 9 Upper Arm, Left B Elbow Region, Right C Elbow Region, Left D Lower Arm, Right F Lower Arm, Left G Wrist Region, Right H Wrist Region, Left J Hand, Right K Hand, Left	Ø Open 3 Percutaneous 4 Percutaneous Endoscopic	1 Radioactive Element 3 Infusion Device Y Other Device	Z No Qualifier

Ø   **Medical and Surgical**
X   **Anatomical Regions, Upper Extremities**
J   **Inspection**   Visually and/or manually exploring a body part

Body Part Character 4	Approach Character 5	Device Character 6	Qualifier Character 7
2 Shoulder Region, Right 3 Shoulder Region, Left 4 Axilla, Right 5 Axilla, Left 6 Upper Extremity, Right 7 Upper Extremity, Left 8 Upper Arm, Right 9 Upper Arm, Left B Elbow Region, Right C Elbow Region, Left D Lower Arm, Right F Lower Arm, Left G Wrist Region, Right H Wrist Region, Left J Hand, Right K Hand, Left	Ø Open 3 Percutaneous 4 Percutaneous Endoscopic X External	Z No Device	Z No Qualifier

     Revised Text in **BLUE**

0   **Medical and Surgical**
X   **Anatomical Regions, Upper Extremities**
M   **Reattachment**   Putting back in or on all or a portion of a separated body part to its normal location or other suitable location

Body Part Character 4	Approach Character 5	Device Character 6	Qualifier Character 7
0 Forequarter, Right **1** Forequarter, Left **2** Shoulder Region, Right **3** Shoulder Region, Left **4** Axilla, Right **5** Axilla, Left **6** Upper Extremity, Right **7** Upper Extremity, Left **8** Upper Arm, Right **9** Upper Arm, Left **B** Elbow Region, Right **C** Elbow Region, Left **D** Lower Arm, Right **F** Lower Arm, Left **G** Wrist Region, Right **H** Wrist Region, Left **J** Hand, Right **K** Hand, Left **L** Thumb, Right **M** Thumb, Left **N** Index Finger, Right **P** Index Finger, Left **Q** Middle Finger, Right **R** Middle Finger, Left **S** Ring Finger, Right **T** Ring Finger, Left **V** Little Finger, Right **W** Little Finger, Left	**0** Open	**Z** No Device	**Z** No Qualifier

0   **Medical and Surgical**
X   **Anatomical Regions, Upper Extremities**
P   **Removal**   Taking out or off a device from a body part

Body Part Character 4	Approach Character 5	Device Character 6	Qualifier Character 7
6 Upper Extremity, Right **7** Upper Extremity, Left	**0** Open **3** Percutaneous **4** Percutaneous Endoscopic **X** External	**0** Drainage Device **1** Radioactive Element **3** Infusion Device **7** Autologous Tissue Substitute **J** Synthetic Substitute **K** Nonautologous Tissue Substitute **Y** Other Device	**Z** No Qualifier

Ø   **Medical and Surgical**
X   **Anatomical Regions, Upper Extremities**
Q   **Repair**   Restoring, to the extent possible, a body part to its normal anatomic structure and function

Body Part Character 4	Approach Character 5	Device Character 6	Qualifier Character 7
2 Shoulder Region, Right **3** Shoulder Region, Left **4** Axilla, Right **5** Axilla, Left **6** Upper Extremity, Right **7** Upper Extremity, Left **8** Upper Arm, Right **9** Upper Arm, Left **B** Elbow Region, Right **C** Elbow Region, Left **D** Lower Arm, Right **F** Lower Arm, Left **G** Wrist Region, Right **H** Wrist Region, Left **J** Hand, Right **K** Hand, Left **L** Thumb, Right **M** Thumb, Left **N** Index Finger, Right **P** Index Finger, Left **Q** Middle Finger, Right **R** Middle Finger, Left **S** Ring Finger, Right **T** Ring Finger, Left **V** Little Finger, Right **W** Little Finger, Left	**Ø** Open **3** Percutaneous **4** Percutaneous Endoscopic **X** External	**Z** No Device	**Z** No Qualifier

Ø   **Medical and Surgical**
X   **Anatomical Regions, Upper Extremities**
R   **Replacement**   Putting in or on biological or synthetic material that physically takes the place and/or function of all or a portion of a body part

Body Part Character 4	Approach Character 5	Device Character 6	Qualifier Character 7
L Thumb, Right **M** Thumb, Left	**Ø** Open **4** Percutaneous Endoscopic	**7** Autologous Tissue Substitute	**N** Toe, Right **P** Toe, Left

Ø   **Medical and Surgical**
X   **Anatomical Regions, Upper Extremities**
U   **Supplement**   Putting in or on biological or synthetic material that physically reinforces and/or augments the function of a portion of a body part

Body Part Character 4	Approach Character 5	Device Character 6	Qualifier Character 7
2 Shoulder Region, Right **3** Shoulder Region, Left **4** Axilla, Right **5** Axilla, Left **6** Upper Extremity, Right **7** Upper Extremity, Left **8** Upper Arm, Right **9** Upper Arm, Left **B** Elbow Region, Right **C** Elbow Region, Left **D** Lower Arm, Right **F** Lower Arm, Left **G** Wrist Region, Right **H** Wrist Region, Left **J** Hand, Right **K** Hand, Left **L** Thumb, Right **M** Thumb, Left **N** Index Finger, Right **P** Index Finger, Left **Q** Middle Finger, Right **R** Middle Finger, Left **S** Ring Finger, Right **T** Ring Finger, Left **V** Little Finger, Right **W** Little Finger, Left	**Ø** Open **4** Percutaneous Endoscopic	**7** Autologous Tissue Substitute **J** Synthetic Substitute **K** Nonautologous Tissue Substitute	**Z** No Qualifier

Ø   **Medical and Surgical**
X   **Anatomical Regions, Upper Extremities**
W   **Revision**   Correcting, to the extent possible, a portion of a malfunctioning device or the position of a displaced device

Body Part Character 4	Approach Character 5	Device Character 6	Qualifier Character 7
6 Upper Extremity, Right **7** Upper Extremity, Left	**Ø** Open **3** Percutaneous **4** Percutaneous Endoscopic **X** External	**Ø** Drainage Device **3** Infusion Device **7** Autologous Tissue Substitute **J** Synthetic Substitute **K** Nonautologous Tissue Substitute **Y** Other Device	**Z** No Qualifier

Ø   **Medical and Surgical**
X   **Anatomical Regions, Upper Extremities**
X   **Transfer**   Moving, without taking out, all or a portion of a body part to another location to take over the function of all or a portion of a body part

Body Part Character 4	Approach Character 5	Device Character 6	Qualifier Character 7
N Index Finger, Right	**Ø** Open	**Z** No Device	**L** Thumb, Right
P Index Finger, Left	**Ø** Open	**Z** No Device	**M** Thumb, Left

Anatomical Regions, Lower Extremities ØYØ–ØYW

Ø   **Medical and Surgical**
Y   **Anatomical Regions, Lower Extremities**
Ø   **Alteration**   Modifying the anatomic structure of a body part without affecting the function of the body part

Body Part Character 4	Approach Character 5	Device Character 6	Qualifier Character 7
Ø Buttock, Right 1 Buttock, Left 9 Lower Extremity, Right B Lower Extremity, Left C Upper Leg, Right D Upper Leg, Left F Knee Region, Right G Knee Region, Left H Lower Leg, Right J Lower Leg, Left K Ankle Region, Right L Ankle Region, Left	Ø Open 3 Percutaneous 4 Percutaneous Endoscopic	7 Autologous Tissue Substitute J Synthetic Substitute K Nonautologous Tissue Substitute Z No Device	Z No Qualifier

Ø   **Medical and Surgical**
Y   **Anatomical Regions, Lower Extremities**
2   **Change**   Taking out or off a device from a body part and putting back an identical or similar device in or on the same body part without cutting or puncturing the skin or a mucous membrane

Body Part Character 4	Approach Character 5	Device Character 6	Qualifier Character 7
9 Lower Extremity, Right B Lower Extremity, Left	X External	Ø Drainage Device Y Other Device	Z No Qualifier

Ø   **Medical and Surgical**
Y   **Anatomical Regions, Lower Extremities**
3   **Control**   Stopping, or attempting to stop, postprocedural bleeding

Body Part Character 4	Approach Character 5	Device Character 6	Qualifier Character 7
Ø Buttock, Right 1 Buttock, Left 5 Inguinal Region, Right 6 Inguinal Region, Left 7 Femoral Region, Right 8 Femoral Region, Left 9 Lower Extremity, Right B Lower Extremity, Left C Upper Leg, Right D Upper Leg, Left F Knee Region, Right G Knee Region, Left H Lower Leg, Right J Lower Leg, Left K Ankle Region, Right L Ankle Region, Left M Foot, Right N Foot, Left	Ø Open 3 Percutaneous 4 Percutaneous Endoscopic	Z No Device	Z No Qualifier

Ø   **Medical and Surgical**
Y   **Anatomical Regions, Lower Extremities**
6   **Detachment**   Cutting off all or a portion of the upper or lower extremities

Body Part Character 4	Approach Character 5	Device Character 6	Qualifier Character 7
2 Hindquarter, Right 3 Hindquarter, Left 4 Hindquarter, Bilateral 7 Femoral Region, Right 8 Femoral Region, Left F Knee Region, Right G Knee Region, Left	Ø Open	Z No Device	Z No Qualifier
C Upper Leg, Right D Upper Leg, Left H Lower Leg, Right J Lower Leg, Left	Ø Open	Z No Device	1 High 2 Mid 3 Low

ØY6 Continued on next page

Ø   **Medical and Surgical**   *ØY6 Continued*
Y   **Anatomical Regions, Lower Extremities**
6   **Detachment**   Cutting off all or a portion of the upper or lower extremities

Body Part Character 4	Approach Character 5	Device Character 6	Qualifier Character 7
M Foot, Right N Foot, Left	Ø Open	Z No Device	Ø Complete 4 Complete 1st Ray 5 Complete 2nd Ray 6 Complete 3rd Ray 7 Complete 4th Ray 8 Complete 5th Ray 9 Partial 1st Ray B Partial 2nd Ray C Partial 3rd Ray D Partial 4th Ray F Partial 5th Ray
P 1st Toe, Right Q 1st Toe, Left R 2nd Toe, Right S 2nd Toe, Left T 3rd Toe, Right U 3rd Toe, Left V 4th Toe, Right W 4th Toe, Left X 5th Toe, Right Y 5th Toe, Left	Ø Open	Z No Device	Ø Complete 1 High 2 Mid 3 Low

Ø   **Medical and Surgical**
Y   **Anatomical Regions, Lower Extremities**
9   **Drainage**   Taking or letting out fluids and/or gases from a body part

Body Part Character 4	Approach Character 5	Device Character 6	Qualifier Character 7
Ø Buttock, Right 1 Buttock, Left 5 Inguinal Region, Right 6 Inguinal Region, Left 7 Femoral Region, Right 8 Femoral Region, Left 9 Lower Extremity, Right B Lower Extremity, Left C Upper Leg, Right D Upper Leg, Left F Knee Region, Right G Knee Region, Left H Lower Leg, Right J Lower Leg, Left K Ankle Region, Right L Ankle Region, Left M Foot, Right N Foot, Left	Ø Open 3 Percutaneous 4 Percutaneous Endoscopic	Ø Drainage Device	Z No Qualifier
Ø Buttock, Right 1 Buttock, Left 5 Inguinal Region, Right 6 Inguinal Region, Left 7 Femoral Region, Right 8 Femoral Region, Left 9 Lower Extremity, Right B Lower Extremity, Left C Upper Leg, Right D Upper Leg, Left F Knee Region, Right G Knee Region, Left H Lower Leg, Right J Lower Leg, Left K Ankle Region, Right L Ankle Region, Left M Foot, Right N Foot, Left	Ø Open 3 Percutaneous 4 Percutaneous Endoscopic	Z No Device	X Diagnostic Z No Qualifier

Anatomical Regions, Lower Extremities

Ø   **Medical and Surgical**
Y   **Anatomical Regions, Lower Extremities**
B   **Excision**   Cutting out or off, without replacement, a portion of a body part

Body Part Character 4	Approach Character 5	Device Character 6	Qualifier Character 7
Ø Buttock, Right 1 Buttock, Left 5 Inguinal Region, Right 6 Inguinal Region, Left 7 Femoral Region, Right 8 Femoral Region, Left 9 Lower Extremity, Right B Lower Extremity, Left C Upper Leg, Right D Upper Leg, Left F Knee Region, Right G Knee Region, Left H Lower Leg, Right J Lower Leg, Left K Ankle Region, Right L Ankle Region, Left M Foot, Right N Foot, Left	Ø Open 3 Percutaneous 4 Percutaneous Endoscopic	Z No Device	X Diagnostic Z No Qualifier

Ø   **Medical and Surgical**
Y   **Anatomical Regions, Lower Extremities**
H   **Insertion**   Putting in a nonbiological appliance that monitors, assists, performs, or prevents a physiological function but does not physically take the place of a body part

Body Part Character 4	Approach Character 5	Device Character 6	Qualifier Character 7
Ø Buttock, Right 1 Buttock, Left 5 Inguinal Region, Right 6 Inguinal Region, Left 7 Femoral Region, Right 8 Femoral Region, Left 9 Lower Extremity, Right B Lower Extremity, Left C Upper Leg, Right D Upper Leg, Left F Knee Region, Right G Knee Region, Left H Lower Leg, Right J Lower Leg, Left K Ankle Region, Right L Ankle Region, Left M Foot, Right N Foot, Left	Ø Open 3 Percutaneous 4 Percutaneous Endoscopic	1 Radioactive Element 3 Infusion Device Y Other Device	Z No Qualifier

Ø   **Medical and Surgical**
Y   **Anatomical Regions, Lower Extremities**
J   **Inspection**   Visually and/or manually exploring a body part

Body Part Character 4	Approach Character 5	Device Character 6	Qualifier Character 7
Ø Buttock, Right 1 Buttock, Left 5 Inguinal Region, Right 6 Inguinal Region, Left 7 Femoral Region, Right 8 Femoral Region, Left 9 Lower Extremity, Right A Inguinal Region, Bilateral B Lower Extremity, Left C Upper Leg, Right D Upper Leg, Left E Femoral Region, Bilateral F Knee Region, Right G Knee Region, Left H Lower Leg, Right J Lower Leg, Left K Ankle Region, Right L Ankle Region, Left M Foot, Right N Foot, Left	Ø Open 3 Percutaneous 4 Percutaneous Endoscopic X External	Z No Device	Z No Qualifier

     Revised Text in **BLUE**   © 2Ø11 Ingenix, Inc

Ø **Medical and Surgical**
Y **Anatomical Regions, Lower Extremities**
M **Reattachment**   Putting back in or on all or a portion of a separated body part to its normal location or other suitable location

Body Part Character 4	Approach Character 5	Device Character 6	Qualifier Character 7
Ø Buttock, Right	**Ø** Open	**Z** No Device	**Z** No Qualifier
1 Buttock, Left			
2 Hindquarter, Right			
3 Hindquarter, Left			
4 Hindquarter, Bilateral			
5 Inguinal Region, Right			
6 Inguinal Region, Left			
7 Femoral Region, Right			
8 Femoral Region, Left			
9 Lower Extremity, Right			
B Lower Extremity, Left			
C Upper Leg, Right			
D Upper Leg, Left			
F Knee Region, Right			
G Knee Region, Left			
H Lower Leg, Right			
J Lower Leg, Left			
K Ankle Region, Right			
L Ankle Region, Left			
M Foot, Right			
N Foot, Left			
P 1st Toe, Right			
Q 1st Toe, Left			
R 2nd Toe, Right			
S 2nd Toe, Left			
T 3rd Toe, Right			
U 3rd Toe, Left			
V 4th Toe, Right			
W 4th Toe, Left			
X 5th Toe, Right			
Y 5th Toe, Left			

Ø **Medical and Surgical**
Y **Anatomical Regions, Lower Extremities**
P **Removal**   Taking out or off a device from a body part

Body Part Character 4	Approach Character 5	Device Character 6	Qualifier Character 7
9 Lower Extremity, Right	**Ø** Open	**Ø** Drainage Device	**Z** No Qualifier
B Lower Extremity, Left	**3** Percutaneous	**1** Radioactive Element	
	4 Percutaneous Endoscopic	**3** Infusion Device	
	X External	**7** Autologous Tissue Substitute	
		J Synthetic Substitute	
		K Nonautologous Tissue Substitute	
		Y Other Device	

Anatomical Regions, Lower Extremities

Ø   **Medical and Surgical**
Y   **Anatomical Regions, Lower Extremities**
Q   **Repair**   Restoring, to the extent possible, a body part to its normal anatomic structure and function

Body Part Character 4	Approach Character 5	Device Character 6	Qualifier Character 7
Ø Buttock, Right **1** Buttock, Left **5** Inguinal Region, Right **6** Inguinal Region, Left **7** Femoral Region, Right **8** Femoral Region, Left **9** Lower Extremity, Right **A** Inguinal Region, Bilateral **B** Lower Extremity, Left **C** Upper Leg, Right **D** Upper Leg, Left **E** Femoral Region, Bilateral **F** Knee Region, Right **G** Knee Region, Left **H** Lower Leg, Right **J** Lower Leg, Left **K** Ankle Region, Right **L** Ankle Region, Left **M** Foot, Right **N** Foot, Left **P** 1st Toe, Right **Q** 1st Toe, Left **R** 2nd Toe, Right **S** 2nd Toe, Left **T** 3rd Toe, Right **U** 3rd Toe, Left **V** 4th Toe, Right **W** 4th Toe, Left **X** 5th Toe, Right **Y** 5th Toe, Left	**Ø** Open **3** Percutaneous **4** Percutaneous Endoscopic **X** External	**Z** No Device	**Z** No Qualifier

Ø   **Medical and Surgical**
Y   **Anatomical Regions, Lower Extremities**
U   **Supplement**   Putting in or on biological or synthetic material that physically reinforces and/or augments the function of a portion of a body part

Body Part Character 4	Approach Character 5	Device Character 6	Qualifier Character 7
Ø Buttock, Right **1** Buttock, Left **5** Inguinal Region, Right **6** Inguinal Region, Left **7** Femoral Region, Right **8** Femoral Region, Left **9** Lower Extremity, Right **A** Inguinal Region, Bilateral **B** Lower Extremity, Left **C** Upper Leg, Right **D** Upper Leg, Left **E** Femoral Region, Bilateral **F** Knee Region, Right **G** Knee Region, Left **H** Lower Leg, Right **J** Lower Leg, Left **K** Ankle Region, Right **L** Ankle Region, Left **M** Foot, Right **N** Foot, Left **P** 1st Toe, Right **Q** 1st Toe, Left **R** 2nd Toe, Right **S** 2nd Toe, Left **T** 3rd Toe, Right **U** 3rd Toe, Left **V** 4th Toe, Right **W** 4th Toe, Left **X** 5th Toe, Right **Y** 5th Toe, Left	**Ø** Open **4** Percutaneous Endoscopic	**7** Autologous Tissue Substitute **J** Synthetic Substitute **K** Nonautologous Tissue Substitute	**Z** No Qualifier

Ø　Medical and Surgical
Y　Anatomical Regions, Lower Extremities
W　Revision　　　Correcting, to the extent possible, a portion of a malfunctioning device or the position of a displaced device

Body Part Character 4	Approach Character 5	Device Character 6	Qualifier Character 7
9　Lower Extremity, Right B　Lower Extremity, Left	Ø　Open 3　Percutaneous 4　Percutaneous Endoscopic X　External	Ø　Drainage Device 3　Infusion Device 7　Autologous Tissue Substitute J　Synthetic Substitute K　Nonautologous Tissue Substitute Y　Other Device	Z　No Qualifier

Obstetrics 102–10Y

1 Obstetrics
Ø Pregnancy
2 Change — Taking out or off a device from a body part and putting back an identical or similar device in or on the same body part without cutting or puncturing the skin or a mucous membrane

Body Part Character 4	Approach Character 5	Device Character 6	Qualifier Character 7
Ø Products of Conception	7 Via Natural or Artificial Opening	3 Monitoring Electrode Y Other Device	Z No Qualifier

1 Obstetrics
Ø Pregnancy
9 Drainage — Taking or letting out fluids and/or gases from a body part

Body Part Character 4	Approach Character 5	Device Character 6	Qualifier Character 7
Ø Products of Conception	Ø Open 3 Percutaneous 4 Percutaneous Endoscopic 7 Via Natural or Artificial Opening 8 Via Natural or Artificial Opening Endoscopic	Z No Device	9 Fetal Blood A Fetal Cerebrospinal Fluid B Fetal Fluid, Other C Amniotic Fluid, Therapeutic D Fluid, Other U Amniotic Fluid, Diagnostic

1 Obstetrics
Ø Pregnancy
A Abortion — Artificially terminating a pregnancy

Body Part Character 4	Approach Character 5	Device Character 6	Qualifier Character 7
Ø Products of Conception	Ø Open 3 Percutaneous 4 Percutaneous Endoscopic 8 Via Natural or Artificial Opening Endoscopic	Z No Device	Z No Qualifier
Ø Products of Conception	7 Via Natural or Artificial Opening	Z No Device	6 Vacuum W Laminaria X Abortifacient Z No Qualifier

1 Obstetrics
Ø Pregnancy
D Extraction — Pulling or stripping out or off all or a portion of a body part

Body Part Character 4	Approach Character 5	Device Character 6	Qualifier Character 7
Ø Products of Conception	Ø Open	Z No Device	Ø Classical 1 Low Cervical 2 Extraperitoneal
Ø Products of Conception	7 Via Natural or Artificial Opening	Z No Device	3 Low Forceps 4 Mid Forceps 5 High Forceps 6 Vacuum 7 Internal Version 8 Other
1 Products of Conception, Retained 2 Products of Conception, Ectopic	7 Via Natural or Artificial Opening 8 Via Natural or Artificial Opening Endoscopic	Z No Device	Z No Qualifier

1 Obstetrics
Ø Pregnancy
E Delivery — Assisting the passage of the products of conception from the genital canal

Body Part Character 4	Approach Character 5	Device Character 6	Qualifier Character 7
Ø Products of Conception	X External	Z No Device	Z No Qualifier

1   Obstetrics
Ø   Pregnancy
H   Insertion   Putting in a nonbiological appliance that monitors, assists, performs, or prevents a physiological function but does not physically take the place of a body part

Body Part Character 4	Approach Character 5	Device Character 6	Qualifier Character 7
Ø Products of Conception	Ø Open 7 Via Natural or Artificial Opening	3 Monitoring Electrode Y Other Device	Z No Qualifier

1   Obstetrics
Ø   Pregnancy
J   Inspection   Visually and/or manually exploring a body part

Body Part Character 4	Approach Character 5	Device Character 6	Qualifier Character 7
Ø Products of Conception 1 Products of Conception, Retained 2 Products of Conception, Ectopic	Ø Open 3 Percutaneous 4 Percutaneous Endoscopic 7 Via Natural or Artificial Opening 8 Via Natural or Artificial Opening Endoscopic X External	Z No Device	Z No Qualifier

1   Obstetrics
Ø   Pregnancy
P   Removal   Taking out or off a device from a body part, region or orifice

Body Part Character 4	Approach Character 5	Device Character 6	Qualifier Character 7
Ø Products of Conception	Ø Open 7 Via Natural or Artificial Opening	3 Monitoring Electrode Y Other Device	Z No Qualifier

1   Obstetrics
Ø   Pregnancy
Q   Repair   Restoring, to the extent possible, a body part to its normal anatomic structure and function

Body Part Character 4	Approach Character 5	Device Character 6	Qualifier Character 7
Ø Products of Conception	Ø Open 3 Percutaneous 4 Percutaneous Endoscopic 7 Via Natural or Artificial Opening 8 Via Natural or Artificial Opening Endoscopic	Y Other Device Z No Device	E Nervous System F Cardiovascular System G Lymphatics and Hemic H Eye J Ear, Nose and Sinus K Respiratory System L Mouth and Throat M Gastrointestinal System N Hepatobiliary and Pancreas P Endocrine System Q Skin R Musculoskeletal System S Urinary System T Female Reproductive System V Male Reproductive System Y Other Body System

1   Obstetrics
Ø   Pregnancy
S   Reposition   Moving to its normal location or other suitable location all or a portion of a body part

Body Part Character 4	Approach Character 5	Device Character 6	Qualifier Character 7
Ø Products of Conception	7 Via Natural or Artificial Opening X External	Z No Device	Z No Qualifier
2 Products of Conception, Ectopic	Ø Open 3 Percutaneous 4 Percutaneous Endoscopic 7 Via Natural or Artificial Opening 8 Via Natural or Artificial Opening Endoscopic	Z No Device	Z No Qualifier

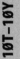

1   Obstetrics
Ø   Pregnancy
T   Resection   Cutting out or off, without replacement, all of a body part

Body Part Character 4	Approach Character 5	Device Character 6	Qualifier Character 7
2 Products of Conception, Ectopic	**Ø** Open **3** Percutaneous **4** Percutaneous Endoscopic **7** Via Natural or Artificial Opening **8** Via Natural or Artificial Opening Endoscopic	**Z** No Device	**Z** No Qualifier

1   Obstetrics
Ø   Pregnancy
Y   Transplantation   Putting in or on all or a portion of a living body part taken from another individual or animal to physically take the place and/or function of all or a portion of a similar body part

Body Part Character 4	Approach Character 5	Device Character 6	Qualifier Character 7
Ø Products of Conception	**3** Percutaneous **4** Percutaneous Endoscopic **7** Via Natural or Artificial Opening	**Z** No Device	**E** Nervous System **F** Cardiovascular System **G** Lymphatics and Hemic **H** Eye **J** Ear, Nose and Sinus **K** Respiratory System **L** Mouth and Throat **M** Gastrointestinal System **N** Hepatobiliary and Pancreas **P** Endocrine System **Q** Skin **R** Musculoskeletal System **S** Urinary System **T** Female Reproductive System **V** Male Reproductive System **Y** Other Body System

Placement—Anatomical Regions 2W0–2W6

2　Placement
W　Anatomical Regions
0　Change　　Taking out or off a device from a body part and putting back an identical or similar device in or on the same body part without cutting or puncturing the skin or a mucous membrane

Body Region Character 4	Approach Character 5	Device Character 6	Qualifier Character 7
0　Head	X　External	0　Traction Apparatus 1　Splint 2　Cast 3　Brace 4　Bandage 5　Packing Material 6　Pressure Dressing 7　Intermittent Pressure Device 8　Stereotactic Apparatus Y　Other Device	Z　No Qualifier
1　Face	X　External	0　Traction Apparatus 1　Splint 2　Cast 3　Brace 4　Bandage 5　Packing Material 6　Pressure Dressing 7　Intermittent Pressure Device 9　Wire Y　Other Device	Z　No Qualifier
2　Neck 3　Abdominal Wall 4　Chest Wall 5　Back 6　Inguinal Region, Right 7　Inguinal Region, Left 8　Upper Extremity, Right 9　Upper Extremity, Left A　Upper Arm, Right B　Upper Arm, Left C　Lower Arm, Right D　Lower Arm, Left E　Hand, Right F　Hand, Left G　Thumb, Right H　Thumb, Left J　Finger, Right K　Finger, Left L　Lower Extremity, Right M　Lower Extremity, Left N　Upper Leg, Right P　Upper Leg, Left Q　Lower Leg, Right R　Lower Leg, Left S　Foot, Right T　Foot, Left U　Toe, Right V　Toe, Left	X　External	0　Traction Apparatus 1　Splint 2　Cast 3　Brace 4　Bandage 5　Packing Material 6　Pressure Dressing 7　Intermittent Pressure Device Y　Other Device	Z　No Qualifier

2   Placement
W   Anatomical Regions
1   Compression   Putting pressure on a body region

Body Region Character 4	Approach Character 5	Device Character 6	Qualifier Character 7
Ø Head 1 Face 2 Neck 3 Abdominal Wall 4 Chest Wall 5 Back 6 Inguinal Region, Right 7 Inguinal Region, Left 8 Upper Extremity, Right 9 Upper Extremity, Left A Upper Arm, Right B Upper Arm, Left C Lower Arm, Right D Lower Arm, Left E Hand, Right F Hand, Left G Thumb, Right H Thumb, Left J Finger, Right K Finger, Left L Lower Extremity, Right M Lower Extremity, Left N Upper Leg, Right P Upper Leg, Left Q Lower Leg, Right R Lower Leg, Left S Foot, Right T Foot, Left U Toe, Right V Toe, Left	X External	6 Pressure Dressing 7 Intermittent Pressure Device	Z No Qualifier

2   Placement
W   Anatomical Regions
2   Dressing   Putting material on a body region for protection

Body Region Character 4	Approach Character 5	Device Character 6	Qualifier Character 7
Ø Head 1 Face 2 Neck 3 Abdominal Wall 4 Chest Wall 5 Back 6 Inguinal Region, Right 7 Inguinal Region, Left 8 Upper Extremity, Right 9 Upper Extremity, Left A Upper Arm, Right B Upper Arm, Left C Lower Arm, Right D Lower Arm, Left E Hand, Right F Hand, Left G Thumb, Right H Thumb, Left J Finger, Right K Finger, Left L Lower Extremity, Right M Lower Extremity, Left N Upper Leg, Right P Upper Leg, Left Q Lower Leg, Right R Lower Leg, Left S Foot, Right T Foot, Left U Toe, Right V Toe, Left	X External	4 Bandage	Z No Qualifier

2　Placement
W　Anatomical Regions
3　Immobilization　Limiting or preventing motion of a body region

Body Region Character 4	Approach Character 5	Device Character 6	Qualifier Character 7
0　Head	X　External	1　Splint 2　Cast 3　Brace 8　Stereotactic Apparatus Y　Other Device	Z　No Qualifier
1　Face	X　External	1　Splint 2　Cast 3　Brace 9　Wire Y　Other Device	Z　No Qualifier
2　Neck 3　Abdominal Wall 4　Chest Wall 5　Back 6　Inguinal Region, Right 7　Inguinal Region, Left 8　Upper Extremity, Right 9　Upper Extremity, Left A　Upper Arm, Right B　Upper Arm, Left C　Lower Arm, Right D　Lower Arm, Left E　Hand, Right F　Hand, Left G　Thumb, Right H　Thumb, Left J　Finger, Right K　Finger, Left L　Lower Extremity, Right M　Lower Extremity, Left N　Upper Leg, Right P　Upper Leg, Left Q　Lower Leg, Right R　Lower Leg, Left S　Foot, Right T　Foot, Left U　Toe, Right V　Toe, Left	X　External	1　Splint 2　Cast 3　Brace Y　Other Device	Z　No Qualifier

2　Placement
W　Anatomical Regions
4　Packing　　Putting material in a body region or orifice

Body Region Character 4	Approach Character 5	Device Character 6	Qualifier Character 7
0　Head 1　Face 2　Neck 3　Abdominal Wall 4　Chest Wall 5　Back 6　Inguinal Region, Right 7　Inguinal Region, Left 8　Upper Extremity, Right 9　Upper Extremity, Left A　Upper Arm, Right B　Upper Arm, Left C　Lower Arm, Right D　Lower Arm, Left E　Hand, Right F　Hand, Left G　Thumb, Right H　Thumb, Left J　Finger, Right K　Finger, Left L　Lower Extremity, Right M　Lower Extremity, Left N　Upper Leg, Right P　Upper Leg, Left Q　Lower Leg, Right R　Lower Leg, Left S　Foot, Right T　Foot, Left U　Toe, Right V　Toe, Left	X　External	5　Packing Material	Z　No Qualifier

2   **Placement**
W   **Anatomical Regions**
5   **Removal**   Taking out or off a device from a body part

Body Region Character 4	Approach Character 5	Device Character 6	Qualifier Character 7
Ø Head	**X** External	**Ø** Traction Apparatus **1** Splint **2** Cast **3** Brace **4** Bandage **5** Packing Material **6** Pressure Dressing **7** Intermittent Pressure Device **8** Stereotactic Apparatus **Y** Other Device	**Z** No Qualifier
1 Face	**X** External	**Ø** Traction Apparatus **1** Splint **2** Cast **3** Brace **4** Bandage **5** Packing Material **6** Pressure Dressing **7** Intermittent Pressure Device **9** Wire **Y** Other Device	**Z** No Qualifier
2 Neck **3** Abdominal Wall **4** Chest Wall **5** Back **6** Inguinal Region, Right **7** Inguinal Region, Left **8** Upper Extremity, Right **9** Upper Extremity, Left **A** Upper Arm, Right **B** Upper Arm, Left **C** Lower Arm, Right **D** Lower Arm, Left **E** Hand, Right **F** Hand, Left **G** Thumb, Right **H** Thumb, Left **J** Finger, Right **K** Finger, Left **L** Lower Extremity, Right **M** Lower Extremity, Left **N** Upper Leg, Right **P** Upper Leg, Left **Q** Lower Leg, Right **R** Lower Leg, Left **S** Foot, Right **T** Foot, Left **U** Toe, Right **V** Toe, Left	**X** External	**Ø** Traction Apparatus **1** Splint **2** Cast **3** Brace **4** Bandage **5** Packing Material **6** Pressure Dressing **7** Intermittent Pressure Device **Y** Other Device	**Z** No Qualifier

2　Placement
W　Anatomical Regions
6　Traction　　　Exerting a pulling force on a body region in a distal direction

Body Region Character 4	Approach Character 5	Device Character 6	Qualifier Character 7
0 Head	**X** External	**0** Traction Apparatus	**Z** No Qualifier
1 Face		**Z** No Device	
2 Neck			
3 Abdominal Wall			
4 Chest Wall			
5 Back			
6 Inguinal Region, Right			
7 Inguinal Region, Left			
8 Upper Extremity, Right			
9 Upper Extremity, Left			
A Upper Arm, Right			
B Upper Arm, Left			
C Lower Arm, Right			
D Lower Arm, Left			
E Hand, Right			
F Hand, Left			
G Thumb, Right			
H Thumb, Left			
J Finger, Right			
K Finger, Left			
L Lower Extremity, Right			
M Lower Extremity, Left			
N Upper Leg, Right			
P Upper Leg, Left			
Q Lower Leg, Right			
R Lower Leg, Left			
S Foot, Right			
T Foot, Left			
U Toe, Right			
V Toe, Left			

Placement—Anatomical Orifices 2Y0–2Y5

2   **Placement**
Y   **Anatomical Orifices**
0   **Change**   Taking out or off a device from a body part and putting back an identical or similar device in or on the same body part without cutting or puncturing the skin or a mucous membrane

Body Region Character 4	Approach Character 5	Device Character 6	Qualifier Character 7
0 Mouth and Pharynx **1** Nasal **2** Ear **3** Anorectal **4** Female Genital Tract **5** Urethra	**X** External	**5** Packing Material	**Z** No Qualifier

2   **Placement**
Y   **Anatomical Orifices**
4   **Packing**   Putting material in a body region or orifice

Body Region Character 4	Approach Character 5	Device Character 6	Qualifier Character 7
0 Mouth and Pharynx **1** Nasal **2** Ear **3** Anorectal **4** Female Genital Tract **5** Urethra	**X** External	**5** Packing Material	**Z** No Qualifier

2   **Placement**
Y   **Anatomical Orifices**
5   **Removal**   Taking out or off a device from a body part

Body Region Character 4	Approach Character 5	Device Character 6	Qualifier Character 7
0 Mouth and Pharynx **1** Nasal **2** Ear **3** Anorectal **4** Female Genital Tract **5** Urethra	**X** External	**5** Packing Material	**Z** No Qualifier

   Revised Text in **BLUE**   © 2011 Ingenix, Inc

Administration 302–3E1

3 Administration
0 Circulatory
2 Transfusion   Putting in blood or blood products

Body System/Region Character 4	Approach Character 5	Substance Character 6	Qualifier Character 7
3 Peripheral Vein 4 Central Vein	0 Open 3 Percutaneous	A Stem Cells, Embryonic	Z No Qualifier
3 Peripheral Vein 4 Central Vein 5 Peripheral Artery 6 Central Artery	0 Open 3 Percutaneous	G Bone Marrow H Whole Blood J Serum Albumin K Frozen Plasma L Fresh Plasma M Plasma Cryoprecipitate N Red Blood Cells P Frozen Red Cells Q White Cells R Platelets S Globulin T Fibrinogen V Antihemophilic Factors W Factor IX X Stem Cells, Cord Blood Y Stem Cells, Hematopoietic	0 Autologous 1 Nonautologous
7 Products of Conception, Circulatory	3 Percutaneous 7 Via Natural or Artificial Opening	H Whole Blood J Serum Albumin K Frozen Plasma L Fresh Plasma M Plasma Cryoprecipitate N Red Blood Cells P Frozen Red Cells Q White Cells R Platelets S Globulin T Fibrinogen V Antihemophilic Factors W Factor IX	1 Nonautologous

3 Administration
C Indwelling Device
1 Irrigation   Putting in or on a cleansing substance

Body System/Region Character 4	Approach Character 5	Substance Character 6	Qualifier Character 7
Z None	X External	8 Irrigating Substance	Z No Qualifier

3 Administration
E Physiological Systems and Anatomical Regions
0 Introduction   Putting in or on a therapeutic, diagnostic, nutritional, physiological, or prophylactic substance except blood or blood products

Body System/Region Character 4	Approach Character 5	Substance Character 6	Qualifier Character 7
0 Skin and Mucous Membranes	X External	0 Antineoplastic	5 Other Antineoplastic M Monoclonal Antibody
0 Skin and Mucous Membranes	X External	2 Anti-infective	8 Oxazolidinones 9 Other Anti-infective
0 Skin and Mucous Membranes	X External	3 Anti-inflammatory 4 Serum, Toxoid and Vaccine B Local Anesthetic K Other Diagnostic Substance M Pigment N Analgesics, Hypnotics, Sedatives T Destructive Agent	Z No Qualifier
0 Skin and Mucous Membranes	X External	G Other Therapeutic Substance	C Other Substance
1 Subcutaneous Tissue	3 Percutaneous	V Hormone	G Insulin J Other Hormone

3E0 Continued on next page

3   Administration
E   Physiological Systems and Anatomical Regions
0   Introduction   Putting in or on a therapeutic, diagnostic, nutritional, physiological, or prophylactic substance except blood or blood products

3E0 Continued

Body System/Region Character 4	Approach Character 5	Substance Character 6	Qualifier Character 7
1 Subcutaneous Tissue **2** Muscle	**3** Percutaneous	**3** Anti-inflammatory **4** Serum, Toxoid and Vaccine **6** Nutritional Substance **7** Electrolytic and Water Balance Substance **B** Local Anesthetic **H** Radioactive Substance **J** Contrast Agent **K** Other Diagnostic Substance **N** Analgesics, Hypnotics, Sedatives **T** Destructive Agent	**Z** No Qualifier
1 Subcutaneous Tissue **2** Muscle **A** Bone Marrow **F** Respiratory Tract **L** Pleural Cavity **M** Peritoneal Cavity **Q** Cranial Cavity and Brain **R** Spinal Canal **S** Epidural Space **T** Peripheral Nerves and Plexi **W** Lymphatics **X** Cranial Nerves **Y** Pericardial Cavity	**3** Percutaneous	**G** Other Therapeutic Substance	**C** Other Substance
1 Subcutaneous Tissue **2** Muscle **A** Bone Marrow **V** Bones **W** Lymphatics	**3** Percutaneous	**0** Antineoplastic	**5** Other Antineoplastic **M** Monoclonal Antibody
1 Subcutaneous Tissue **2** Muscle **F** Respiratory Tract **L** Pleural Cavity **M** Peritoneal Cavity **Q** Cranial Cavity and Brain **R** Spinal Canal **S** Epidural Space **U** Joints **V** Bones **W** Lymphatics **Y** Pericardial Cavity	**3** Percutaneous	**2** Anti-infective	**8** Oxazolidinones **9** Other Anti-infective
3 Peripheral Vein	**0** Open **3** Percutaneous	**U** Pancreatic Islet Cells	**0** Autologous **1** Nonautologous
3 Peripheral Vein **4** Central Vein **5** Peripheral Artery **6** Central Artery	**0** Open **3** Percutaneous	**0** Antineoplastic	**2** High-dose Interleukin-2 **3** Low-dose Interleukin-2 **5** Other Antineoplastic **M** Monoclonal Antibody **P** Clofarabine
3 Peripheral Vein **4** Central Vein **5** Peripheral Artery **6** Central Artery	**0** Open **3** Percutaneous	**2** Anti-infective	**8** Oxazolidinones **9** Other Anti-infective
3 Peripheral Vein **4** Central Vein **5** Peripheral Artery **6** Central Artery	**0** Open **3** Percutaneous	**3** Anti-inflammatory **4** Serum, Toxoid and Vaccine **6** Nutritional Substance **7** Electrolytic and Water Balance Substance **F** Intracirculatory Anesthetic **H** Radioactive Substance **J** Contrast Agent **K** Other Diagnostic Substance **N** Analgesics, Hypnotics, Sedatives **P** Platelet Inhibitor **R** Antiarrhythmic **T** Destructive Agent **X** Vasopressor	**Z** No Qualifier
3 Peripheral Vein **4** Central Vein **5** Peripheral Artery **6** Central Artery	**0** Open **3** Percutaneous	**G** Other Therapeutic Substance	**C** Other Substance **N** Blood Brain Barrier Disruption
3 Peripheral Vein **4** Central Vein **5** Peripheral Artery **6** Central Artery	**0** Open **3** Percutaneous	**V** Hormone	**G** Insulin **H** Human B-type Natriuretic Peptide **J** Other Hormone

3E0 Continued on next page

       Revised Text in **BLUE**

3　**Administration**
E　**Physiological Systems and Anatomical Regions**
Ø　**Introduction**　　Putting in or on a therapeutic, diagnostic, nutritional, physiological, or prophylactic substance except blood or blood products

Body System/Region Character 4	Approach Character 5	Substance Character 6	Qualifier Character 7
3 Peripheral Vein 4 Central Vein 5 Peripheral Artery 6 Central Artery	Ø Open 3 Percutaneous	W Immunotherapeutic	K Immunostimulator L Immunosuppressive
3 Peripheral Vein 4 Central Vein 5 Peripheral Artery 6 Central Artery 7 Coronary Artery 8 Heart	Ø Open 3 Percutaneous	1 Thrombolytic	6 Recombinant Human-activated Protein C 7 Other Thrombolytic
7 Coronary Artery 8 Heart	Ø Open 3 Percutaneous	G Other Therapeutic Substance	C Other Substance
7 Coronary Artery 8 Heart	Ø Open 3 Percutaneous	J Contrast Agent K Other Diagnostic Substance P Platelet Inhibitor	Z No Qualifier
9 Nose	3 Percutaneous 7 Via Natural or Artificial Opening X External	Ø Antineoplastic	5 Other Antineoplastic M Monoclonal Antibody
9 Nose	3 Percutaneous 7 Via Natural or Artificial Opening X External	3 Anti-inflammatory 4 Serum, Toxoid and Vaccine B Local Anesthetic H Radioactive Substance J Contrast Agent K Other Diagnostic Substance N Analgesics, Hypnotics, Sedatives T Destructive Agent	Z No Qualifier
9 Nose B Ear C Eye D Mouth and Pharynx	3 Percutaneous 7 Via Natural or Artificial Opening X External	2 Anti-infective	8 Oxazolidinones 9 Other Anti-infective
9 Nose B Ear C Eye D Mouth and Pharynx	3 Percutaneous 7 Via Natural or Artificial Opening X External	G Other Therapeutic Substance	C Other Substance
B Ear	3 Percutaneous 7 Via Natural or Artificial Opening X External	3 Anti-inflammatory B Local Anesthetic H Radioactive Substance J Contrast Agent K Other Diagnostic Substance N Analgesics, Hypnotics, Sedatives T Destructive Agent	Z No Qualifier
B Ear C Eye D Mouth and Pharynx	3 Percutaneous 7 Via Natural or Artificial Opening X External	Ø Antineoplastic	4 Liquid Brachytherapy Radioisotope 5 Other Antineoplastic M Monoclonal Antibody
C Eye	3 Percutaneous 7 Via Natural or Artificial Opening X External	3 Anti-inflammatory B Local Anesthetic H Radioactive Substance K Other Diagnostic Substance M Pigment N Analgesics, Hypnotics, Sedatives T Destructive Agent	Z No Qualifier
C Eye	3 Percutaneous 7 Via Natural or Artificial Opening X External	S Gas	F Other Gas
D Mouth and Pharynx	3 Percutaneous 7 Via Natural or Artificial Opening X External	3 Anti-inflammatory 4 Serum, Toxoid and Vaccine 6 Nutritional Substance 7 Electrolytic and Water Balance Substance B Local Anesthetic H Radioactive Substance J Contrast Agent K Other Diagnostic Substance N Analgesics, Hypnotics, Sedatives R Antiarrhythmic T Destructive Agent	Z No Qualifier

3EØ Continued on next page

　　　　Revised Text in **BLUE**

Administration

3E0 Continued

3   **Administration**
E   **Physiological Systems and Anatomical Regions**
0   **Introduction**   Putting in or on a therapeutic, diagnostic, nutritional, physiological, or prophylactic substance except blood or blood products

Body System/Region Character 4	Approach Character 5	Substance Character 6	Qualifier Character 7
E Products of Conception F Respiratory Tract G Upper GI H Lower GI J Biliary and Pancreatic Tract K Genitourinary Tract N Male Reproductive P Female Reproductive	3 Percutaneous 7 Via Natural or Artificial Opening 8 Via Natural or Artificial Opening Endoscopic	0 Antineoplastic	4 Liquid Brachytherapy Radioisotope 5 Other Antineoplastic M Monoclonal Antibody
E Products of Conception F Respiratory Tract G Upper GI H Lower GI J Biliary and Pancreatic Tract K Genitourinary Tract N Male Reproductive P Female Reproductive	3 Percutaneous 7 Via Natural or Artificial Opening 8 Via Natural or Artificial Opening Endoscopic	2 Anti-infective	8 Oxazolidinones 9 Other Anti-infective
E Products of Conception F Respiratory Tract G Upper GI H Lower GI J Biliary and Pancreatic Tract K Genitourinary Tract N Male Reproductive P Female Reproductive	3 Percutaneous 7 Via Natural or Artificial Opening 8 Via Natural or Artificial Opening Endoscopic	G Other Therapeutic Substance	C Other Substance
E Products of Conception G Upper GI H Lower GI J Biliary and Pancreatic Tract K Genitourinary Tract N Male Reproductive	3 Percutaneous 7 Via Natural or Artificial Opening 8 Via Natural or Artificial Opening Endoscopic	3 Anti-inflammatory 6 Nutritional Substance 7 Electrolytic and Water Balance Substance B Local Anesthetic H Radioactive Substance J Contrast Agent K Other Diagnostic Substance N Analgesics, Hypnotics, Sedatives T Destructive Agent	Z No Qualifier
E Products of Conception G Upper GI H Lower GI J Biliary and Pancreatic Tract K Genitourinary Tract N Male Reproductive P Female Reproductive	3 Percutaneous 7 Via Natural or Artificial Opening 8 Via Natural or Artificial Opening Endoscopic	S Gas	F Other Gas
F Respiratory Tract	3 Percutaneous 7 Via Natural or Artificial Opening 8 Via Natural or Artificial Opening Endoscopic	S Gas	D Nitric Oxide F Other Gas
F Respiratory Tract	7 Via Natural or Artificial Opening 8 Via Natural or Artificial Opening Endoscopic	3 Anti-inflammatory 6 Nutritional Substance 7 Electrolytic and Water Balance Substance B Local Anesthetic D Inhalation Anesthetic H Radioactive Substance J Contrast Agent K Other Diagnostic Substance N Analgesics, Hypnotics, Sedatives T Destructive Agent	Z No Qualifier
F Respiratory Tract L Pleural Cavity M Peritoneal Cavity U Joints V Bones W Lymphatics Y Pericardial Cavity	3 Percutaneous	3 Anti-inflammatory 6 Nutritional Substance 7 Electrolytic and Water Balance Substance B Local Anesthetic H Radioactive Substance J Contrast Agent K Other Diagnostic Substance N Analgesics, Hypnotics, Sedatives T Destructive Agent	Z No Qualifier
J Biliary and Pancreatic Tract	3 Percutaneous 7 Via Natural or Artificial Opening 8 Via Natural or Artificial Opening Endoscopic	U Pancreatic Islet Cells	0 Autologous 1 Nonautologous
L Pleural Cavity M Peritoneal Cavity P Female Reproductive	0 Open	5 Adhesion Barrier	Z No Qualifier

3E0 Continued on next page

     Revised Text in **BLUE**   © 2011 Ingenix, Inc

3   **Administration**   *3E0 Continued*
E   **Physiological Systems and Anatomical Regions**
0   **Introduction**   Putting in or on a therapeutic, diagnostic, nutritional, physiological, or prophylactic substance except blood or blood products

Body System/Region Character 4	Approach Character 5	Substance Character 6	Qualifier Character 7
L Pleural Cavity M Peritoneal Cavity Q Cranial Cavity and Brain R Spinal Canal S Epidural Space U Joints Y Pericardial Cavity	3 Percutaneous 7 Via Natural or Artificial Opening	S Gas	F Other Gas
L Pleural Cavity M Peritoneal Cavity Q Cranial Cavity and Brain U Joints Y Pericardial Cavity	3 Percutaneous 7 Via Natural or Artificial Opening	0 Antineoplastic	4 Liquid Brachytherapy Radioisotope 5 Other Antineoplastic M Monoclonal Antibody
P Female Reproductive	3 Percutaneous 7 Via Natural or Artificial Opening	3 Anti-inflammatory 6 Nutritional Substance 7 Electrolytic and Water Balance Substance B Local Anesthetic H Radioactive Substance J Contrast Agent K Other Diagnostic Substance L Sperm N Analgesics, Hypnotics, Sedatives T Destructive Agent	Z No Qualifier
P Female Reproductive	3 Percutaneous 7 Via Natural or Artificial Opening	Q Fertilized Ovum	0 Autologous 1 Nonautologous
P Female Reproductive	8 Via Natural or Artificial Opening Endoscopic	3 Anti-inflammatory 6 Nutritional Substance 7 Electrolytic and Water Balance Substance B Local Anesthetic H Radioactive Substance J Contrast Agent K Other Diagnostic Substance N Analgesics, Hypnotics, Sedatives T Destructive Agent	Z No Qualifier
Q Cranial Cavity and Brain	3 Percutaneous	3 Anti-inflammatory 6 Nutritional Substance 7 Electrolytic and Water Balance Substance A Stem Cells, Embryonic B Local Anesthetic H Radioactive Substance J Contrast Agent K Other Diagnostic Substance N Analgesics, Hypnotics, Sedatives T Destructive Agent	Z No Qualifier
Q Cranial Cavity and Brain R Spinal Canal	0 Open	A Stem Cells, Embryonic	Z No Qualifier
Q Cranial Cavity and Brain R Spinal Canal	0 Open 3 Percutaneous	E Stem Cells, Somatic	0 Autologous 1 Nonautologous
R Spinal Canal	3 Percutaneous	3 Anti-inflammatory 6 Nutritional Substance 7 Electrolytic and Water Balance Substance A Stem Cells, Embryonic B Local Anesthetic C Regional Anesthetic H Radioactive Substance J Contrast Agent K Other Diagnostic Substance N Analgesics, Hypnotics, Sedatives T Destructive Agent	Z No Qualifier
R Spinal Canal S Epidural Space	3 Percutaneous	0 Antineoplastic	2 High-dose Interleukin-2 3 Low-dose Interleukin-2 4 Liquid Brachytherapy Radioisotope 5 Other Antineoplastic M Monoclonal Antibody

3E0 Continued on next page

Administration

3 Administration
E Physiological Systems and Anatomical Regions
0 Introduction   Putting in or on a therapeutic, diagnostic, nutritional, physiological, or prophylactic substance except blood or blood products

3E0 Continued

Body System/Region Character 4	Approach Character 5	Substance Character 6	Qualifier Character 7
S Epidural Space	**3** Percutaneous	**3** Anti-inflammatory **6** Nutritional Substance **7** Electrolytic and Water Balance Substance **B** Local Anesthetic **C** Regional Anesthetic **H** Radioactive Substance **J** Contrast Agent **K** Other Diagnostic Substance **N** Analgesics, Hypnotics, Sedatives **T** Destructive Agent	**Z** No Qualifier
T Peripheral Nerves and Plexi **X** Cranial Nerves	**3** Percutaneous	**3** Anti-inflammatory **C** Regional Anesthetic **T** Destructive Agent	**Z** No Qualifier
U Joints **V** Bones	**3** Percutaneous	**G** Other Therapeutic Substance	**B** Recombinant Bone Morphogenetic Protein **C** Other Substance
U **Joints** **V** **Bones**	**Ø** **Open**	**G** **Other Therapeutic Substance**	**B** **Recombinant Bone Morphogenetic Protein**

3 Administration
E Physiological Systems and Anatomical Regions
1 Irrigation   Putting in or on a cleansing substance

Body System/Region Character 4	Approach Character 5	Substance Character 6	Qualifier Character 7
Ø Skin and Mucous Membranes **C** Eye	**3** Percutaneous **X** External	**8** Irrigating Substance	**X** Diagnostic **Z** No Qualifier
9 Nose **B** Ear **F** Respiratory Tract **G** Upper GI **H** Lower GI **J** Biliary and Pancreatic Tract **K** Genitourinary Tract **N** Male Reproductive **P** Female Reproductive	**3** Percutaneous **7** Via Natural or Artificial Opening **8** Via Natural or Artificial Opening Endoscopic	**8** Irrigating Substance	**X** Diagnostic **Z** No Qualifier
L Pleural Cavity **M** Peritoneal Cavity **Q** Cranial Cavity and Brain **R** Spinal Canal **S** Epidural Space **U** Joints **Y** Pericardial Cavity	**3** Percutaneous	**8** Irrigating Substance	**X** Diagnostic **Z** No Qualifier
M Peritoneal Cavity	**3** Percutaneous	**9** Dialysate	**Z** No Qualifier

Measurement and Monitoring 4AØ–4BØ

4　**Measurement and Monitoring**
A　**Physiological Systems**
Ø　**Measurement**　　Determining the level of a physiological or physical function at a point in time

Body System Character 4	Approach Character 5	Function/Device Character 6	Qualifier Character 7
Ø Central Nervous	Ø Open	2 Conductivity 4 Electrical Activity B Pressure	Z No Qualifier
Ø Central Nervous	3 Percutaneous 7 Via Natural or Artificial Opening	B Pressure K Temperature R Saturation	D Intracranial
Ø Central Nervous	X External	2 Conductivity 4 Electrical Activity	Z No Qualifier
1 Peripheral Nervous	Ø Open 3 Percutaneous X External	2 Conductivity	9 Sensory B Motor
2 Cardiac	Ø Open 3 Percutaneous	N Sampling and Pressure	6 Right Heart 7 Left Heart 8 Bilateral
2 Cardiac	Ø Open 3 Percutaneous	4 Electrical Activity 9 Output C Rate F Rhythm H Sound P Action Currents	Z No Qualifier
2 Cardiac	X External	9 Output C Rate F Rhythm H Sound P Action Currents	Z No Qualifier
2 Cardiac	X External	M Total Activity	4 Stress
2 Cardiac	X External	4 Electrical Activity	**A Guidance** **Z No Qualifier**
3 Arterial	Ø Open 3 Percutaneous	5 Flow J Pulse	1 Peripheral 3 Pulmonary C Coronary
3 Arterial	Ø Open 3 Percutaneous	B Pressure	1 Peripheral 3 Pulmonary C Coronary F Other Thoracic
3 Arterial	Ø Open 3 Percutaneous	H Sound R Saturation	1 Peripheral
3 Arterial	X External	5 Flow B Pressure H Sound J Pulse R Saturation	1 Peripheral
4 Venous	Ø Open 3 Percutaneous	5 Flow B Pressure J Pulse	Ø Central 1 Peripheral 2 Portal 3 Pulmonary
4 Venous	Ø Open 3 Percutaneous	R Saturation	1 Peripheral
4 Venous	X External	5 Flow B Pressure J Pulse R Saturation	1 Peripheral
5 Circulatory	X External	L Volume	Z No Qualifier
6 Lymphatic	Ø Open 3 Percutaneous	5 Flow B Pressure	Z No Qualifier
7 Visual	X External	Ø Acuity 7 Mobility B Pressure	Z No Qualifier
8 Olfactory	X External	Ø Acuity	Z No Qualifier

4AØ Continued on next page

4A0 Continued

4   **Measurement and Monitoring**
A   **Physiological Systems**
0   **Measurement**   Determining the level of a physiological or physical function at a point in time

Body System Character 4	Approach Character 5	Function/Device Character 6	Qualifier Character 7
9 Respiratory	7 Via Natural or Artificial Opening 8 Via Natural or Artificial Opening Endoscopic X External	1 Capacity 5 Flow C Rate D Resistance L Volume M Total Activity	Z No Qualifier
B Gastrointestinal	7 Via Natural or Artificial Opening 8 Via Natural or Artificial Opening Endoscopic	8 Motility B Pressure G Secretion	Z No Qualifier
C Biliary	3 Percutaneous 4 Percutaneous Endoscopic 7 Via Natural or Artificial Opening 8 Via Natural or Artificial Opening Endoscopic	5 Flow B Pressure	Z No Qualifier
D Urinary	7 Via Natural or Artificial Opening	3 Contractility 5 Flow B Pressure D Resistance L Volume	Z No Qualifier
F Musculoskeletal	3 Percutaneous X External	3 Contractility	Z No Qualifier
H Products of Conception, Cardiac	7 Via Natural or Artificial Opening 8 Via Natural or Artificial Opening Endoscopic X External	4 Electrical Activity C Rate F Rhythm H Sound	Z No Qualifier
J Products of Conception, Nervous	7 Via Natural or Artificial Opening 8 Via Natural or Artificial Opening Endoscopic X External	2 Conductivity 4 Electrical Activity B Pressure	Z No Qualifier
Z None	7 Via Natural or Artificial Opening	6 Metabolism K Temperature	Z No Qualifier
Z None	X External	6 Metabolism K Temperature Q Sleep	Z No Qualifier

4   **Measurement and Monitoring**
A   **Physiological Systems**
1   **Monitoring**   Determining the level of a physiological or physical function repetitively over a period of time

Body System Character 4	Approach Character 5	Function/Device Character 6	Qualifier Character 7
0 Central Nervous	0 Open	2 Conductivity B Pressure	Z No Qualifier
0 Central Nervous	0 Open X External	4 Electrical Activity	G Intraoperative Z No Qualifier
0 Central Nervous	3 Percutaneous 7 Via Natural or Artificial Opening	B Pressure K Temperature R Saturation	D Intracranial
0 Central Nervous	X External	2 Conductivity	Z No Qualifier
1 Peripheral Nervous	0 Open 3 Percutaneous X External	2 Conductivity	9 Sensory B Motor
2 Cardiac	0 Open 3 Percutaneous	4 Electrical Activity 9 Output C Rate F Rhythm H Sound	Z No Qualifier
2 Cardiac	X External	4 Electrical Activity	5 Ambulatory Z No Qualifier
2 Cardiac	X External	9 Output C Rate F Rhythm H Sound	Z No Qualifier
2 Cardiac	X External	M Total Activity	4 Stress
3 Arterial	0 Open 3 Percutaneous	5 Flow B Pressure J Pulse	1 Peripheral 3 Pulmonary C Coronary

4A1 Continued on next page

     Revised Text in **BLUE**   © 2011 Ingenix, Inc

4   Measurement and Monitoring
A   Physiological Systems
1   Monitoring   Determining the level of a physiological or physical function repetitively over a period of time

4A1 Continued

Body System Character 4	Approach Character 5	Function/Device Character 6	Qualifier Character 7
3 Arterial	**Ø** Open **3** Percutaneous	**H** Sound **R** Saturation	**1** Peripheral
3 Arterial	**X** External	**5** Flow **B** Pressure **H** Sound **J** Pulse **R** Saturation	**1** Peripheral
4 Venous	**Ø** Open **3** Percutaneous	**5** Flow **B** Pressure **J** Pulse	**Ø** Central **1** Peripheral **2** Portal **3** Pulmonary
4 Venous	**Ø** Open **3** Percutaneous	**R** Saturation	**Ø** Central **2** Portal **3** Pulmonary
4 Venous	**X** External	**5** Flow **B** Pressure **J** Pulse	**1** Peripheral
6 Lymphatic	**Ø** Open **3** Percutaneous	**5** Flow **B** Pressure	**Z** No Qualifier
9 Respiratory	**7** Via Natural or Artificial Opening **X** External	**1** Capacity **5** Flow **C** Rate **D** Resistance **L** Volume	**Z** No Qualifier
B Gastrointestinal	**7** Via Natural or Artificial Opening **8** Via Natural or Artificial Opening Endoscopic	**8** Motility **B** Pressure **G** Secretion	**Z** No Qualifier
D Urinary	**7** Via Natural or Artificial Opening	**3** Contractility **5** Flow **B** Pressure **D** Resistance **L** Volume	**Z** No Qualifier
H Products of Conception, Cardiac	**7** Via Natural or Artificial Opening **8** Via Natural or Artificial Opening Endoscopic **X** External	**4** Electrical Activity **C** Rate **F** Rhythm **H** Sound	**Z** No Qualifier
J Products of Conception, Nervous	**7** Via Natural or Artificial Opening **8** Via Natural or Artificial Opening Endoscopic **X** External	**2** Conductivity **4** Electrical Activity **B** Pressure	**Z** No Qualifier
Z None	**7** Via Natural or Artificial Opening	**K** Temperature	**Z** No Qualifier
Z None	**X** External	**K** Temperature **Q** Sleep	**Z** No Qualifier

4   Measurement and Monitoring
B   Physiological Devices
Ø   Measurement   Determining the level of a physiological or physical function repetitively over a period of time

Body System Character 4	Approach Character 5	Function/Device Character 6	Qualifier Character 7
Ø Central Nervous **1** Peripheral Nervous **F** Musculoskeletal	**X** External	**V** Stimulator	**Z** No Qualifier
2 Cardiac	**X** External	**S** Pacemaker **T** Defibrillator	**Z** No Qualifier
9 Respiratory	**X** External	**S** Pacemaker	**Z** No Qualifier

Extracorporeal Assistance and Performance 5A0–5A2

5 Extracorporeal Assistance and Performance
A Physiological Systems
0 Assistance   Taking over a portion of a physiological function by extracorporeal means

Body System Character 4	Duration Character 5	Function Character 6	Qualifier Character 7
2 Cardiac	1 Intermittent 2 Continuous	1 Output	0 Balloon Pump 5 Pulsatile Compression 6 Other Pump D Impeller Pump
5 Circulatory	1 Intermittent 2 Continuous	2 Oxygenation	1 Hyperbaric C Supersaturated
9 Respiratory	3 Less than 24 Consecutive Hours 4 24-96 Consecutive Hours 5 Greater than 96 Consecutive Hours	5 Ventilation	7 Continuous Positive Airway Pressure 8 Intermittent Positive Airway Pressure 9 Continuous Negative Airway Pressure B Intermittent Negative Airway Pressure Z No Qualifier

5 Extracorporeal Assistance and Performance
A Physiological Systems
1 Performance   Completely taking over a physiological function by extracorporeal means

Body System Character 4	Duration Character 5	Function Character 6	Qualifier Character 7
2 Cardiac	0 Single	1 Output	2 Manual
2 Cardiac	1 Intermittent	3 Pacing	Z No Qualifier
2 Cardiac	2 Continuous	1 Output 3 Pacing	Z No Qualifier
5 Circulatory	2 Continuous	2 Oxygenation	3 Membrane
9 Respiratory	0 Single	5 Ventilation	4 Nonmechanical
9 Respiratory	3 Less than 24 Consecutive Hours 4 24-96 Consecutive Hours 5 Greater than 96 Consecutive Hours	5 Ventilation	Z No Qualifier
C Biliary D Urinary	0 Single 6 Multiple	0 Filtration	Z No Qualifier

5 Extracorporeal Assistance and Performance
A Physiological Systems
2 Restoration   Returning, or attempting to return, a physiological function to its original state by extracorporeal means.

Body System Character 4	Duration Character 5	Function Character 6	Qualifier Character 7
2 Cardiac	0 Single	4 Rhythm	Z No Qualifier

Revised Text in **BLUE**

Extracorporeal Therapies 6A0–6A9

6 **Extracorporeal Therapies**
A **Physiological Systems**
0 **Atmospheric Control**　　Extracorporeal control of atmospheric pressure and composition

Body System Character 4	Duration Character 5	Qualifier Character 6	Qualifier Character 7
Z　None	0　Single 1　Multiple	Z　No Qualifier	Z　No Qualifier

6 **Extracorporeal Therapies**
A **Physiological Systems**
1 **Decompression**　　Extracorporeal elimination of undissolved gas from body fluids

Body System Character 4	Duration Character 5	Qualifier Character 6	Qualifier Character 7
5　Circulatory	0　Single 1　Multiple	Z　No Qualifier	Z　No Qualifier

6 **Extracorporeal Therapies**
A **Physiological Systems**
2 **Electromagnetic Therapy**　　Extracorporeal treatment by electromagnetic rays

Body System Character 4	Duration Character 5	Qualifier Character 6	Qualifier Character 7
1　Urinary 2　Central Nervous	0　Single 1　Multiple	Z　No Qualifier	Z　No Qualifier

6 **Extracorporeal Therapies**
A **Physiological Systems**
3 **Hyperthermia**　　Extracorporeal raising of body temperature

Body System Character 4	Duration Character 5	Qualifier Character 6	Qualifier Character 7
Z　None	0　Single 1　Multiple	Z　No Qualifier	Z　No Qualifier

6 **Extracorporeal Therapies**
A **Physiological Systems**
4 **Hypothermia**　　Extracorporeal lowering of body temperature

Body System Character 4	Duration Character 5	Qualifier Character 6	Qualifier Character 7
Z　None	0　Single 1　Multiple	Z　No Qualifier	Z　No Qualifier

6 **Extracorporeal Therapies**
A **Physiological Systems**
5 **Pheresis**　　Extracorporeal separation of blood products

Body System Character 4	Duration Character 5	Qualifier Character 6	Qualifier Character 7
5　Circulatory	0　Single 1　Multiple	Z　No Qualifier	0　Erythrocytes 1　Leukocytes 2　Platelets 3　Plasma T　Stem Cells, Cord Blood V　Stem Cells, Hematopoietic

6 **Extracorporeal Therapies**
A **Physiological Systems**
6 **Phototherapy**　　Extracorporeal treatment by light rays

Body System Character 4	Duration Character 5	Qualifier Character 6	Qualifier Character 7
0　Skin 5　Circulatory	0　Single 1　Multiple	Z　No Qualifier	Z　No Qualifier

Extracorporeal Therapies (side tab)

6A7–6A9 (side tab)

6   **Extracorporeal Therapies**
A   **Physiological Systems**
7   **Ultrasound Therapy**   Extracorporeal treatment by ultrasound

Body System Character 4	Duration Character 5	Qualifier Character 6	Qualifier Character 7
5 Circulatory	**Ø** Single **1** Multiple	**Z** No Qualifier	**4** Head and Neck Vessels **5** Heart **6** Peripheral Vessels **7** Other Vessels **Z** No Qualifier

6   **Extracorporeal Therapies**
A   **Physiological Systems**
8   **Ultraviolet Light Therapy**   Extracorporeal treatment by ultraviolet light

Body System Character 4	Duration Character 5	Qualifier Character 6	Qualifier Character 7
Ø Skin	**Ø** Single **1** Multiple	**Z** No Qualifier	**Z** No Qualifier

6   **Extracorporeal Therapies**
A   **Physiological Systems**
9   **Shock Wave Therapy**   Extracorporeal treatment by shock waves

Body System Character 4	Duration Character 5	Qualifier Character 6	Qualifier Character 7
3 Musculoskeletal	**Ø** Single **1** Multiple	**Z** No Qualifier	**Z** No Qualifier

Osteopathic 7W0

7　Osteopathic
W　Anatomical Regions
0　Treatment　　Manual treatment to eliminate or alleviate somatic dysfunction and related disorders

Body Region Character 4	Approach Character 5	Method Character 6	Qualifier Character 7
0　Head 1　Cervical 2　Thoracic 3　Lumbar 4　Sacrum 5　Pelvis 6　Lower Extremities 7　Upper Extremities 8　Rib Cage 9　Abdomen	X　External	0　Articulatory-Raising 1　Fascial Release 2　General Mobilization 3　High Velocity-Low Amplitude 4　Indirect 5　Low Velocity-High Amplitude 6　Lymphatic Pump 7　Muscle Energy-Isometric 8　Muscle Energy-Isotonic 9　Other Method	Z　None

Other Procedures 8C0–8E0

8   **Other Procedures**
C   **Indwelling Device**
Ø   **Other Procedures**   Methodologies which attempt to remediate or cure a disorder or disease

Body Region Character 4	Approach Character 5	Method Character 6	Qualifier Character 7
1 Nervous System	**X** External	**6** Collection	**J** Cerebrospinal Fluid **L** Other Fluid
2 Circulatory System	**X** External	**6** Collection	**K** Blood **L** Other Fluid

8   **Other Procedures**
E   **Physiological Systems and Anatomical Regions**
Ø   **Other Procedures**   Methodologies which attempt to remediate or cure a disorder or disease

Body Region Character 4	Approach Character 5	Method Character 6	Qualifier Character 7
1 Nervous System **K** Musculoskeletal System **U** Female Reproductive System	**X** External	**Y** Other Method	**7** Examination
2 Circulatory System	**3** Percutaneous	**D** Near Infrared Spectroscopy	**Z** No Qualifier
9 Head and Neck Region **W** Trunk Region	**Ø** Open **3** Percutaneous **4** Percutaneous Endoscopic **7** Via Natural or Artificial Opening **8** Via Natural or Artificial Opening Endoscopic **X** External	**C** Robotic Assisted Procedure	**Z** No Qualifier
9 Head and Neck Region **W** Trunk Region **X** Upper Extremity **Y** Lower Extremity	**X** External	**B** Computer Assisted Procedure	**F** With Fluoroscopy **G** With Computerized Tomography **H** With Magnetic Resonance Imaging **Z** No Qualifier
9 Head and Neck Region **W** Trunk Region **X** Upper Extremity **Y** Lower Extremity	**X** External	**Y** Other Method	**8** Suture Removal
H Integumentary System and Breast	**3** Percutaneous	**Ø** Acupuncture	**Ø** Anesthesia **Z** No Qualifier
H Integumentary System and Breast	**X** External	**6** Collection	**2** Breast Milk
H Integumentary System and Breast	**X** External	**Y** Other Method	**9** Piercing
K Musculoskeletal System	**X** External	**1** Therapeutic Massage	**Z** No Qualifier
V Male Reproductive System	**X** External	**1** Therapeutic Massage	**C** Prostate **D** Rectum
V Male Reproductive System	**X** External	**6** Collection	**3** Sperm
X Upper Extremity **Y** Lower Extremity	**Ø** Open **3** Percutaneous **4** Percutaneous Endoscopic **X** External	**C** Robotic Assisted Procedure	**Z** No Qualifier
Z None	**X** External	**Y** Other Method	**1** In Vitro Fertilization **4** Yoga Therapy **5** Meditation **6** Isolation

Chiropractic 9WB

9　**Chiropractic**
W　**Anatomical Regions**
B　**Manipulation**　　Manual procedure that involves a directed thrust to move a joint past the physiological range of motion, without exceeding the anatomical limit

Body Region Character 4	Approach Character 5	Method Character 6	Qualifier Character 7
Ø Head	X External	B Non-Manual	Z None
1 Cervical		C Indirect Visceral	
2 Thoracic		D Extra-Articular	
3 Lumbar		F Direct Visceral	
4 Sacrum		G Long Lever Specific Contact	
5 Pelvis		H Short Lever Specific Contact	
6 Lower Extremities		J Long and Short Lever Specific Contact	
7 Upper Extremities		K Mechanically Assisted	
8 Rib Cage		L Other Method	
9 Abdomen			

Imaging B00–BY4

B   **Imaging**
0   **Central Nervous System**
0   **Plain Radiography**   Planar display of an image developed from the capture of external ionizing radiation on photographic or photoconductive plate

Body Part Character 4	Contrast Character 5	Qualifier Character 6	Qualifier Character 7
B Spinal Cord	**0** High Osmolar **1** Low Osmolar **Y** Other Contrast **Z** None	**Z** None	**Z** None

B   **Imaging**
0   **Central Nervous System**
1   **Fluoroscopy**   Single plane or bi-plane real time display of an image developed from the capture of external ionizing radioation on a fluorescent screen. The image may also be stored by either digital or analog means

Body Part Character 4	Contrast Character 5	Qualifier Character 6	Qualifier Character 7
B Spinal Cord	**0** High Osmolar **1** Low Osmolar **Y** Other Contrast **Z** None	**Z** None	**Z** None

B   **Imaging**
0   **Central Nervous System**
2   **Computerized Tomography (CT Scan)**   Computer reformatted digital display of multiplanar images developed from the capture of multiple exposures of external ionizing radiation

Body Part Character 4	Contrast Character 5	Qualifier Character 6	Qualifier Character 7
0 Brain **7** Cisterna **8** Cerebral Ventricle(s) **9** Sella Turcica/Pituitary Gland **B** Spinal Cord	**0** High Osmolar **1** Low Osmolar **Y** Other Contrast	**0** Unenhanced and Enhanced **Z** None	**Z** None
0 Brain **7** Cisterna **8** Cerebral Ventricle(s) **9** Sella Turcica/Pituitary Gland **B** Spinal Cord	**Z** None	**Z** None	**Z** None

B   **Imaging**
0   **Central Nervous System**
3   **Magnetic Resonance Imaging (MRI)**   Computer reformatted digital display of multiplanar images developed from the capture of radio-frequency signals emitted by nuclei in a body site excited within a magnetic field

Body Part Character 4	Contrast Character 5	Qualifier Character 6	Qualifier Character 7
0 Brain **9** Sella Turcica/Pituitary Gland **B** Spinal Cord **C** Acoustic Nerves	**Y** Other Contrast	**0** Unenhanced and Enhanced **Z** None	**Z** None
0 Brain **9** Sella Turcica/Pituitary Gland **B** Spinal Cord **C** Acoustic Nerves	**Z** None	**Z** None	**Z** None

B   **Imaging**
0   **Central Nervous System**
4   **Ultrasonography**   Real time display of images of anatomy or flow information developed from the capture of relected and attenuated high frequency sound waves

Body Part Character 4	Contrast Character 5	Qualifier Character 6	Qualifier Character 7
0 Brain **B** Spinal Cord	**Z** None	**Z** None	**Z** None

B　Imaging
2　Heart
Ø　Plain Radiography　Planar display of an image developed from the capture of external ionizing radiation on photographic or photoconductive plate

Body Part Character 4	Contrast Character 5	Qualifier Character 6	Qualifier Character 7
Ø Coronary Artery, Single 1 Coronary Arteries, Multiple 2 Coronary Artery Bypass Graft, Single 3 Coronary Artery Bypass Grafts, Multiple 4 Heart, Right 5 Heart, Left 6 Heart, Right and Left 7 Internal Mammary Bypass Graft, Right 8 Internal Mammary Bypass Graft, Left F Bypass Graft, Other	Ø High Osmolar 1 Low Osmolar Y Other Contrast	Z None	Z None

B　Imaging
2　Heart
1　Fluoroscopy　Single plane or bi-plane real time display of an image developed from the capture of external ionizing radioation on a fluorescent screen. The image may also be stored by either digital or analog means

Body Part Character 4	Contrast Character 5	Qualifier Character 6	Qualifier Character 7
Ø Coronary Artery, Single 1 Coronary Arteries, Multiple 2 Coronary Artery Bypass Graft, Single 3 Coronary Artery Bypass Grafts, Multiple	Ø High Osmolar 1 Low Osmolar Y Other Contrast	1 Laser	Ø Intraoperative
Ø Coronary Artery, Single 1 Coronary Arteries, Multiple 2 Coronary Artery Bypass Graft, Single 3 Coronary Artery Bypass Grafts, Multiple 4 Heart, Right 5 Heart, Left 6 Heart, Right and Left 7 Internal Mammary Bypass Graft, Right 8 Internal Mammary Bypass Graft, Left F Bypass Graft, Other	Ø High Osmolar 1 Low Osmolar Y Other Contrast	Z None	Z None

B　Imaging
2　Heart
2　Computerized Tomography (CT Scan)　Computer reformatted digital display of multiplanar images developed from the capture of multiple exposures of external ionizing radiation

Body Part Character 4	Contrast Character 5	Qualifier Character 6	Qualifier Character 7
1 Coronary Arteries, Multiple 3 Coronary Artery Bypass Grafts, Multiple 6 Heart, Right and Left	Ø High Osmolar 1 Low Osmolar Y Other Contrast	Ø Unenhanced and Enhanced Z None	Z None
1 Coronary Arteries, Multiple 3 Coronary Artery Bypass Grafts, Multiple 6 Heart, Right and Left	Z None	2 Intravascular Optical Coherence Z None	Z None

B　Imaging
2　Heart
3　Magnetic Resonance Imaging (MRI)　Computer reformatted digital display of multiplanar images developed from the capture of radio-frequency signals emitted by nuclei in a body site excited within a magnetic field

Body Part Character 4	Contrast Character 5	Qualifier Character 6	Qualifier Character 7
1 Coronary Arteries, Multiple 3 Coronary Artery Bypass Grafts, Multiple 6 Heart, Right and Left	Y Other Contrast	Ø Unenhanced and Enhanced Z None	Z None
1 Coronary Arteries, Multiple 3 Coronary Artery Bypass Grafts, Multiple 6 Heart, Right and Left	Z None	Z None	Z None

B   **Imaging**
2   **Heart**
4   **Ultrasonography**   Real time display of images of anatomy or flow information developed from the capture of relected and attenuated high frequency sound waves

Body Part Character 4	Contrast Character 5	Qualifier Character 6	Qualifier Character 7
Ø Coronary Artery, Single 1 Coronary Arteries, Multiple 4 Heart, Right 5 Heart, Left 6 Heart, Right and Left B Heart with Aorta C Pericardium D Pediatric Heart	Y Other Contrast	Z None	Z None
Ø Coronary Artery, Single 1 Coronary Arteries, Multiple 4 Heart, Right 5 Heart, Left 6 Heart, Right and Left B Heart with Aorta C Pericardium D Pediatric Heart	Z None	Z None	3 Intravascular 4 **Transesophageal** Z None

B   **Imaging**
3   **Upper Arteries**
Ø   **Plain Radiography**   Planar display of an image developed from the capture of external ionizing radiation on photographic or photoconductive plate

Body Part Character 4	Contrast Character 5	Qualifier Character 6	Qualifier Character 7
Ø Thoracic Aorta 1 Brachiocephalic-Subclavian Artery, Right 2 Subclavian Artery, Left 3 Common Carotid Artery, Right 4 Common Carotid Artery, Left 5 Common Carotid Arteries, Bilateral 6 Internal Carotid Artery, Right 7 Internal Carotid Artery, Left 8 Internal Carotid Arteries, Bilateral 9 External Carotid Artery, Right B External Carotid Artery, Left C External Carotid Arteries, Bilateral D Vertebral Artery, Right F Vertebral Artery, Left G Vertebral Arteries, Bilateral H Upper Extremity Arteries, Right J Upper Extremity Arteries, Left K Upper Extremity Arteries, Bilateral L Intercostal and Bronchial Arteries M Spinal Arteries N Upper Arteries, Other P Thoraco-Abdominal Aorta Q Cervico-Cerebral Arch R Intracranial Arteries S Pulmonary Artery, Right T Pulmonary Artery, Left	Ø High Osmolar 1 Low Osmolar Y Other Contrast Z None	Z None	Z None

B　Imaging
3　Upper Arteries
1　Fluoroscopy　　Fluoroscopy: Single plane or bi-plane real time display of an image developed from the capture of external ionizing radiation on a fluorescent screen. The image may also be stored by either digital or analog means

Body Part Character 4	Contrast Character 5	Qualifier Character 6	Qualifier Character 7
0 Thoracic Aorta 1 Brachiocephalic-Subclavian Artery, Right 2 Subclavian Artery, Left 3 Common Carotid Artery, Right 4 Common Carotid Artery, Left 5 Common Carotid Arteries, Bilateral 6 Internal Carotid Artery, Right 7 Internal Carotid Artery, Left 8 Internal Carotid Arteries, Bilateral 9 External Carotid Artery, Right B External Carotid Artery, Left C External Carotid Arteries, Bilateral D Vertebral Artery, Right F Vertebral Artery, Left G Vertebral Arteries, Bilateral H Upper Extremity Arteries, Right J Upper Extremity Arteries, Left K Upper Extremity Arteries, Bilateral L Intercostal and Bronchial Arteries M Spinal Arteries N Upper Arteries, Other P Thoraco-Abdominal Aorta Q Cervico-Cerebral Arch R Intracranial Arteries S Pulmonary Artery, Right T Pulmonary Artery, Left	0 High Osmolar 1 Low Osmolar Y Other Contrast	1 Laser	0 Intraoperative
0 Thoracic Aorta 1 Brachiocephalic-Subclavian Artery, Right 2 Subclavian Artery, Left 3 Common Carotid Artery, Right 4 Common Carotid Artery, Left 5 Common Carotid Arteries, Bilateral 6 Internal Carotid Artery, Right 7 Internal Carotid Artery, Left 8 Internal Carotid Arteries, Bilateral 9 External Carotid Artery, Right B External Carotid Artery, Left C External Carotid Arteries, Bilateral D Vertebral Artery, Right F Vertebral Artery, Left G Vertebral Arteries, Bilateral H Upper Extremity Arteries, Right J Upper Extremity Arteries, Left K Upper Extremity Arteries, Bilateral L Intercostal and Bronchial Arteries M Spinal Arteries N Upper Arteries, Other P Thoraco-Abdominal Aorta Q Cervico-Cerebral Arch R Intracranial Arteries S Pulmonary Artery, Right T Pulmonary Artery, Left	0 High Osmolar 1 Low Osmolar Y Other Contrast	Z None	Z None

B31 Continued on next page

Imaging

B   **Imaging**
3   **Upper Arteries**
1   **Fluoroscopy**   Fluoroscopy: Single plane or bi-plane real time display of an image developed from the capture of external ionizing radiation on a fluorescent screen. The image may also be stored by either digital or analog means

Body Part Character 4	Contrast Character 5	Qualifier Character 6	Qualifier Character 7
Ø Thoracic Aorta **1** Brachiocephalic-Subclavian Artery, Right **2** Subclavian Artery, Left **3** Common Carotid Artery, Right **4** Common Carotid Artery, Left **5** Common Carotid Arteries, Bilateral **6** Internal Carotid Artery, Right **7** Internal Carotid Artery, Left **8** Internal Carotid Arteries, Bilateral **9** External Carotid Artery, Right **B** External Carotid Artery, Left **C** External Carotid Arteries, Bilateral **D** Vertebral Artery, Right **F** Vertebral Artery, Left **G** Vertebral Arteries, Bilateral **H** Upper Extremity Arteries, Right **J** Upper Extremity Arteries, Left **K** Upper Extremity Arteries, Bilateral **L** Intercostal and Bronchial Arteries **M** Spinal Arteries **N** Upper Arteries, Other **P** Thoraco-Abdominal Aorta **Q** Cervico-Cerebral Arch **R** Intracranial Arteries **S** Pulmonary Artery, Right **T** Pulmonary Artery, Left	**Z** None	**Z** None	**Z** None

B   **Imaging**
3   **Upper Arteries**
2   **Computerized Tomography (CT Scan)**   Computer reformatted digital display of multiplanar images developed from the capture of multiple exposures of external ionizing radiation

Body Part Character 4	Contrast Character 5	Qualifier Character 6	Qualifier Character 7
Ø Thoracic Aorta **5** Common Carotid Arteries, Bilateral **8** Internal Carotid Arteries, Bilateral **G** Vertebral Arteries, Bilateral **R** Intracranial Arteries **S** Pulmonary Artery, Right **T** Pulmonary Artery, Left	**Ø** High Osmolar **1** Low Osmolar **Y** Other Contrast	**Z** None	**Z** None
Ø Thoracic Aorta **5** Common Carotid Arteries, Bilateral **8** Internal Carotid Arteries, Bilateral **G** Vertebral Arteries, Bilateral **R** Intracranial Arteries **S** Pulmonary Artery, Right **T** Pulmonary Artery, Left	**Z** None	**2** Intravascular Optical Coherence **Z** None	**Z** None

     Revised Text in **BLUE**

B　Imaging
3　Upper Arteries
3　Magnetic Resonance Imaging (MRI)　Computer reformatted digital display of multiplanar images developed from the capture of radio-frequency signals emitted by nuclei in a body site excited within a magnetic field

Body Part Character 4	Contrast Character 5	Qualifier Character 6	Qualifier Character 7
Ø Thoracic Aorta 5 Common Carotid Arteries, Bilateral 8 Internal Carotid Arteries, Bilateral G Vertebral Arteries, Bilateral H Upper Extremity Arteries, Right J Upper Extremity Arteries, Left K Upper Extremity Arteries, Bilateral M Spinal Arteries Q Cervico-Cerebral Arch R Intracranial Arteries	Y Other Contrast	Ø Unenhanced and Enhanced Z None	Z None
Ø Thoracic Aorta 5 Common Carotid Arteries, Bilateral 8 Internal Carotid Arteries, Bilateral G Vertebral Arteries, Bilateral H Upper Extremity Arteries, Right J Upper Extremity Arteries, Left K Upper Extremity Arteries, Bilateral M Spinal Arteries Q Cervico-Cerebral Arch R Intracranial Arteries	Z None	Z None	Z None

B　Imaging
3　Upper Arteries
4　Ultrasonography　Real time display of images of anatomy or flow information developed from the capture of relected and attenuated high frequency sound waves

Body Part Character 4	Contrast Character 5	Qualifier Character 6	Qualifier Character 7
Ø Thoracic Aorta 1 Brachiocephalic-Subclavian Artery, Right 2 Subclavian Artery, Left 3 Common Carotid Artery, Right 4 Common Carotid Artery, Left 5 Common Carotid Arteries, Bilateral 6 Internal Carotid Artery, Right 7 Internal Carotid Artery, Left 8 Internal Carotid Arteries, Bilateral H Upper Extremity Arteries, Right J Upper Extremity Arteries, Left K Upper Extremity Arteries, Bilateral R Intracranial Arteries S Pulmonary Artery, Right T Pulmonary Artery, Left V Ophthalmic Arteries	Z None	Z None	3 Intravascular Z None

B　Imaging
4　Lower Arteries
Ø　Plain Radiography　Planar display of an image developed from the capture of external ionizing radiation on photographic or photoconductive plate

Body Part Character 4	Contrast Character 5	Qualifier Character 6	Qualifier Character 7
Ø Abdominal Aorta 2 Hepatic Artery 3 Splenic Arteries 4 Superior Mesenteric Artery 5 Inferior Mesenteric Artery 6 Renal Artery, Right 7 Renal Artery, Left 8 Renal Arteries, Bilateral 9 Lumbar Arteries B Intra-Abdominal Arteries, Other C Pelvic Arteries D Aorta and Bilateral Lower Extremity Arteries F Lower Extremity Arteries, Right G Lower Extremity Arteries, Left J Lower Arteries, Other M Renal Artery Transplant	Ø High Osmolar 1 Low Osmolar Y Other Contrast	Z None	Z None

B   **Imaging**
4   **Lower Arteries**
1   **Fluoroscopy**   Single plane or bi-plane real time display of an image developed from the capture of external ionizing radiation on a fluorescent screen. The image may also be stored by either digital or analog means

Body Part Character 4	Contrast Character 5	Qualifier Character 6	Qualifier Character 7
Ø Abdominal Aorta **2** Hepatic Artery **3** Splenic Arteries **4** Superior Mesenteric Artery **5** Inferior Mesenteric Artery **6** Renal Artery, Right **7** Renal Artery, Left **8** Renal Arteries, Bilateral **9** Lumbar Arteries **B** Intra-Abdominal Arteries, Other **C** Pelvic Arteries **D** Aorta and Bilateral Lower Extremity Arteries **F** Lower Extremity Arteries, Right **G** Lower Extremity Arteries, Left **J** Lower Arteries, Other	**Ø** High Osmolar **1** Low Osmolar **Y** Other Contrast	**1** Laser	**Ø** Intraoperative
Ø Abdominal Aorta **2** Hepatic Artery **3** Splenic Arteries **4** Superior Mesenteric Artery **5** Inferior Mesenteric Artery **6** Renal Artery, Right **7** Renal Artery, Left **8** Renal Arteries, Bilateral **9** Lumbar Arteries **B** Intra-Abdominal Arteries, Other **C** Pelvic Arteries **D** Aorta and Bilateral Lower Extremity Arteries **F** Lower Extremity Arteries, Right **G** Lower Extremity Arteries, Left **J** Lower Arteries, Other	**Ø** High Osmolar **1** Low Osmolar **Y** Other Contrast	**Z** None	**Z** None
Ø Abdominal Aorta **2** Hepatic Artery **3** Splenic Arteries **4** Superior Mesenteric Artery **5** Inferior Mesenteric Artery **6** Renal Artery, Right **7** Renal Artery, Left **8** Renal Arteries, Bilateral **9** Lumbar Arteries **B** Intra-Abdominal Arteries, Other **C** Pelvic Arteries **D** Aorta and Bilateral Lower Extremity Arteries **F** Lower Extremity Arteries, Right **G** Lower Extremity Arteries, Left **J** Lower Arteries, Other	**Z** None	**Z** None	**Z** None

B   **Imaging**
4   **Lower Arteries**
2   **Computerized Tomography (CT Scan)**   Computer reformatted digital display of multiplanar images developed from the capture of multiple exposures of external ionizing radiation

Body Part Character 4	Contrast Character 5	Qualifier Character 6	Qualifier Character 7
Ø Abdominal Aorta **1** Celiac Artery **4** Superior Mesenteric Artery **8** Renal Arteries, Bilateral **C** Pelvic Arteries **F** Lower Extremity Arteries, Right **G** Lower Extremity Arteries, Left **H** Lower Extremity Arteries, Bilateral **M** Renal Artery Transplant	**Ø** High Osmolar **1** Low Osmolar **Y** Other Contrast	**Z** None	**Z** None
Ø Abdominal Aorta **1** Celiac Artery **4** Superior Mesenteric Artery **8** Renal Arteries, Bilateral **C** Pelvic Arteries **F** Lower Extremity Arteries, Right **G** Lower Extremity Arteries, Left **H** Lower Extremity Arteries, Bilateral **M** Renal Artery Transplant	**Z** None	**2** Intravascular Optical Coherence **Z** None	**Z** None

B　Imaging
4　Lower Arteries
3　Magnetic Resonance Imaging (MRI)　Computer reformatted digital display of multiplanar images developed from the capture of radio-frequency signals emitted by nuclei in a body site excited within a magnetic field

Body Part Character 4	Contrast Character 5	Qualifier Character 6	Qualifier Character 7
0 Abdominal Aorta 1 Celiac Artery 4 Superior Mesenteric Artery 8 Renal Arteries, Bilateral C Pelvic Arteries F Lower Extremity Arteries, Right G Lower Extremity Arteries, Left H Lower Extremity Arteries, Bilateral	Y Other Contrast	0 Unenhanced and Enhanced Z None	Z None
0 Abdominal Aorta 1 Celiac Artery 4 Superior Mesenteric Artery 8 Renal Arteries, Bilateral C Pelvic Arteries F Lower Extremity Arteries, Right G Lower Extremity Arteries, Left H Lower Extremity Arteries, Bilateral	Z None	Z None	Z None

B　Imaging
4　Lower Arteries
4　Ultrasonography　Real time display of images of anatomy or flow information developed from the capture of relected and attenuated high frequency sound waves

Body Part Character 4	Contrast Character 5	Qualifier Character 6	Qualifier Character 7
0 Abdominal Aorta 4 Superior Mesenteric Artery 5 Inferior Mesenteric Artery 6 Renal Artery, Right 7 Renal Artery, Left 8 Renal Arteries, Bilateral B Intra-Abdominal Arteries, Other F Lower Extremity Arteries, Right G Lower Extremity Arteries, Left H Lower Extremity Arteries, Bilateral K Celiac and Mesenteric Arteries L Femoral Artery N Penile Arteries	Z None	Z None	3 Intravascular Z None

B　Imaging
5　Veins
0　Plain Radiography　Planar display of an image developed from the capture of external ionizing radiation on photographic or photoconductive plate

Body Part Character 4	Contrast Character 5	Qualifier Character 6	Qualifier Character 7
0 Epidural Veins 1 Cerebral and Cerebellar Veins 2 Intracranial Sinuses 3 Jugular Veins, Right 4 Jugular Veins, Left 5 Jugular Veins, Bilateral 6 Subclavian Vein, Right 7 Subclavian Vein, Left 8 Superior Vena Cava 9 Inferior Vena Cava B Lower Extremity Veins, Right C Lower Extremity Veins, Left D Lower Extremity Veins, Bilateral F Pelvic (Iliac) Veins, Right G Pelvic (Iliac) Veins, Left H Pelvic (Iliac) Veins, Bilateral J Renal Vein, Right K Renal Vein, Left L Renal Veins, Bilateral M Upper Extremity Veins, Right N Upper Extremity Veins, Left P Upper Extremity Veins, Bilateral Q Pulmonary Vein, Right R Pulmonary Vein, Left S Pulmonary Veins, Bilateral T Portal and Splanchnic Veins V Veins, Other W Dialysis Shunt/Fistula	0 High Osmolar 1 Low Osmolar Y Other Contrast	Z None	Z None

Imaging

B51–B52

B Imaging
5 Veins
1 Fluoroscopy Single plane or bi-plane real time display of an image developed from the capture of external ionizing radioation on a fluorescent screen. The image may also be stored by either digital or analog means

Body Part Character 4	Contrast Character 5	Qualifier Character 6	Qualifier Character 7
0 Epidural Veins	0 High Osmolar	Z None	A Guidance
1 Cerebral and Cerebellar Veins	1 Low Osmolar		Z None
2 Intracranial Sinuses	Y Other Contrast		
3 Jugular Veins, Right	Z None		
4 Jugular Veins, Left			
5 Jugular Veins, Bilateral			
6 Subclavian Vein, Right			
7 Subclavian Vein, Left			
8 Superior Vena Cava			
9 Inferior Vena Cava			
B Lower Extremity Veins, Right			
C Lower Extremity Veins, Left			
D Lower Extremity Veins, Bilateral			
F Pelvic (Iliac) Veins, Right			
G Pelvic (Iliac) Veins, Left			
H Pelvic (Iliac) Veins, Bilateral			
J Renal Vein, Right			
K Renal Vein, Left			
L Renal Veins, Bilateral			
M Upper Extremity Veins, Right			
N Upper Extremity Veins, Left			
P Upper Extremity Veins, Bilateral			
Q Pulmonary Vein, Right			
R Pulmonary Vein, Left			
S Pulmonary Veins, Bilateral			
T Portal and Splanchnic Veins			
V Veins, Other			
W Dialysis Shunt/Fistula			

B Imaging
5 Veins
2 Computerized Tomography (CT Scan) Computer reformatted digital display of multiplanar images developed from the capture of multiple exposures of external ionizing radiation

Body Part Character 4	Contrast Character 5	Qualifier Character 6	Qualifier Character 7
2 Intracranial Sinuses	0 High Osmolar	0 Unenhanced and Enhanced	Z None
8 Superior Vena Cava	1 Low Osmolar	Z None	
9 Inferior Vena Cava	Y Other Contrast		
F Pelvic (Iliac) Veins, Right			
G Pelvic (Iliac) Veins, Left			
H Pelvic (Iliac) Veins, Bilateral			
J Renal Vein, Right			
K Renal Vein, Left			
L Renal Veins, Bilateral			
Q Pulmonary Vein, Right			
R Pulmonary Vein, Left			
S Pulmonary Veins, Bilateral			
T Portal and Splanchnic Veins			
2 Intracranial Sinuses	Z None	2 Intravascular Optical Coherence	Z None
8 Superior Vena Cava		Z None	
9 Inferior Vena Cava			
F Pelvic (Iliac) Veins, Right			
G Pelvic (Iliac) Veins, Left			
H Pelvic (Iliac) Veins, Bilateral			
J Renal Vein, Right			
K Renal Vein, Left			
L Renal Veins, Bilateral			
Q Pulmonary Vein, Right			
R Pulmonary Vein, Left			
S Pulmonary Veins, Bilateral			
T Portal and Splanchnic Veins			

B   Imaging
5   Veins
3   Magnetic Resonance Imaging (MRI)   Computer reformatted digital display of multiplanar images developed from the capture of radio-frequency signals emitted by nuclei in a body site excited within a magnetic field

Body Part Character 4	Contrast Character 5	Qualifier Character 6	Qualifier Character 7
1 Cerebral and Cerebellar Veins 2 Intracranial Sinuses 5 Jugular Veins, Bilateral 8 Superior Vena Cava 9 Inferior Vena Cava B Lower Extremity Veins, Right C Lower Extremity Veins, Left D Lower Extremity Veins, Bilateral H Pelvic (Iliac) Veins, Bilateral L Renal Veins, Bilateral M Upper Extremity Veins, Right N Upper Extremity Veins, Left P Upper Extremity Veins, Bilateral S Pulmonary Veins, Bilateral T Portal and Splanchnic Veins V Veins, Other	Y Other Contrast	Ø Unenhanced and Enhanced Z None	Z None
1 Cerebral and Cerebellar Veins 2 Intracranial Sinuses 5 Jugular Veins, Bilateral 8 Superior Vena Cava 9 Inferior Vena Cava B Lower Extremity Veins, Right C Lower Extremity Veins, Left D Lower Extremity Veins, Bilateral H Pelvic (Iliac) Veins, Bilateral L Renal Veins, Bilateral M Upper Extremity Veins, Right N Upper Extremity Veins, Left P Upper Extremity Veins, Bilateral S Pulmonary Veins, Bilateral T Portal and Splanchnic Veins V Veins, Other	Z None	Z None	Z None

B   Imaging
5   Veins
4   Ultrasonography   Real time display of images of anatomy or flow information developed from the capture of relected and attenuated high frequency sound waves

Body Part Character 4	Contrast Character 5	Qualifier Character 6	Qualifier Character 7
3 Jugular Veins, Right 4 Jugular Veins, Left 6 Subclavian Vein, Right 7 Subclavian Vein, Left 9 Inferior Vena Cava B Lower Extremity Veins, Right C Lower Extremity Veins, Left D Lower Extremity Veins, Bilateral J Renal Vein, Right K Renal Vein, Left L Renal Veins, Bilateral M Upper Extremity Veins, Right N Upper Extremity Veins, Left P Upper Extremity Veins, Bilateral T Portal and Splanchnic Veins	Z None	Z None	3 Intravascular A **Guidance** Z None

B **Imaging**
7 **Lymphatic System**
Ø **Plain Radiography**   Planar display of an image developed from the capture of external ionizing radiation on photographic or photoconductive plate

Body Part Character 4	Contrast Character 5	Qualifier Character 6	Qualifier Character 7
Ø Abdominal/Retroperitoneal 　Lymphatics, Unilateral 1 Abdominal/Retroperitoneal 　Lymphatics, Bilateral 4 Lymphatics, Head and Neck 5 Upper Extremity Lymphatics, Right 6 Upper Extremity Lymphatics, Left 7 Upper Extremity Lymphatics, 　Bilateral 8 Lower Extremity Lymphatics, Right 9 Lower Extremity Lymphatics, Left B Lower Extremity Lymphatics, 　Bilateral C Lymphatics, Pelvic	Ø High Osmolar 1 Low Osmolar Y Other Contrast	Z None	Z None

B **Imaging**
8 **Eye**
Ø **Plain Radiography**   Planar display of an image developed from the capture of external ionizing radiation on photographic or photoconductive plate

Body Part Character 4	Contrast Character 5	Qualifier Character 6	Qualifier Character 7
Ø Lacrimal Duct, Right 1 Lacrimal Duct, Left 2 Lacrimal Ducts, Bilateral	Ø High Osmolar 1 Low Osmolar Y Other Contrast	Z None	Z None
3 Optic Foramina, Right 4 Optic Foramina, Left 5 Eye, Right 6 Eye, Left 7 Eyes, Bilateral	Z None	Z None	Z None

B **Imaging**
8 **Eye**
2 **Computerized Tomography (CT Scan)**   Computer reformatted digital display of multiplanar images developed from the capture of multiple exposures of external ionizing radiation

Body Part Character 4	Contrast Character 5	Qualifier Character 6	Qualifier Character 7
5 Eye, Right 6 Eye, Left 7 Eyes, Bilateral	Ø High Osmolar 1 Low Osmolar Y Other Contrast	Ø Unenhanced and Enhanced Z None	Z None
5 Eye, Right 6 Eye, Left 7 Eyes, Bilateral	Z None	Z None	Z None

B **Imaging**
8 **Eye**
3 **Magnetic Resonance Imaging (MRI)**   Computer reformatted digital display of multiplanar images developed from the capture of radio-frequency signals emitted by nuclei in a body site excited within a magnetic field

Body Part Character 4	Contrast Character 5	Qualifier Character 6	Qualifier Character 7
5 Eye, Right 6 Eye, Left 7 Eyes, Bilateral	Y Other Contrast	Ø Unenhanced and Enhanced Z None	Z None
5 Eye, Right 6 Eye, Left 7 Eyes, Bilateral	Z None	Z None	Z None

B **Imaging**
8 **Eye**
4 **Ultrasonography**   Real time display of images of anatomy or flow information developed from the capture of relected and attenuated high frequency sound waves

Body Part Character 4	Contrast Character 5	Qualifier Character 6	Qualifier Character 7
5 Eye, Right 6 Eye, Left 7 Eyes, Bilateral	Z None	Z None	Z None

Revised Text in **BLUE**

B Imaging
9 Ear, Nose, Mouth and Throat
0 Plain Radiography   Planar display of an image developed from the capture of external ionizing radiation on photographic or photoconductive plate

Body Part Character 4	Contrast Character 5	Qualifier Character 6	Qualifier Character 7
2 Paranasal Sinuses F Nasopharynx/Oropharynx H Mastoids	Z None	Z None	Z None
4 Parotid Gland, Right 5 Parotid Gland, Left 6 Parotid Glands, Bilateral 7 Submandibular Gland, Right 8 Submandibular Gland, Left 9 Submandibular Glands, Bilateral B Salivary Gland, Right C Salivary Gland, Left D Salivary Glands, Bilateral	0 High Osmolar 1 Low Osmolar Y Other Contrast	Z None	Z None

B Imaging
9 Ear, Nose, Mouth and Throat
1 Fluoroscopy   Single plane or bi-plane real time display of an image developed from the capture of external ionizing radioation on a fluorescent screen. The image may also be stored by either digital or analog means

Body Part Character 4	Contrast Character 5	Qualifier Character 6	Qualifier Character 7
G Pharynx and Epiglottis J Larynx	Y Other Contrast Z None	Z None	Z None

B Imaging
9 Ear, Nose, Mouth and Throat
2 Computerized Tomography (CT Scan)   Computer reformatted digital display of multiplanar images developed from the capture of multiple exposures of external ionizing radiation

Body Part Character 4	Contrast Character 5	Qualifier Character 6	Qualifier Character 7
0 Ear 2 Paranasal Sinuses 6 Parotid Glands, Bilateral 9 Submandibular Glands, Bilateral D Salivary Glands, Bilateral F Nasopharynx/Oropharynx J Larynx	0 High Osmolar 1 Low Osmolar Y Other Contrast	0 Unenhanced and Enhanced Z None	Z None
0 Ear 2 Paranasal Sinuses 6 Parotid Glands, Bilateral 9 Submandibular Glands, Bilateral D Salivary Glands, Bilateral F Nasopharynx/Oropharynx J Larynx	Z None	Z None	Z None

B Imaging
9 Ear, Nose, Mouth and Throat
3 Magnetic Resonance Imaging (MRI)   Computer reformatted digital display of multiplanar images developed from the capture of radio-frequency signals emitted by nuclei in a body site excited within a magnetic field

Body Part Character 4	Contrast Character 5	Qualifier Character 6	Qualifier Character 7
0 Ear 2 Paranasal Sinuses 6 Parotid Glands, Bilateral 9 Submandibular Glands, Bilateral D Salivary Glands, Bilateral F Nasopharynx/Oropharynx J Larynx	Y Other Contrast	0 Unenhanced and Enhanced Z None	Z None
0 Ear 2 Paranasal Sinuses 6 Parotid Glands, Bilateral 9 Submandibular Glands, Bilateral D Salivary Glands, Bilateral F Nasopharynx/Oropharynx J Larynx	Z None	Z None	Z None

B Imaging
B Respiratory System
0 Plain Radiography — Planar display of an image developed from the capture of external ionizing radiation on photographic or photoconductive plate

Body Part Character 4	Contrast Character 5	Qualifier Character 6	Qualifier Character 7
7 Tracheobronchial Tree, Right 8 Tracheobronchial Tree, Left 9 Tracheobronchial Trees, Bilateral	Y Other Contrast	Z None	Z None
D Upper Airways	Z None	Z None	Z None

B Imaging
B Respiratory System
1 Fluoroscopy — Single plane or bi-plane real time display of an image developed from the capture of external ionizing radioation on a fluorescent screen. The image may also be stored by either digital or analog means

Body Part Character 4	Contrast Character 5	Qualifier Character 6	Qualifier Character 7
2 Lung, Right 3 Lung, Left 4 Lungs, Bilateral 6 Diaphragm C Mediastinum D Upper Airways	Z None	Z None	Z None
7 Tracheobronchial Tree, Right 8 Tracheobronchial Tree, Left 9 Tracheobronchial Trees, Bilateral	Y Other Contrast	Z None	Z None

B Imaging
B Respiratory System
2 Computerized Tomography (CT Scan) — Computer reformatted digital display of multiplanar images developed from the capture of multiple exposures of external ionizing radiation

Body Part Character 4	Contrast Character 5	Qualifier Character 6	Qualifier Character 7
4 Lungs, Bilateral 7 Tracheobronchial Tree, Right 8 Tracheobronchial Tree, Left 9 Tracheobronchial Trees, Bilateral F Trachea/Airways	0 High Osmolar 1 Low Osmolar Y Other Contrast	0 Unenhanced and Enhanced Z None	Z None
4 Lungs, Bilateral 7 Tracheobronchial Tree, Right 8 Tracheobronchial Tree, Left 9 Tracheobronchial Trees, Bilateral F Trachea/Airways	Z None	Z None	Z None

B Imaging
B Respiratory System
3 Magnetic Resonance Imaging (MRI) — Computer reformatted digital display of multiplanar images developed from the capture of radio-frequency signals emitted by nuclei in a body site excited within a magnetic field

Body Part Character 4	Contrast Character 5	Qualifier Character 6	Qualifier Character 7
G Lung Apices	Y Other Contrast	0 Unenhanced and Enhanced Z None	Z None
G Lung Apices	Z None	Z None	Z None

B Imaging
B Respiratory System
4 Ultrasonography — Real time display of images of anatomy or flow information developed from the capture of relected and attenuated high frequency sound waves

Body Part Character 4	Contrast Character 5	Qualifier Character 6	Qualifier Character 7
B Pleura C Mediastinum	Z None	Z None	Z None

 © 2011 Ingenix, Inc

B   **Imaging**
D   **Gastrointestinal System**
1   **Fluoroscopy**   Single plane or bi-plane real time display of an image developed from the capture of external ionizing radioation on a fluorescent screen. The image may also be stored by either digital or analog means

Body Part Character 4	Contrast Character 5	Qualifier Character 6	Qualifier Character 7
1 Esophagus **2** Stomach **3** Small Bowel **4** Colon **5** Upper GI **6** Upper GI and Small Bowel **9** Duodenum **B** Mouth/Oropharynx	**Y** Other Contrast **Z** None	**Z** None	**Z** None

B   **Imaging**
D   **Gastrointestinal System**
2   **Computerized Tomography (CT Scan)**   Computer reformatted digital display of multiplanar images developed from the capture of multiple exposures of external ionizing radiation

Body Part Character 4	Contrast Character 5	Qualifier Character 6	Qualifier Character 7
4 Colon	**Ø** High Osmolar **1** Low Osmolar **Y** Other Contrast	**Ø** Unenhanced and Enhanced **Z** None	**Z** None
4 Colon	**Z** None	**Z** None	**Z** None

B   **Imaging**
D   **Gastrointestinal System**
4   **Ultrasonography**   Real time display of images of anatomy or flow information developed from the capture of relected and attenuated high frequency sound waves

Body Part Character 4	Contrast Character 5	Qualifier Character 6	Qualifier Character 7
1 Esophagus **2** Stomach **7** Gastrointestinal Tract **8** Appendix **9** Duodenum **C** Rectum	**Z** None	**Z** None	**Z** None

B   **Imaging**
F   **Hepatobiliary System and Pancreas**
Ø   **Plain Radiography**   Planar display of an image developed from the capture of external ionizing radiation on photographic or photoconductive plate

Body Part Character 4	Contrast Character 5	Qualifier Character 6	Qualifier Character 7
Ø Bile Ducts **3** Gallbladder and Bile Ducts **C** Hepatobiliary System, All	**Ø** High Osmolar **1** Low Osmolar **Y** Other Contrast	**Z** None	**Z** None

B   **Imaging**
F   **Hepatobiliary System and Pancreas**
1   **Fluoroscopy**   Single plane or bi-plane real time display of an image developed from the capture of external ionizing radioation on a fluorescent screen. The image may also be stored by either digital or analog means

Body Part Character 4	Contrast Character 5	Qualifier Character 6	Qualifier Character 7
Ø Bile Ducts **1** Biliary and Pancreatic Ducts **2** Gallbladder **3** Gallbladder and Bile Ducts **4** Gallbladder, Bile Ducts and Pancreatic Ducts **8** Pancreatic Ducts	**Ø** High Osmolar **1** Low Osmolar **Y** Other Contrast	**Z** None	**Z** None

B   **Imaging**
F   **Hepatobiliary System and Pancreas**
2   **Computerized Tomography (CT Scan)** Computer reformatted digital display of multiplanar images developed from the capture of multiple exposures of external ionizing radiation

Body Part Character 4	Contrast Character 5	Qualifier Character 6	Qualifier Character 7
5 Liver **6** Liver and Spleen **7** Pancreas **C** Hepatobiliary System, All	**Ø** High Osmolar **1** Low Osmolar **Y** Other Contrast	**Ø** Unenhanced and Enhanced **Z** None	**Z** None
5 Liver **6** Liver and Spleen **7** Pancreas **C** Hepatobiliary System, All	**Z** None	**Z** None	**Z** None

B   **Imaging**
F   **Hepatobiliary System and Pancreas**
3   **Magnetic Resonance Imaging (MRI)** Computer reformatted digital display of multiplanar images developed from the capture of radio-frequency signals emitted by nuclei in a body site excited within a magnetic field

Body Part Character 4	Contrast Character 5	Qualifier Character 6	Qualifier Character 7
5 Liver **6** Liver and Spleen **7** Pancreas	**Y** Other Contrast	**Ø** Unenhanced and Enhanced **Z** None	**Z** None
5 Liver **6** Liver and Spleen **7** Pancreas	**Z** None	**Z** None	**Z** None

B   **Imaging**
F   **Hepatobiliary System and Pancreas**
4   **Ultrasonography** Real time display of images of anatomy or flow information developed from the capture of relected and attenuated high frequency sound waves

Body Part Character 4	Contrast Character 5	Qualifier Character 6	Qualifier Character 7
Ø Bile Ducts **2** Gallbladder **3** Gallbladder and Bile Ducts **5** Liver **6** Liver and Spleen **7** Pancreas **C** Hepatobiliary System, All	**Z** None	**Z** None	**Z** None

B   **Imaging**
G   **Endocrine System**
2   **Computerized Tomography (CT Scan)** Computer reformatted digital display of multiplanar images developed from the capture of multiple exposures of external ionizing radiation

Body Part Character 4	Contrast Character 5	Qualifier Character 6	Qualifier Character 7
2 Adrenal Glands, Bilateral **3** Parathyroid Glands **4** Thyroid Gland	**Ø** High Osmolar **1** Low Osmolar **Y** Other Contrast	**Ø** Unenhanced and Enhanced **Z** None	**Z** None
2 Adrenal Glands, Bilateral **3** Parathyroid Glands **4** Thyroid Gland	**Z** None	**Z** None	**Z** None

B   **Imaging**
G   **Endocrine System**
3   **Magnetic Resonance Imaging (MRI)** Computer reformatted digital display of multiplanar images developed from the capture of radio-frequency signals emitted by nuclei in a body site excited within a magnetic field

Body Part Character 4	Contrast Character 5	Qualifier Character 6	Qualifier Character 7
2 Adrenal Glands, Bilateral **3** Parathyroid Glands **4** Thyroid Gland	**Y** Other Contrast	**Ø** Unenhanced and Enhanced **Z** None	**Z** None
2 Adrenal Glands, Bilateral **3** Parathyroid Glands **4** Thyroid Gland	**Z** None	**Z** None	**Z** None

                       Revised Text in **BLUE**

B   **Imaging**
G   **Endocrine System**
4   **Ultrasonography**   Real time display of images of anatomy or flow information developed from the capture of relected and attenuated high frequency sound waves

Body Part Character 4	Contrast Character 5	Qualifier Character 6	Qualifier Character 7
Ø Adrenal Gland, Right **1** Adrenal Gland, Left **2** Adrenal Glands, Bilateral **3** Parathyroid Glands **4** Thyroid Gland	**Z** None	**Z** None	**Z** None

B   **Imaging**
H   **Skin, Subcutaneous Tissue and Breast**
Ø   **Plain Radiography**   Planar display of an image developed from the capture of external ionizing radiation on photographic or photoconductive plate

Body Part Character 4	Contrast Character 5	Qualifier Character 6	Qualifier Character 7
Ø Breast, Right **1** Breast, Left **2** Breasts, Bilateral	**Z** None	**Z** None	**Z** None
3 Single Mammary Duct, Right **4** Single Mammary Duct, Left **5** Multiple Mammary Ducts, Right **6** Multiple Mammary Ducts, Left	**Ø** High Osmolar **1** Low Osmolar **Y** Other Contrast **Z** None	**Z** None	**Z** None

B   **Imaging**
H   **Skin, Subcutaneous Tissue and Breast**
3   **Magnetic Resonance Imaging (MRI)**   Computer reformatted digital display of multiplanar images developed from the capture of radio-frequency signals emitted by nuclei in a body site excited within a magnetic field

Body Part Character 4	Contrast Character 5	Qualifier Character 6	Qualifier Character 7
Ø Breast, Right **1** Breast, Left **2** Breasts, Bilateral **D** Subcutaneous Tissue, Head/Neck **F** Subcutaneous Tissue, Upper Extremity **G** Subcutaneous Tissue, Thorax **H** Subcutaneous Tissue, Abdomen and Pelvis **J** Subcutaneous Tissue, Lower Extremity	**Y** Other Contrast	**Ø** Unenhanced and Enhanced **Z** None	**Z** None
Ø Breast, Right **1** Breast, Left **2** Breasts, Bilateral **D** Subcutaneous Tissue, Head/Neck **F** Subcutaneous Tissue, Upper Extremity **G** Subcutaneous Tissue, Thorax **H** Subcutaneous Tissue, Abdomen and Pelvis **J** Subcutaneous Tissue, Lower Extremity	**Z** None	**Z** None	**Z** None

B   **Imaging**
H   **Skin, Subcutaneous Tissue and Breast**
4   **Ultrasonography**   Real time display of images of anatomy or flow information developed from the capture of relected and attenuated high frequency sound waves

Body Part Character 4	Contrast Character 5	Qualifier Character 6	Qualifier Character 7
Ø Breast, Right **1** Breast, Left **2** Breasts, Bilateral **7** Extremity, Upper **8** Extremity, Lower **9** Abdominal Wall **B** Chest Wall **C** Head and Neck	**Z** None	**Z** None	**Z** None

Revised Text in **BLUE**

B   **Imaging**
L   **Connective Tissue**
3   **Magnetic Resonance Imaging (MRI)**   Computer reformatted digital display of multiplanar images developed from the capture of radio-frequency signals emitted by nuclei in a body site excited within a magnetic field

Body Part Character 4	Contrast Character 5	Qualifier Character 6	Qualifier Character 7
Ø Connective Tissue, Upper Extremity **1** Connective Tissue, Lower Extremity **2** Tendons, Upper Extremity **3** Tendons, Lower Extremity	**Y** Other Contrast	**Ø** Unenhanced and Enhanced **Z** None	**Z** None
Ø Connective Tissue, Upper Extremity **1** Connective Tissue, Lower Extremity **2** Tendons, Upper Extremity **3** Tendons, Lower Extremity	**Z** None	**Z** None	**Z** None

B   **Imaging**
L   **Connective Tissue**
4   **Ultrasonography**   Real time display of images of anatomy or flow information developed from the capture of relected and attenuated high frequency sound waves

Body Part Character 4	Contrast Character 5	Qualifier Character 6	Qualifier Character 7
Ø Connective Tissue, Upper Extremity **1** Connective Tissue, Lower Extremity **2** Tendons, Upper Extremity **3** Tendons, Lower Extremity	**Z** None	**Z** None	**Z** None

B   **Imaging**
N   **Skull and Facial Bones**
Ø   **Plain Radiography**   Planar display of an image developed from the capture of external ionizing radiation on photographic or photoconductive plate

Body Part Character 4	Contrast Character 5	Qualifier Character 6	Qualifier Character 7
Ø Skull **1** Orbit, Right **2** Orbit, Left **3** Orbits, Bilateral **4** Nasal Bones **5** Facial Bones **6** Mandible **B** Zygomatic Arch, Right **C** Zygomatic Arch, Left **D** Zygomatic Arches, Bilateral **G** Tooth, Single **H** Teeth, Multiple **J** Teeth, All	**Z** None	**Z** None	**Z** None
7 Temporomandibular Joint, Right **8** Temporomandibular Joint, Left **9** Temporomandibular Joints, Bilateral	**Ø** High Osmolar **1** Low Osmolar **Y** Other Contrast **Z** None	**Z** None	**Z** None

B   **Imaging**
N   **Skull and Facial Bones**
1   **Fluoroscopy**   Single plane or bi-plane real time display of an image developed from the capture of external ionizing radioation on a fluorescent screen. The image may also be stored by either digital or analog means

Body Part Character 4	Contrast Character 5	Qualifier Character 6	Qualifier Character 7
7 Temporomandibular Joint, Right **8** Temporomandibular Joint, Left **9** Temporomandibular Joints, Bilateral	**Ø** High Osmolar **1** Low Osmolar **Y** Other Contrast **Z** None	**Z** None	**Z** None

B   **Imaging**
N   **Skull and Facial Bones**
2   **Computerized Tomography (CT Scan)**   Computer reformatted digital display of multiplanar images developed from the capture of multiple exposures of external ionizing radiation

Body Part Character 4	Contrast Character 5	Qualifier Character 6	Qualifier Character 7
Ø Skull 3 Orbits, Bilateral 5 Facial Bones 6 Mandible 9 Temporomandibular Joints, Bilateral F Temporal Bones	Ø High Osmolar 1 Low Osmolar Y Other Contrast Z None	Z None	Z None

B   **Imaging**
N   **Skull and Facial Bones**
3   **Magnetic Resonance Imaging (MRI)**   Computer reformatted digital display of multiplanar images developed from the capture of radio-frequency signals emitted by nuclei in a body site excited within a magnetic field

Body Part Character 4	Contrast Character 5	Qualifier Character 6	Qualifier Character 7
9 Temporomandibular Joints, Bilateral	Y Other Contrast Z None	Z None	Z None

B   **Imaging**
P   **Non-Axial Upper Bones**
Ø   **Plain Radiography**   Planar display of an image developed from the capture of external ionizing radiation on photographic or photoconductive plate

Body Part Character 4	Contrast Character 5	Qualifier Character 6	Qualifier Character 7
Ø Sternoclavicular Joint, Right 1 Sternoclavicular Joint, Left 2 Sternoclavicular Joints, Bilateral 3 Acromioclavicular Joints, Bilateral 4 Clavicle, Right 5 Clavicle, Left 6 Scapula, Right 7 Scapula, Left A Humerus, Right B Humerus, Left E Upper Arm, Right F Upper Arm, Left J Forearm, Right K Forearm, Left N Hand, Right P Hand, Left R Finger(s), Right S Finger(s), Left X Ribs, Right Y Ribs, Left	Z None	Z None	Z None
8 Shoulder, Right 9 Shoulder, Left C Hand/Finger Joint, Right D Hand/Finger Joint, Left G Elbow, Right H Elbow, Left L Wrist, Right M Wrist, Left	Ø High Osmolar 1 Low Osmolar Y Other Contrast Z None	Z None	Z None

Imaging

B   **Imaging**
P   **Non-Axial Upper Bones**
1   **Fluoroscopy**   Single plane or bi-plane real time display of an image developed from the capture of external ionizing radioation on a fluorescent screen. The image may also be stored by either digital or analog means

Body Part Character 4	Contrast Character 5	Qualifier Character 6	Qualifier Character 7
0 Sternoclavicular Joint, Right 1 Sternoclavicular Joint, Left 2 Sternoclavicular Joints, Bilateral 3 Acromioclavicular Joints, Bilateral 4 Clavicle, Right 5 Clavicle, Left 6 Scapula, Right 7 Scapula, Left A Humerus, Right B Humerus, Left E Upper Arm, Right F Upper Arm, Left J Forearm, Right K Forearm, Left N Hand, Right P Hand, Left R Finger(s), Right S Finger(s), Left X Ribs, Right Y Ribs, Left	Z None	Z None	Z None
8 Shoulder, Right 9 Shoulder, Left L Wrist, Right M Wrist, Left	0 High Osmolar 1 Low Osmolar Y Other Contrast Z None	Z None	Z None
C Hand/Finger Joint, Right D Hand/Finger Joint, Left G Elbow, Right H Elbow, Left	0 High Osmolar 1 Low Osmolar Y Other Contrast	Z None	Z None

B   **Imaging**
P   **Non-Axial Upper Bones**
2   **Computerized Tomography (CT Scan)**   Computer reformatted digital display of multiplanar images developed from the capture of multiple exposures of external ionizing radiation

Body Part Character 4	Contrast Character 5	Qualifier Character 6	Qualifier Character 7
0 Sternoclavicular Joint, Right 1 Sternoclavicular Joint, Left W Thorax	0 High Osmolar 1 Low Osmolar Y Other Contrast	Z None	Z None
2 Sternoclavicular Joints, Bilateral 3 Acromioclavicular Joints, Bilateral 4 Clavicle, Right 5 Clavicle, Left 6 Scapula, Right 7 Scapula, Left 8 Shoulder, Right 9 Shoulder, Left A Humerus, Right B Humerus, Left E Upper Arm, Right F Upper Arm, Left G Elbow, Right H Elbow, Left J Forearm, Right K Forearm, Left L Wrist, Right M Wrist, Left N Hand, Right P Hand, Left Q Hands and Wrists, Bilateral R Finger(s), Right S Finger(s), Left T Upper Extremity, Right U Upper Extremity, Left V Upper Extremities, Bilateral X Ribs, Right Y Ribs, Left	0 High Osmolar 1 Low Osmolar Y Other Contrast Z None	Z None	Z None
C Hand/Finger Joint, Right D Hand/Finger Joint, Left	Z None	Z None	Z None

B　Imaging
P　Non-Axial Upper Bones
3　Magnetic Resonance Imaging (MRI) Computer reformatted digital display of multiplanar images developed from the capture of radio-frequency signals emitted by nuclei in a body site excited within a magnetic field

Body Part Character 4	Contrast Character 5	Qualifier Character 6	Qualifier Character 7
8　Shoulder, Right 9　Shoulder, Left C　Hand/Finger Joint, Right D　Hand/Finger Joint, Left E　Upper Arm, Right F　Upper Arm, Left G　Elbow, Right H　Elbow, Left J　Forearm, Right K　Forearm, Left L　Wrist, Right M　Wrist, Left	Y　Other Contrast	0　Unenhanced and Enhanced Z　None	Z　None
8　Shoulder, Right 9　Shoulder, Left C　Hand/Finger Joint, Right D　Hand/Finger Joint, Left E　Upper Arm, Right F　Upper Arm, Left G　Elbow, Right H　Elbow, Left J　Forearm, Right K　Forearm, Left L　Wrist, Right M　Wrist, Left	Z　None	Z　None	Z　None

B　Imaging
P　Non-Axial Upper Bones
4　Ultrasonography Real time display of images of anatomy or flow information developed from the capture of relected and attenuated high frequency sound waves

Body Part Character 4	Contrast Character 5	Qualifier Character 6	Qualifier Character 7
8　Shoulder, Right 9　Shoulder, Left G　Elbow, Right H　Elbow, Left L　Wrist, Right M　Wrist, Left N　Hand, Right P　Hand, Left	Z　None	Z　None	1　Densitometry Z　None

B　Imaging
Q　Non-Axial Lower Bones
0　Plain Radiography Planar display of an image developed from the capture of external ionizing radiation on photographic or photoconductive plate

Body Part Character 4	Contrast Character 5	Qualifier Character 6	Qualifier Character 7
0　Hip, Right 1　Hip, Left 3　Femur, Right 4　Femur, Left	Z　None	Z　None	1　Densitometry Z　None
0　Hip, Right 1　Hip, Left X　Foot/Toe Joint, Right Y　Foot/Toe Joint, Left	0　High Osmolar 1　Low Osmolar Y　Other Contrast	Z　None	Z　None
7　Knee, Right 8　Knee, Left G　Ankle, Right H　Ankle, Left	0　High Osmolar 1　Low Osmolar Y　Other Contrast Z　None	Z　None	Z　None
D　Lower Leg, Right F　Lower Leg, Left J　Calcaneus, Right K　Calcaneus, Left L　Foot, Right M　Foot, Left P　Toe(s), Right Q　Toe(s), Left V　Patella, Right W　Patella, Left	Z　None	Z　None	Z　None

B   Imaging
Q   Non-Axial Lower Bones
1   Fluoroscopy   Single plane or bi-plane real time display of an image developed from the capture of external ionizing radiation on a fluorescent screen. The image may also be stored by either digital or analog means

Body Part Character 4	Contrast Character 5	Qualifier Character 6	Qualifier Character 7
Ø Hip, Right 1 Hip, Left 7 Knee, Right 8 Knee, Left G Ankle, Right H Ankle, Left X Foot/Toe Joint, Right Y Foot/Toe Joint, Left	Ø High Osmolar 1 Low Osmolar Y Other Contrast Z None	Z None	Z None
3 Femur, Right 4 Femur, Left D Lower Leg, Right F Lower Leg, Left J Calcaneus, Right K Calcaneus, Left L Foot, Right M Foot, Left P Toe(s), Right Q Toe(s), Left V Patella, Right W Patella, Left	Z None	Z None	Z None

B   Imaging
Q   Non-Axial Lower Bones
2   Computerized Tomography (CT Scan)   Computer reformatted digital display of multiplanar images developed from the capture of multiple exposures of external ionizing radiation

Body Part Character 4	Contrast Character 5	Qualifier Character 6	Qualifier Character 7
Ø Hip, Right 1 Hip, Left 3 Femur, Right 4 Femur, Left 7 Knee, Right 8 Knee, Left D Lower Leg, Right F Lower Leg, Left G Ankle, Right H Ankle, Left J Calcaneus, Right K Calcaneus, Left L Foot, Right M Foot, Left P Toe(s), Right Q Toe(s), Left R Lower Extremity, Right S Lower Extremity, Left V Patella, Right W Patella, Left X Foot/Toe Joint, Right Y Foot/Toe Joint, Left	Ø High Osmolar 1 Low Osmolar Y Other Contrast Z None	Z None	Z None
B Tibia/Fibula, Right C Tibia/Fibula, Left	Ø High Osmolar 1 Low Osmolar Y Other Contrast	Z None	Z None

B   Imaging
Q   Non-Axial Lower Bones
3   Magnetic Resonance Imaging (MRI)   Computer reformatted digital display of multiplanar images developed from the capture of radio-frequency signals emitted by nuclei in a body site excited within a magnetic field

Body Part Character 4	Contrast Character 5	Qualifier Character 6	Qualifier Character 7
Ø Hip, Right 1 Hip, Left 3 Femur, Right 4 Femur, Left 7 Knee, Right 8 Knee, Left D Lower Leg, Right F Lower Leg, Left G Ankle, Right H Ankle, Left J Calcaneus, Right K Calcaneus, Left L Foot, Right M Foot, Left P Toe(s), Right Q Toe(s), Left V Patella, Right W Patella, Left	Y Other Contrast	Ø Unenhanced and Enhanced Z None	Z None
Ø Hip, Right 1 Hip, Left 3 Femur, Right 4 Femur, Left 7 Knee, Right 8 Knee, Left D Lower Leg, Right F Lower Leg, Left G Ankle, Right H Ankle, Left J Calcaneus, Right K Calcaneus, Left L Foot, Right M Foot, Left P Toe(s), Right Q Toe(s), Left V Patella, Right W Patella, Left	Z None	Z None	Z None

B   Imaging
Q   Non-Axial Lower Bones
4   Ultrasonography   Real time display of images of anatomy or flow information developed from the capture of relected and attenuated high frequency sound waves

Body Part Character 4	Contrast Character 5	Qualifier Character 6	Qualifier Character 7
Ø Hip, Right 1 Hip, Left 2 Hips, Bilateral 7 Knee, Right 8 Knee, Left 9 Knees, Bilateral	Z None	Z None	Z None

B   **Imaging**
R   **Axial Skeleton, Except Skull and Facial Bones**
0   **Plain Radiography**   Planar display of an image developed from the capture of external ionizing radiation on photographic or photoconductive plate

Body Part Character 4	Contrast Character 5	Qualifier Character 6	Qualifier Character 7
0 Cervical Spine **7** Thoracic Spine **9** Lumbar Spine **G** Whole Spine	**Z** None	**Z** None	**1** Densitometry **Z** None
1 Cervical Disc(s) **2** Thoracic Disc(s) **3** Lumbar Disc(s) **4** Cervical Facet Joint(s) **5** Thoracic Facet Joint(s) **6** Lumbar Facet Joint(s) **D** Sacroiliac Joints	**0** High Osmolar **1** Low Osmolar **Y** Other Contrast **Z** None	**Z** None	**Z** None
8 Thoracolumbar Joint **B** Lumbosacral Joint **C** Pelvis **F** Sacrum and Coccyx **H** Sternum	**Z** None	**Z** None	**Z** None

B   **Imaging**
R   **Axial Skeleton, Except Skull and Facial Bones**
1   **Fluoroscopy**   Single plane or bi-plane real time display of an image developed from the capture of external ionizing radioation on a fluorescent screen. The image may also be stored by either digital or analog means

Body Part Character 4	Contrast Character 5	Qualifier Character 6	Qualifier Character 7
0 Cervical Spine **1** Cervical Disc(s) **2** Thoracic Disc(s) **3** Lumbar Disc(s) **4** Cervical Facet Joint(s) **5** Thoracic Facet Joint(s) **6** Lumbar Facet Joint(s) **7** Thoracic Spine **8** Thoracolumbar Joint **9** Lumbar Spine **B** Lumbosacral Joint **C** Pelvis **D** Sacroiliac Joints **F** Sacrum and Coccyx **G** Whole Spine **H** Sternum	**0** High Osmolar **1** Low Osmolar **Y** Other Contrast **Z** None	**Z** None	**Z** None

B   **Imaging**
R   **Axial Skeleton, Except Skull and Facial Bones**
2   **Computerized Tomography (CT Scan)**   Computer reformatted digital display of multiplanar images developed from the capture of multiple exposures of external ionizing radiation

Body Part Character 4	Contrast Character 5	Qualifier Character 6	Qualifier Character 7
0 Cervical Spine **7** Thoracic Spine **9** Lumbar Spine **C** Pelvis **D** Sacroiliac Joints **F** Sacrum and Coccyx	**0** High Osmolar **1** Low Osmolar **Y** Other Contrast **Z** None	**Z** None	**Z** None

B　Imaging
R　Axial Skeleton, Except Skull and Facial Bones
3　Magnetic Resonance Imaging (MRI)　Computer reformatted digital display of multiplanar images developed from the capture of radio-frequency signals emitted by nuclei in a body site excited within a magnetic field

Body Part Character 4	Contrast Character 5	Qualifier Character 6	Qualifier Character 7
Ø Cervical Spine 1 Cervical Disc(s) 2 Thoracic Disc(s) 3 Lumbar Disc(s) 7 Thoracic Spine 9 Lumbar Spine C Pelvis F Sacrum and Coccyx	Y Other Contrast	Ø Unenhanced and Enhanced Z None	Z None
Ø Cervical Spine 1 Cervical Disc(s) 2 Thoracic Disc(s) 3 Lumbar Disc(s) 7 Thoracic Spine 9 Lumbar Spine C Pelvis F Sacrum and Coccyx	Z None	Z None	Z None

B　Imaging
R　Axial Skeleton, Except Skull and Facial Bones
4　Ultrasonography　Real time display of images of anatomy or flow information developed from the capture of relected and attenuated high frequency sound waves

Body Part Character 4	Contrast Character 5	Qualifier Character 6	Qualifier Character 7
Ø Cervical Spine 7 Thoracic Spine 9 Lumbar Spine F Sacrum and Coccyx	Z None	Z None	Z None

B　Imaging
T　Urinary System
Ø　Plain Radiography　Planar display of an image developed from the capture of external ionizing radiation on photographic or photoconductive plate

Body Part Character 4	Contrast Character 5	Qualifier Character 6	Qualifier Character 7
Ø Bladder 1 Kidney, Right 2 Kidney, Left 3 Kidneys, Bilateral 4 Kidneys, Ureters and Bladder 5 Urethra 6 Ureter, Right 7 Ureter, Left 8 Ureters, Bilateral B Bladder and Urethra C Ileal Diversion Loop	Ø High Osmolar 1 Low Osmolar Y Other Contrast Z None	Z None	Z None

B　Imaging
T　Urinary System
1　Fluoroscopy　Single plane or bi-plane real time display of an image developed from the capture of external ionizing radioation on a fluorescent screen. The image may also be stored by either digital or analog means

Body Part Character 4	Contrast Character 5	Qualifier Character 6	Qualifier Character 7
Ø Bladder 1 Kidney, Right 2 Kidney, Left 3 Kidneys, Bilateral 4 Kidneys, Ureters and Bladder 5 Urethra 6 Ureter, Right 7 Ureter, Left B Bladder and Urethra C Ileal Diversion Loop D Kidney, Ureter and Bladder, Right F Kidney, Ureter and Bladder, Left G Ileal Loop, Ureters and Kidneys	Ø High Osmolar 1 Low Osmolar Y Other Contrast Z None	Z None	Z None

B   **Imaging**
T   **Urinary System**
2   **Computerized Tomography (CT Scan)**   Computer reformatted digital display of multiplanar images developed from the capture of multiple exposures of external ionizing radiation

Body Part Character 4	Contrast Character 5	Qualifier Character 6	Qualifier Character 7
0 Bladder 1 Kidney, Right 2 Kidney, Left 3 Kidneys, Bilateral 9 Kidney Transplant	0 High Osmolar 1 Low Osmolar Y Other Contrast	0 Unenhanced and Enhanced Z None	Z None
0 Bladder 1 Kidney, Right 2 Kidney, Left 3 Kidneys, Bilateral 9 Kidney Transplant	Z None	Z None	Z None

B   **Imaging**
T   **Urinary System**
3   **Magnetic Resonance Imaging (MRI)**   Computer reformatted digital display of multiplanar images developed from the capture of radio-frequency signals emitted by nuclei in a body site excited within a magnetic field

Body Part Character 4	Contrast Character 5	Qualifier Character 6	Qualifier Character 7
0 Bladder 1 Kidney, Right 2 Kidney, Left 3 Kidneys, Bilateral 9 Kidney Transplant	Y Other Contrast	0 Unenhanced and Enhanced Z None	Z None
0 Bladder 1 Kidney, Right 2 Kidney, Left 3 Kidneys, Bilateral 9 Kidney Transplant	Z None	Z None	Z None

B   **Imaging**
T   **Urinary System**
4   **Ultrasonography**   Real time display of images of anatomy or flow information developed from the capture of relected and attenuated high frequency sound waves

Body Part Character 4	Contrast Character 5	Qualifier Character 6	Qualifier Character 7
0 Bladder 1 Kidney, Right 2 Kidney, Left 3 Kidneys, Bilateral 5 Urethra 6 Ureter, Right 7 Ureter, Left 8 Ureters, Bilateral 9 Kidney Transplant J Kidneys and Bladder	Z None	Z None	Z None

B   **Imaging**
U   **Female Reproductive System**
0   **Plain Radiography**   Planar display of an image developed from the capture of external ionizing radiation on photographic or photoconductive plate

Body Part Character 4	Contrast Character 5	Qualifier Character 6	Qualifier Character 7
0 Fallopian Tube, Right 1 Fallopian Tube, Left 2 Fallopian Tubes, Bilateral 6 Uterus 8 Uterus and Fallopian Tubes 9 Vagina	0 High Osmolar 1 Low Osmolar Y Other Contrast	Z None	Z None

B   Imaging
U   Female Reproductive System
1   Fluoroscopy   Single plane or bi-plane real time display of an image developed from the capture of external ionizing radioation on a fluorescent screen. The image may also be stored by either digital or analog means

Body Part Character 4	Contrast Character 5	Qualifier Character 6	Qualifier Character 7
0 Fallopian Tube, Right 1 Fallopian Tube, Left 2 Fallopian Tubes, Bilateral 6 Uterus 8 Uterus and Fallopian Tubes 9 Vagina	0 High Osmolar 1 Low Osmolar Y Other Contrast Z None	Z None	Z None

B   Imaging
U   Female Reproductive System
3   Magnetic Resonance Imaging (MRI)   Computer reformatted digital display of multiplanar images developed from the capture of radio-frequency signals emitted by nuclei in a body site excited within a magnetic field

Body Part Character 4	Contrast Character 5	Qualifier Character 6	Qualifier Character 7
3 Ovary, Right 4 Ovary, Left 5 Ovaries, Bilateral 6 Uterus 9 Vagina B Pregnant Uterus C Uterus and Ovaries	Y Other Contrast	0 Unenhanced and Enhanced Z None	Z None
3 Ovary, Right 4 Ovary, Left 5 Ovaries, Bilateral 6 Uterus 9 Vagina B Pregnant Uterus C Uterus and Ovaries	Z None	Z None	Z None

B   Imaging
U   Female Reproductive System
4   Ultrasonography   Real time display of images of anatomy or flow information developed from the capture of relected and attenuated high frequency sound waves

Body Part Character 4	Contrast Character 5	Qualifier Character 6	Qualifier Character 7
0 Fallopian Tube, Right 1 Fallopian Tube, Left 2 Fallopian Tubes, Bilateral 3 Ovary, Right 4 Ovary, Left 5 Ovaries, Bilateral 6 Uterus C Uterus and Ovaries	Y Other Contrast Z None	Z None	Z None

B   Imaging
V   Male Reproductive System
0   Plain Radiography   Planar display of an image developed from the capture of external ionizing radiation on photographic or photoconductive plate

Body Part Character 4	Contrast Character 5	Qualifier Character 6	Qualifier Character 7
0 Corpora Cavernosa 1 Epididymis, Right 2 Epididymis, Left 3 Prostate 5 Testicle, Right 6 Testicle, Left 8 Vasa Vasorum	0 High Osmolar 1 Low Osmolar Y Other Contrast	Z None	Z None

B   Imaging
V   Male Reproductive System
1   Fluoroscopy   Single plane or bi-plane real time display of an image developed from the capture of external ionizing radioation on a fluorescent screen. The image may also be stored by either digital or analog means

Body Part Character 4	Contrast Character 5	Qualifier Character 6	Qualifier Character 7
0 Corpora Cavernosa 8 Vasa Vasorum	0 High Osmolar 1 Low Osmolar Y Other Contrast Z None	Z None	Z None

B   Imaging
V   Male Reproductive System
2   **Computerized Tomography (CT Scan)** Computer reformatted digital display of multiplanar images developed from the capture of multiple exposures of external ionizing radiation

Body Part Character 4	Contrast Character 5	Qualifier Character 6	Qualifier Character 7
3 Prostate	0 High Osmolar 1 Low Osmolar Y Other Contrast	0 Unenhanced and Enhanced Z None	Z None
3 Prostate	Z None	Z None	Z None

B   Imaging
V   Male Reproductive System
3   **Magnetic Resonance Imaging (MRI)** Computer reformatted digital display of multiplanar images developed from the capture of radio-frequency signals emitted by nuclei in a body site excited within a magnetic field

Body Part Character 4	Contrast Character 5	Qualifier Character 6	Qualifier Character 7
0 Corpora Cavernosa 3 Prostate 4 Scrotum 5 Testicle, Right 6 Testicle, Left 7 Testicles, Bilateral	Y Other Contrast	0 Unenhanced and Enhanced Z None	Z None
0 Corpora Cavernosa 3 Prostate 4 Scrotum 5 Testicle, Right 6 Testicle, Left 7 Testicles, Bilateral	Z None	Z None	Z None

B   Imaging
V   Male Reproductive System
4   **Ultrasonography** Real time display of images of anatomy or flow information developed from the capture of relected and attenuated high frequency sound waves

Body Part Character 4	Contrast Character 5	Qualifier Character 6	Qualifier Character 7
4 Scrotum 9 Prostate and Seminal Vesicles B Penis	Z None	Z None	Z None

B   Imaging
W   Anatomical Regions
0   **Plain Radiography** Planar display of an image developed from the capture of external ionizing radiation on photographic or photoconductive plate

Body Part Character 4	Contrast Character 5	Qualifier Character 6	Qualifier Character 7
0 Abdomen 1 Abdomen and Pelvis 3 Chest B Long Bones, All C Lower Extremity J Upper Extremity K Whole Body L Whole Skeleton M Whole Body, Infant	Z None	Z None	Z None

B   Imaging
W   Anatomical Regions
1   **Fluoroscopy** Single plane or bi-plane real time display of an image developed from the capture of external ionizing radioation on a fluorescent screen. The image may also be stored by either digital or analog means

Body Part Character 4	Contrast Character 5	Qualifier Character 6	Qualifier Character 7
1 Abdomen and Pelvis 9 Head and Neck C Lower Extremity J Upper Extremity	0 High Osmolar 1 Low Osmolar Y Other Contrast Z None	Z None	Z None

B   **Imaging**
W   **Anatomical Regions**
2   **Computerized Tomography (CT Scan)** Computer reformatted digital display of multiplanar images developed from the capture of multiple exposures of external ionizing radiation

Body Part Character 4	Contrast Character 5	Qualifier Character 6	Qualifier Character 7
Ø Abdomen **1** Abdomen and Pelvis **4** Chest and Abdomen **5** Chest, Abdomen and Pelvis **8** Head **9** Head and Neck **F** Neck **G** Pelvic Region	**Ø** High Osmolar **1** Low Osmolar **Y** Other Contrast	**Ø** Unenhanced and Enhanced **Z** None	**Z** None
Ø Abdomen **1** Abdomen and Pelvis **4** Chest and Abdomen **5** Chest, Abdomen and Pelvis **8** Head **9** Head and Neck **F** Neck **G** Pelvic Region	**Z** None	**Z** None	**Z** None

B   **Imaging**
W   **Anatomical Regions**
3   **Magnetic Resonance Imaging (MRI)** Computer reformatted digital display of multiplanar images developed from the capture of radio-frequency signals emitted by nuclei in a body site excited within a magnetic field

Body Part Character 4	Contrast Character 5	Qualifier Character 6	Qualifier Character 7
Ø Abdomen **3** Chest **8** Head **F** Neck **G** Pelvic Region **H** Retroperitoneum **P** Brachial Plexus	**Y** Other Contrast	**Ø** Unenhanced and Enhanced **Z** None	**Z** None
Ø Abdomen **8** Head **F** Neck **G** Pelvic Region **H** Retroperitoneum **P** Brachial Plexus	**Z** None	**Z** None	**Z** None

B   **Imaging**
W   **Anatomical Regions**
4   **Ultrasonography** Real time display of images of anatomy or flow information developed from the capture of relected and attenuated high frequency sound waves

Body Part Character 4	Contrast Character 5	Qualifier Character 6	Qualifier Character 7
Ø Abdomen **1** Abdomen and Pelvis **F** Neck **G** Pelvic Region	**Z** None	**Z** None	**Z** None

B   Imaging
Y   Fetus and Obstetrical
3   Magnetic Resonance Imaging (MRI)   Computer reformatted digital display of multiplanar images developed from the capture of radio-frequency signals emitted by nuclei in a body site excited within a magnetic field

Body Part Character 4	Contrast Character 5	Qualifier Character 6	Qualifier Character 7
Ø Fetal Head 1 Fetal Heart 2 Fetal Thorax 3 Fetal Abdomen 4 Fetal Spine 5 Fetal Extremities 6 Whole Fetus	Y Other Contrast	Ø Unenhanced and Enhanced Z None	Z None
Ø Fetal Head 1 Fetal Heart 2 Fetal Thorax 3 Fetal Abdomen 4 Fetal Spine 5 Fetal Extremities 6 Whole Fetus	Z None	Z None	Z None

B   Imaging
Y   Fetus and Obstetrical
4   Ultrasonography   Real time display of images of anatomy or flow information developed from the capture of relected and attenuated high frequency sound waves

Body Part Character 4	Contrast Character 5	Qualifier Character 6	Qualifier Character 7
7 Fetal Umbilical Cord 8 Placenta 9 First Trimester, Single Fetus B First Trimester, Multiple Gestation C Second Trimester, Single Fetus D Second Trimester, Multiple Gestation F Third Trimester, Single Fetus G Third Trimester, Multiple Gestation	Z None	Z None	Z None

Revised Text in **BLUE**

Nuclear Medicine C01–CW7

C **Nuclear Medicine**
0 **Central Nervous System**
1 **Planar Nuclear Medicine Imaging**　Introduction of radioactive materials into the body for single plane display of images developed from the capture of radioactive emissions

Body Part Character 4	Radionuclide Character 5	Qualifier Character 6	Qualifier Character 7
0 Brain	**1** Technetium 99m (Tc-99m) **Y** Other Radionuclide	**Z** None	**Z** None
5 Cerebrospinal Fluid	**D** Indium 111 (In-111) **Y** Other Radionuclide	**Z** None	**Z** None
Y Central Nervous System	**Y** Other Radionuclide	**Z** None	**Z** None

C **Nuclear Medicine**
0 **Central Nervous System**
2 **Tomographic (Tomo) Nuclear Medicine Imaging**　Introduction of radioactive materials into the body for three dimensional display of images developed from the capture of radioactive emissions

Body Part Character 4	Radionuclide Character 5	Qualifier Character 6	Qualifier Character 7
0 Brain	**1** Technetium 99m (Tc-99m) **F** Iodine 123 (I-123) **S** Thallium 201 (Tl-201) **Y** Other Radionuclide	**Z** None	**Z** None
5 Cerebrospinal Fluid	**D** Indium 111 (In-111) **Y** Other Radionuclide	**Z** None	**Z** None
Y Central Nervous System	**Y** Other Radionuclide	**Z** None	**Z** None

C **Nuclear Medicine**
0 **Central Nervous System**
3 **Positron Emission Tomographic (PET) Imaging**　Introduction of radioactive materials into the body for three dimensional display of images developed from the simultaneous capture, 180 degrees apart, of radioactive emissions

Body Part Character 4	Radionuclide Character 5	Qualifier Character 6	Qualifier Character 7
0 Brain	**B** Carbon 11 (C-11) **K** Fluorine 18 (F-18) **M** Oxygen 15 (O-15) **Y** Other Radionuclide	**Z** None	**Z** None
Y Central Nervous System	**Y** Other Radionuclide	**Z** None	**Z** None

C **Nuclear Medicine**
0 **Central Nervous System**
5 **Nonimaging Nuclear Medicine Probe**　Introduction of radioactive materials into the body for the study of distribution and fate of certain substances by the detection of radioactive emissions; or, alternatively, measurement of absorption of radioactive emissions from an external source

Body Part Character 4	Radionuclide Character 5	Qualifier Character 6	Qualifier Character 7
0 Brain	**V** Xenon 133 (Xe-133) **Y** Other Radionuclide	**Z** None	**Z** None
Y Central Nervous System	**Y** Other Radionuclide	**Z** None	**Z** None

C **Nuclear Medicine**
2 **Heart**
1 **Planar Nuclear Medicine Imaging**　Introduction of radioactive materials into the body for single plane display of images developed from the capture of radioactive emissions

Body Part Character 4	Radionuclide Character 5	Qualifier Character 6	Qualifier Character 7
6 Heart, Right and Left	**1** Technetium 99m (Tc-99m) **Y** Other Radionuclide	**Z** None	**Z** None
G Myocardium	**1** Technetium 99m (Tc-99m) **D** Indium 111 (In-111) **S** Thallium 201 (Tl-201) **Y** Other Radionuclide **Z** None	**Z** None	**Z** None
Y Heart	**Y** Other Radionuclide	**Z** None	**Z** None

C   **Nuclear Medicine**
2   **Heart**
2   **Tomographic (Tomo) Nuclear Medicine Imaging**   Introduction of radioactive materials into the body for three dimensional display of images developed from the capture of radioactive emissions

Body Part Character 4	Radionuclide Character 5	Qualifier Character 6	Qualifier Character 7
6 Heart, Right and Left	**1** Technetium 99m (Tc-99m) **Y** Other Radionuclide	**Z** None	**Z** None
G Myocardium	**1** Technetium 99m (Tc-99m) **D** Indium 111 (In-111) **K** Fluorine 18 (F-18) **S** Thallium 201 (Tl-201) **Y** Other Radionuclide **Z** None	**Z** None	**Z** None
Y Heart	**Y** Other Radionuclide	**Z** None	**Z** None

C   **Nuclear Medicine**
2   **Heart**
3   **Positron Emission Tomographic (PET) Imaging**   Introduction of radioactive materials into the body for three dimensional display of images developed from the simultaneous capture, 180 degrees apart, of radioactive emissions

Body Part Character 4	Radionuclide Character 5	Qualifier Character 6	Qualifier Character 7
G Myocardium	**K** Fluorine 18 (F-18) **M** Oxygen 15 (O-15) **Q** Rubidium 82 (Rb-82) **R** Nitrogen 13 (N-13) **Y** Other Radionuclide	**Z** None	**Z** None
Y Heart	**Y** Other Radionuclide	**Z** None	**Z** None

C   **Nuclear Medicine**
2   **Heart**
5   **Nonimaging Nuclear Medicine Probe**   Introduction of radioactive materials into the body for the study of distribution and fate of certain substances by the detection of radioactive emissions; or, alternatively, measurement of absorption of radioactive emissions from an external source

Body Part Character 4	Radionuclide Character 5	Qualifier Character 6	Qualifier Character 7
6 Heart, Right and Left	**1** Technetium 99m (Tc-99m) **Y** Other Radionuclide	**Z** None	**Z** None
Y Heart	**Y** Other Radionuclide	**Z** None	**Z** None

C   **Nuclear Medicine**
5   **Veins**
1   **Planar Nuclear Medicine Imaging**   Introduction of radioactive materials into the body for single plane display of images developed from the capture of radioactive emissions

Body Part Character 4	Radionuclide Character 5	Qualifier Character 6	Qualifier Character 7
B Lower Extremity Veins, Right **C** Lower Extremity Veins, Left **D** Lower Extremity Veins, Bilateral **N** Upper Extremity Veins, Right **P** Upper Extremity Veins, Left **Q** Upper Extremity Veins, Bilateral **R** Central Veins	**1** Technetium 99m (Tc-99m) **Y** Other Radionuclide	**Z** None	**Z** None
Y Veins	**Y** Other Radionuclide	**Z** None	**Z** None

C　Nuclear Medicine
7　Lymphatic and Hematologic System
1　Planar Nuclear Medicine Imaging　Introduction of radioactive materials into the body for single plane display of images developed from the capture of radioactive emissions

Body Part Character 4	Radionuclide Character 5	Qualifier Character 6	Qualifier Character 7
Ø　Bone Marrow	1　Technetium 99m (Tc-99m) D　Indium 111 (In-111) Y　Other Radionuclide	Z　None	Z　None
2　Spleen 5　Lymphatics, Head and Neck D　Lymphatics, Pelvic J　Lymphatics, Head K　Lymphatics, Neck L　Lymphatics, Upper Chest M　Lymphatics, Trunk N　Lymphatics, Upper Extremity P　Lymphatics, Lower Extremity	1　Technetium 99m (Tc-99m) Y　Other Radionuclide	Z　None	Z　None
3　Blood	D　Indium 111 (In-111) Y　Other Radionuclide	Z　None	Z　None
Y　Lymphatic and Hematologic System	Y　Other Radionuclide	Z　None	Z　None

C　Nuclear Medicine
7　Lymphatic and Hematologic System
2　Tomographic (Tomo) Nuclear Medicine Imaging　Introduction of radioactive materials into the body for three dimensional display of images developed from the capture of radioactive emissions

Body Part Character 4	Radionuclide Character 5	Qualifier Character 6	Qualifier Character 7
2　Spleen	1　Technetium 99m (Tc-99m) Y　Other Radionuclide	Z　None	Z　None
Y　Lymphatic and Hematologic System	Y　Other Radionuclide	Z　None	Z　None

C　Nuclear Medicine
7　Lymphatic and Hematologic System
5　Nonimaging Nuclear Medicine Probe　Introduction of radioactive materials into the body for the study of distribution and fate of certain substances by the detection of radioactive emissions; or, alternatively, measurement of absorption of radioactive emissions from an external source

Body Part Character 4	Radionuclide Character 5	Qualifier Character 6	Qualifier Character 7
5　Lymphatics, Head and Neck D　Lymphatics, Pelvic J　Lymphatics, Head K　Lymphatics, Neck L　Lymphatics, Upper Chest M　Lymphatics, Trunk N　Lymphatics, Upper Extremity P　Lymphatics, Lower Extremity	1　Technetium 99m (Tc-99m) Y　Other Radionuclide	Z　None	Z　None
Y　Lymphatic and Hematologic System	Y　Other Radionuclide	Z　None	Z　None

C　Nuclear Medicine
7　Lymphatic and Hematologic System
6　Nonimaging Nuclear Medicine Assay　Introduction of radioactive materials into the body for the study of body fluids and blood elements, by the detection of radioactive emissions

Body Part Character 4	Radionuclide Character 5	Qualifier Character 6	Qualifier Character 7
3　Blood	1　Technetium 99m (Tc-99m) 7　Cobalt 58 (Co-58) C　Cobalt 57 (Co-57) D　Indium 111 (In-111) H　Iodine 125 (I-125) W　Chromium (Cr-51) Y　Other Radionuclide	Z　None	Z　None
Y　Lymphatic and Hematologic System	Y　Other Radionuclide	Z　None	Z　None

C   Nuclear Medicine
8   Eye
1   Planar Nuclear Medicine Imaging   Introduction of radioactive materials into the body for single plane display of images developed from the capture of radioactive emissions

Body Part Character 4	Radionuclide Character 5	Qualifier Character 6	Qualifier Character 7
9 Lacrimal Ducts, Bilateral	1 Technetium 99m (Tc-99m) Y Other Radionuclide	Z None	Z None
Y Eye	Y Other Radionuclide	Z None	Z None

C   Nuclear Medicine
9   Ear, Nose, Mouth and Throat
1   Planar Nuclear Medicine Imaging   Introduction of radioactive materials into the body for single plane display of images developed from the capture of radioactive emissions

Body Part Character 4	Radionuclide Character 5	Qualifier Character 6	Qualifier Character 7
B Salivary Glands, Bilateral	1 Technetium 99m (Tc-99m) Y Other Radionuclide	Z None	Z None
Y Ear, Nose, Mouth and Throat	Y Other Radionuclide	Z None	Z None

C   Nuclear Medicine
B   Respiratory System
1   Planar Nuclear Medicine Imaging   Introduction of radioactive materials into the body for single plane display of images developed from the capture of radioactive emissions

Body Part Character 4	Radionuclide Character 5	Qualifier Character 6	Qualifier Character 7
2 Lungs and Bronchi	1 Technetium 99m (Tc-99m) 9 Krypton (Kr-81m) T Xenon 127 (Xe-127) V Xenon 133 (Xe-133) Y Other Radionuclide	Z None	Z None
Y Respiratory System	Y Other Radionuclide	Z None	Z None

C   Nuclear Medicine
B   Respiratory System
2   Tomographic (Tomo) Nuclear Medicine Imaging   Introduction of radioactive materials into the body for three dimensional display of images developed from the capture of radioactive emissions

Body Part Character 4	Radionuclide Character 5	Qualifier Character 6	Qualifier Character 7
2 Lungs and Bronchi	1 Technetium 99m (Tc-99m) 9 Krypton (Kr-81m) Y Other Radionuclide	Z None	Z None
Y Respiratory System	Y Other Radionuclide	Z None	Z None

C   Nuclear Medicine
B   Respiratory System
3   Positron Emission Tomographic (PET) Imaging   Introduction of radioactive materials into the body for three dimensional display of images developed from the simultaneous capture, 180 degrees apart, of radioactive emissions

Body Part Character 4	Radionuclide Character 5	Qualifier Character 6	Qualifier Character 7
2 Lungs and Bronchi	K Fluorine 18 (F-18) Y Other Radionuclide	Z None	Z None
Y Respiratory System	Y Other Radionuclide	Z None	Z None

C   Nuclear Medicine
D   Gastrointestinal System
1   Planar Nuclear Medicine Imaging   Introduction of radioactive materials into the body for single plane display of images developed from the capture of radioactive emissions

Body Part Character 4	Radionuclide Character 5	Qualifier Character 6	Qualifier Character 7
5 Upper Gastrointestinal Tract 7 Gastrointestinal Tract	1 Technetium 99m (Tc-99m) D Indium 111 (In-111) Y Other Radionuclide	Z None	Z None
Y Digestive System	Y Other Radionuclide	Z None	Z None

C Nuclear Medicine
D Gastrointestinal System
2 Tomographic (Tomo) Nuclear Medicine Imaging Introduction of radioactive materials into the body for three dimensional display of images developed from the capture of radioactive emissions

Body Part Character 4	Radionuclide Character 5	Qualifier Character 6	Qualifier Character 7
7 Gastrointestinal Tract	1 Technetium 99m (Tc-99m) D Indium 111 (In-111) Y Other Radionuclide	Z None	Z None
Y Digestive System	Y Other Radionuclide	Z None	Z None

C Nuclear Medicine
F Hepatobiliary System and Pancreas
1 Planar Nuclear Medicine Imaging Introduction of radioactive materials into the body for single plane display of images developed from the capture of radioactive emissions

Body Part Character 4	Radionuclide Character 5	Qualifier Character 6	Qualifier Character 7
4 Gallbladder 5 Liver 6 Liver and Spleen C Hepatobiliary System, All	1 Technetium 99m (Tc-99m) Y Other Radionuclide	Z None	Z None
Y Hepatobiliary System and Pancreas	Y Other Radionuclide	Z None	Z None

C Nuclear Medicine
F Hepatobiliary System and Pancreas
2 Tomographic (Tomo) Nuclear Medicine Imaging Introduction of radioactive materials into the body for three dimensional display of images developed from the capture of radioactive emissions

Body Part Character 4	Radionuclide Character 5	Qualifier Character 6	Qualifier Character 7
4 Gallbladder 5 Liver 6 Liver and Spleen	1 Technetium 99m (Tc-99m) Y Other Radionuclide	Z None	Z None
Y Hepatobiliary System and Pancreas	Y Other Radionuclide	Z None	Z None

C Nuclear Medicine
G Endocrine System
1 Planar Nuclear Medicine Imaging Introduction of radioactive materials into the body for single plane display of images developed from the capture of radioactive emissions

Body Part Character 4	Radionuclide Character 5	Qualifier Character 6	Qualifier Character 7
1 Parathyroid Glands	1 Technetium 99m (Tc-99m) S Thallium 201 (Tl-201) Y Other Radionuclide	Z None	Z None
2 Thyroid Gland	1 Technetium 99m (Tc-99m) F Iodine 123 (I-123) G Iodine 131 (I-131) Y Other Radionuclide	Z None	Z None
4 Adrenal Glands, Bilateral	G Iodine 131 (I-131) Y Other Radionuclide	Z None	Z None
Y Endocrine System	Y Other Radionuclide	Z None	Z None

C Nuclear Medicine
G Endocrine System
2 Tomographic (Tomo) Nuclear Medicine Imaging Introduction of radioactive materials into the body for three dimensional display of images developed from the capture of radioactive emissions

Body Part Character 4	Radionuclide Character 5	Qualifier Character 6	Qualifier Character 7
1 Parathyroid Glands	1 Technetium 99m (Tc-99m) S Thallium 201 (Tl-201) Y Other Radionuclide	Z None	Z None
Y Endocrine System	Y Other Radionuclide	Z None	Z None

C   **Nuclear Medicine**
G   **Endocrine System**
4   **Nonimaging Nuclear Medicine Uptake**   Introduction of radioactive materials into the body for measurements of organ function, from the detection of radioactive emmissions

Body Part Character 4	Radionuclide Character 5	Qualifier Character 6	Qualifier Character 7
2 Thyroid Gland	**1** Technetium 99m (Tc-99m) **F** Iodine 123 (I-123) **G** Iodine 131 (I-131) **Y** Other Radionuclide	**Z** None	**Z** None
Y Endocrine System	**Y** Other Radionuclide	**Z** None	**Z** None

C   **Nuclear Medicine**
H   **Skin, Subcutaneous Tissue and Breast**
1   **Planar Nuclear Medicine Imaging**   Introduction of radioactive materials into the body for single plane display of images developed from the capture of radioactive emissions

Body Part Character 4	Radionuclide Character 5	Qualifier Character 6	Qualifier Character 7
0 Breast, Right **1** Breast, Left **2** Breasts, Bilateral	**1** Technetium 99m (Tc-99m) **S** Thallium 201 (Tl-201) **Y** Other Radionuclide	**Z** None	**Z** None
Y Skin, Subcutaneous Tissue and Breast	**Y** Other Radionuclide	**Z** None	**Z** None

C   **Nuclear Medicine**
H   **Skin, Subcutaneous Tissue and Breast**
2   **Tomographic (Tomo) Nuclear Medicine Imaging**   Introduction of radioactive materials into the body for three dimensional display of images developed from the capture of radioactive emissions

Body Part Character 4	Radionuclide Character 5	Qualifier Character 6	Qualifier Character 7
0 Breast, Right **1** Breast, Left **2** Breasts, Bilateral	**1** Technetium 99m (Tc-99m) **S** Thallium 201 (Tl-201) **Y** Other Radionuclide	**Z** None	**Z** None
Y Skin, Subcutaneous Tissue and Breast	**Y** Other Radionuclide	**Z** None	**Z** None

C   **Nuclear Medicine**
P   **Musculoskeletal System**
1   **Planar Nuclear Medicine Imaging**   Introduction of radioactive materials into the body for single plane display of images developed from the capture of radioactive emissions

Body Part Character 4	Radionuclide Character 5	Qualifier Character 6	Qualifier Character 7
1 Skull **4** Thorax **5** Spine **6** Pelvis **7** Spine and Pelvis **8** Upper Extremity, Right **9** Upper Extremity, Left **B** Upper Extremities, Bilateral **C** Lower Extremity, Right **D** Lower Extremity, Left **F** Lower Extremities, Bilateral **Z** Musculoskeletal System, All	**1** Technetium 99m (Tc-99m) **Y** Other Radionuclide	**Z** None	**Z** None
Y Musculoskeletal System, Other	**Y** Other Radionuclide	**Z** None	**Z** None

   Revised Text in **BLUE**   © 2011 Ingenix, Inc

C **Nuclear Medicine**
P **Musculoskeletal System**
2 **Tomographic (Tomo) Nuclear Medicine Imaging** Introduction of radioactive materials into the body for three dimensional display of images developed from the capture of radioactive emissions

Body Part Character 4	Radionuclide Character 5	Qualifier Character 6	Qualifier Character 7
1 Skull **2** Cervical Spine **3** Skull and Cervical Spine **4** Thorax **6** Pelvis **7** Spine and Pelvis **8** Upper Extremity, Right **9** Upper Extremity, Left **B** Upper Extremities, Bilateral **C** Lower Extremity, Right **D** Lower Extremity, Left **F** Lower Extremities, Bilateral **G** Thoracic Spine **H** Lumbar Spine **J** Thoracolumbar Spine	**1** Technetium 99m (Tc-99m) **Y** Other Radionuclide	**Z** None	**Z** None
Y Musculoskeletal System, Other	**Y** Other Radionuclide	**Z** None	**Z** None

C **Nuclear Medicine**
P **Musculoskeletal System**
5 **Nonimaging Nuclear Medicine Probe** Introduction of radioactive materials into the body for the study of distribution and fate of certain substances by the detection of radioactive emissions; or, alternatively, measurement of absorption of radioactive emissions from an external source

Body Part Character 4	Radionuclide Character 5	Qualifier Character 6	Qualifier Character 7
5 Spine **N** Upper Extremities **P** Lower Extremities	**Z** None	**Z** None	**Z** None
Y Musculoskeletal System, Other	**Y** Other Radionuclide	**Z** None	**Z** None

C **Nuclear Medicine**
T **Urinary System**
1 **Planar Nuclear Medicine Imaging** Introduction of radioactive materials into the body for single plane display of images developed from the capture of radioactive emissions

Body Part Character 4	Radionuclide Character 5	Qualifier Character 6	Qualifier Character 7
3 Kidneys, Ureters and Bladder	**1** Technetium 99m (Tc-99m) **F** Iodine 123 (I-123) **G** Iodine 131 (I-131) **Y** Other Radionuclide	**Z** None	**Z** None
H Bladder and Ureters	**1** Technetium 99m (Tc-99m) **Y** Other Radionuclide	**Z** None	**Z** None
Y Urinary System	**Y** Other Radionuclide	**Z** None	**Z** None

C **Nuclear Medicine**
T **Urinary System**
2 **Tomographic (Tomo) Nuclear Medicine Imaging** Introduction of radioactive materials into the body for three dimensional display of images developed from the capture of radioactive emissions

Body Part Character 4	Radionuclide Character 5	Qualifier Character 6	Qualifier Character 7
3 Kidneys, Ureters and Bladder	**1** Technetium 99m (Tc-99m) **Y** Other Radionuclide	**Z** None	**Z** None
Y Urinary System	**Y** Other Radionuclide	**Z** None	**Z** None

C   **Nuclear Medicine**
T   **Urinary System**
6   **Nonimaging Nuclear Medicine Assay**   Introduction of radioactive materials into the body for the study of body fluids and blood elements, by the detection of radioactive emissions

Body Part Character 4	Radionuclide Character 5	Qualifier Character 6	Qualifier Character 7
3 Kidneys, Ureters and Bladder	**1** Technetium 99m (Tc-99m) **F** Iodine 123 (I-123) **G** Iodine 131 (I-131) **H** Iodine 125 (I-125) **Y** Other Radionuclide	**Z** None	**Z** None
Y Urinary System	**Y** Other Radionuclide	**Z** None	**Z** None

C   **Nuclear Medicine**
V   **Male Reproductive System**
1   **Planar Nuclear Medicine Imaging**   Introduction of radioactive materials into the body for single plane display of images developed from the capture of radioactive emissions

Body Part Character 4	Radionuclide Character 5	Qualifier Character 6	Qualifier Character 7
9 Testicles, Bilateral	**1** Technetium 99m (Tc-99m) **Y** Other Radionuclide	**Z** None	**Z** None
Y Male Reproductive System	**Y** Other Radionuclide	**Z** None	**Z** None

C   **Nuclear Medicine**
W   **Anatomical Regions**
1   **Planar Nuclear Medicine Imaging**   Introduction of radioactive materials into the body for single plane display of images developed from the capture of radioactive emissions

Body Part Character 4	Radionuclide Character 5	Qualifier Character 6	Qualifier Character 7
Ø Abdomen **1** Abdomen and Pelvis **4** Chest and Abdomen **6** Chest and Neck **B** Head and Neck **D** Lower Extremity **J** Pelvic Region **M** Upper Extremity **N** Whole Body	**1** Technetium 99m (Tc-99m) **D** Indium 111 (In-111) **F** Iodine 123 (I-123) **G** Iodine 131 (I-131) **L** Gallium 67 (Ga-67) **S** Thallium 201 (Tl-201) **Y** Other Radionuclide	**Z** None	**Z** None
3 Chest	**1** Technetium 99m (Tc-99m) **D** Indium 111 (In-111) **F** Iodine 123 (I-123) **G** Iodine 131 (I-131) **K** Fluorine 18 (F-18) **L** Gallium 67 (Ga-67) **S** Thallium 201 (Tl-201) **Y** Other Radionuclide	**Z** None	**Z** None
Y Anatomical Regions, Multiple	**Y** Other Radionuclide	**Z** None	**Z** None
Z Anatomical Region, Other	**Z** None	**Z** None	**Z** None

C   **Nuclear Medicine**
W   **Anatomical Regions**
2   **Tomographic (Tomo) Nuclear Medicine Imaging**   Introduction of radioactive materials into the body for three dimensional display of images developed from the capture of radioactive emissions

Body Part Character 4	Radionuclide Character 5	Qualifier Character 6	Qualifier Character 7
Ø Abdomen **1** Abdomen and Pelvis **3** Chest **4** Chest and Abdomen **6** Chest and Neck **B** Head and Neck **D** Lower Extremity **J** Pelvic Region **M** Upper Extremity	**1** Technetium 99m (Tc-99m) **D** Indium 111 (In-111) **F** Iodine 123 (I-123) **G** Iodine 131 (I-131) **K** Fluorine 18 (F-18) **L** Gallium 67 (Ga-67) **S** Thallium 201 (Tl-201) **Y** Other Radionuclide	**Z** None	**Z** None
Y Anatomical Regions, Multiple	**Y** Other Radionuclide	**Z** None	**Z** None

     Revised Text in **BLUE**   © 2011 Ingenix, Inc

C   Nuclear Medicine
W   Anatomical Regions
3   Positron Emission Tomographic (PET) Imaging   Introduction of radioactive materials into the body for three dimensional display of images developed from the simultaneous capture, 180 degrees apart, of radioactive emissions

Body Part Character 4	Radionuclide Character 5	Qualifier Character 6	Qualifier Character 7
N Whole Body	**Y** Other Radionuclide	**Z** None	**Z** None

C   Nuclear Medicine
W   Anatomical Regions
5   Nonimaging Nuclear Medicine Probe   Introduction of radioactive materials into the body for the study of distribution and fate of certain substances by the detection of radioactive emissions; or, alternatively, measurement of absorption of radioactive emissions from an external source

Body Part Character 4	Radionuclide Character 5	Qualifier Character 6	Qualifier Character 7
0 Abdomen **1** Abdomen and Pelvis **3** Chest **4** Chest and Abdomen **6** Chest and Neck **B** Head and Neck **D** Lower Extremity **J** Pelvic Region **M** Upper Extremity	**1** Technetium 99m (Tc-99m) **D** Indium 111 (In-111) **Y** Other Radionuclide	**Z** None	**Z** None

C   Nuclear Medicine
W   Anatomical Regions
7   Systemic Nuclear Medicine Therapy   Introduction of radioactive materials into the body for treatment

Body Part Character 4	Radionuclide Character 5	Qualifier Character 6	Qualifier Character 7
0 Abdomen **3** Chest	**N** Phosphorus 32 (P-32) **Y** Other Radionuclide	**Z** None	**Z** None
G Thyroid	**G** Iodine 131 (I-131) **Y** Other Radionuclide	**Z** None	**Z** None
N Whole Body	**8** Samarium 153 (Sm-153) **G** Iodine 131 (I-131) **N** Phosphorus 32 (P-32) **P** Strontium 89 (Sr-89) **Y** Other Radionuclide	**Z** None	**Z** None
Y Anatomical Regions, Multiple	**Y** Other Radionuclide	**Z** None	**Z** None

Radiation Oncology DØØ–DWY

D Radiation Oncology
Ø Central and Peripheral Nervous System
Ø Beam Radiation

Treatment Site Character 4	Modal. Qualifier Character 5	Isotope Character 6	Qualifier Character 7
Ø Brain **1** Brain Stem **6** Spinal Cord **7** Peripheral Nerve	**Ø** Photons <1 MeV **1** Photons 1- 1Ø MeV **2** Photons >1Ø MeV **4** Heavy Particles (Protons, Ions) **5** Neutrons **6** Neutron Capture	**Z** None	**Z** None
Ø Brain **1** Brain Stem **6** Spinal Cord **7** Peripheral Nerve	**3** Electrons	**Z** None	**Ø** Intraoperative **Z** None

D Radiation Oncology
Ø Central and Peripheral Nervous System
1 Brachytherapy

Treatment Site Character 4	Modal. Qualifier Character 5	Isotope Character 6	Qualifier Character 7
Ø Brain **1** Brain Stem **6** Spinal Cord **7** Peripheral Nerve	**9** High Dose Rate (HDR) **B** Low Dose Rate (LDR)	**7** Cesium 137 (Cs-137) **8** Iridium 192 (Ir-192) **9** Iodine 125 (I-125) **B** Palladium 1Ø3 (Pd-1Ø3) **C** Californium 252 (Cf-252) **Y** Other Isotope	**Z** None

D Radiation Oncology
Ø Central and Peripheral Nervous System
2 Stereotactic Radiosurgery

Treatment Site Character 4	Modal. Qualifier Character 5	Isotope Character 6	Qualifier Character 7
Ø Brain **1** Brain Stem **6** Spinal Cord **7** Peripheral Nerve	**D** Stereotactic Other Photon Radiosurgery **H** Stereotactic Particulate Radiosurgery **J** Stereotactic Gamma Beam Radiosurgery	**Z** None	**Z** None

D Radiation Oncology
Ø Central and Peripheral Nervous System
Y Other Radiation

Treatment Site Character 4	Modal. Qualifier Character 5	Isotope Character 6	Qualifier Character 7
Ø Brain **1** Brain Stem **6** Spinal Cord **7** Peripheral Nerve	**7** Contact Radiation **8** Hyperthermia **F** Plaque Radiation **K** Laser Interstitial Thermal Therapy	**Z** None	**Z** None

D Radiation Oncology
7 Lymphatic and Hematologic System
Ø Beam Radiation

Treatment Site Character 4	Modal. Qualifier Character 5	Isotope Character 6	Qualifier Character 7
Ø Bone Marrow 1 Thymus 2 Spleen 3 Lymphatics, Neck 4 Lymphatics, Axillary 5 Lymphatics, Thorax 6 Lymphatics, Abdomen 7 Lymphatics, Pelvis 8 Lymphatics, Inguinal	Ø Photons <1 MeV 1 Photons 1- 1Ø MeV 2 Photons >1Ø MeV 4 Heavy Particles (Protons, Ions) 5 Neutrons 6 Neutron Capture	Z None	Z None
Ø Bone Marrow 1 Thymus 2 Spleen 3 Lymphatics, Neck 4 Lymphatics, Axillary 5 Lymphatics, Thorax 6 Lymphatics, Abdomen 7 Lymphatics, Pelvis 8 Lymphatics, Inguinal	3 Electrons	Z None	Ø Intraoperative Z None

D Radiation Oncology
7 Lymphatic and Hematologic System
1 Brachytherapy

Treatment Site Character 4	Modal. Qualifier Character 5	Isotope Character 6	Qualifier Character 7
Ø Bone Marrow 1 Thymus 2 Spleen 3 Lymphatics, Neck 4 Lymphatics, Axillary 5 Lymphatics, Thorax 6 Lymphatics, Abdomen 7 Lymphatics, Pelvis 8 Lymphatics, Inguinal	9 High Dose Rate (HDR) B Low Dose Rate (LDR)	7 Cesium 137 (Cs-137) 8 Iridium 192 (Ir-192) 9 Iodine 125 (I-125) B Palladium 1Ø3 (Pd-1Ø3) C Californium 252 (Cf-252) Y Other Isotope	Z None

D Radiation Oncology
7 Lymphatic and Hematologic System
2 Stereotactic Radiosurgery

Treatment Site Character 4	Modal. Qualifier Character 5	Isotope Character 6	Qualifier Character 7
Ø Bone Marrow 1 Thymus 2 Spleen 3 Lymphatics, Neck 4 Lymphatics, Axillary 5 Lymphatics, Thorax 6 Lymphatics, Abdomen 7 Lymphatics, Pelvis 8 Lymphatics, Inguinal	D Stereotactic Other Photon Radiosurgery H Stereotactic Particulate Radiosurgery J Stereotactic Gamma Beam Radiosurgery	Z None	Z None

D Radiation Oncology
7 Lymphatic and Hematologic System
Y Other Radiation

Treatment Site Character 4	Modal. Qualifier Character 5	Isotope Character 6	Qualifier Character 7
Ø Bone Marrow 1 Thymus 2 Spleen 3 Lymphatics, Neck 4 Lymphatics, Axillary 5 Lymphatics, Thorax 6 Lymphatics, Abdomen 7 Lymphatics, Pelvis 8 Lymphatics, Inguinal	8 Hyperthermia F Plaque Radiation	Z None	Z None

D Radiation Oncology
8 Eye
Ø Beam Radiation

Treatment Site Character 4	Modal. Qualifier Character 5	Isotope Character 6	Qualifier Character 7
Ø Eye	Ø Photons <1 MeV 1 Photons 1- 1Ø MeV 2 Photons >1Ø MeV 4 Heavy Particles (Protons, Ions) 5 Neutrons 6 Neutron Capture	Z None	Z None
Ø Eye	3 Electrons	Z None	Ø Intraoperative Z None

D Radiation Oncology
8 Eye
1 Brachytherapy

Treatment Site Character 4	Modal. Qualifier Character 5	Isotope Character 6	Qualifier Character 7
Ø Eye	9 High Dose Rate (HDR) B Low Dose Rate (LDR)	7 Cesium 137 (Cs-137) 8 Iridium 192 (Ir-192) 9 Iodine 125 (I-125) B Palladium 1Ø3 (Pd-1Ø3) C Californium 252 (Cf-252) Y Other Isotope	Z None

D Radiation Oncology
8 Eye
2 Stereotactic Radiosurgery

Treatment Site Character 4	Modal. Qualifier Character 5	Isotope Character 6	Qualifier Character 7
Ø Eye	D Stereotactic Other Photon Radiosurgery H Stereotactic Particulate Radiosurgery J Stereotactic Gamma Beam Radiosurgery	Z None	Z None

D Radiation Oncology
8 Eye
Y Other Radiation

Treatment Site Character 4	Modal. Qualifier Character 5	Isotope Character 6	Qualifier Character 7
Ø Eye	7 Contact Radiation 8 Hyperthermia F Plaque Radiation	Z None	Z None

Revised Text in **BLUE**   © 2Ø11 Ingenix, Inc

Radiation Oncology

D   Radiation Oncology
9   Ear, Nose, Mouth and Throat
Ø   Beam Radiation

Treatment Site Character 4	Modal. Qualifier Character 5	Isotope Character 6	Qualifier Character 7
Ø Ear 1 Nose 3 Hypopharynx 4 Mouth 5 Tongue 6 Salivary Glands 7 Sinuses 8 Hard Palate 9 Soft Palate B Larynx D Nasopharynx F Oropharynx	Ø Photons <1 MeV 1 Photons 1- 1Ø MeV 2 Photons >1Ø MeV 4 Heavy Particles (Protons, Ions) 5 Neutrons 6 Neutron Capture	Z None	Z None
Ø Ear 1 Nose 3 Hypopharynx 4 Mouth 5 Tongue 6 Salivary Glands 7 Sinuses 8 Hard Palate 9 Soft Palate B Larynx D Nasopharynx F Oropharynx	3 Electrons	Z None	Ø Intraoperative Z None

D   Radiation Oncology
9   Ear, Nose, Mouth and Throat
1   Brachytherapy

Treatment Site Character 4	Modal. Qualifier Character 5	Isotope Character 6	Qualifier Character 7
Ø Ear 1 Nose 3 Hypopharynx 4 Mouth 5 Tongue 6 Salivary Glands 7 Sinuses 8 Hard Palate 9 Soft Palate B Larynx D Nasopharynx F Oropharynx	9 High Dose Rate (HDR) B Low Dose Rate (LDR)	7 Cesium 137 (Cs-137) 8 Iridium 192 (Ir-192) 9 Iodine 125 (I-125) B Palladium 1Ø3 (Pd-1Ø3) C Californium 252 (Cf-252) Y Other Isotope	Z None

D   Radiation Oncology
9   Ear, Nose, Mouth and Throat
2   Stereotactic Radiosurgery

Treatment Site Character 4	Modal. Qualifier Character 5	Isotope Character 6	Qualifier Character 7

Ø Ear
1 Nose
4 Mouth
5 Tongue
6 Salivary Glands
7 Sinuses
8 Hard Palate
9 Soft Palate
B Larynx
C Pharynx
D Nasopharynx
	D Stereotactic Other Photon
	   Radiosurgery
	H Stereotactic Particulate
	   Radiosurgery
	J Stereotactic Gamma Beam
	   Radiosurgery
		Z None	Z None

D   **Radiation Oncology**
9   **Ear, Nose, Mouth and Throat**
Y   **Other Radiation**

Treatment Site Character 4	Modal. Qualifier Character 5	Isotope Character 6	Qualifier Character 7
0 Ear **1** Nose **5** Tongue **6** Salivary Glands **7** Sinuses **8** Hard Palate **9** Soft Palate	**7** Contact Radiation **8** Hyperthermia **F** Plaque Radiation	**Z** None	**Z** None
3 Hypopharynx **F** Oropharynx	**7** Contact Radiation **8** Hyperthermia	**Z** None	**Z** None
4 Mouth **B** Larynx **D** Nasopharynx	**7** Contact Radiation **8** Hyperthermia **C** Intraoperative Radiation Therapy (IORT) **F** Plaque Radiation	**Z** None	**Z** None
C Pharynx	**C** Intraoperative Radiation Therapy (IORT) **F** Plaque Radiation	**Z** None	**Z** None

D   **Radiation Oncology**
B   **Respiratory System**
0   **Beam Radiation**

Treatment Site Character 4	Modal. Qualifier Character 5	Isotope Character 6	Qualifier Character 7
0 Trachea **1** Bronchus **2** Lung **5** Pleura **6** Mediastinum **7** Chest Wall **8** Diaphragm	**0** Photons <1 MeV **1** Photons 1- 10 MeV **2** Photons >10 MeV **4** Heavy Particles (Protons, Ions) **5** Neutrons **6** Neutron Capture	**Z** None	**Z** None
0 Trachea **1** Bronchus **2** Lung **5** Pleura **6** Mediastinum **7** Chest Wall **8** Diaphragm	**3** Electrons	**Z** None	**0** Intraoperative **Z** None

D   **Radiation Oncology**
B   **Respiratory System**
1   **Brachytherapy**

Treatment Site Character 4	Modal. Qualifier Character 5	Isotope Character 6	Qualifier Character 7
0 Trachea **1** Bronchus **2** Lung **5** Pleura **6** Mediastinum **7** Chest Wall **8** Diaphragm	**9** High Dose Rate (HDR) **B** Low Dose Rate (LDR)	**7** Cesium 137 (Cs-137) **8** Iridium 192 (Ir-192) **9** Iodine 125 (I-125) **B** Palladium 103 (Pd-103) **C** Californium 252 (Cf-252) **Y** Other Isotope	**Z** None

D   **Radiation Oncology**
B   **Respiratory System**
2   **Stereotactic Radiosurgery**

Treatment Site Character 4	Modal. Qualifier Character 5	Isotope Character 6	Qualifier Character 7
0 Trachea **1** Bronchus **2** Lung **5** Pleura **6** Mediastinum **7** Chest Wall **8** Diaphragm	**D** Stereotactic Other Photon Radiosurgery **H** Stereotactic Particulate Radiosurgery **J** Stereotactic Gamma Beam Radiosurgery	**Z** None	**Z** None

D　Radiation Oncology
B　Respiratory System
Y　Other Radiation

Treatment Site Character 4	Modal. Qualifier Character 5	Isotope Character 6	Qualifier Character 7
0　Trachea 1　Bronchus 2　Lung 5　Pleura 6　Mediastinum 7　Chest Wall 8　Diaphragm	7　Contact Radiation 8　Hyperthermia F　Plaque Radiation	Z　None	Z　None

D　Radiation Oncology
D　Gastrointestinal System
0　Beam Radiation

Treatment Site Character 4	Modal. Qualifier Character 5	Isotope Character 6	Qualifier Character 7
0　Esophagus 1　Stomach 2　Duodenum 3　Jejunum 4　Ileum 5　Colon 7　Rectum	0　Photons <1 MeV 1　Photons 1- 10 MeV 2　Photons >10 MeV 4　Heavy Particles (Protons, Ions) 5　Neutrons 6　Neutron Capture	Z　None	Z　None
0　Esophagus 1　Stomach 2　Duodenum 3　Jejunum 4　Ileum 5　Colon 7　Rectum	3　Electrons	Z　None	0　Intraoperative Z　None

D　Radiation Oncology
D　Gastrointestinal System
1　Brachytherapy

Treatment Site Character 4	Modal. Qualifier Character 5	Isotope Character 6	Qualifier Character 7
0　Esophagus 1　Stomach 2　Duodenum 3　Jejunum 4　Ileum 5　Colon 7　Rectum	9　High Dose Rate (HDR) B　Low Dose Rate (LDR)	7　Cesium 137 (Cs-137) 8　Iridium 192 (Ir-192) 9　Iodine 125 (I-125) B　Palladium 103 (Pd-103) C　Californium 252 (Cf-252) Y　Other Isotope	Z　None

D　Radiation Oncology
D　Gastrointestinal System
2　Stereotactic Radiosurgery

Treatment Site Character 4	Modal. Qualifier Character 5	Isotope Character 6	Qualifier Character 7
0　Esophagus 1　Stomach 2　Duodenum 3　Jejunum 4　Ileum 5　Colon 7　Rectum	D　Stereotactic Other Photon Radiosurgery H　Stereotactic Particulate Radiosurgery J　Stereotactic Gamma Beam Radiosurgery	Z　None	Z　None

D Radiation Oncology
D Gastrointestinal System
Y Other Radiation

Treatment Site Character 4	Modal. Qualifier Character 5	Isotope Character 6	Qualifier Character 7
0 Esophagus	**7** Contact Radiation **8** Hyperthermia **F** Plaque Radiation **K** Laser Interstitial Thermal Therapy	**Z** None	**Z** None
1 Stomach **2** Duodenum **3** Jejunum **4** Ileum **5** Colon **7** Rectum	**7** Contact Radiation **8** Hyperthermia **C** Intraoperative Radiation Therapy (IORT) **F** Plaque Radiation **K** Laser Interstitial Thermal Therapy	**Z** None	**Z** None
8 Anus	**C** Intraoperative Radiation Therapy (IORT) **F** Plaque Radiation **K** Laser Interstitial Thermal Therapy	**Z** None	**Z** None

D Radiation Oncology
F Hepatobiliary System and Pancreas
0 Beam Radiation

Treatment Site Character 4	Modal. Qualifier Character 5	Isotope Character 6	Qualifier Character 7
0 Liver **1** Gallbladder **2** Bile Ducts **3** Pancreas	**0** Photons <1 MeV **1** Photons 1- 10 MeV **2** Photons >10 MeV **4** Heavy Particles (Protons, Ions) **5** Neutrons **6** Neutron Capture	**Z** None	**Z** None
0 Liver **1** Gallbladder **2** Bile Ducts **3** Pancreas	**3** Electrons	**Z** None	**0** Intraoperative **Z** None

D Radiation Oncology
F Hepatobiliary System and Pancreas
1 Brachytherapy

Treatment Site Character 4	Modal. Qualifier Character 5	Isotope Character 6	Qualifier Character 7
0 Liver **1** Gallbladder **2** Bile Ducts **3** Pancreas	**9** High Dose Rate (HDR) **B** Low Dose Rate (LDR)	**7** Cesium 137 (Cs-137) **8** Iridium 192 (Ir-192) **9** Iodine 125 (I-125) **B** Palladium 103 (Pd-103) **C** Californium 252 (Cf-252) **Y** Other Isotope	**Z** None

D Radiation Oncology
F Hepatobiliary System and Pancreas
2 Stereotactic Radiosurgery

Treatment Site Character 4	Modal. Qualifier Character 5	Isotope Character 6	Qualifier Character 7
0 Liver **1** Gallbladder **2** Bile Ducts **3** Pancreas	**D** Stereotactic Other Photon Radiosurgery **H** Stereotactic Particulate Radiosurgery **J** Stereotactic Gamma Beam Radiosurgery	**Z** None	**Z** None

D Radiation Oncology
F Hepatobiliary System and Pancreas
Y Other Radiation

Treatment Site Character 4	Modal. Qualifier Character 5	Isotope Character 6	Qualifier Character 7
0 Liver **1** Gallbladder **2** Bile Ducts **3** Pancreas	**7** Contact Radiation **8** Hyperthermia **C** Intraoperative Radiation Therapy (IORT) **F** Plaque Radiation **K** Laser Interstitial Thermal Therapy	**Z** None	**Z** None

Revised Text in **BLUE**

D   Radiation Oncology
G   Endocrine System
0   Beam Radiation

Treatment Site Character 4	Modal. Qualifier Character 5	Isotope Character 6	Qualifier Character 7
0 Pituitary Gland 1 Pineal Body 2 Adrenal Glands 4 Parathyroid Glands 5 Thyroid	0 Photons <1 MeV 1 Photons 1- 10 MeV 2 Photons >10 MeV 5 Neutrons 6 Neutron Capture	Z None	Z None
0 Pituitary Gland 1 Pineal Body 2 Adrenal Glands 4 Parathyroid Glands 5 Thyroid	3 Electrons	Z None	0 Intraoperative Z None

D   Radiation Oncology
G   Endocrine System
1   Brachytherapy

Treatment Site Character 4	Modal. Qualifier Character 5	Isotope Character 6	Qualifier Character 7
0 Pituitary Gland 1 Pineal Body 2 Adrenal Glands 4 Parathyroid Glands 5 Thyroid	9 High Dose Rate (HDR) B Low Dose Rate (LDR)	7 Cesium 137 (Cs-137) 8 Iridium 192 (Ir-192) 9 Iodine 125 (I-125) B Palladium 103 (Pd-103) C Californium 252 (Cf-252) Y Other Isotope	Z None

D   Radiation Oncology
G   Endocrine System
2   Stereotactic Radiosurgery

Treatment Site Character 4	Modal. Qualifier Character 5	Isotope Character 6	Qualifier Character 7

0 Pituitary Gland
1 Pineal Body
2 Adrenal Glands
4 Parathyroid Glands
5 Thyroid
	D Stereotactic Other Photon
	   Radiosurgery
	H Stereotactic Particulate
	   Radiosurgery
	J Stereotactic Gamma Beam
	   Radiosurgery
		Z None	Z None

D   Radiation Oncology
G   Endocrine System
Y   Other Radiation

Treatment Site Character 4	Modal. Qualifier Character 5	Isotope Character 6	Qualifier Character 7
0 Pituitary Gland 1 Pineal Body 2 Adrenal Glands 4 Parathyroid Glands 5 Thyroid	7 Contact Radiation 8 Hyperthermia F Plaque Radiation K Laser Interstitial Thermal Therapy	Z None	Z None

D   **Radiation Oncology**
H   **Skin**
0   **Beam Radiation**

Treatment Site Character 4	Modal. Qualifier Character 5	Isotope Character 6	Qualifier Character 7
2 Skin, Face 3 Skin, Neck 4 Skin, Arm 6 Skin, Chest 7 Skin, Back 8 Skin, Abdomen 9 Skin, Buttock B Skin, Leg	0 Photons <1 MeV 1 Photons 1- 10 MeV 2 Photons >10 MeV 4 Heavy Particles (Protons, Ions) 5 Neutrons 6 Neutron Capture	Z None	Z None
2 Skin, Face 3 Skin, Neck 4 Skin, Arm 6 Skin, Chest 7 Skin, Back 8 Skin, Abdomen 9 Skin, Buttock B Skin, Leg	3 Electrons	Z None	0 Intraoperative Z None

D   **Radiation Oncology**
H   **Skin**
Y   **Other Radiation**

Treatment Site Character 4	Modal. Qualifier Character 5	Isotope Character 6	Qualifier Character 7
2 Skin, Face 3 Skin, Neck 4 Skin, Arm 6 Skin, Chest 7 Skin, Back 8 Skin, Abdomen 9 Skin, Buttock B Skin, Leg	7 Contact Radiation 8 Hyperthermia F Plaque Radiation	Z None	Z None
5 Skin, Hand C Skin, Foot	F Plaque Radiation	Z None	Z None

D   **Radiation Oncology**
M   **Breast**
0   **Beam Radiation**

Treatment Site Character 4	Modal. Qualifier Character 5	Isotope Character 6	Qualifier Character 7
0 Breast, Left 1 Breast, Right	0 Photons <1 MeV 1 Photons 1- 10 MeV 2 Photons >10 MeV 4 Heavy Particles (Protons, Ions) 5 Neutrons 6 Neutron Capture	Z None	Z None
0 Breast, Left 1 Breast, Right	3 Electrons	Z None	0 Intraoperative Z None

D   **Radiation Oncology**
M   **Breast**
1   **Brachytherapy**

Treatment Site Character 4	Modal. Qualifier Character 5	Isotope Character 6	Qualifier Character 7
0 Breast, Left 1 Breast, Right	9 High Dose Rate (HDR) B Low Dose Rate (LDR)	7 Cesium 137 (Cs-137) 8 Iridium 192 (Ir-192) 9 Iodine 125 (I-125) B Palladium 103 (Pd-103) C Californium 252 (Cf-252) Y Other Isotope	Z None

D   **Radiation Oncology**
M   **Breast**
2   **Stereotactic Radiosurgery**

Treatment Site Character 4	Modal. Qualifier Character 5	Isotope Character 6	Qualifier Character 7

Ø Breast, Left
1 Breast, Right
	D Stereotactic Other Photon
	   Radiosurgery
	H Stereotactic Particulate
	   Radiosurgery
	J Stereotactic Gamma Beam
	   Radiosurgery
		Z None	Z None

D   **Radiation Oncology**
M   **Breast**
Y   **Other Radiation**

Treatment Site Character 4	Modal. Qualifier Character 5	Isotope Character 6	Qualifier Character 7
Ø Breast, Left 1 Breast, Right	7 Contact Radiation 8 Hyperthermia F Plaque Radiation	Z None	Z None

D   **Radiation Oncology**
P   **Musculoskeletal System**
Ø   **Beam Radiation**

Treatment Site Character 4	Modal. Qualifier Character 5	Isotope Character 6	Qualifier Character 7
Ø Skull 2 Maxilla 3 Mandible 4 Sternum 5 Rib(s) 6 Humerus 7 Radius/Ulna 8 Pelvic Bones 9 Femur B Tibia/Fibula C Other Bone	Ø Photons <1 MeV 1 Photons 1- 1Ø MeV 2 Photons >1Ø MeV 4 Heavy Particles (Protons, Ions) 5 Neutrons 6 Neutron Capture	Z None	Z None
Ø Skull 2 Maxilla 3 Mandible 4 Sternum 5 Rib(s) 6 Humerus 7 Radius/Ulna 8 Pelvic Bones 9 Femur B Tibia/Fibula C Other Bone	3 Electrons	Z None	Ø Intraoperative Z None

D   **Radiation Oncology**
P   **Musculoskeletal System**
Y   **Other Radiation**

Treatment Site Character 4	Modal. Qualifier Character 5	Isotope Character 6	Qualifier Character 7
Ø Skull 2 Maxilla 3 Mandible 4 Sternum 5 Rib(s) 6 Humerus 7 Radius/Ulna 8 Pelvic Bones 9 Femur B Tibia/Fibula C Other Bone	7 Contact Radiation 8 Hyperthermia F Plaque Radiation	Z None	Z None

Revised Text in **BLUE**

Radiation Oncology

DT0–DU0

D Radiation Oncology
T Urinary System
0 Beam Radiation

Treatment Site Character 4	Modal. Qualifier Character 5	Isotope Character 6	Qualifier Character 7
0 Kidney 1 Ureter 2 Bladder 3 Urethra	0 Photons <1 MeV 1 Photons 1- 10 MeV 2 Photons >10 MeV 4 Heavy Particles (Protons, Ions) 5 Neutrons 6 Neutron Capture	Z None	Z None
0 Kidney 1 Ureter 2 Bladder 3 Urethra	3 Electrons	Z None	0 Intraoperative Z None

D Radiation Oncology
T Urinary System
1 Brachytherapy

Treatment Site Character 4	Modal. Qualifier Character 5	Isotope Character 6	Qualifier Character 7
0 Kidney 1 Ureter 2 Bladder 3 Urethra	9 High Dose Rate (HDR) B Low Dose Rate (LDR)	7 Cesium 137 (Cs-137) 8 Iridium 192 (Ir-192) 9 Iodine 125 (I-125) B Palladium 103 (Pd-103) C Californium 252 (Cf-252) Y Other Isotope	Z None

D Radiation Oncology
T Urinary System
2 Stereotactic Radiosurgery

Treatment Site Character 4	Modal. Qualifier Character 5	Isotope Character 6	Qualifier Character 7
0 Kidney 1 Ureter 2 Bladder 3 Urethra	D Stereotactic Other Photon Radiosurgery H Stereotactic Particulate Radiosurgery J Stereotactic Gamma Beam Radiosurgery	Z None	Z None

D Radiation Oncology
T Urinary System
Y Other Radiation

Treatment Site Character 4	Modal. Qualifier Character 5	Isotope Character 6	Qualifier Character 7
0 Kidney 1 Ureter 2 Bladder 3 Urethra	7 Contact Radiation 8 Hyperthermia C Intraoperative Radiation Therapy (IORT) F Plaque Radiation	Z None	Z None

D Radiation Oncology
U Female Reproductive System
0 Beam Radiation

Treatment Site Character 4	Modal. Qualifier Character 5	Isotope Character 6	Qualifier Character 7
0 Ovary 1 Cervix 2 Uterus	0 Photons <1 MeV 1 Photons 1- 10 MeV 2 Photons >10 MeV 4 Heavy Particles (Protons, Ions) 5 Neutrons 6 Neutron Capture	Z None	Z None
0 Ovary 1 Cervix 2 Uterus	3 Electrons	Z None	0 Intraoperative Z None

D Radiation Oncology
U Female Reproductive System
1 Brachytherapy

Treatment Site Character 4	Modal. Qualifier Character 5	Isotope Character 6	Qualifier Character 7
0 Ovary 1 Cervix 2 Uterus	9 High Dose Rate (HDR) B Low Dose Rate (LDR)	7 Cesium 137 (Cs-137) 8 Iridium 192 (Ir-192) 9 Iodine 125 (I-125) B Palladium 103 (Pd-103) C Californium 252 (Cf-252) Y Other Isotope	Z None

D Radiation Oncology
U Female Reproductive System
2 Stereotactic Radiosurgery

Treatment Site Character 4	Modal. Qualifier Character 5	Isotope Character 6	Qualifier Character 7
0 Ovary 1 Cervix 2 Uterus	D Stereotactic Other Photon Radiosurgery H Stereotactic Particulate Radiosurgery J Stereotactic Gamma Beam Radiosurgery	Z None	Z None

D Radiation Oncology
U Female Reproductive System
Y Other Radiation

Treatment Site Character 4	Modal. Qualifier Character 5	Isotope Character 6	Qualifier Character 7
0 Ovary 1 Cervix 2 Uterus	7 Contact Radiation 8 Hyperthermia C Intraoperative Radiation Therapy (IORT) F Plaque Radiation	Z None	Z None

D Radiation Oncology
V Male Reproductive System
0 Beam Radiation

Treatment Site Character 4	Modal. Qualifier Character 5	Isotope Character 6	Qualifier Character 7
0 Prostate 1 Testis	0 Photons <1 MeV 1 Photons 1- 10 MeV 2 Photons >10 MeV 4 Heavy Particles (Protons, Ions) 5 Neutrons 6 Neutron Capture	Z None	Z None
0 Prostate 1 Testis	3 Electrons	Z None	0 Intraoperative Z None

D Radiation Oncology
V Male Reproductive System
1 Brachytherapy

Treatment Site Character 4	Modal. Qualifier Character 5	Isotope Character 6	Qualifier Character 7
0 Prostate 1 Testis	9 High Dose Rate (HDR) B Low Dose Rate (LDR)	7 Cesium 137 (Cs-137) 8 Iridium 192 (Ir-192) 9 Iodine 125 (I-125) B Palladium 103 (Pd-103) C Californium 252 (Cf-252) Y Other Isotope	Z None

        Revised Text in **BLUE**

Radiation Oncology

D   Radiation Oncology
V   Male Reproductive System
2   Stereotactic Radiosurgery

Treatment Site Character 4	Modal. Qualifier Character 5	Isotope Character 6	Qualifier Character 7
Ø Prostate **1** Testis	**D** Stereotactic Other Photon Radiosurgery **H** Stereotactic Particulate Radiosurgery **J** Stereotactic Gamma Beam Radiosurgery	**Z** None	**Z** None

D   Radiation Oncology
V   Male Reproductive System
Y   Other Radiation

Treatment Site Character 4	Modal. Qualifier Character 5	Isotope Character 6	Qualifier Character 7
Ø Prostate	**7** Contact Radiation **8** Hyperthermia **C** Intraoperative Radiation Therapy (IORT) **F** Plaque Radiation	**Z** None	**Z** None
1 Testis	**7** Contact Radiation **8** Hyperthermia **F** Plaque Radiation	**Z** None	**Z** None

D   Radiation Oncology
W   Anatomical Regions
Ø   Beam Radiation

Treatment Site Character 4	Modal. Qualifier Character 5	Isotope Character 6	Qualifier Character 7
1 Head and Neck **2** Chest **3** Abdomen **4** Hemibody **5** Whole Body **6** Pelvic Region	**Ø** Photons <1 MeV **1** Photons 1- 1Ø MeV **2** Photons >1Ø MeV **4** Heavy Particles (Protons, Ions) **5** Neutrons **6** Neutron Capture	**Z** None	**Z** None
1 Head and Neck **2** Chest **3** Abdomen **4** Hemibody **5** Whole Body **6** Pelvic Region	**3** Electrons	**Z** None	**Ø** Intraoperative **Z** None

D   Radiation Oncology
W   Anatomical Regions
1   Brachytherapy

Treatment Site Character 4	Modal. Qualifier Character 5	Isotope Character 6	Qualifier Character 7
1 Head and Neck **2** Chest **3** Abdomen **6** Pelvic Region	**9** High Dose Rate (HDR) **B** Low Dose Rate (LDR)	**7** Cesium 137 (Cs-137) **8** Iridium 192 (Ir-192) **9** Iodine 125 (I-125) **B** Palladium 1Ø3 (Pd-1Ø3) **C** Californium 252 (Cf-252) **Y** Other Isotope	**Z** None

D   Radiation Oncology
W   Anatomical Regions
2   Stereotactic Radiosurgery

Treatment Site Character 4	Modal. Qualifier Character 5	Isotope Character 6	Qualifier Character 7
1 Head and Neck **2** Chest **3** Abdomen **6** Pelvic Region	**D** Stereotactic Other Photon Radiosurgery **H** Stereotactic Particulate Radiosurgery **J** Stereotactic Gamma Beam Radiosurgery	**Z** None	**Z** None

D   Radiation Oncology
W   Anatomical Regions
Y   Other Radiation

Treatment Site Character 4	Modal. Qualifier Character 5	Isotope Character 6	Qualifier Character 7
1 Head and Neck **2** Chest **3** Abdomen **4** Hemibody **5** Whole Body **6** Pelvic Region	**7** Contact Radiation **8** Hyperthermia **F** Plaque Radiation	**Z** None	**Z** None
5 Whole Body	**G** Isotope Administration	**D** Iodine 131 (I-131) **F** Phosphorus 32 (P-32) **G** Strontium 89 (Sr-89) **H** Strontium 90 (Sr-90) **Y** Other Isotope	**Z** None

Physical Rehabilitation and Diagnostic Audiology F00–F15

F   Physical Rehabilitation and Diagnostic Audiology
0   Rehabilitation
0   Speech Assessment   Measurement of speech and related functions

Body System/Region Character 4	Type Qualifier Character 5	Equipment Character 6	Qualifier Character 7
3 Neurological System - Whole Body	G Communicative/Cognitive Integration Skills	K Audiovisual M Augmentative / Alternative Communication P Computer Y Other Equipment Z None	Z None
Z None	0 Filtered Speech 3 Staggered Spondaic Word Q Performance Intensity Phonetically Balanced Speech Discrimination R Brief Tone Stimuli S Distorted Speech T Dichotic Stimuli V Temporal Ordering of Stimuli W Masking Patterns	1 Audiometer 2 Sound Field / Booth K Audiovisual Z None	Z None
Z None	1 Speech Threshold 2 Speech/Word Recognition	1 Audiometer 2 Sound Field / Booth 9 Cochlear Implant K Audiovisual Z None	Z None
Z None	4 Sensorineural Acuity Level	1 Audiometer 2 Sound Field / Booth Z None	Z None
Z None	5 Synthetic Sentence Identification	1 Audiometer 2 Sound Field / Booth 9 Cochlear Implant K Audiovisual	Z None
Z None	6 Speech and/or Language Screening 7 Nonspoken Language 8 Receptive/Expressive Language C Aphasia G Communicative/Cognitive Integration Skills L Augmentative/Alternative Communication System	K Audiovisual M Augmentative / Alternative Communication P Computer Y Other Equipment Z None	Z None
Z None	9 Articulation/Phonology	K Audiovisual P Computer Q Speech Analysis Y Other Equipment Z None	Z None
Z None	B Motor Speech	K Audiovisual N Biosensory Feedback P Computer Q Speech Analysis T Aerodynamic Function Y Other Equipment Z None	Z None
Z None	D Fluency	K Audiovisual N Biosensory Feedback P Computer Q Speech Analysis S Voice Analysis T Aerodynamic Function Y Other Equipment Z None	Z None
Z None	F Voice	K Audiovisual N Biosensory Feedback P Computer S Voice Analysis T Aerodynamic Function Y Other Equipment Z None	Z None
Z None	H Bedside Swallowing and Oral Function P Oral Peripheral Mechanism	Y Other Equipment Z None	Z None
Z None	J Instrumental Swallowing and Oral Function	T Aerodynamic Function W Swallowing Y Other Equipment	Z None

F00 Continued on next page

    Revised Text in **BLUE**   © 2011 Ingenix, Inc

F Physical Rehabilitation and Diagnostic Audiology
Ø Rehabilitation
Ø Speech Assessment Measurement of speech and related functions

F00 Continued

Body System/Region Character 4	Type Qualifier Character 5	Equipment Character 6	Qualifier Character 7
Z None	K Orofacial Myofunctional	K Audiovisual P Computer Y Other Equipment Z None	Z None
Z None	M Voice Prosthetic	K Audiovisual P Computer S Voice Analysis V Speech Prosthesis Y Other Equipment Z None	Z None
Z None	N Non-invasive Instrumental Status	N Biosensory Feedback P Computer Q Speech Analysis S Voice Analysis T Aerodynamic Function Y Other Equipment	Z None
Z None	X Other Specified Central Auditory Processing	Z None	Z None

F Physical Rehabilitation and Diagnostic Audiology
Ø Rehabilitation
1 Motor and/or Nerve Function Assessment Measurement of motor, nerve, and related functions

Body System/Region Character 4	Type Qualifier Character 5	Equipment Character 6	Qualifier Character 7
Ø Neurological System - Head and Neck 1 Neurological System - Upper Back / Upper Extremity 2 Neurological System - Lower Back / Lower Extremity 3 Neurological System - Whole Body	1 Integumentary Integrity 3 Coordination/Dexterity 4 Motor Function G Reflex Integrity	Z None	Z None
Ø Neurological System - Head and Neck 1 Neurological System - Upper Back / Upper Extremity 2 Neurological System - Lower Back / Lower Extremity 3 Neurological System - Whole Body D Integumentary System - Head and Neck F Integumentary System - Upper Back / Upper Extremity G Integumentary System - Lower Back / Lower Extremity H Integumentary System - Whole Body J Musculoskeletal System - Head and Neck K Musculoskeletal System - Upper Back / Upper Extremity L Musculoskeletal System - Lower Back / Lower Extremity M Musculoskeletal System - Whole Body	5 Range of Motion and Joint Integrity 6 Sensory Awareness/Processing/Integrity	Y Other Equipment Z None	Z None
Ø Neurological System - Head and Neck 1 Neurological System - Upper Back / Upper Extremity 2 Neurological System - Lower Back / Lower Extremity 3 Neurological System - Whole Body D Integumentary System - Head and Neck F Integumentary System - Upper Back / Upper Extremity G Integumentary System - Lower Back / Lower Extremity H Integumentary System - Whole Body J Musculoskeletal System - Head and Neck K Musculoskeletal System - Upper Back / Upper Extremity L Musculoskeletal System - Lower Back / Lower Extremity M Musculoskeletal System - Whole Body N Genitourinary System	Ø Muscle Performance	E Orthosis F Assistive, Adaptive, Supportive or Protective U Prosthesis Y Other Equipment Z None	Z None

F01 Continued on next page

F   **Physical Rehabilitation and Diagnostic Audiology**   *F01 Continued*
0   **Rehabilitation**
1   **Motor and/or Nerve Function Assessment**   Measurement of motor, nerve, and related functions

Body System/Region Character 4	Type Qualifier Character 5	Equipment Character 6	Qualifier Character 7
D Integumentary System - Head and Neck **F** Integumentary System - Upper Back / Upper Extremity **G** Integumentary System - Lower Back / Lower Extremity **H** Integumentary System - Whole Body **J** Musculoskeletal System - Head and Neck **K** Musculoskeletal System - Upper Back / Upper Extremity **L** Musculoskeletal System - Lower Back / Lower Extremity **M** Musculoskeletal System - Whole Body	**1** Integumentary Integrity	**Z** None	**Z** None
Z None	**2** Visual Motor Integration	**K** Audiovisual **M** Augmentative / Alternative Communication **N** Biosensory Feedback **P** Computer **Q** Speech Analysis **S** Voice Analysis **Y** Other Equipment **Z** None	**Z** None
Z None	**7** Facial Nerve Function	**7** Electrophysiologic	**Z** None
Z None	**8** Neurophysiologic Intraoperative	**7** Electrophysiologic **J** Somatosensory	**Z** None
Z None	**9** Somatosensory Evoked Potentials	**J** Somatosensory	**Z** None
Z None	**B** Bed Mobility **C** Transfer **F** Wheelchair Mobility	**E** Orthosis **F** Assistive, Adaptive, Supportive or Protective **U** Prosthesis **Z** None	**Z** None
Z None	**D** Gait and/or Balance	**E** Orthosis **F** Assistive, Adaptive, Supportive or Protective **U** Prosthesis **Y** Other Equipment **Z** None	**Z** None

F   **Physical Rehabilitation and Diagnostic Audiology**
0   **Rehabilitation**
2   **Activities of Daily Living Assessment**   Measurement of functional level for activities of daily living

Body System/Region Character 4	Type Qualifier Character 5	Equipment Character 6	Qualifier Character 7
0 Neurological System - Head and Neck	**9** Cranial Nerve Integrity **D** Neuromotor Development	**Y** Other Equipment **Z** None	**Z** None
1 Neurological System - Upper Back / Upper Extremity **2** Neurological System - Lower Back / Lower Extremity **3** Neurological System - Whole Body	**D** Neuromotor Development	**Y** Other Equipment **Z** None	**Z** None
4 Circulatory System - Head and Neck **5** Circulatory System - Upper Back / Upper Extremity **6** Circulatory System - Lower Back / Lower Extremity **7** Circulatory System - Whole Body **8** Respiratory System - Head and Neck **9** Respiratory System - Upper Back / Upper Extremity **B** Respiratory System - Lower Back / Lower Extremity **C** Respiratory System - Whole Body	**G** Ventilation, Respiration and Circulation	**C** Mechanical **G** Aerobic Endurance and Conditioning **Y** Other Equipment **Z** None	**Z** None
7 Circulatory System - Whole Body **C** Respiratory System - Whole Body	**7** Aerobic Capacity and Endurance	**E** Orthosis **G** Aerobic Endurance and Conditioning **U** Prosthesis **Y** Other Equipment **Z** None	**Z** None

F02 Continued on next page

        Revised Text in **BLUE**   © 2011 Ingenix, Inc

F02 Continued

F   Physical Rehabilitation and Diagnostic Audiology
Ø   Rehabilitation
2   Activities of Daily Living Assessment Measurement of functional level for activities of daily living

Body System/Region Character 4	Type Qualifier Character 5	Equipment Character 6	Qualifier Character 7
Z None	Ø Bathing/Showering 1 Dressing 3 Grooming/Personal Hygiene 4 Home Management	E Orthosis F Assistive, Adaptive, Supportive or Protective U Prosthesis Z None	Z None
Z None	2 Feeding/Eating 8 Anthropometric Characteristics F Pain	Y Other Equipment Z None	Z None
Z None	5 Perceptual Processing	K Audiovisual M Augmentative / Alternative Communication N Biosensory Feedback P Computer Q Speech Analysis S Voice Analysis Y Other Equipment Z None	Z None
Z None	6 Psychosocial Skills	Z None	Z None
Z None	B Environmental, Home and Work Barriers C Ergonomics and Body Mechanics	E Orthosis F Assistive, Adaptive, Supportive or Protective U Prosthesis Y Other Equipment Z None	Z None
Z None	H Vocational Activities and Functional Community or Work Reintegration Skills	E Orthosis F Assistive, Adaptive, Supportive or Protective G Aerobic Endurance and Conditioning U Prosthesis Y Other Equipment Z None	Z None

F   Physical Rehabilitation and Diagnostic Audiology
Ø   Rehabilitation
6   Speech Treatment Application of techniques to improve, augment, or compensate for speech and related functional impairment

Body System/Region Character 4	Type Qualifier Character 5	Equipment Character 6	Qualifier Character 7
3 Neurological System - Whole Body	6 Communicative/Cognitive Integration Skills	K Audiovisual M Augmentative / Alternative Communication P Computer Y Other Equipment Z None	Z None
Z None	Ø Nonspoken Language 3 Aphasia 6 Communicative/Cognitive Integration Skills	K Audiovisual M Augmentative / Alternative Communication P Computer Y Other Equipment Z None	Z None
Z None	1 Speech-Language Pathology and Related Disorders Counseling 2 Speech-Language Pathology and Related Disorders Prevention	K Audiovisual Z None	Z None
Z None	4 Articulation/Phonology	K Audiovisual P Computer Q Speech Analysis T Aerodynamic Function Y Other Equipment Z None	Z None
Z None	5 Aural Rehabilitation	K Audiovisual L Assistive Listening M Augmentative / Alternative Communication N Biosensory Feedback P Computer Q Speech Analysis S Voice Analysis Y Other Equipment Z None	Z None

F06 Continued on next page

F   **Physical Rehabilitation and Diagnostic Audiology**   *F06 Continued*
0   **Rehabilitation**
6   **Speech Treatment**   Application of techniques to improve, augment, or compensate for speech and related functional impairment

Body System/Region Character 4	Type Qualifier Character 5	Equipment Character 6	Qualifier Character 7
Z None	**7** Fluency	**4** Electroacoustic Immitance / Acoustic Reflex **K** Audiovisual **N** Biosensory Feedback **Q** Speech Analysis **S** Voice Analysis **T** Aerodynamic Function **Y** Other Equipment **Z** None	**Z** None
Z None	**8** Motor Speech	**K** Audiovisual **N** Biosensory Feedback **P** Computer **Q** Speech Analysis **S** Voice Analysis **T** Aerodynamic Function **Y** Other Equipment **Z** None	**Z** None
Z None	**9** Orofacial Myofunctional	**K** Audiovisual **P** Computer **Y** Other Equipment **Z** None	**Z** None
Z None	**B** Receptive/Expressive Language	**K** Audiovisual **L** Assistive Listening **M** Augmentative / Alternative Communication **P** Computer **Y** Other Equipment **Z** None	**Z** None
Z None	**C** Voice	**K** Audiovisual **N** Biosensory Feedback **P** Computer **S** Voice Analysis **T** Aerodynamic Function **V** Speech Prosthesis **Y** Other Equipment **Z** None	**Z** None
Z None	**D** Swallowing Dysfunction	**M** Augmentative / Alternative Communication **T** Aerodynamic Function **V** Speech Prosthesis **Y** Other Equipment **Z** None	**Z** None

Revised Text in **BLUE**

F   Physical Rehabilitation and Diagnostic Audiology
0   Rehabilitation
7   Motor Treatment   Exercise or activities to increase or facilitate motor function

Body System/Region Character 4	Type Qualifier Character 5	Equipment Character 6	Qualifier Character 7
0 Neurological System - Head and Neck **1** Neurological System - Upper Back / Upper Extremity **2** Neurological System - Lower Back / Lower Extremity **3** Neurological System - Whole Body **4** Circulatory System - Head and Neck **5** Circulatory System - Upper Back / Upper Extremity **6** Circulatory System - Lower Back / Lower Extremity **7** Circulatory System - Whole Body **8** Respiratory System - Head and Neck **9** Respiratory System - Upper Back / Upper Extremity **B** Respiratory System - Lower Back / Lower Extremity **C** Respiratory System - Whole Body **D** Integumentary System - Head and Neck **F** Integumentary System - Upper Back / Upper Extremity **G** Integumentary System - Lower Back / Lower Extremity **H** Integumentary System - Whole Body **J** Musculoskeletal System - Head and Neck **K** Musculoskeletal System - Upper Back / Upper Extremity **L** Musculoskeletal System - Lower Back / Lower Extremity **M** Musculoskeletal System - Whole Body **N** Genitourinary System	**6** Therapeutic Exercise	**B** Physical Agents **C** Mechanical **D** Electrotherapeutic **E** Orthosis **F** Assistive, Adaptive, Supportive or Protective **G** Aerobic Endurance and Conditioning **H** Mechanical or Electromechanical **U** Prosthesis **Y** Other Equipment **Z** None	**Z** None
0 Neurological System - Head and Neck **1** Neurological System - Upper Back / Upper Extremity **2** Neurological System - Lower Back / Lower Extremity **3** Neurological System - Whole Body **D** Integumentary System - Head and Neck **F** Integumentary System - Upper Back / Upper Extremity **G** Integumentary System - Lower Back / Lower Extremity **H** Integumentary System - Whole Body **J** Musculoskeletal System - Head and Neck **K** Musculoskeletal System - Upper Back / Upper Extremity **L** Musculoskeletal System - Lower Back / Lower Extremity **M** Musculoskeletal System - Whole Body	**0** Range of Motion and Joint Mobility **1** Muscle Performance **2** Coordination/Dexterity **3** Motor Function	**E** Orthosis **F** Assistive, Adaptive, Supportive or Protective **U** Prosthesis **Y** Other Equipment **Z** None	**Z** None
0 Neurological System - Head and Neck **1** Neurological System - Upper Back / Upper Extremity **2** Neurological System - Lower Back / Lower Extremity **3** Neurological System - Whole Body **D** Integumentary System - Head and Neck **F** Integumentary System - Upper Back / Upper Extremity **G** Integumentary System - Lower Back / Lower Extremity **H** Integumentary System - Whole Body **J** Musculoskeletal System - Head and Neck **K** Musculoskeletal System - Upper Back / Upper Extremity **L** Musculoskeletal System - Lower Back / Lower Extremity **M** Musculoskeletal System - Whole Body	**7** Manual Therapy Techniques	**Z** None	**Z** None

F07 Continued on next page

F Physical Rehabilitation and Diagnostic Audiology
0 Rehabilitation
7 Motor Treatment   Exercise or activities to increase or facilitate motor function

F07 Continued

Body System/Region Character 4	Type Qualifier Character 5	Equipment Character 6	Qualifier Character 7
N Genitourinary System	1 Muscle Performance	E Orthosis F Assistive, Adaptive, Supportive or Protective U Prosthesis Y Other Equipment Z None	Z None
Z None	4 Wheelchair Mobility	D Electrotherapeutic E Orthosis F Assistive, Adaptive, Supportive or Protective U Prosthesis Y Other Equipment Z None	Z None
Z None	5 Bed Mobility	C Mechanical E Orthosis F Assistive, Adaptive, Supportive or Protective U Prosthesis Y Other Equipment Z None	Z None
Z None	8 Transfer Training	C Mechanical D Electrotherapeutic E Orthosis F Assistive, Adaptive, Supportive or Protective U Prosthesis Y Other Equipment Z None	Z None
Z None	9 Gait Training/Functional Ambulation	C Mechanical D Electrotherapeutic E Orthosis F Assistive, Adaptive, Supportive or Protective G Aerobic Endurance and Conditioning U Prosthesis Y Other Equipment Z None	Z None

F Physical Rehabilitation and Diagnostic Audiology
0 Rehabilitation
8 Activities of Daily Living Treatment   Exercise or activities to facilitate functional competence for activities of daily living

Body System/Region Character 4	Type Qualifier Character 5	Equipment Character 6	Qualifier Character 7
D Integumentary System - Head and Neck F Integumentary System - Upper Back / Upper Extremity G Integumentary System - Lower Back / Lower Extremity H Integumentary System - Whole Body J Musculoskeletal System - Head and Neck K Musculoskeletal System - Upper Back / Upper Extremity L Musculoskeletal System - Lower Back / Lower Extremity M Musculoskeletal System - Whole Body	5 Wound Management	B Physical Agents C Mechanical D Electrotherapeutic E Orthosis F Assistive, Adaptive, Supportive or Protective U Prosthesis Y Other Equipment Z None	Z None
Z None	0 Bathing/Showering Techniques 1 Dressing Techniques 2 Grooming/Personal Hygiene	E Orthosis F Assistive, Adaptive, Supportive or Protective U Prosthesis Y Other Equipment Z None	Z None
Z None	3 Feeding/Eating	C Mechanical D Electrotherapeutic E Orthosis F Assistive, Adaptive, Supportive or Protective U Prosthesis Y Other Equipment Z None	Z None

F08 Continued on next page

 © 2011 Ingenix, Inc

F   **Physical Rehabilitation and Diagnostic Audiology**   *F08 Continued*
0   **Rehabilitation**
8   **Activities of Daily Living Treatment**   Exercise or activities to facilitate functional competence for activities of daily living

Body System/Region Character 4	Type Qualifier Character 5	Equipment Character 6	Qualifier Character 7
Z None	4 Home Management	D Electrotherapeutic E Orthosis F Assistive, Adaptive, Supportive or Protective U Prosthesis Y Other Equipment Z None	Z None
Z None	6 Psychosocial Skills	Z None	Z None
Z None	7 Vocational Activities and Functional Community or Work Reintegration Skills	B Physical Agents C Mechanical D Electrotherapeutic E Orthosis F Assistive, Adaptive, Supportive or Protective G Aerobic Endurance and Conditioning U Prosthesis Y Other Equipment Z None	Z None

F   **Physical Rehabilitation and Diagnostic Audiology**
0   **Rehabilitation**
9   **Hearing Treatment**   Application of techniques to improve, augment, or compensate for hearing and related functional impairment

Body System/Region Character 4	Type Qualifier Character 5	Equipment Character 6	Qualifier Character 7
Z None	0 Hearing and Related Disorders Counseling 1 Hearing and Related Disorders Prevention	K Audiovisual Z None	Z None
Z None	2 Auditory Processing	K Audiovisual L Assistive Listening P Computer Y Other Equipment Z None	Z None
Z None	3 Cerumen Management	X Cerumen Management Z None	Z None

F   **Physical Rehabilitation and Diagnostic Audiology**
0   **Rehabilitation**
B   **Cochlear Implant Treatment**   Application of techniques to improve the communication abilities of individuals with cochlear implant

Body System/Region Character 4	Type Qualifier Character 5	Equipment Character 6	Qualifier Character 7
Z None	0 Cochlear Implant Rehabilitation	1 Audiometer 2 Sound Field / Booth 9 Cochlear Implant K Audiovisual P Computer Y Other Equipment	Z None

F   **Physical Rehabilitation and Diagnostic Audiology**
Ø   **Rehabilitation**
C   **Vestibular Treatment**   Application of techniques to improve, augment, or compensate for vestibular and related functional impairment

Body System/Region Character 4	Type Qualifier Character 5	Equipment Character 6	Qualifier Character 7
3 Neurological System - Whole Body **H** Integumentary System - Whole Body **M** Musculoskeletal System - Whole Body	**3** Postural Control	**E** Orthosis **F** Assistive, Adaptive, Supportive or Protective **U** Prosthesis **Y** Other Equipment **Z** None	**Z** None
Z None	**Ø** Vestibular	**8** Vestibular / Balance **Z** None	**Z** None
Z None	**1** Perceptual Processing **2** Visual Motor Integration	**K** Audiovisual **L** Assistive Listening **N** Biosensory Feedback **P** Computer **Q** Speech Analysis **S** Voice Analysis **T** Aerodynamic Function **Y** Other Equipment **Z** None	**Z** None

F   **Physical Rehabilitation and Diagnostic Audiology**
Ø   **Rehabilitation**
D   **Device Fitting**   Fitting of a device designed to facilitate or support achievement of a higher level of function

Body System/Region Character 4	Type Qualifier Character 5	Equipment Character 6	Qualifier Character 7
Z None	**Ø** Tinnitus Masker	**5** Hearing Aid Selection / Fitting / Test **Z** None	**Z** None
Z None	**1** Monaural Hearing Aid **2** Binaural Hearing Aid **5** Assistive Listening Device	**1** Audiometer **2** Sound Field / Booth **5** Hearing Aid Selection / Fitting / Test **K** Audiovisual **L** Assistive Listening **Z** None	**Z** None
Z None	**3** Augmentative/Alternative Communication System	**M** Augmentative / Alternative Communication	**Z** None
Z None	**4** Voice Prosthetic	**S** Voice Analysis **V** Speech Prosthesis	**Z** None
Z None	**6** Dynamic Orthosis **7** Static Orthosis **8** Prosthesis **9** Assistive, Adaptive, Supportive or Protective Devices	**E** Orthosis **F** Assistive, Adaptive, Supportive or Protective **U** Prosthesis **Z** None	**Z** None

F   Physical Rehabilitation and Diagnostic Audiology
Ø   Rehabilitation
F   Caregiver Training   Training in activities to support patient's optimal level of function

Body System/Region Character 4	Type Qualifier Character 5	Equipment Character 6	Qualifier Character 7
Z None	Ø Bathing/Showering Technique 1 Dressing 2 Feeding and Eating 3 Grooming/Personal Hygiene 4 Bed Mobility 5 Transfer 6 Wheelchair Mobility 7 Therapeutic Exercise 8 Airway Clearance Techniques 9 Wound Management B Vocational Activities and Functional Community or Work Reintegration Skills C Gait Training/Functional Ambulation D Application, Proper Use and Care of Assistive, Adaptive, Supportive or Protective Devices F Application, Proper Use and Care of Orthoses G Application, Proper Use and Care of Prosthesis H Home Management	E Orthosis F Assistive, Adaptive, Supportive or Protective U Prosthesis Z None	Z None
Z None	J Communication Skills	K Audiovisual L Assistive Listening M Augmentative / Alternative Communication P Computer Z None	Z None

F   Physical Rehabilitation and Diagnostic Audiology
1   Diagnostic Audiology
3   Hearing Assessment   Measurement of hearing and related functions

Body System/Region Character 4	Type Qualifier Character 5	Equipment Character 6	Qualifier Character 7
Z None	Ø Hearing Screening	Ø Occupational Hearing 1 Audiometer 2 Sound Field / Booth 3 Tympanometer 8 Vestibular / Balance 9 Cochlear Implant Z None	Z None
Z None	1 Pure Tone Audiometry, Air 2 Pure Tone Audiometry, Air and Bone	Ø Occupational Hearing 1 Audiometer 2 Sound Field / Booth Z None	Z None
Z None	3 Bekesy Audiometry 6 Visual Reinforcement Audiometry 9 Short Increment Sensitivity Index B Stenger C Pure Tone Stenger	1 Audiometer 2 Sound Field / Booth Z None	Z None
Z None	4 Conditioned Play Audiometry 5 Select Picture Audiometry	1 Audiometer 2 Sound Field / Booth K Audiovisual Z None	Z None
Z None	7 Alternate Binaural or Monaural Loudness Balance	1 Audiometer K Audiovisual Z None	Z None
Z None	8 Tone Decay D Tympanometry F Eustachian Tube Function G Acoustic Reflex Patterns H Acoustic Reflex Threshold J Acoustic Reflex Decay	3 Tympanometer 4 Electroacoustic Immitance / Acoustic Reflex Z None	Z None
Z None	K Electrocochleography L Auditory Evoked Potentials	7 Electrophysiologic Z None	Z None
Z None	M Evoked Otoacoustic Emissions, Screening N Evoked Otoacoustic Emissions, Diagnostic	6 Otoacoustic Emission (OAE) Z None	Z None

F13 Continued on next page

F13 Continued

F   **Physical Rehabilitation and Diagnostic Audiology**
1   **Diagnostic Audiology**
3   **Hearing Assessment**   Measurement of hearing and related functions

Body System/Region Character 4	Type Qualifier Character 5	Equipment Character 6	Qualifier Character 7
Z None	**P** Aural Rehabilitation Status	**1** Audiometer **2** Sound Field / Booth **4** Electroacoustic Immitance / Acoustic Reflex **9** Cochlear Implant **K** Audiovisual **L** Assistive Listening **P** Computer **Z** None	**Z** None
Z None	**Q** Auditory Processing	**K** Audiovisual **P** Computer **Y** Other Equipment **Z** None	**Z** None

F   **Physical Rehabilitation and Diagnostic Audiology**
1   **Diagnostic Audiology**
4   **Hearing Aid Assessment**   Measurement of the appropriateness and/or effectiveness of a hearing device

Body System/Region Character 4	Type Qualifier Character 5	Equipment Character 6	Qualifier Character 7
Z None	**Ø** Cochlear Implant	**1** Audiometer **2** Sound Field / Booth **3** Tympanometer **4** Electroacoustic Immitance / Acoustic Reflex **5** Hearing Aid Selection / Fitting / Test **7** Electrophysiologic **9** Cochlear Implant **K** Audiovisual **L** Assistive Listening **P** Computer **Y** Other Equipment **Z** None	**Z** None
Z None	**1** Ear Canal Probe Microphone **6** Binaural Electroacoustic Hearing Aid Check **8** Monaural Electroacoustic Hearing Aid Check	**5** Hearing Aid Selection / Fitting / Test **Z** None	**Z** None
Z None	**2** Monaural Hearing Aid **3** Binaural Hearing Aid	**1** Audiometer **2** Sound Field / Booth **3** Tympanometer **4** Electroacoustic Immitance / Acoustic Reflex **5** Hearing Aid Selection / Fitting / Test **K** Audiovisual **L** Assistive Listening **P** Computer **Z** None	**Z** None
Z None	**4** Assistive Listening System/Device Selection	**1** Audiometer **2** Sound Field / Booth **3** Tympanometer **4** Electroacoustic Immitance / Acoustic Reflex **K** Audiovisual **L** Assistive Listening **Z** None	**Z** None
Z None	**5** Sensory Aids	**1** Audiometer **2** Sound Field / Booth **3** Tympanometer **4** Electroacoustic Immitance / Acoustic Reflex **5** Hearing Aid Selection / Fitting / Test **K** Audiovisual **L** Assistive Listening **Z** None	**Z** None
Z None	**7** Ear Protector Attentuation	**Ø** Occupational Hearing **Z** None	**Z** None

Revised Text in **BLUE**   © 2011 Ingenix, Inc

F　Physical Rehabilitation and Diagnostic Audiology
1　Diagnostic Audiology
5　Vestibular Assessment　　Measurement of the vestibular system and related functions

Body System/Region Character 4	Type Qualifier Character 5	Equipment Character 6	Qualifier Character 7
Z None	**Ø** Bithermal, Binaural Caloric Irrigation **1** Bithermal, Monaural Caloric Irrigation **2** Unithermal Binaural Screen **3** Oscillating Tracking **4** Sinusoidal Vertical Axis Rotational **5** Dix-Hallpike Dynamic **6** Computerized Dynamic Posturography	**8** Vestibular / Balance **Z** None	**Z** None
Z None	**7** Tinnitus Masker	**5** Hearing Aid Selection / Fitting / Test **Z** None	**Z** None

Mental Health GZ1–GZJ

G **Mental Health**
Z **None**
1 **Psychological Tests** The administration and interpretation of standardized psychological tests and measurement instruments for the assessment of psychological function

Type Qualifier Character 4	Qualifier Character 5	Qualifier Character 6	Qualifier Character 7
Ø Developmental **1** Personality and Behavioral **2** Intellectual and Psychoeducational **3** Neuropsychological **4** Neurobehavioral and Cognitive Status	**Z** None	**Z** None	**Z** None

G **Mental Health**
Z **None**
2 **Crisis Intervention** Treatment of a traumatized, acutely disturbed or distressed individual for the purpose of short-term stabilization

Type Qualifier Character 4	Qualifier Character 5	Qualifier Character 6	Qualifier Character 7
Z None	**Z** None	**Z** None	**Z** None

G **Mental Health**
Z **None**
3 **Medication Management** Monitoring and adjusting the use of medications for the treatment of a mental health disorder

Type Qualifier Character 4	Qualifier Character 5	Qualifier Character 6	Qualifier Character 7
Z None	**Z** None	**Z** None	**Z** None

G **Mental Health**
Z **None**
5 **Individual Psychotherapy** Treatment of an individual with a mental health disorder by behavioral, cognitive, psychoanalytic, psychodynamic or psychophysiological means to improve functioning or well-being

Type Qualifier Character 4	Qualifier Character 5	Qualifier Character 6	Qualifier Character 7
Ø Interactive **1** Behavioral **2** Cognitive **3** Interpersonal **4** Psychoanalysis **5** Psychodynamic **6** Supportive **8** Cognitive-Behavioral **9** Psychophysiological	**Z** None	**Z** None	**Z** None

G **Mental Health**
Z **None**
6 **Counseling** The application of psychological methods to treat an individual with normal developmental issues and psychological problems in order to increase function, improve well-being, alleviate distress, maladjustment or resolve crises

Type Qualifier Character 4	Qualifier Character 5	Qualifier Character 6	Qualifier Character 7
Ø Educational **1** Vocational **3** Other Counseling	**Z** None	**Z** None	**Z** None

G **Mental Health**
Z **None**
7 **Family Psychotherapy** Treatment that includes one or more family members of an individual with a mental health disorder by behavioral, cognitive, psychoanalytic, psychodynamic or psychophysiological means to improve functioning or well-being

Type Qualifier Character 4	Qualifier Character 5	Qualifier Character 6	Qualifier Character 7
2 Other Family Psychotherapy	**Z** None	**Z** None	**Z** None

　　　　　　　　　Revised Text in **BLUE**　　　　　　　　　© 2011 Ingenix, Inc

G   Mental Health
Z   None
B   Electroconvulsive Therapy   The application of controlled electrical voltages to treat a mental health disorder

Type Qualifier Character 4	Qualifier Character 5	Qualifier Character 6	Qualifier Character 7
Ø Unilateral-Single Seizure	Z None	Z None	Z None
1 Unilateral-Multiple Seizure			
2 Bilateral-Single Seizure			
3 Bilateral-Multiple Seizure			
4 Other Electroconvulsive Therapy			

G   Mental Health
Z   None
C   Biofeedback   Provision of information from the monitoring and regulating of physiological processes in conjunction with cognitive-behavioral techniques to improve patient functioning or well-being

Type Qualifier Character 4	Qualifier Character 5	Qualifier Character 6	Qualifier Character 7
9 Other Biofeedback	Z None	Z None	Z None

G   Mental Health
Z   None
F   Hypnosis   Induction of a state of heightened suggestibility by auditory, visual and tactile techniques to elicit an emotional or behavioral response

Type Qualifier Character 4	Qualifier Character 5	Qualifier Character 6	Qualifier Character 7
Z None	Z None	Z None	Z None

G   Mental Health
Z   None
G   Narcosynthesis   Administration of intravenous barbiturates in order to release suppressed or repressed thoughts

Type Qualifier Character 4	Qualifier Character 5	Qualifier Character 6	Qualifier Character 7
Z None	Z None	Z None	Z None

G   Mental Health
Z   None
H   Group Psychotherapy   Treatment of two or more individuals with a mental health disorder by behavioral, cognitive, psychoanalytic, psychodynamic or psychophysiological means to improve functioning or well-being

Type Qualifier Character 4	Qualifier Character 5	Qualifier Character 6	Qualifier Character 7
Z None	Z None	Z None	Z None

G   Mental Health
Z   None
J   Light Therapy   Application of specialized light treatments to improve functioning or well-being

Type Qualifier Character 4	Qualifier Character 5	Qualifier Character 6	Qualifier Character 7
Z None	Z None	Z None	Z None

Substance Abuse HZ2–HZ9

H   **Substance Abuse Treatment**
Z   **None**
2   **Detoxification Services**   Detoxification from alcohol and/or drugs

Type Qualifier Character 4	Qualifier Character 5	Qualifier Character 6	Qualifier Character 7
Z None	**Z** None	**Z** None	**Z** None

H   **Substance Abuse Treatment**
Z   **None**
3   **Individual Counseling**   The application of psychological methods to treat an individual with addictive behavior

Type Qualifier Character 4	Qualifier Character 5	Qualifier Character 6	Qualifier Character 7
Ø Cognitive **1** Behavioral **2** Cognitive-Behavioral **3** 12-Step **4** Interpersonal **5** Vocational **6** Psychoeducation **7** Motivational Enhancement **8** Confrontational **9** Continuing Care **B** Spiritual **C** Pre/Post-Test Infectious Disease	**Z** None	**Z** None	**Z** None

H   **Substance Abuse Treatment**
Z   **None**
4   **Group Counseling**   The application of psychological methods to treat two or more individuals with addictive behavior

Type Qualifier Character 4	Qualifier Character 5	Qualifier Character 6	Qualifier Character 7
Ø Cognitive **1** Behavioral **2** Cognitive-Behavioral **3** 12-Step **4** Interpersonal **5** Vocational **6** Psychoeducation **7** Motivational Enhancement **8** Confrontational **9** Continuing Care **B** Spiritual **C** Pre/Post-Test Infectious Disease	**Z** None	**Z** None	**Z** None

H   **Substance Abuse Treatment**
Z   **None**
5   **Individual Psychotherapy**   Treatment of an individual with addictive behavior by behavioral, cognitive, psychoanalytic, psychodynamic or psychophysiological means

Type Qualifier Character 4	Qualifier Character 5	Qualifier Character 6	Qualifier Character 7
Ø Cognitive **1** Behavioral **2** Cognitive-Behavioral **3** 12-Step **4** Interpersonal **5** Interactive **6** Psychoeducation **7** Motivational Enhancement **8** Confrontational **9** Supportive **B** Psychoanalysis **C** Psychodynamic **D** Psychophysiological	**Z** None	**Z** None	**Z** None

H **Substance Abuse Treatment**
Z **None**
6 **Family Counseling**　　The application of psychological methods that includes one or more family members to treat an individual with addictive behavior

Type Qualifier Character 4	Qualifier Character 5	Qualifier Character 6	Qualifier Character 7
3　Other Family Counseling	Z　None	Z　None	Z　None

H **Substance Abuse Treatment**
Z **None**
8 **Medication Management**　　Monitoring or adjusting the use of replacment medications for the treatment of addiction

Type Qualifier Character 4	Qualifier Character 5	Qualifier Character 6	Qualifier Character 7
Ø　Nicotine Replacement 1　Methadone Maintenance 2　Levo-alpha-acetyl-methadol (LAAM) 3　Antabuse 4　Naltrexone 5　Naloxone 6　Clonidine 7　Bupropion 8　Psychiatric Medication 9　Other Replacement Medication	Z　None	Z　None	Z　None

H **Substance Abuse Treatment**
Z **None**
9 **Pharmacotherapy**　　The use of replacement medications for the treatment of addiction

Type Qualifier Character 4	Qualifier Character 5	Qualifier Character 6	Qualifier Character 7
Ø　Nicotine Replacement 1　Methadone Maintenance 2　Levo-alpha-acetyl-methadol (LAAM) 3　Antabuse 4　Naltrexone 5　Naloxone 6　Clonidine 7　Bupropion 8　Psychiatric Medication 9　Other Replacement Medication	Z　None	Z　None	Z　None

Appendix A: Root Operations Definitions

0		**Medical and Surgical**		
Ø	Alteration	Definition:	Modifying the natural anatomic structure of a body part without affecting the function of the body part	
		Explanation:	Principal purpose is to improve appearance	
		Examples:	Face lift, breast augmentation	
1	Bypass	Definition:	Altering the route of passage of the contents of a tubular body part	
		Explanation:	Rerouting contents of a body part to a downstream area of the normal route, to a similar route and body part, or to an abnormal route and dissimilar body part. Includes one or more anastomoses, with or without the use of a device	
		Examples:	Coronary artery bypass, colostomy formation	
2	Change	Definition:	Taking out or off a device from a body part and putting back an identical or similar device in or on the same body part without cutting or puncturing the skin or a mucous membrane	
		Explanation:	All CHANGE procedures are coded using the approach EXTERNAL	
		Example:	Urinary catheter change, gastrostomy tube change	
3	Control	Definition:	Stopping, or attempting to stop, postprocedural bleeding	
		Explanation:	The site of the bleeding is coded as an anatomical region and not to a specific body part.	
		Examples:	Control of post-prostatectomy hemorrhage, control of post-tonsillectomy hemorrhage	
4	Creation	Definition:	Making a new genital structure that does not take over the function of a body part	
		Explanation:	Used only for sex change operations	
		Examples:	Creation of vagina in a male, creation of penis in a female	
5	Destruction	Definition:	Physical eradication of all or a portion of a body part by the direct use of energy, force, or a destructive agent	
		Explanation:	None of the body part is physically taken out.	
		Examples:	Fulguration of rectal polyp, cautery of skin lesion	
6	Detachment	Definition:	Cutting off all or part of the upper or lower extremities	
		Explanation:	The body part value is the site of the detachment, with a qualifier if applicable to further specify the level where the extremity was detached	
		Examples:	Below knee amputation, disarticulation of shoulder	
7	Dilation	Definition:	Expanding an orifice or the lumen of a tubular body part	
		Explanation:	The orifice can be a natural orifice or an artificially created orifice. Accomplished by stretching a tubular body part using intraluminal pressure or by cutting part of the orifice or wall of the tubular body part.	
		Examples:	Percutaneous transluminal angioplasty, pyloromyotomy	
8	Division	Definition:	Cutting into a body part without draining fluids and/or gases from the body part in order to separate or transect a body part	
		Explanation:	All or a portion of the body part is separated into two or more portions.	
		Examples:	Spinal cordotomy, osteotomy	
9	Drainage	Definition:	Taking or letting out fluids and/or gases from a body part	
		Explanation:	The qualifier *diagnostic* is used to identify drainage procedures that are biopsies.	
		Examples:	Thoracentesis, incision and drainage	
B	Excision	Definition:	Cutting out or off, without replacement, a portion of a body part	
		Explanation:	The qualifier *diagnostic* is used to identify excision procedures that are biopsies.	
		Examples:	Partial nephrectomy, liver biopsy	
C	Extirpation	Definition:	Taking or cutting out solid matter from a body part	
		Explanation:	The solid matter may be an abnormal byproduct of a biological function or a foreign body; it may be imbedded in a body part or in the lumen of a tubular body part. The solid matter may or may not have been previously broken into pieces.	
		Examples:	Thrombectomy, choledocholithotomy, endarterectomy	

Continued on next page

0	Medical and Surgical		*Continued from previous page*
D	Extraction	Definition:	Pulling or stripping out or off all or a portion of a body part by the use of force
		Explanation:	The qualifier *Diagnostic* is used to identify extractions that are biopsies.
		Examples:	Dilation and curettage, vein stripping
F	Fragmentation	Definition:	Breaking solid matter in a body part into pieces
		Explanation:	Physical force (e.g., manual, ultrasonic) applied directly or indirectly through intervening body parts are used to break the solid matter into pieces. The solid matter may be an abnormal byproduct of a biological function or a foreign body. The pieces of solid matter are not taken out, but are eliminated or absorbed through normal biological functions.
		Examples:	Extracorporeal shockwave lithotripsy, transurethral lithotripsy
G	Fusion	Definition:	Joining together portions of an articular body part, rendering the articular body part immobile
		Explanation:	The body part is joined together by fixation device, bone graft, or other means.
		Examples:	Spinal fusion, ankle arthrodesis
H	Insertion	Definition:	Putting in a nonbiological appliance that monitors, assists, performs, or prevents a physiological function but does not physically take the place of a body part
		Explanation:	None
		Examples:	Insertion of radioactive implant, insertion of central venous catheter
J	Inspection	Definition:	Visually and/or manually exploring a body part
		Explanation:	Visual exploration may be performed with or without optical instrumentation. Manual exploration may be performed directly or through intervening body layers.
		Examples:	Diagnostic arthroscopy, exploratory laparotomy
K	Map	Definition:	Locating the route of passage of electrical impulses and/or locating functional areas in a body part
		Explanation:	Applicable only to the cardiac conduction mechanism and the central nervous system
		Examples:	Cardiac mapping, cortical mapping
L	Occlusion	Definition:	Completely closing an orifice or lumen of a tubular body part
		Explanation:	The orifice can be a natural orifice or an artificially created orifice.
		Examples:	Fallopian tube ligation, ligation of inferior vena cava
M	Reattachment	Definition:	Putting back in or on all or a portion of a separated body part to its normal location or other suitable location
		Explanation:	Vascular circulation and nervous pathways may or may not be reestablished.
		Examples:	Reattachment of hand, reattachment of avulsed kidney
N	Release	Definition:	Freeing a body part from an abnormal physical constraint by cutting or by use of force
		Explanation:	Some of the restraining tissue may be taken out but none of the body part is taken out.
		Examples:	Adhesiolysis, carpal tunnel release
P	Removal	Definition:	Taking out or off a device from a body part
		Explanation:	If a device is taken out and a similar device put in without cutting or puncturing the skin or mucous membrane, the procedure is coded to the root operation *Change*. Otherwise, the procedure for taking out the device is coded to the root operation *Removal*, and the procedure for putting in the new device is coded to the root operation performed.
		Examples:	Drainage tube removal, cardiac pacemaker removal
Q	Repair	Definition:	Restoring, to the extent possible, a body part to its normal anatomic structure and function
		Explanation:	Used only when the method to accomplish the repair is not one of the other root operations
		Examples:	Colostomy takedown, herniorrhaphy, suture of laceration
R	Replacement	Definition:	Putting in or on a biological or synthetic material that physically takes the place and/or function of all or a portion of a body part
		Explanation:	The body part may have been taken out or replaced, or may be taken out, physically eradicated, or rendered nonfunctional during the REPLACEMENT procedure. A REMOVAL procedure is coded for taking out the device used in a previous replacement procedure
		Examples:	Total hip replacement, free skin graft
S	Reposition	Definition:	Moving to its normal location or other suitable location all or a portion of a body part
		Explanation:	The body part is moved to a new location from an abnormal location, or from a normal location where it is not functioning correctly. The body part may or may not be cut out or off to be moved to the new location.
		Examples:	Reposition of undescended testicle, fracture reduction

Continued on next page

0	**Medical and Surgical**		*Continued from previous page*
T	Resection	Definition:	Cutting out or off, without replacement, all of a body part
		Explanation:	None
		Examples:	Total nephrectomy, total lobectomy of lung
V	Restriction	Definition:	Partially closing an orifice or the lumen of a tubular body part
		Explanation:	The orifice can be a natural orifice or an artificially created orifice.
		Examples:	Esophagogastric fundoplication, cervical cerclage
W	Revision	Definition:	Correcting, to the extent possible, a portion of a malfunctioning device or the position of a displaced device
		Explanation:	Revision can include correcting a malfunctioning or displaced device by taking out or putting in components of the device such as a screw or pin.
		Examples:	Adjustment of pacemaker lead, adjustment of hip prosthesis
U	Supplement	Definition:	Putting in or on biological or synthetic material that physically reinforces and/or augments the function of a portion of a body part
		Explanation:	The biological material is non-living, or is living and from the same individual. The body part may have been previously replaced, and the SUPPLEMENT procedure is performed to physically reinforce and/or augment the function of the replaced body part
		Examples:	Herniorrhaphy using mesh, free nerve graft, mitral valve ring annuloplasty, put a new acetabular liner in a previous hip replacement
X	Transfer	Definition:	Moving, without taking out, all or a portion of a body part to another location to take over the function of all or a portion of a body part
		Explanation:	The body part transferred remains connected to its vascular and nervous supply.
		Examples:	Tendon transfer, skin pedicle flap transfer
Y	Transplantation	Definition:	Putting in or on all or a portion of a living body part taken from another individual or animal to physically take the place and/or function of all or a portion of a similar body part
		Explanation:	The native body part may or may not be taken out, and the transplanted body part may take over all or a portion of its function.
		Examples:	Kidney transplant, heart transplant

Root Operation Definitions for Other Sections

1	**Obstetrics**		
A	Abortion	Definition:	Artificially terminating a pregnancy
		Explanation:	Subdivided according to whether an additional device such as a laminaria or abortifacient is used, or whether the abortion was performed by mechanical means
		Examples:	Transvaginal abortion using vacuum aspiration technique
E	Delivery	Definition:	Assisting the passage of the products of conception from the genital canal
		Explanation:	Applies only to manually-assisted, vaginal delivery
		Examples:	Manually-assisted delivery

2	**Placement**		
Ø	Change	Definition:	Taking out or off a device from a body region and putting back an identical or similar device in or on the same body region without cutting or puncturing the skin or a mucous membrane
		Explanation:	Procedures performed without making an incision or a puncture.
		Examples:	Change of vaginal packing
1	Compression	Definition:	Putting pressure on a body region
		Explanation:	Procedures performed without making an incision or a puncture
		Examples:	Placement of pressure dressing on abdominal wall
2	Dressing	Definition:	Putting material on a body region for protection
		Explanation:	Procedures performed without making an incision or a puncture
		Examples:	Application of sterile dressing to head wound

Continued on next page

2	Placement			*Continued from previous page*
3	Immobilization	Definition:	Limiting or preventing motion of a body region	
		Explanation:	Procedures to fit a device, such as splints and braces, as described in FØDZ6EZ and FØDZ7EZ, apply only to the rehabilitation setting.	
		Examples:	Placement of splint on left finger	
4	Packing	Definition:	Putting material in a body region or orifice	
		Explanation:	Procedures performed without making an incision or a puncture	
		Examples:	Placement of nasal packing	
5	Removal	Definition:	Taking out or off a device from a body region	
		Explanation:	Procedures performed without making an incision or a puncture	
		Examples:	Removal of stereotactic head frame	
6	Traction	Definition:	Exerting a pulling force on a body region in a distal direction	
		Explanation:	Traction in this section includes only the task performed using a mechanical traction apparatus.	
		Examples:	Lumbar traction using motorized split-traction table	

3	Administration		
Ø	Introduction	Definition:	Putting in or on a therapeutic, diagnostic, nutritional, physiological, or prophylactic substance except blood or blood products
		Explanation:	All other substances administered, such as antineoplastic substance
		Examples:	Nerve block injection to median nerve
1	Irrigation	Definition:	Putting in or on a cleansing substance
		Explanation:	Substance given is a cleansing substance or dialysate
		Examples:	Flushing of eye
2	Transfusion	Definition:	Putting in blood or blood products
		Explanation:	Substance given is a blood product or a stem cell substance
		Examples:	Transfusion of cell saver red cells into central venous line

4	Measurement and Monitoring		
Ø	Measurement	Definition:	Determining the level of a physiological or physical function at a point in time
		Explanation:	A single temperature reading is considered measurement.
		Examples:	External electrocardiogram(EKG), single reading
1	Monitoring	Definition:	Determining the level of a physiological or physical function repetitively over a period of time
		Explanation:	Temperature taken every half hour for 8 hours is considered monitoring
		Examples:	Urinary pressure monitoring

5	Extracorporeal Assistance and Performance		
Ø	Assistance	Definition:	Taking over a portion of a physiological function by extracorporeal means
		Explanation:	Procedures that support a physiological function but do not take complete control of it, such as intra-aortic balloon pump to support cardiac output and hyperbaric oxygen treatment
		Examples:	Hyperbaric oxygenation of wound
1	Performance	Definition:	Completely taking over a physiological function by extracorporeal means
		Explanation:	Procedures in which complete control is exercised over a physiological function, such as total mechanical ventilation, cardiac pacing, and cardiopulmonary bypass
		Examples:	Cardiopulmonary bypass in conjunction with CABG
2	Restoration	Definition:	Returning, or attempting to return, a physiological function to its original state by extracorporeal means
		Explanation:	Only external cardioversion and defibrillation procedures. Failed cardioversion procedures are also included in the definition of restoration, and are coded the same as successful procedures
		Examples:	Attempted cardiac defibrillation, unsuccessful

6   Extracorporeal Therapies

Ø	Atmospheric Control	Definition:	Extracorporeal control of atmospheric pressure and composition
		Explanation:	None
		Examples:	Antigen-free air conditioning, series treatment
1	Decompression	Definition:	Extracorporeal elimination of undissolved gas from body fluids
		Explanation:	A single type of procedure—treatment for decompression sickness (the bends) in a hyperbaric chamber
		Examples:	Hyperbaric decompression treatment, single
2	Electromagnetic Therapy	Definition:	Extracorporeal treatment by electromagnetic rays
		Explanation:	None
		Examples:	TMS (transcranial magnetic stimulation), series treatment
3	Hyperthermia	Definition:	Extracorporeal raising of body temperature
		Explanation:	To treat temperature imbalance, and as an adjunct radiation treatment for cancer. When performed to treat temperature imbalance, the procedure is coded to this section. When performed for cancer treatment, whole-body hyperthermia is classified as a modality qualifier in section D, "Radiation Oncology."
		Examples:	None
4	Hypothermia	Definition:	Extracorporeal lowering of body temperature
		Explanation:	None
		Examples:	Whole body hypothermia treatment for temperature imbalances, series
5	Pheresis	Definition:	Extracorporeal separation of blood products
		Explanation:	Used in medical practice for two main purposes: to treat diseases where too much of a blood component is produced, such as leukemia, or to remove a blood product such as platelets from a donor, for transfusion into a patient who needs them
		Examples:	Therapeutic leukopheresis, single treatment
6	Phototherapy	Definition:	Extracorporeal treatment by light rays
		Explanation:	Phototherapy to the circulatory system means exposing the blood to light rays outside the body, using a machine that recirculates the blood and returns it to the body after phototherapy.
		Examples:	Phototherapy of circulatory system, series treatment
7	Ultrasound Therapy	Definition:	Extracorporeal treatment by ultrasound
		Explanation:	None
		Examples:	Therapeutic ultrasound of peripheral vessels, single treatment
8	Ultraviolet Light Therapy	Definition:	Extracorporeal treatment by ultraviolet light
		Explanation:	None
		Examples:	Ultraviolet light phototherapy, series treatment
9	Shock Wave Therapy	Definition:	Extracorporeal treatment by shockwaves
		Explanation:	None
		Examples:	Shockwave therapy of plantar fascia, single treatment

7   Osteopathic

Ø	Treatment	Definition:	Manual treatment to eliminate or alleviate somatic dysfunction and related disorders
		Explanation:	None
		Examples:	Fascial release of abdomen, osteopathic treatment

8   Other Procedures

Ø	Other Procedures	Definition:	Methodologies that attempt to remediate or cure a disorder or disease
		Explanation:	For nontraditional, whole-body therapies including acupuncture and meditation
		Examples:	Acupuncture

9	Chiropractic		
B	Manipulation	Definition:	Manual procedure that involves a directed thrust to move a joint past the physiological range of motion, without exceeding the anatomical limit
		Explanation:	None
		Examples:	Chiropractic treatment of cervical spine, short lever specific contact

Note: Sections B-H (Imaging through Substance Abuse Treatment) do not include root operations. Character 3 position represents type of procedure, therefore those definitions are not included in this appendix. See appendix D for definitions of the type (character 3) or type qualifiers (character 5) that provide details of the procedures performed.

Appendix B: Comparison of Medical and Surgical Root Operations

Note: the character associated with each operation appears in parentheses after its title.

Procedures That Take Out or Eliminate Some or All of a Body Part

Operation	Action	Target	Clarification	Example
Excision (B)	Cutting out or off	Portion of a body part	Without replacing body part	Breast lumpectomy
Resection (T)	Cutting out or off	All of a body part	Without replacing body part	Total nephrectomy
Extraction (D)	Pulling out or off	All or a portion of a body part	Without replacing body part	Suction D&C
Destruction (5)	Eradicating	All or a portion of a body part	Without taking out or replacing body part	Rectal polyp fulguration
Detachment (6)	Cutting out/off	All or a portion of an extremity	Without replacing extremity	Below knee amputation

Procedures That Put in/Put Back or Move Some/All of a Body Part

Operation	Action	Target	Clarification	Example
Transplantation (Y)	Putting in	All or a portion of a living body part from other individual or animal	Physically takes the place and/or function of all or a portion of a body part	Heart transplant, kidney transplant
Reattachment (M)	Putting back in or on	All or a portion of a separated body part	Put in its normal or other suitable location. The vascular circulation and nervous pathways may or may not be reestablished.	Finger reattachment
Reposition (S)	Moving	All or a portion of a body part	Put in its normal or other suitable location. Body part may or may not be cut out or off	Reposition undescended testicle
Transfer (X)	Moving ; to function for a similar body part	All or a portion of a body part	Without taking out body part; assumes function of similar body part and remains connected to its vascular and nervous supply	Tendon transfer, skin transfer flap

Procedures That Take Out or Eliminate Solid Matter, Fluids, or Gases From a Body Part

Operation	Action	Target	Clarification	Example
Drainage (9)	Taking or letting out	Fluids and/or gases from a body part	Without taking out any of the body part. The qualifier DIAGNOSTIC is used to identify drainage procedures that are biopsies.	Incision and drainage
Extirpation (C)	Taking or cutting out	Solid matter in a body part	Without taking out any of the body part. The solid matter may be an abnormal byproduct of a biological function or a foreign body; it may be imbedded in a body part or in the lumen of a tubular body part. The solid matter may or may not have been previously broken into pieces.	Thrombectomy
Fragmentation (F)	Breaking down	Solid matter into pieces within a body part	The physical force (e.g., manual, ultrasonic) is applied directly or indirectly, without taking out any of the body part or any solid matter. The solid matter may be an abnormal byproduct of a biological function or a foreign body. The pieces of solid matter are not taken out.	Lithotripsy

Procedures That Involve Only Examination of Body Parts and Regions

Operation	Action	Target	Clarification	Example
Inspection (J)	Visual and/or manual exploration	Some or all of a body part	Performed with or without optical instrumentation, directly or through body layers	Diagnostic arthroscopy, diagnostic cystoscopy
Map (K)	Locating	Route of passage of electrical impulses or functional areas in a body part	Applicable only to cardiac conduction mechanism and central nervous system	Cardiac mapping

Procedures That Alter the Diameter/Route of a Tubular Body Part

Operation	Action	Target	Clarification	Example
Bypass (1)	Altering the route of passage	Contents of tubular body part	May include use of living tissue, nonliving biological material or synthetic material which does not take the place of the body part. Includes one or more anastomoses, with or without the use of a device.	Gastrojejunal bypass, coronary artery bypass (CABG)
Dilation (7)	Expanding	Orifice or lumen of tubular body part	By application of intraluminal pressure or by cutting the wall of the orifice	Percutaneous transluminal angioplasty
Occlusion (L)	Completely closing	Orifice or lumen of tubular body part	Orifice may be natural or artificially created	Fallopian tube ligation
Restriction (V)	Partially closing	Orifice or lumen of tubular body part	Orifice may be natural or artificially created	Cervical cerclage, gastroesophageal fundoplication

Procedures That Always Involve Devices

Operation		Action	Target	Clarification	Example
Insertion (H)	DVC	Putting in non-biological device	Device in or on a body part	Putting in a non-biological device that monitors, performs, assists, or prevents a physical function, does not physically take the place of a body part	Pacemaker insertion, central line insertion
Replacement (R)	DVC	Putting in or on	Biological or synthetic material; living tissue taken from same individual	Physically takes the place of all or a portion of a body part. A REMOVAL procedure is assigned for taking out the device used in a previous replacement procedure.	Total hip replacement
Supplement (U)	DVC	Putting in or on	Device that reinforces or augments a body part	Biological material is nonliving or living and from the same individual	Herniorrhaphy using mesh
Removal (P)	DVC	Taking a device out or off	Device from a body part	If a new device is inserted via an incision or puncture, that procedure is coded separately	Cardiac pacemaker removal, central line removal
Change (2)	DVC	Taking a device out or off and putting back an indentical or similar device	Identical or similar device in or on a body part	Without cutting or puncturing skin or mucous membrane; all *change* procedures are coded using the *External* approach	Drainage tube change
Revision (W)	DVC	Correcting	Malfunctioning or displaced device in or on a body part	To the extent possible	Hip prosthesis adjustment, revision of pacemaker lead

Procedures Involving Cutting or Separation Only

Operation	Action	Target	Clarification	Example
Division (8)	Cutting into/Separating	A body part	Without taking out any of the body part or draining fluids and/or gases. All or a portion of the body part is separated into two or more portions.	Osteotomy, neurotomy
Release (N)	Freeing, by cutting or by the use of force	A body part	Eliminating abnormal constraint without taking out any of the body part. Some of the restraining tissue may be taken out, but none of the body part is taken out.	Peritoneal adhesiolysis

Procedures Involving Other Repairs

Operation	Action	Target	Clarification	Example
Control (3)	Stopping or attempting to stop	Postprocedural bleeding	Limited to anatomic regions not specific body parts	Control of postprostatectomy bleeding
Repair (Q)	Restoring	A body part to its natural anatomic structure and function	To the extent possible	Hernia repair, suture laceration

Procedures with Other Objectives

Operation	Action	Target	Clarification	Example
Alteration (Ø)	Modifying	Natural anatomical structure of a body part	Without affecting function of body part, performed for cosmetic purposes	Face lift
Creation (4)	Making	New genital structure	Does not physically take the place of a body part, used only for sex change operations	Artificial vagina creation
Fusion (G)	Unification and immobilization	Joint or articular body part	Stabilization of damaged joints by graft and/or fixation	Spinal fusion

Appendix C: Body Part Key

Anatomical Term	PCS Description
Abdominal aortic plexus	Abdominal Sympathetic Nerve
Abdominal esophagus	Esophagus, Lower
Abductor hallucis muscle	Foot Muscle, Right
	Foot Muscle, Left
Abductor hallucis tendon	Foot Tendon, Right
	Foot Tendon, Left
Accessory cephalic vein	Cephalic Vein, Right
	Cephalic Vein, Left
Accessory obturator nerve	Lumbar Plexus
Accessory phrenic nerve	Phrenic nerve
Accessory spleen	Spleen
Acetabulofemoral joint	Hip Joint, Left
	Hip Joint, Right
Achilles tendon	Lower Leg Tendon, Right
	Lower Leg Tendon, Left
Acromioclavicular ligament	Shoulder Bursa and Ligament, Right
	Shoulder Bursa and Ligament, Left
Acromion (process)	Scapula, Left
	Scapula, Right
Acute margin	Ventricle, Right
Adductor brevis muscle	Upper Leg Muscle, Right
	Upper Leg Muscle, Left
Adductor brevis tendon	Upper Leg Tendon, Right
	Upper Leg Tendon, Left
Adductor hallucis muscle	Foot Muscle, Right
	Foot Muscle, Left
Adductor hallucis tendon	Foot Tendon, Right
	Foot Tendon, Left
Adductor longus muscle	Upper Leg Muscle, Right
	Upper Leg Muscle, Left
Adductor longus tendon	Upper Leg Tendon, Right
	Upper Leg Tendon, Left
Adductor magnus muscle	Upper Leg Muscle, Right
	Upper Leg Muscle, Left
Adductor magnus tendon	Upper Leg Tendon, Right
	Upper Leg Tendon, Left
Adenohypophysis	Pituitary Gland
Alar ligament of axis	Head and Neck Bursa and Ligament
Alveolar process of mandible	Mandible, Left
	Mandible, Right
Alveolar process of maxilla	Maxilla, Left
	Maxilla, Right
Anal orifice (syn)	Anus
Anatomical snuffbox	Lower Arm and Wrist Tendon, Right
	Lower Arm and Wrist Tendon, Left
Angular artery	Face Artery

Anatomical Term	PCS Description
Angular vein	Face Vein, Left
	Face Vein, Right
Annular ligament	Elbow Bursa and Ligament, Right
	Elbow Bursa and Ligament, Left
Anorectal junction	Rectum
Ansa cervicalis	Cervical Plexus
Antebrachial fascia	Subcutaneous Tissue and Fascia, Right Lower Arm
	Subcutaneous Tissue and Fascia, Left Lower Arm
Anterior (pectoral) lymph node	Lymphatic, Left Axillary
	Lymphatic, Right Axillary
Anterior cerebral artery	Intracranial Artery
Anterior cerebral vein	Intracranial Vein
Anterior choroidal artery	Intracranial Artery
Anterior circumflex humeral artery	Axillary Artery, Right
	Axillary Artery, Left
Anterior communicating artery	Intracranial Artery
Anterior crural nerve	Femoral Nerve
Anterior cruciate ligament (ACL)	Knee Bursa and Ligament, Right
	Knee Bursa and Ligament, Left
Anterior facial vein	Face Vein, Left
	Face Vein, Right
Anterior intercostal artery	Internal Mammary Artery, Right
	Internal Mammary Artery, Left
Anterior interosseous nerve	Median Nerve
Anterior lateral malleolar artery	Anterior Tibial Artery, Right
	Anterior Tibial Artery, Left
Anterior lingual gland	Minor Salivary Gland
Anterior medial malleolar artery	Anterior Tibial Artery, Right
	Anterior Tibial Artery, Left
Anterior spinal artery	Vertebral Artery, Right
	Vertebral Artery, Left
Anterior tibial recurrent artery	Anterior Tibial Artery, Right
	Anterior Tibial Artery, Left
Anterior ulnar recurrent artery	Ulnar Artery, Right
	Ulnar Artery, Left
Anterior vagal trunk	Vagus Nerve
Anterior vertebral tendon	Head and Neck Tendon
Anterior vertebral muscle	Neck Muscle, Right
	Neck Muscle, Left
Antihelix	External Ear, Right
	External Ear, Left
	External Ear, Bilateral

Anatomical Term	PCS Description
Antitragus	External Ear, Right
	External Ear, Left
	External Ear, Bilateral
Antrum of Highmore	Maxillary Sinus, Right
	Maxillary Sinus, Left
Aortic annulus	Aortic Valve
Aortic arch (syn)	Thoracic Aorta
Aortic intercostal artery	Thoracic Aorta
Apical (subclavicular) lymph node	Lymphatic, Left Axillary
	Lymphatic, Right Axillary
Apneustic center	Pons
Aqueduct of Sylvius	Cerebral Ventricle
Aqueous humour	Anterior Chamber, Right
	Anterior Chamber, Left
Arachnoid mater	Cerebral Meninges
	Spinal Meninges
Arcuate artery	Foot Artery, Right
	Foot Artery, Right
Areola	Nipple, Left
	Nipple, Right
Aryepiglottic fold	Larynx
Arytenoid cartilage	Larynx
Arytenoid muscle	Neck Muscle, Right
	Neck Muscle, Left
Arytenoid tendon	Head and Neck Tendon
Ascending aorta	Thoracic Aorta
Ascending palatine artery	Face Artery
Ascending pharyngeal artery	External Carotid Artery, Right
	External Carotid Artery, Left
Atlantoaxial joint	Cervical Vertebral Joint
Atrioventricular node	Conduction Mechanism
Atrium dextrum cordis	Atrium, Right
Atrium pulmonale	Atrium, Left
Auditory tube	Eustachian Tube, Right
	Eustachian Tube, Left
Auerbach's (myenteric) plexus	Abdominal Sympathetic Nerve
Auricle	External Ear, Right
	External Ear, Left
	External Ear, Bilateral
Auricularis tendon	Head and Neck Tendon
Auricularis muscle	Head Muscle
Axillary fascia	Subcutaneous Tissue and Fascia, Right Upper Arm
	Subcutaneous Tissue and Fascia, Left Upper Arm
Axillary nerve	Brachial Plexus
Bartholin's (greater vestibular) gland	Vestibular Gland
Basal (internal) cerebral vein	Intracranial Vein
Basal nuclei	Basal Ganglia

Anatomical Term	PCS Description
Basilar artery	Intracranial Artery
Basis pontis	Pons
Biceps brachii muscle	Upper Arm Muscle, Right
	Upper Arm Muscle, Left
Biceps brachii tendon	Upper Arm Tendon, Right
	Upper Arm Tendon, Left
Biceps femoris muscle	Upper Leg Muscle, Right
	Upper Leg Muscle, Left
Biceps femoris tendon	Upper Leg Tendon, Right
	Upper Leg Tendon, Left
Bicipital aponeurosis	Subcutaneous Tissue and Fascia, Right Lower Arm
	Subcutaneous Tissue and Fascia, Left Lower Arm
Bicuspid valve	Mitral Valve
Body of femur	Femoral Shaft, Right
	Femoral Shaft, Left
Body of fibula	Fibula, Left
	Fibula, Right
Bony labyrinth	Inner Ear, Left
	Inner Ear, Right
Bony orbit	Orbit, Left
	Orbit, Right
Bony vestibule	Inner Ear, Left
	Inner Ear, Right
Brachial (lateral) lymph node	Lymphatic, Left Axillary
	Lymphatic, Right Axillary
Brachialis muscle	Upper Arm Muscle, Right
	Upper Arm Muscle, Left
Brachialis tendon	Upper Arm Tendon, Right
	Upper Arm Tendon, Left
Brachiocephalic trunk or artery	Innominate Artery
	Innominate Artery
Brachiocephalic vein (syn)	Innominate Vein, Right
	Innominate Vein, Left
Brachioradialis tendon	Lower Arm and Wrist Tendon, Right
	Lower Arm and Wrist Tendon, Left
Brachioradialis muscle	Lower Arm and Wrist Muscle, Right
	Lower Arm and Wrist Muscle, Left
Broad ligament	Uterine Supporting Structure
Bronchial artery	Thoracic Aorta
Buccal gland	Buccal Mucosa
Buccinator lymph node	Lymphatic, Head
Buccinator muscle	Facial Muscle
Bulbospongiosus muscle	Perineum Muscle
Bulbospongiosus tendon	Perineum Tendon
Bulbourethral (Cowper's) gland	Urethra
Bundle of His	Conduction Mechanism
Bundle of Kent	Conduction Mechanism
Calcaneocuboid ligament	Foot Bursa and Ligament, Right
	Foot Bursa and Ligament, Left

Anatomical Term	PCS Description
Calcaneocuboid joint	Tarsal Joint, Right
	Tarsal Joint, Left
Calcaneofibular ligament	Ankle Bursa and Ligament, Right
	Ankle Bursa and Ligament, Left
Calcaneus	Tarsal, Left
	Tarsal, Right
Capitate bone	Carpal, Left
	Carpal, Right
Cardia	Esophagogastric Junction
Cardiac plexus	Thoracic Sympathetic Nerve
Cardioesophageal junction	Esophagogastric Junction
Caroticotympanic artery	Internal Carotid Artery, Right
	Internal Carotid Artery, Left
Carotid glomus	Carotid Bodies, Bilateral
	Carotid Body, Right
	Carotid Body, Left
Carotid sinus nerve	Glossopharyngeal Nerve
Carotid sinus	Internal Carotid Artery, Right
	Internal Carotid Artery, Left
Carpometacarpal ligament	Hand Bursa and Ligament, Right
	Hand Bursa and Ligament, Left
Carpometacarpal (CMC) joint	Metacarpocarpal Joint, Right
	Metacarpocarpal Joint, Left
Cauda equina	Lumbar Spinal Cord
Cavernous plexus	Head and Neck Sympathetic Nerve
Celiac (solar) plexus	Abdominal Sympathetic Nerve
Celiac ganglion	Abdominal Sympathetic Nerve
Celiac lymph node	Lymphatic, Aortic
Celiac trunk	Celiac Artery
Central axillary lymph node	Lymphatic, Left Axillary
	Lymphatic, Right Axillary
Cerebral aqueduct (Sylvius)	Cerebral Ventricle
Cerebrum (syn)	Brain
Cervical esophagus	Esophagus, Upper
Cervical facet joint	Cervical Vertebral Joints, 2 or more
	Cervical Vertebral Joint
Cervical ganglion	Head and Neck Sympathetic Nerve
Cervical intertransverse ligament	Head and Neck Bursa and Ligament
Cervical interspinous ligament	Head and Neck Bursa and Ligament
Cervical ligamentum flavum	Head and Neck Bursa and Ligament
Cervical lymph node	Lymphatic, Left Neck
	Lymphatic, Right Neck
Cervicothoracic facet joint	Cervicothoracic Vertebral Joint
Choana	Nasopharynx
Chondroglossus muscle	Tongue, Palate, Pharynx Muscle
Chorda tympani	Facial Nerve
Choroid plexus	Cerebral Ventricle

Anatomical Term	PCS Description
Ciliary body	Eye, Left
	Eye, Right
Ciliary ganglion	Head and Neck Sympathetic Nerve
Circle of Willis	Intracranial Artery
Circumflex illiac artery	Femoral Artery, Right
	Femoral Artery, Left
Claustrum	Basal Ganglia
Coccygeal body	Coccygeal Glomus
Coccygeus muscle	Trunk Muscle, Left
Coccygeus tendon	Trunk Tendon, Left
Cochlea	Inner Ear, Left
	Inner Ear, Right
Cochlear nerve	Acoustic Nerve
Columella	Nose
Common digital vein	Foot Vein, Left
	Foot Vein, Right
Common facial vein	Face Vein, Left
	Face Vein, Right
Common fibular nerve	Peroneal Nerve
Common hepatic artery	Hepatic Artery
Common iliac (subaortic) lymph node	Lymphatic, Pelvis
Common interosseous artery	Ulnar Artery, Right
	Ulnar Artery, Left
Common peroneal nerve (syn)	Peroneal Nerve
Condyloid process	Mandible, Left
	Mandible, Right
Conus arteriosus	Ventricle, Right
Conus medullaris	Lumbar Spinal Cord
Coracoacromial ligament	Shoulder Bursa and Ligament, Right
	Shoulder Bursa and Ligament, Left
Coracobrachialis muscle	Upper Arm Muscle, Right
	Upper Arm Muscle, Left
Coracobrachialis tendon	Upper Arm Tendon, Right
	Upper Arm Tendon, Left
Coracoclavicular ligament	Shoulder Bursa and Ligament, Right
	Shoulder Bursa and Ligament, Left
Coracohumeral ligament	Shoulder Bursa and Ligament, Right
	Shoulder Bursa and Ligament, Left
Coracoid process	Scapula, Left
	Scapula, Right
Corniculate cartilage	Larynx
Corpus callosum	Brain
Corpus cavernosum	Penis
Corpus spongiosum	Penis
Corpus striatum	Basal Ganglia
Corrugator supercilii muscle	Facial Muscle
Costocervical trunk	Subclavian Artery, Right
	Subclavian Artery, Left

Anatomical Term	PCS Description
Costoclavicular ligament	Shoulder Bursa and Ligament, Right
	Shoulder Bursa and Ligament, Left
Costotransverse joint	Thoracic Vertebral Joints, 8 or more
	Thoracic Vertebral Joints, 2 to 7
	Thoracic Vertebral Joint
Costotransverse ligament	Thorax Bursa and Ligament, Right
	Thorax Bursa and Ligament, Left
Costovertebral joint	Thoracic Vertebral Joints, 8 or more
	Thoracic Vertebral Joints, 2 to 7
	Thoracic Vertebral Joint
Costoxiphoid ligament	Thorax Bursa and Ligament, Right
	Thorax Bursa and Ligament, Left
Cowper's (bulbourethral) gland	Urethra
Cranial dura mater	Dura Mater
Cranial epidural space	Epidural Space
Cranial subarachnoid space	Subarachnoid Space
Cranial subdural space	Subdural Space
Cremaster muscle	Perineum Muscle
Cremaster tendon	Perineum Tendon
Cribriform plate	Ethmoid Bone, Right
	Ethmoid Bone, Left
Cricoid cartilage	Larynx
Cricothyroid tendon	Head and Neck Tendon
Cricothyroid muscle	Neck Muscle, Right
	Neck Muscle, Left
Cricothyroid artery	Thyroid Artery, Right
	Thyroid Artery, Left
Crural fascia	Subcutaneous Tissue and Fascia, Right Upper Leg
	Subcutaneous Tissue and Fascia, Left Upper Leg
Cubital lymph node	Lymphatic, Left Upper Extremity
	Lymphatic, Right Upper Extremity
Cubital nerve	Ulnar Nerve
Cuboid bone	Tarsal, Left
	Tarsal, Right
Cuboideonavicular joint	Tarsal Joint, Right
	Tarsal Joint, Left
Culmen	Cerebellum
Cuneiform cartilage	Larynx
Cuneonavicular ligament	Foot Bursa and Ligament, Right
	Foot Bursa and Ligament, Left
Cuneonavicular joint	Tarsal Joint, Right
	Tarsal Joint, Left
Cutaneous (transverse) cervical nerve	Cervical Plexus
Deep cervical fascia	Subcutaneous Tissue and Fascia, Anterior Neck
Deep cervical vein	Vertebral Vein, Right
	Vertebral Vein, Left

Anatomical Term	PCS Description
Deep circumflex iliac artery	External Iliac Artery, Right
	External Iliac Artery, Left
Deep facial vein	Face Vein, Left
	Face Vein, Right
Deep femoral artery	Femoral Artery, Right
	Femoral Artery, Left
Deep femoral (profunda femoris) vein	Femoral Vein, Right
	Femoral Vein, Left
Deep palmar arch	Hand Artery, Right
	Hand Artery, Left
Deep transverse perineal muscle	Perineum Muscle
Deep transverse perineal tendon	Perineum Tendon
Deferential artery	Internal Iliac Artery, Right
	Internal Iliac Artery, Left
Deltoid fascia	Subcutaneous Tissue and Fascia, Right Upper Arm
	Subcutaneous Tissue and Fascia, Left Upper Arm
Deltoid ligament	Ankle Bursa and Ligament, Right
	Ankle Bursa and Ligament, Left
Deltoid muscle	Shoulder Muscle, Right
	Shoulder Muscle, Left
Deltoid tendon	Shoulder Tendon, Right
	Shoulder Tendon, Left
Deltopectoral (infraclavicular) lymph node	Lymphatic, Left Upper Extremity
	Lymphatic, Right Upper Extremity
Dentate ligament	Dura Mater
Denticulate ligament	Spinal Cord
Depressor anguli oris muscle	Facial Muscle
Depressor labii inferioris muscle	Facial Muscle
Depressor septi nasi muscle	Facial Muscle
Depressor supercilii muscle	Facial Muscle
Dermis	Skin
Descending genicular artery	Femoral Artery, Right
	Femoral Artery, Left
Diaphragma sellae	Dura Mater
Distal radioulnar joint	Wrist Joint, Right
	Wrist Joint, Left
Dorsal digital nerve	Radial Nerve
Dorsal metacarpal vein	Hand Vein, Left
	Hand Vein, Right
Dorsal metatarsal artery	Foot Artery, Right
	Foot Artery, Left
Dorsal metatarsal vein	Foot Vein, Left
	Foot Vein, Right
Dorsal scapular nerve	Brachial Plexus

Anatomical Term	PCS Description
Dorsal scapular artery	Subclavian Artery, Right
	Subclavian Artery, Left
Dorsal venous arch	Foot Vein, Left
	Foot Vein, Right
Dorsalis pedis artery	Anterior Tibial Artery, Right
	Anterior Tibial Artery, Left
Duct of Santorini	Pancreatic Duct, Accessory
Duct of Wirsung	Pancreatic Duct
Ductus deferens	Vas Deferens, Right
	Vas Deferens, Left
	Vas Deferens, Bilateral
	Vas Deferens
Duodenal ampulla	Ampulla of Vater
Duodenojejunal flexure	Jejunum
Dural venous sinus	Intracranial Vein
Earlobe	External Ear, Right
	External Ear, Left
	External Ear, Bilateral
Eighth cranial nerve	Acoustic Nerve
Ejaculatory duct	Vas Deferens, Right
	Vas Deferens, Left
	Vas Deferens, Bilateral
	Vas Deferens
Eleventh cranial nerve	Accessory Nerve
Encephalon	Brain
Ependyma	Cerebral Ventricle
Epidermis	Skin
Epiploic foramen	Peritoneum
Epithalamus	Thalamus
Epitroclear lymph node	Lymphatic, Left Upper Extremity
	Lymphatic, Right Upper Extremity
Erector spinae muscle	Trunk Muscle, Right
	Trunk Muscle, Left
Erector spinae tendon	Trunk Tendon, Right
	Trunk Tendon, Left
Esophageal artery	Thoracic Aorta
Esophageal plexus	Thoracic Sympathetic Nerve
Ethmoidal air cell	Ethmoid Sinus, Right
	Ethmoid Sinus, Left
Extensor carpi ulnaris tendon	Lower Arm and Wrist Tendon, Right
Extensor carpi radialis tendon	Lower Arm and Wrist Tendon, Right
Extensor carpi ulnaris	Lower Arm and Wrist Tendon, Left
Extensor carpi radialis	Lower Arm and Wrist Tendon, Left
Extensor carpi ulnaris muscle	Lower Arm and Wrist Muscle, Right
Extensor carpi radialis muscle	Lower Arm and Wrist Muscle, Right
Extensor carpi ulnaris	Lower Arm and Wrist Muscle, Left
Extensor carpi radialis	Lower Arm and Wrist Muscle, Left

Anatomical Term	PCS Description
Extensor digitorum brevis muscle	Foot Muscle, Right
	Foot Muscle, Left
Extensor digitorum brevis tendon	Foot Tendon, Right
	Foot Tendon, Left
Extensor digitorum longus muscle	Lower Leg Muscle, Right
	Lower Leg Muscle, Left
Extensor digitorum longus tendon	Lower Leg Tendon, Right
	Lower Leg Tendon, Left
Extensor hallucis brevis muscle	Foot Muscle, Right
	Foot Muscle, Left
Extensor hallucis brevis tendon	Foot Tendon, Right
	Foot Tendon, Left
Extensor hallucis longus muscle	Lower Leg Muscle, Right
	Lower Leg Muscle, Left
Extensor hallucis longus tendon	Lower Leg Tendon, Right
	Lower Leg Tendon, Left
External anal sphincter	Anal Sphincter
External auditory meatus (syn)	External Auditory Canal, Right
	External Auditory Canal, Left
External maxillary artery	Face Artery
External naris	Nose
External oblique muscle	Abdomen Muscle, Right
	Abdomen Muscle, Left
External oblique tendon	Abdomen Tendon, Right
	Abdomen Tendon, Left
External oblique aponeurosis	Subcutaneous Tissue and Fascia, Trunk
External popliteal nerve	Peroneal Nerve
External pudendal artery	Femoral Artery, Right
	Femoral Artery, Left
External pudendal vein	Greater Saphenous Vein, Right
	Greater Saphenous Vein, Left
External urethral sphincter	Urethra
Extradural space	Epidural Space
Facial artery	Face Artery
False vocal cord	Larynx
Falx cerebri	Dura Mater
Fascia lata	Subcutaneous Tissue and Fascia, Right Upper Leg
	Subcutaneous Tissue and Fascia, Left Upper Leg
Femoral head	Upper Femur, Right
	Upper Femur, Left
Femoral lymph node	Lymphatic, Left Lower Extremity
	Lymphatic, Right Lower Extremity
Femoropatellar joint	Knee Joint, Right
	Knee Joint, Left
Femorotibial joint	Knee Joint, Right
	Knee Joint, Left
Fibular artery	Peroneal Artery, Right
	Peroneal Artery, Left

Anatomical Term	PCS Description
Fibularis brevis muscle	Lower Leg Muscle, Right
	Lower Leg Muscle, Left
Fibularis brevis tendon	Lower Leg Tendon, Right
	Lower Leg Tendon, Left
Fibularis longus muscle	Lower Leg Muscle, Right
	Lower Leg Muscle, Left
Fibularis longus tendon	Lower Leg Tendon, Right
	Lower Leg Tendon, Left
Fifth cranial nerve	Trigeminal Nerve
First cranial nerve	Olfactory Nerve
First intercostal nerve	Brachial Plexus
Flexor carpi ulnaris tendon	Lower Arm and Wrist Tendon, Left
	Lower Arm and Wrist Tendon, Right
Flexor carpi ulnaris muscle	Lower Arm and Wrist Muscle, Left
	Lower Arm and Wrist Muscle, Right
Flexor digitorum brevis muscle	Foot Muscle, Right
	Foot Muscle, Left
Flexor digitorum brevis tendon	Foot Tendon, Right
	Foot Tendon, Left
Flexor digitorum longus muscle	Lower Leg Muscle, Right
	Lower Leg Muscle, Left
Flexor digitorum longus tendon	Lower Leg Tendon, Right
	Lower Leg Tendon, Left
Flexor hallucis brevis muscle	Foot Muscle, Right
	Foot Muscle, Left
Flexor hallucis brevis tendon	Foot Tendon, Right
	Foot Tendon, Left
Flexor hallucis longus muscle	Lower Leg Muscle, Right
	Lower Leg Muscle, Left
Flexor hallucis longus tendon	Lower Leg Tendon, Right
	Lower Leg Tendon, Left
Flexor pollicis longus tendon	Lower Arm and Wrist Tendon, Right
	Lower Arm and Wrist Tendon, Left
Flexor pollicis longus muscle	Lower Arm and Wrist Muscle, Right
	Lower Arm and Wrist Muscle, Left
Foramen magnum	Occipital Bone, Right
	Occipital Bone, Left
Foramen of Monro (intraventricular)	Cerebral Ventricle
Foreskin	Prepuce
Fossa of Rosenmuller	Nasopharynx
Fourth cranial nerve	Trochlear Nerve
Fourth ventricle	Cerebral Ventricle
Fovea	Retina, Left
	Retina, Right
Frenulum labii inferioris	Lower Lip
Frenulum labii superioris	Upper Lip
Frenulum linguae	Tongue
Frontal lobe	Cerebral Hemisphere
Frontal vein	Face Vein, Left
	Face Vein, Right
Fundus uteri	Uterus

Anatomical Term	PCS Description
Galea aponeurotica	Subcutaneous Tissue and Fascia, Scalp
Ganglion impar (ganglion of Walther)	Sacral Sympathetic Nerve
Gasserian ganglion	Trigeminal Nerve
Gastric lymph node	Lymphatic, Aortic
Gastric plexus	Abdominal Sympathetic Nerve
Gastrocnemius muscle	Lower Leg Muscle, Right
	Lower Leg Muscle, Left
Gastrocnemius tendon	Lower Leg Tendon, Right
	Lower Leg Tendon, Left
Gastrocolic omentum	Greater Omentum
Gastrocolic ligament	Greater Omentum
Gastroduodenal artery	Hepatic Artery
Gastroesophageal (GE) junction	Esophagogastric Junction
Gastrohepatic omentum	Lesser Omentum
Gastrophrenic ligament	Greater Omentum
Gastrosplenic ligament	Greater Omentum
Gemellus muscle	Hip Muscle, Right
	Hip Muscle, Left
Gemellus tendon	Hip Tendon, Right
	Hip Tendon, Left
Geniculate ganglion	Facial Nerve
Geniculate nucleus	Thalamus
Genioglossus muscle	Tongue, Palate, Pharynx Muscle
Genitofemoral nerve	Lumbar Plexus
Glans penis	Prepuce
Glenohumeral ligament	Shoulder Bursa and Ligament, Right
	Shoulder Bursa and Ligament, Left
Glenohumeral joint	Shoulder Joint, Right
	Shoulder Joint, Left
Glenoid fossa (of scapula) (syn)	Glenoid Cavity, Right
	Glenoid Cavity, Left
Glenoid ligament (labrum)	Shoulder Bursa and Ligament, Right
	Shoulder Bursa and Ligament, Left
Globus pallidus	Basal Ganglia
Glossoepiglottic fold	Epiglottis
Glottis	Larynx
Gluteal lymph node	Lymphatic, Pelvis
Gluteal vein	Hypogastric Vein, Right
	Hypogastric Vein, Left
Gluteus maximus muscle	Hip Muscle, Right
	Hip Muscle, Left
Gluteus maximus tendon	Hip Tendon, Right
	Hip Tendon, Left
Gluteus medius muscle	Hip Muscle, Right
	Hip Muscle, Left
Gluteus medius tendon	Hip Tendon, Right
	Hip Tendon, Left
Gluteus minimus muscle	Hip Muscle, Right
	Hip Muscle, Left

Anatomical Term	PCS Description
Gluteus minimus tendon	Hip Tendon, Right
	Hip Tendon, Left
Gracilis muscle	Upper Leg Muscle, Right
	Upper Leg Muscle, Left
Gracilis tendon	Upper Leg Tendon, Right
	Upper Leg Tendon, Left
Great auricular nerve	Cervical Plexus
Great cerebral vein	Intracranial Vein
Great saphenous vein	Greater Saphenous Vein, Right
	Greater Saphenous Vein, Left
Greater alar cartilage	Nose
Greater occipital nerve	Cervical Nerve
Greater splanchnic nerve	Thoracic Sympathetic Nerve
Greater superficial petrosal nerve	Facial Nerve
Greater trochanter	Upper Femur, Right
	Upper Femur, Left
Greater tuberosity	Humeral Head, Right
	Humeral Head, Left
Greater vestibular (Bartholin's) gland	Vestibular Gland
Greater wing	Sphenoid Bone, Right
	Sphenoid Bone, Left
Hallux	1st Toe, Left
	1st Toe, Right
Hamate bone	Carpal, Left
	Carpal, Right
Head of fibula	Fibula, Left
	Fibula, Right
Helix	External Ear, Right
	External Ear, Left
	External Ear, Bilateral
Hepatic artery proper	Hepatic Artery
Hepatic flexure	Ascending Colon
Hepatic lymph node	Lymphatic, Aortic
Hepatic plexus	Abdominal Sympathetic Nerve
Hepatic portal vein	Portal Vein
Hepatogastric ligament	Lesser Omentum
Hepatopancreatic ampulla	Ampulla of Vater
Humeroradial joint	Elbow Joint, Right
	Elbow Joint, Left
Humeroulnar joint	Elbow Joint, Right
	Elbow Joint, Left
Hyoglossus muscle	Tongue, Palate, Pharynx Muscle
Hyoid artery	Thyroid Artery, Right
	Thyroid Artery, Left
Hypogastric artery	Internal Iliac Artery, Right
	Internal Iliac Artery, Left
Hypopharynx	Pharynx
Hypophysis	Pituitary Gland

Anatomical Term	PCS Description
Hypothenar muscle	Hand Muscle, Right
	Hand Muscle, Left
Hypothenar tendon	Hand Tendon, Right
	Hand Tendon, Left
Ileal artery	Superior Mesenteric Artery
Ileocolic artery	Superior Mesenteric Artery
Ileocolic vein	Colic Vein
Iliac crest	Pelvic Bone, Right
	Pelvic Bone, Left
Iliac fascia	Subcutaneous Tissue and Fascia, Right Upper Leg
	Subcutaneous Tissue and Fascia, Left Upper Leg
Iliac lymph node	Lymphatic, Pelvis
Iliacus muscle	Hip Muscle, Right
	Hip Muscle, Left
Iliacus tendon	Hip Tendon, Right
	Hip Tendon, Left
Iliofemoral ligament	Hip Bursa and Ligament, Right
	Hip Bursa and Ligament, Left
Iliohypogastric nerve	Lumbar Plexus
Ilioinguinal nerve	Lumbar Plexus
Iliolumbar artery	Internal Iliac Artery, Right
	Internal Iliac Artery, Left
Iliolumbar ligament	Trunk Bursa and Ligament, Right
	Trunk Bursa and Ligament, Left
Iliotibial tract (band)	Subcutaneous Tissue and Fascia, Right Upper Leg
	Subcutaneous Tissue and Fascia, Left Upper Leg
Ilium	Pelvic Bone, Right
	Pelvic Bone, Left
Incus	Auditory Ossicle, Right
	Auditory Ossicle, Left
Inferior cardiac nerve	Thoracic Sympathetic Nerve
Inferior cerebral vein	Intracranial Vein
Inferior cerebellar vein	Intracranial Vein
Inferior epigastric artery	External Iliac Artery, Right
	External Iliac Artery, Left
Inferior epigastric lymph node	Lymphatic, Pelvis
Inferior genicular artery	Popliteal Artery, Right
	Popliteal Artery, Left
Inferior gluteal artery	Internal Iliac Artery, Right
	Internal Iliac Artery, Left
Inferior gluteal nerve	Sacral Plexus
Inferior hypogastric plexus	Abdominal Sympathetic Nerve
Inferior labial artery	Face Artery
Inferior longitudinal muscle	Tongue, Palate, Pharynx Muscle
Inferior mesenteric plexus	Abdominal Sympathetic Nerve

Anatomical Term	PCS Description
Inferior mesenteric ganglion	Abdominal Sympathetic Nerve
Inferior mesenteric lymph node	Lymphatic, Mesenteric
Inferior oblique muscle	Extraocular Muscle, Right
	Extraocular Muscle, Left
Inferior pancreaticoduo-denal artery	Superior Mesenteric Artery
Inferior phrenic artery	Abdominal Aorta
Inferior rectus muscle	Extraocular Muscle, Right
	Extraocular Muscle, Left
Inferior suprarenal artery	Renal Artery, Right
	Renal Artery, Left
Inferior tarsal plate	Lower Eyelid, Right
	Lower Eyelid, Left
Inferior thyroid vein	Innominate Vein, Right
	Innominate Vein, Left
Inferior tibiofibular joint	Ankle Joint, Right
	Ankle Joint, Left
Inferior turbinate	Nasal Turbinate
Inferior ulnar collateral artery	Brachial Artery, Right
	Brachial Artery, Left
Inferior vesical artery	Internal Iliac Artery, Right
	Internal Iliac Artery, Left
Infraauricular lymph node	Lymphatic, Head
Infraclavicular (deltopectoral) lymph node	Lymphatic, Left Upper Extremity
	Lymphatic, Right Upper Extremity
Infrahyoid muscle	Neck Muscle, Right
	Neck Muscle, Left
Infrahyoid tendon	Head and Neck Tendon
Infraparotid lymph node	Lymphatic, Head
Infraspinatus muscle	Shoulder Muscle, Right
	Shoulder Muscle, Left
Infraspinatus tendon	Shoulder Tendon, Right
	Shoulder Tendon, Left
Infraspinatus fascia	Subcutaneous Tissue and Fascia, Right Upper Arm
	Subcutaneous Tissue and Fascia, Left Upper Arm
Infundibulopelvic ligament	Uterine Supporting Structure
Inguinal canal	Inguinal Region, Right
	Inguinal Region, Left
	Inguinal Region, Bilateral
Inguinal triangle	Inguinal Region, Right
	Inguinal Region, Left
	Inguinal Region, Bilateral
Interatrial septum	Atrial Septum
Interatrial septum	Heart
Intercarpal joint	Carpal Joint, Right
	Carpal Joint, Left

Anatomical Term	PCS Description
Intercarpal ligament	Hand Bursa and Ligament, Right
	Hand Bursa and Ligament, Left
Interclavicular ligament	Shoulder Bursa and Ligament, Right
	Shoulder Bursa and Ligament, Left
Intercostal lymph node	Lymphatic, Thorax
Intercostal nerve	Thoracic Nerve
Intercostal muscle	Thorax Muscle, Right
	Thorax Muscle, Left
Intercostal tendon	Thorax Tendon, Right
	Thorax Tendon, Left
Intercostobrachial nerve	Thoracic Nerve
Intercuneiform ligament	Foot Bursa and Ligament, Right
	Foot Bursa and Ligament, Left
Intercuneiform joint	Tarsal Joint, Right
	Tarsal Joint, Left
Intermediate cuneiform bone	Tarsal, Left
	Tarsal, Right
Internal (basal) cerebral vein	Intracranial Vein
Internal anal sphincter	Anal Sphincter
Internal carotid plexus	Head and Neck Sympathetic Nerve
Internal iliac vein	Hypogastric Vein, Right
	Hypogastric Vein, Left
Internal maxillary artery	External Carotid Artery, Right
	External Carotid Artery, Left
Internal naris	Nose
Internal oblique muscle	Abdomen Muscle, Right
	Abdomen Muscle, Left
Internal oblique tendon	Abdomen Tendon, Right
	Abdomen Tendon, Left
Internal pudendal vein	Hypogastric Vein, Right
	Hypogastric Vein, Left
Internal pudendal artery	Internal Iliac Artery, Left
	Internal Iliac Artery, Right
Internal thoracic artery	Internal Mammary Artery, Right
	Internal Mammary Artery, Left
Internal thoracic artery	Subclavian Artery, Right
	Subclavian Artery, Left
Internal urethral sphincter	Urethra
Interphalangeal (IP) joint	Finger Phalangeal Joint, Right
	Finger Phalangeal Joint, Left
	Toe Phalangeal Joint, Right
	Toe Phalangeal Joint, Left
Interphalangeal ligament	Foot Bursa and Ligament, Right
	Foot Bursa and Ligament, Left
	Hand Bursa and Ligament, Right
	Hand Bursa and Ligament, Left
Interspinalis muscle	Trunk Muscle, Right
	Trunk Muscle, Left
Interspinalis tendon	Trunk Tendon, Right
	Trunk Tendon, Left

Anatomical Term	PCS Description
Interspinous ligament	Trunk Bursa and Ligament, Right
	Trunk Bursa and Ligament, Left
Intertransverse ligament	Trunk Bursa and Ligament, Right
	Trunk Bursa and Ligament, Left
Intertransversarius muscle	Trunk Muscle, Right
	Trunk Muscle, Left
Intertransversarius tendon	Trunk Tendon, Right
	Trunk Tendon, Left
Interventricular foramen (Monro)	Cerebral Ventricle
Interventricular septum	Ventricular Septum
Intestinal lymphatic trunk	Cisterna Chyli
Ischiatic nerve	Sciatic Nerve
Ischiocavernosus muscle	Perineum Muscle
Ischiocavernosus tendon	Perineum Tendon
Ischiofemoral ligament	Hip Bursa and Ligament, Right
	Hip Bursa and Ligament, Left
Ischium	Pelvic Bone, Right
	Pelvic Bone, Left
Jejunal artery	Superior Mesenteric Artery
Jugular body	Glomus Jugulare
Jugular lymph node	Lymphatic, Left Neck
	Lymphatic, Right Neck
Labia majora	Vulva
Labia minora	Vulva
Labial gland	Buccal Mucosa
Lacrimal canaliculus	Lacrimal Duct, Right
	Lacrimal Duct, Left
Lacrimal punctum	Lacrimal Duct, Right
	Lacrimal Duct, Left
Lacrimal sac	Lacrimal Duct, Right
	Lacrimal Duct, Left
Laryngopharynx	Pharynx
Lateral (brachial) lymph node	Lymphatic, Left Axillary
	Lymphatic, Right Axillary
Lateral canthus	Upper Eyelid, Right
	Upper Eyelid, Left
Lateral collateral ligament (LCL)	Knee Bursa and Ligament, Right
	Knee Bursa and Ligament, Left
Lateral condyle of femur	Lower Femur, Right
	Lower Femur, Left
Lateral condyle of tibia	Tibia, Left
	Tibia, Right
Lateral cuneiform bone	Tarsal, Left
	Tarsal, Right
Lateral epicondyle of humerus	Humeral Shaft, Right
	Humeral Shaft, Left
Lateral epicondyle of femur	Lower Femur, Right
	Lower Femur, Left
Lateral femoral cutaneous nerve	Lumbar Plexus

Anatomical Term	PCS Description
Lateral malleolus	Fibula, Left
	Fibula, Right
Lateral meniscus	Knee Joint, Right
	Knee Joint, Left
Lateral nasal cartilage	Nose
Lateral plantar artery	Foot Artery, Right
	Foot Artery, Left
Lateral plantar nerve	Tibial Nerve
Lateral rectus muscle	Extraocular Muscle, Right
	Extraocular Muscle, Left
Lateral sacral vein	Hypogastric Vein, Right
	Hypogastric Vein, Left
Lateral sacral artery	Internal Iliac Artery, Right
	Internal Iliac Artery, Left
Lateral sural cutaneous nerve	Peroneal Nerve
Lateral tarsal artery	Foot Artery, Right
	Foot Artery, Left
Lateral temporomandibular ligament	Head and Neck Bursa and Ligament
Lateral thoracic artery	Axillary Artery, Right
	Axillary Artery, Left
Latissimus dorsi muscle	Trunk Muscle, Right
	Trunk Muscle, Left
Latissimus dorsi tendon	Trunk Tendon, Right
	Trunk Tendon, Left
Least splanchnic nerve	Thoracic Sympathetic Nerve
Left ascending lumbar vein	Hemiazygos Vein
Left atrioventricular valve (syn)	Mitral Valve
Left auricular appendix	Atrium, Left
Left colic vein	Colic Vein
Left coronary sulcus	Heart, Left
Left gastric artery	Gastric Artery
Left gastroepiploic artery	Splenic Artery
Left gastroepiploic vein	Splenic Vein
Left inferior pulmonary vein	Pulmonary Vein, Left
Left inferior phrenic vein	Renal Vein, Left
Left jugular trunk	Thoracic Duct
Left lateral ventricle	Cerebral Ventricle
Left ovarian vein	Renal Vein, Left
Left second lumbar vein	Renal Vein, Left
Left subclavian trunk	Thoracic Duct
Left subcostal vein	Hemiazygos Vein
Left superior pulmonary vein	Pulmonary Vein, Left
Left suprarenal vein	Renal Vein, Left
Left testicular vein	Renal Vein, Left
Leptomeninges	Cerebral Meninges
	Spinal Meninges
Lesser alar cartilage	Nose

Anatomical Term	PCS Description
Lesser occipital nerve	Cervical Plexus
Lesser splanchnic nerve	Thoracic Sympathetic Nerve
Lesser trochanter	Upper Femur, Right
	Upper Femur, Left
Lesser tuberosity	Humeral Head, Right
	Humeral Head, Left
Lesser wing	Sphenoid Bone, Right
	Sphenoid Bone, Left
Levator anguli oris muscle	Facial Muscle
Levator ani muscle	Trunk Muscle, Left
Levator ani tendon	Trunk Tendon, Left
Levator labii superioris muscle	Facial Muscle
Levator labii superioris alaeque nasi muscle	Facial Muscle
Levator palpebrae superioris muscle	Upper Eyelid, Right
	Upper Eyelid, Left
Levator scapulae tendon	Head and Neck Tendon
Levator scapulae muscle	Neck Muscle, Right
	Neck Muscle, Left
Levator veli palatini muscle	Tongue, Palate, Pharynx Muscle
Levatores costarum muscle	Thorax Muscle, Right
	Thorax Muscle, Left
Levatores costarum tendon	Thorax Tendon, Right
	Thorax Tendon, Left
Ligament of the lateral malleolus	Ankle Bursa and Ligament, Right
	Ankle Bursa and Ligament, Left
Ligament of head of fibula	Knee Bursa and Ligament, Right
	Knee Bursa and Ligament, Left
Ligamentum flavum	Trunk Bursa and Ligament, Right
	Trunk Bursa and Ligament, Left
Lingual artery	External Carotid Artery, Right
	External Carotid Artery, Left
Lingual tonsil	Tongue
Locus ceruleus	Pons
Long thoracic nerve	Brachial Plexus
Lumbar artery	Abdominal Aorta
Lumbar facet joint	Lumbar Vertebral Joints, 2 or more
	Lumbar Vertebral Joint
Lumbar ganglion	Lumbar Sympathetic Nerve
Lumbar lymphatic trunk	Cisterna Chyli
Lumbar lymph node	Lymphatic, Aortic
Lumbar splanchnic nerve	Lumbar Sympathetic Nerve
Lumbosacral trunk	Lumbar Nerve
Lumbosacral facet joint	Lumbosacral Joint
Lunate bone	Carpal, Left
	Carpal, Right
Lunotriquetral ligament	Hand Bursa and Ligament, Right
	Hand Bursa and Ligament, Left

Anatomical Term	PCS Description
Macula	Retina, Left
	Retina, Right
Malleus	Auditory Ossicle, Right
	Auditory Ossicle, Left
Mammary duct	Breast, Bilateral
	Breast, Left
	Breast, Right
Mammary gland	Breast, Bilateral
	Breast, Left
	Breast, Right
Mammillary body	Hypothalamus
Mandibular notch	Mandible, Left
	Mandible, Right
Mandibular nerve	Trigeminal Nerve
Manubrium	Sternum
Masseter muscle	Head Muscle
Masseter tendon	Head and Neck Tendon
Masseteric fascia	Subcutaneous Tissue and Fascia, Face
Mastoid (postauricular) lymph node	Lymphatic, Left Neck
	Lymphatic, Right Neck
Mastoid air cells	Mastoid Sinus, Right
	Mastoid Sinus, Left
Mastoid process	Temporal Bone, Right
	Temporal Bone, Left
Maxillary artery	External Carotid Artery, Right
	External Carotid Artery, Left
Maxillary nerve	Trigeminal Nerve
Medial canthus	Lower Eyelid, Right
	Lower Eyelid, Left
Medial collateral ligament (MCL)	Knee Bursa and Ligament, Right
	Knee Bursa and Ligament, Left
Medial condyle of femur	Lower Femur, Right
	Lower Femur, Left
Medial condyle of tibia	Tibia, Left
	Tibia, Right
Medial cuneiform bone	Tarsal, Left
	Tarsal, Right
Medial epicondyle of humerus	Humeral Shaft, Right
	Humeral Shaft, Left
Medial epicondyle of femur	Lower Femur, Right
	Lower Femur, Left
Medial malleolus	Tibia, Left
	Tibia, Right
Medial meniscus	Knee Joint, Right
	Knee Joint, Left
Medial plantar artery	Foot Artery, Right
	Foot Artery, Left
Medial plantar nerve	Tibial Nerve
Medial popliteal nerve	Tibial Nerve
Medial rectus muscle	Extraocular Muscle, Right
	Extraocular Muscle, Left

Anatomical Term	PCS Description
Medial sural cutaneous nerve	Tibial Nerve
Median antebrachial vein	Basilic Vein, Right
	Basilic Vein, Left
Median cubital vein	Basilic Vein, Right
	Basilic Vein, Left
Median sacral artery	Abdominal Aorta
Mediastinal lymph node	Lymphatic, Thorax
Meissner's (submucous) plexus	Abdominal Sympathetic Nerve
Membranous urethra	Urethra
Mental foramen	Mandible, Left
	Mandible, Right
Mentalis muscle	Facial Muscle
Mesoappendix	Mesentery
Mesocolon	Mesentery
Metacarpal ligament	Hand Bursa and Ligament, Right
	Hand Bursa and Ligament, Left
Metacarpophalan-geal ligament	Hand Bursa and Ligament, Right
	Hand Bursa and Ligament, Left
Metatarsal ligament	Foot Bursa and Ligament, Right
	Foot Bursa and Ligament, Left
Metatarsophalan-geal ligament	Foot Bursa and Ligament, Right
	Foot Bursa and Ligament, Left
Metatarsophalan-geal (MTP) joint	Metatarsal-Phalangeal Joint, Right
	Metatarsal-Phalangeal Joint, Left
Metathalamus	Thalamus
Midcarpal joint	Carpal Joint, Right
	Carpal Joint, Left
Middle cardiac nerve	Thoracic Sympathetic Nerve
Middle cerebral artery	Intracranial Artery
Middle cerebral vein	Intracranial Vein
Middle colic vein	Colic Vein
Middle genicular artery	Popliteal Artery, Right
	Popliteal Artery, Left
Middle hemorrhoidal vein	Hypogastric Vein, Right
	Hypogastric Vein, Left
Middle rectal artery	Internal Iliac Artery, Right
	Internal Iliac Artery, Left
Middle suprarenal artery	Abdominal Aorta
Middle temporal artery	Temporal Artery, Right
	Temporal Artery, Left
Middle turbinate	Nasal Turbinate
Mitral annulus	Mitral Valve
Molar gland	Buccal Mucosa
Musculocutaneous nerve	Brachial Plexus
Musculophrenic artery	Internal Mammary Artery, Right
	Internal Mammary Artery, Left
Musculospiral nerve	Radial Nerve
Myelencephalon	Medulla Oblongata
Myenteric (Auerbach's) plexus	Abdominal Sympathetic Nerve

Anatomical Term	PCS Description
Myometrium	Uterus
Nail bed	Finger Nail
	Toe Nail
Nail plate	Finger Nail
	Toe Nail
Nasal cavity	Nose
Nasal concha	Nasal Turbinate
Nasalis muscle	Facial Muscle
Nasolacrimal duct	Lacrimal Duct, Right
	Lacrimal Duct, Left
Navicular bone	Tarsal, Left
	Tarsal, Right
Neck of femur	Upper Femur, Right
	Upper Femur, Left
Neck of humerus (anatomical) (surgical)	Humeral Head, Right
	Humeral Head, Left
Nerve to the stapedius	Facial Nerve
Neurohypophysis	Pituitary Gland
Ninth cranial nerve	Glossopharyngeal Nerve
Nostril	Nose
Obturator artery	Internal Iliac Artery, Right
	Internal Iliac Artery, Left
Obturator lymph node	Lymphatic, Pelvis
Obturator muscle	Hip Muscle, Right
	Hip Muscle, Left
Obturator nerve	Lumbar Plexus
Obturator tendon	Hip Tendon, Right
	Hip Tendon, Left
Obturator vein	Hypogastric Vein, Right
	Hypogastric Vein, Left
Obtuse margin	Heart, Left
Occipital artery	External Carotid Artery, Right
	External Carotid Artery, Left
Occipital lobe	Cerebral Hemisphere
Occipital lymph node	Lymphatic, Left Neck
	Lymphatic, Right Neck
Occipitofrontalis muscle	Facial Muscle
Olecranon bursa	Elbow Bursa and Ligament, Right
	Elbow Bursa and Ligament, Left
Olecranon process	Ulna, Left
	Ulna, Right
Olfactory bulb	Olfactory Nerve
Ophthalmic artery	Internal Carotid Artery, Right
	Internal Carotid Artery, Left
Ophthalmic nerve	Trigeminal Nerve
Ophthalmic vein	Intracranial Vein
Optic chiasma	Optic Nerve
Optic disc	Retina, Left
	Retina, Right
Optic foramen	Sphenoid Bone, Right
	Sphenoid Bone, Left

Anatomical Term	PCS Description
Orbicularis oris muscle	Facial Muscle
Orbicularis oculi muscle	Upper Eyelid, Right
	Upper Eyelid, Left
Orbital fascia	Subcutaneous Tissue and Fascia, Face
Orbital portion of ethmoid bone	Orbit, Left
	Orbit, Right
Orbital portion of frontal bone	Orbit, Left
	Orbit, Right
Orbital portion of lacrimal bone	Orbit, Left
	Orbit, Right
Orbital portion of maxilla	Orbit, Left
	Orbit, Right
Orbital portion of palatine bone	Orbit, Left
	Orbit, Right
Orbital portion of sphenoid bone	Orbit, Left
	Orbit, Right
Orbital portion of zygomatic bone	Orbit, Left
	Orbit, Right
Oropharynx	Pharynx
Ossicular chain	Auditory Ossicle, Right
	Auditory Ossicle, Left
Otic ganglion	Head and Neck Sympathetic Nerve
Oval window	Inner Ear, Left
	Inner Ear, Right
Ovarian artery	Abdominal Aorta
Ovarian ligament	Uterine Supporting Structure
Oviduct	Fallopian Tube, Right
	Fallopian Tube, Left
Palatine gland	Buccal Mucosa
Palatine tonsil	Tonsils
Palatine uvula	Uvula
Palatoglossal muscle	Tongue, Palate, Pharynx Muscle
Palatopharyngeal muscle	Tongue, Palate, Pharynx Muscle
Palmar (volar) metacarpal vein	Hand Vein, Right
	Hand Vein, Left
Palmar (volar) digital vein	Hand Vein, Left
	Hand Vein, Right
Palmar cutaneous nerve	Median Nerve
	Radial Nerve
Palmar fascia (aponeurosis)	Subcutaneous Tissue and Fascia, Right Hand
	Subcutaneous Tissue and Fascia, Left Hand
Palmar interosseous muscle	Hand Muscle, Right
	Hand Muscle, Left
Palmar interosseous tendon	Hand Tendon, Right
	Hand Tendon, Left
Palmar ulnocarpal ligament	Wrist Bursa and Ligament, Right
	Wrist Bursa and Ligament, Left
Palmaris longus tendon	Lower Arm and Wrist Tendon, Right
	Lower Arm and Wrist Tendon, Left

Anatomical Term	PCS Description
Palmaris longus muscle	Lower Arm and Wrist Muscle, Right
	Lower Arm and Wrist Muscle, Left
Pancreatic artery	Splenic Artery
Pancreatic plexus	Abdominal Sympathetic Nerve
Pancreatic vein	Splenic Vein
Pancreaticosplenic lymph node	Lymphatic, Aortic
Paraaortic lymph node	Lymphatic, Aortic
Pararectal lymph node	Lymphatic, Mesenteric
Parasternal lymph node	Lymphatic, Thorax
Paratracheal lymph node	Lymphatic, Thorax
Paraurethral (Skene's) gland	Vestibular Gland
Parietal lobe	Cerebral Hemisphere
Parotid lymph node	Lymphatic, Head
Parotid plexus	Facial Nerve
Pars flaccida	Tympanic Membrane, Right
	Tympanic Membrane, Left
Patellar ligament	Knee Bursa and Ligament, Right
	Knee Bursa and Ligament, Left
Patellar tendon	Knee Tendon, Right
	Knee Tendon, Left
Pectineus muscle	Upper Leg Muscle, Right
	Upper Leg Muscle, Left
Pectineus tendon	Upper Leg Tendon, Right
	Upper Leg Tendon, Left
Pectoral (anterior) lymph node	Lymphatic, Left Axillary
	Lymphatic, Right Axillary
Pectoral fascia	Subcutaneous Tissue and Fascia, Chest
Pectoralis major muscle	Thorax Muscle, Left
	Thorax Muscle, Right
Pectoralis minor muscle	Thorax Muscle, Left
	Thorax Muscle, Right
Pectoralis minor tendon	Thorax Tendon, Left
	Thorax Tendon, Right
Pectoralis major tendon	Thorax Tendon, Left
	Thorax Tendon, Right
Pelvic fascia	Subcutaneous Tissue and Fascia, Trunk
Pelvic splanchnic nerve	Abdominal Sympathetic Nerve
	Sacral Sympathetic Nerve
Penile urethra	Urethra
Pericardiophrenic artery	Internal Mammary Artery, Right
	Internal Mammary Artery, Left
Perimetrium	Uterus
Peroneus brevis muscle	Lower Leg Muscle, Right
	Lower Leg Muscle, Left
Peroneus brevis tendon	Lower Leg Tendon, Right
	Lower Leg Tendon, Left
Peroneus longus muscle	Lower Leg Muscle, Right
	Lower Leg Muscle, Left
Peroneus longus tendon	Lower Leg Tendon, Right
	Lower Leg Tendon, Left

Anatomical Term	PCS Description	Anatomical Term	PCS Description
Petrous part of temoporal bone	Temporal Bone, Right	Popliteus tendon	Lower Leg Tendon, Right
	Temporal Bone, Left		Lower Leg Tendon, Left
Pharyngeal constrictor muscle	Tongue, Palate, Pharynx Muscle	Postauricular (mastoid) lymph node	Lymphatic, Left Neck
			Lymphatic, Right Neck
Pharyngeal plexus	Vagus Nerve	Postcava (syn)	Inferior Vena Cava
Pharyngeal recess	Nasopharynx	Posterior (subscapular) lymph node	Lymphatic, Left Axillary
Pharyngeal tonsil	Adenoids		Lymphatic, Right Axillary
Pharyngotym-panic tube	Eustachian Tube, Right	Posterior auricular artery	External Carotid Artery, Right
	Eustachian Tube, Left		External Carotid Artery, Left
Pia mater	Cerebral Meninges	Posterior auricular vein	External Jugular Vein, Right
	Spinal Meninges		External Jugular Vein, Left
Pinna	External Ear, Right	Posterior auricular nerve	Facial Nerve
	External Ear, Left	Posterior cerebral artery	Intracranial Artery
	External Ear, Bilateral	Posterior chamber	Eye, Left
Piriform recess (sinus)	Pharynx		Eye, Right
Piriformis muscle	Hip Muscle, Right	Posterior circumflex humeral artery	Axillary Artery, Right
	Hip Muscle, Left		Axillary Artery, Left
Piriformis tendon	Hip Tendon, Right	Posterior communicating artery	Intracranial Artery
	Hip Tendon, Left		
Pisiform bone	Carpal, Left	Posterior cruciate ligament (PCL)	Knee Bursa and Ligament, Right
	Carpal, Right		Knee Bursa and Ligament, Left
Pisohamate ligament	Hand Bursa and Ligament, Right	Posterior facial (retromandibular) vein	Face Vein, Left
	Hand Bursa and Ligament, Left		Face Vein, Right
Pisometacarpal ligament	Hand Bursa and Ligament, Right	Posterior femoral cutaneous nerve	Sacral Plexus
	Hand Bursa and Ligament, Left		
Plantar digital vein	Foot Vein, Left	Posterior inferior cerebellar artery (PICA)	Intracranial Artery
	Foot Vein, Right		
Plantar fascia (aponeurosis)	Subcutaneous Tissue and Fascia, Right Foot	Posterior interosseous nerve	Radial Nerve
	Subcutaneous Tissue and Fascia, Left Foot	Posterior labial nerve	Pudendal Nerve
		Posterior scrotal nerve	Pudendal Nerve
Plantar metatarsal vein	Foot Vein, Left	Posterior spinal artery	Vertebral Artery, Right
	Foot Vein, Right		Vertebral Artery, Left
Plantar venous arch	Foot Vein, Left	Posterior tibial recurrent artery	Anterior Tibial Artery, Right
	Foot Vein, Right		Anterior Tibial Artery, Left
Platysma muscle	Neck Muscle, Right	Posterior ulnar recurrent artery	Ulnar Artery, Right
	Neck Muscle, Left		Ulnar Artery, Left
Platysma tendon	Head and Neck Tendon	Posterior vagal trunk	Vagus Nerve
Plica semilunaris	Conjunctiva, Right	Preauricular lymph node	Lymphatic, Head
	Conjunctiva, Left	Precava	Superior Vena Cava
Pneumogastric nerve	Vagus Nerve	Prepatellar bursa	Knee Bursa and Ligament, Right
Pneumotaxic center	Pons		Knee Bursa and Ligament, Left
Pontine tegmentum	Pons	Pretracheal fascia	Subcutaneous Tissue and Fascia, Anterior Neck
Popliteal lymph node	Lymphatic, Left Lower Extremity	Prevertebral fascia	Subcutaneous Tissue and Fascia, Posterior Neck
	Lymphatic, Right Lower Extremity		
Popliteal ligament	Knee Bursa and Ligament, Right	Princeps pollicis artery	Hand Artery, Right
	Knee Bursa and Ligament, Left		Hand Artery, Left
Popliteal vein	Femoral Vein, Right	Procerus muscle	Facial Muscle
	Femoral Vein, Left	Profunda brachii	Brachial Artery, Right
Popliteus muscle	Lower Leg Muscle, Right		Brachial Artery, Left
	Lower Leg Muscle, Left		

Anatomical Term	PCS Description
Profunda femoris (deep femoral) vein	Femoral Vein, Right
	Femoral Vein, Left
Pronator quadratus tendon	Lower Arm and Wrist Tendon, Right
	Lower Arm and Wrist Tendon, Left
Pronator quadratus muscle	Lower Arm and Wrist Muscle, Right
	Lower Arm and Wrist Muscle, Left
Pronator teres tendon	Lower Arm and Wrist Tendon, Right
	Lower Arm and Wrist Tendon, Left
Pronator teres muscle	Lower Arm and Wrist Muscle, Right
	Lower Arm and Wrist Muscle, Left
Prostatic urethra	Urethra
Proximal radioulnar joint	Elbow Joint, Right
	Elbow Joint, Left
Psoas muscle	Hip Muscle, Right
	Hip Muscle, Left
Psoas tendon	Hip Tendon, Right
	Hip Tendon, Left
Pterygoid muscle	Head Muscle
Pterygoid process	Sphenoid Bone, Right
	Sphenoid Bone, Left
Pterygoid tendon	Head and Neck Tendon
Pterygopalatine (sphenopalatine) ganglion	Head and Neck Sympathetic Nerve
Pubic ligament	Trunk Bursa and Ligament, Right
	Trunk Bursa and Ligament, Left
Pubis	Pelvic Bone, Right
	Pelvic Bone, Left
Pubofemoral ligament	Hip Bursa and Ligament, Right
	Hip Bursa and Ligament, Left
Pudendal nerve	Sacral Plexus
Pulmonary annulus	Pulmonary Valve
Pulmonary plexus	Thoracic Sympathetic Nerve
	Vagus Nerve
Pulmonic valve	Pulmonary Valve
Pulvinar	Thalamus
Pyloric antrum	Stomach, Pylorus
Pyloric canal	Stomach, Pylorus
Pyloric sphincter	Stomach, Pylorus
Pyramidalis muscle	Abdomen Muscle, Right
	Abdomen Muscle, Left
Pyramidalis tendon	Abdomen Tendon, Right
	Abdomen Tendon, Left
Quadrangular cartilage	Nasal Septum
Quadrate lobe	Liver
Quadratus femoris muscle	Hip Muscle, Right
	Hip Muscle, Left
Quadratus femoris tendon	Hip Tendon, Right
	Hip Tendon, Left
Quadratus lumborum muscle	Trunk Muscle, Right
	Trunk Muscle, Left

Anatomical Term	PCS Description
Quadratus lumborum tendon	Trunk Tendon, Right
	Trunk Tendon, Left
Quadratus plantae muscle	Foot Muscle, Right
	Foot Muscle, Left
Quadratus plantae tendon	Foot Tendon, Right
	Foot Tendon, Left
Quadriceps (femoris)	Upper Leg Muscle, Right
	Upper Leg Muscle, Left
	Upper Leg Tendon, Right
	Upper Leg Tendon, Left
Radial collateral ligament	Elbow Bursa and Ligament, Right
	Elbow Bursa and Ligament, Left
Radial collateral carpal ligament	Wrist Bursa and Ligament, Right
	Wrist Bursa and Ligament, Left
Radial notch	Ulna, Left
	Ulna, Right
Radial recurrent artery	Radial Artery, Right
	Radial Artery, Left
Radial vein	Brachial Vein, Right
	Brachial Vein, Left
Radialis indicis	Hand Artery, Right
	Hand Artery, Left
Radiocarpal ligament	Wrist Bursa and Ligament, Right
	Wrist Bursa and Ligament, Left
Radiocarpal joint	Wrist Joint, Right
	Wrist Joint, Left
Radioulnar ligament	Wrist Bursa and Ligament, Right
	Wrist Bursa and Ligament, Left
Rectosigmoid junction	Sigmoid Colon
Rectus abdominis muscle	Abdomen Muscle, Right
	Abdomen Muscle, Left
Rectus abdominis tendon	Abdomen Tendon, Right
	Abdomen Tendon, Left
Rectus femoris muscle	Upper Leg Muscle, Right
	Upper Leg Muscle, Left
Rectus femoris tendon	Upper Leg Tendon, Right
	Upper Leg Tendon, Left
Recurrent laryngeal nerve	Vagus Nerve
Renal calyx	Kidney
	Kidney, Left
	Kidney, Right
	Kidneys, Bilateral
Renal capsule	Kidney
	Kidney, Left
	Kidney, Right
	Kidneys, Bilateral
Renal cortex	Kidney
	Kidney, Left
	Kidney, Right
	Kidneys, Bilateral
Renal plexus	Abdominal Sympathetic Nerve

 Draft (2011)

Anatomical Term	PCS Description
Renal segment	Kidney
	Kidney, Left
	Kidney, Right
	Kidneys, Bilateral
Renal segmental artery	Renal Artery, Right
	Renal Artery, Left
Retroperitoneal lymph node	Lymphatic, Aortic
Retroperitoneal space	Retroperitoneum
Retropharyngeal lymph node	Lymphatic, Left Neck
	Lymphatic, Right Neck
Retropubic space	Pelvic Cavity
Rhinopharynx	Nasopharynx
Rhomboid major muscle	Trunk Muscle, Right
	Trunk Muscle, Left
Rhomboid major tendon	Trunk Tendon, Right
	Trunk Tendon, Left
Rhomboid minor muscle	Trunk Muscle, Right
	Trunk Muscle, Left
Rhomboid minor tendon	Trunk Tendon, Right
	Trunk Tendon, Left
Right ascending lumbar vein	Azygos Vein
Right atrioventricular valve (syn)	Tricuspid Valve
Right auricular appendix	Atrium, Right
Right colic vein	Colic Vein
Right coronary sulcus	Heart, Right
Right gastric artery	Gastric Artery
Right gastroepiploic vein	Superior Mesenteric Vein
Right inferior phrenic vein	Inferior Vena Cava
Right inferior pulmonary vein	Pulmonary Vein, Right
Right jugular trunk	Lymphatic, Right Neck
Right lateral ventricle	Cerebral Ventricle
Right lymphatic duct	Lymphatic, Right Neck
Right ovarian vein	Inferior Vena Cava
Right second lumbar vein	Inferior Vena Cava
Right subclavian trunk	Lymphatic, Right Neck
Right subcostal vein	Azygos Vein
Right superior pulmonary vein	Pulmonary Vein, Right
Right suprarenal vein	Inferior Vena Cava
Right testicular vein	Inferior Vena Cava
Rima glottidis	Larynx
Risorius muscle	Facial Muscle
Round ligament of uterus	Uterine Supporting Structure
Round window	Inner Ear, Left
	Inner Ear, Right
Sacral ganglion	Sacral Sympathetic Nerve
Sacral lymph node	Lymphatic, Pelvis
Sacral splanchnic nerve	Sacral Sympathetic Nerve

Anatomical Term	PCS Description
Sacrococcygeal symphysis	Sacrococcygeal Joint
Sacrococcygeal ligament	Trunk Bursa and Ligament, Right
	Trunk Bursa and Ligament, Left
Sacroiliac ligament	Trunk Bursa and Ligament, Right
	Trunk Bursa and Ligament, Left
Sacrospinous ligament	Trunk Bursa and Ligament, Right
	Trunk Bursa and Ligament, Left
Sacrotuberous ligament	Trunk Bursa and Ligament, Right
	Trunk Bursa and Ligament, Left
Salpingopharyngeus muscle	Tongue, Palate, Pharynx Muscle
Salpinx	Fallopian Tube, Left
	Fallopian Tube, Right
Saphenous nerve	Femoral Nerve
Sartorius muscle	Upper Leg Muscle, Right
	Upper Leg Muscle, Left
Sartorius tendon	Upper Leg Tendon, Right
	Upper Leg Tendon, Left
Scalene muscle	Neck Muscle, Right
	Neck Muscle, Left
Scalene tendon	Head and Neck Tendon
Scaphoid bone	Carpal, Left
	Carpal, Right
Scapholunate ligament	Hand Bursa and Ligament, Right
	Hand Bursa and Ligament, Left
Scaphotrapezium ligament	Hand Bursa and Ligament, Right
	Hand Bursa and Ligament, Left
Scarpa's (vestibular) ganglion	Acoustic Nerve
Sebaceous gland	Skin
Second cranial nerve	Optic Nerve
Sella turcica	Sphenoid Bone, Right
	Sphenoid Bone, Left
Semicircular canal	Inner Ear, Left
	Inner Ear, Right
Semimembranosus muscle	Upper Leg Muscle, Right
	Upper Leg Muscle, Left
Semimembranosus tendon	Upper Leg Tendon, Right
	Upper Leg Tendon, Left
Semitendinosus muscle	Upper Leg Muscle, Right
	Upper Leg Muscle, Left
Semitendinosus tendon	Upper Leg Tendon, Right
	Upper Leg Tendon, Left
Septal cartilage	Nasal Septum
Serratus anterior muscle	Thorax Muscle, Right
	Thorax Muscle, Left
Serratus anterior tendon	Thorax Tendon, Right
	Thorax Tendon, Left
Serratus posterior muscle	Trunk Muscle, Right
	Trunk Muscle, Left

Anatomical Term	PCS Description
Serratus posterior tendon	Trunk Tendon, Right
	Trunk Tendon, Left
Seventh cranial nerve	Facial Nerve
Short gastric artery	Splenic Artery
Sigmoid artery	Inferior Mesenteric Artery
Sigmoid flexure	Sigmoid Colon
Sigmoid vein	Inferior Mesenteric Vein
Sinoatrial node	Conduction Mechanism
Sinus venosus	Atrium, Right
Sixth cranial nerve	Abducens Nerve
Skene's (paraurethral) gland	Vestibular Gland
Small saphenous vein	Lesser Saphenous Vein, Right
	Lesser Saphenous Vein, Left
Solar (celiac) plexus	Abdominal Sympathetic Nerve
Soleus muscle	Lower Leg Muscle, Right
	Lower Leg Muscle, Left
Soleus tendon	Lower Leg Tendon, Right
	Lower Leg Tendon, Left
Sphenomand-ibular ligament	Head and Neck Bursa and Ligament
Sphenopalatine (pterygopalatine) ganglion	Head and Neck Sympathetic Nerve
Spinal dura mater	Dura Mater
Spinal epidural space	Epidural Space
Spinal subarachnoid space	Subarachnoid Space
Spinal subdural space	Subdural Space
Spinous process	Cervical Vertebra
	Lumbar Vertebra
	Thoracic Vertebra
Spiral ganglion	Acoustic Nerve
Splenic flexure	Transverse Colon
Splenic plexus	Abdominal Sympathetic Nerve
Splenius capitis tendon	Head and Neck Tendon
Splenius capitis muscle	Head Muscle
Splenius cervicis tendon	Head and Neck Tendon
Splenius cervicis muscle	Neck Muscle, Right
	Neck Muscle, Left
Stapes	Auditory Ossicle, Right
	Auditory Ossicle, Left
Stellate ganglion	Head and Neck Sympathetic Nerve
Stensen's duct	Parotid Duct, Right
	Parotid Duct, Left
Sternoclavicular ligament	Shoulder Bursa and Ligament, Right
	Shoulder Bursa and Ligament, Left
Sternocleido-mastoid artery	Thyroid Artery, Right
	Thyroid Artery, Left
Sternocleido-mastoid muscle	Neck Muscle, Right
	Neck Muscle, Left
Sternocleido-mastoid tendon	Head and Neck Tendon

Anatomical Term	PCS Description
Sternocostal ligament	Thorax Bursa and Ligament, Right
	Thorax Bursa and Ligament, Left
Styloglossus muscle	Tongue, Palate, Pharynx Muscle
Stylomandibular ligament	Head and Neck Bursa and Ligament
Stylopharyngeus muscle	Tongue, Palate, Pharynx Muscle
Subacromial bursa	Shoulder Bursa and Ligament, Right
	Shoulder Bursa and Ligament, Left
Subaortic (common iliac) lymph node	Lymphatic, Pelvis
Subclavicular (apical) lymph node	Lymphatic, Left Axillary
	Lymphatic, Right Axillary
Subclavius muscle	Thorax Muscle, Right
	Thorax Muscle, Left
Subclavius nerve	Brachial Plexus
Subclavius tendon	Thorax Tendon, Right
	Thorax Tendon, Left
Subcostal artery	Thoracic Aorta
Subcostal muscle	Thorax Muscle, Right
	Thorax Muscle, Left
Subcostal nerve	Thoracic Nerve
Subcostal tendon	Thorax Tendon, Right
	Thorax Tendon, Left
Submandibular ganglion	Facial Nerve
	Head and Neck Sympathetic Nerve
Submandibular gland	Submaxillary Gland, Right
	Submaxillary Gland, Left
Submandibular lymph node	Lymphatic, Head
Submaxillary ganglion	Head and Neck Sympathetic Nerve
Submaxillary lymph node	Lymphatic, Head
Submental artery	Face Artery
Submental lymph node	Lymphatic, Head
Submucous (Meissner's) plexus	Abdominal Sympathetic Nerve
Suboccipital nerve	Cervical Nerve
Suboccipital venous plexus	Vertebral Vein, Right
	Vertebral Vein, Left
Subparotid lymph node	Lymphatic, Head
Subscapular artery	Axillary Artery, Right
	Axillary Artery, Left
Subscapular (posterior) lymph node	Lymphatic, Left Axillary
	Lymphatic, Right Axillary
Subscapular aponeurosis	Subcutaneous Tissue and Fascia, Right Upper Arm
	Subcutaneous Tissue and Fascia, Left Upper Arm
Subscapularis muscle	Shoulder Muscle, Right
	Shoulder Muscle, Left
Subscapularis tendon	Shoulder Tendon, Right
	Shoulder Tendon, Left
Substantia nigra	Basal Ganglia

Anatomical Term	PCS Description
Subtalar (talocalcaneal) joint	Tarsal Joint, Right
	Tarsal Joint, Left
Subtalar ligament	Foot Bursa and Ligament, Right
	Foot Bursa and Ligament, Left
Subthalamic nucleus	Basal Ganglia
Superficial epigastric artery	Femoral Artery, Left
	Femoral Artery, Right
Superficial epigastric vein	Greater Saphenous Vein, Left
	Greater Saphenous Vein, Right
Superficial circumflex iliac vein	Greater Saphenous Vein, Left
	Greater Saphenous Vein, Right
Superficial palmar arch	Hand Artery, Right
	Hand Artery, Left
Superficial palmar venous arch	Hand Vein, Left
	Hand Vein, Right
Superficial transverse perineal muscle	Perineum Muscle
Superficial transverse perineal tendon	Peritoneum Tendon
Superficial temporal artery	Temporal Artery, Right
	Temporal Artery, Left
Superior cardiac nerve	Thoracic Sympathetic Nerve
Superior cerebral vein	Intracranial Vein
Superior cerebellar vein	Intracranial Vein
Superior clunic (cluneal) nerve	Lumbar Nerve
Superior epigastric artery	Internal Mammary Artery, Right
	Internal Mammary Artery, Left
Superior genicular artery	Popliteal Artery, Right
	Popliteal Artery, Left
Superior gluteal artery	Internal Iliac Artery, Right
	Internal Iliac Artery, Left
Superior gluteal nerve	Lumbar Plexus
Superior hypogastric plexus	Abdominal Sympathetic Nerve
Superior labial artery	Face Artery
Superior laryngeal artery	Thyroid Artery, Right
	Thyroid Artery, Left
Superior laryngeal nerve	Vagus Nerve
Superior longitudinal muscle	Tongue, Palate, Pharynx Muscle
Superior mesenteric ganglion	Abdominal Sympathetic Nerve
Superior mesenteric lymph node	Lymphatic, Mesenteric
Superior mesenteric plexus	Abdominal Sympathetic Nerve
Superior oblique muscle	Extraocular Muscle, Right
	Extraocular Muscle, Left
Superior olivary nucleus	Pons
Superior rectal artery	Inferior Mesenteric Artery

Anatomical Term	PCS Description
Superior rectal muscle	Extraocular Muscle, Right
	Extraocular Muscle, Left
Superior rectal vein	Inferior Mesenteric Vein
Superior tarsal plate	Upper Eyelid, Right
	Upper Eyelid, Left
Superior thoracic artery	Axillary Artery, Right
	Axillary Artery, Left
Superior thyroid artery	External Carotid Artery, Right
	External Carotid Artery, Left
	Thyroid Artery, Right
	Thyroid Artery, Left
Superior turbinate	Nasal Turbinate
Superior ulnar collateral artery	Brachial Artery, Right
	Brachial Artery, Left
Supraclavicular nerve	Cervical Plexus
Supraclavicular (Virchow's) lymph node	Lymphatic, Left Neck
	Lymphatic, Right Neck
Suprahyoid lymph node	Lymphatic, Head
Suprahyoid muscle	Neck Muscle, Right
	Neck Muscle, Left
Suprahyoid tendon	Head and Neck Tendon
Suprainguinal lymph node	Lymphatic, Pelvis
Supraorbital vein	Face Vein, Left
	Face Vein, Right
Suprarenal gland	Adrenal Glands, Bilateral
	Adrenal Gland, Right
	Adrenal Gland, Left
	Adrenal Gland
Suprarenal plexus	Abdominal Sympathetic Nerve
Suprascapular nerve	Brachial Plexus
Supraspinatus fascia	Subcutaneous Tissue and Fascia, Right Upper Arm
	Subcutaneous Tissue and Fascia, Left Upper Arm
Supraspinatus muscle	Shoulder Muscle, Right
	Shoulder Muscle, Left
Supraspinatus tendon	Shoulder Tendon, Right
	Shoulder Tendon, Left
Supraspinous ligament	Trunk Bursa and Ligament, Right
	Trunk Bursa and Ligament, Left
Suprasternal notch	Sternum
Supratrochlear lymph node	Lymphatic, Left Upper Extremity
	Lymphatic, Right Upper Extremity
Sural artery	Popliteal Artery, Right
	Popliteal Artery, Left
Sweat gland	Skin
Talocalcaneal ligament	Foot Bursa and Ligament, Right
	Foot Bursa and Ligament, Left
Talocalcaneal (subtalar) joint	Tarsal Joint, Right
	Tarsal Joint, Left

Anatomical Term	PCS Description
Talocalcaneonavicular ligament	Foot Bursa and Ligament, Right
	Foot Bursa and Ligament, Left
Talocalcaneonavicular joint	Tarsal Joint, Right
	Tarsal Joint, Left
Talocrural joint	Ankle Joint, Right
	Ankle Joint, Left
Talofibular ligament	Ankle Bursa and Ligament, Right
	Ankle Bursa and Ligament, Left
Talus bone	Tarsal, Left
	Tarsal, Right
Tarsometatarsal joint	Metatarsal-Tarsal Joint, Right
	Metatarsal-Tarsal Joint, Left
Tarsometatarsal ligament	Foot Bursa and Ligament, Right
	Foot Bursa and Ligament, Left
Temporal lobe	Cerebral Hemisphere
Temporalis muscle	Head Muscle
Temporalis tendon	Head and Neck Tendon
Temporoparietalis muscle	Head Muscle
Temporoparietalis tendon	Head and Neck Tendon
Tensor fasciae latae muscle	Hip Muscle, Right
	Hip Muscle, Left
Tensor fasciae latae tendon	Hip Tendon, Right
	Hip Tendon, Left
Tensor veli palatini muscle	Tongue, Palate, Pharynx Muscle
Tenth cranial nerve	Vagus Nerve
Tentorium cerebelli	Dura Mater
Teres major muscle	Shoulder Muscle, Right
	Shoulder Muscle, Left
Teres major tendon	Shoulder Tendon, Right
	Shoulder Tendon, Left
Teres minor muscle	Shoulder Muscle, Right
	Shoulder Muscle, Left
Teres minor tendon	Shoulder Tendon, Right
	Shoulder Tendon, Left
Testicular artery	Abdominal Aorta
Thenar muscle	Hand Muscle, Right
	Hand Muscle, Left
Thenar tendon	Hand Tendon, Right
	Hand Tendon, Left
Third cranial nerve	Oculomotor Nerve
Third occipital nerve	Cervical Nerve
Third ventricle	Cerebral Ventricle
Thoracic aortic plexus	Thoracic Sympathetic Nerve
Thoracic esophagus	Esophagus, Middle
Thoracic facet joint	Thoracic Vertebral Joints, 8 or more
	Thoracic Vertebral Joints, 2 to 7
	Thoracic Vertebral Joint
Thoracic ganglion	Thoracic Sympathetic Nerve

Anatomical Term	PCS Description
Thoracoacromial artery	Axillary Artery, Right
	Axillary Artery, Left
Thoracolumbar facet joint	Thoracolumbar Vertebral Joint
Thymus gland	Thymus
Thyroarytenoid tendon	Head and Neck Tendon
Thyroarytenoid muscle	Neck Muscle, Right
	Neck Muscle, Left
Thyrocervical trunk	Thyroid Artery, Right
	Thyroid Artery, Left
Thyroid cartilage	Larynx
Tibialis anterior muscle	Lower Leg Muscle, Right
	Lower Leg Muscle, Left
Tibialis anterior tendon	Lower Leg Tendon, Right
	Lower Leg Tendon, Left
Tibialis posterior muscle	Lower Leg Muscle, Right
	Lower Leg Muscle, Left
Tibialis posterior tendon	Lower Leg Tendon, Right
	Lower Leg Tendon, Left
Tracheobronchial lymph node	Lymphatic, Thorax
Tragus	External Ear, Right
	External Ear, Left
	External Ear, Bilateral
Transversalis fascia	Subcutaneous Tissue and Fascia, Trunk
Transverse acetabular ligament	Hip Bursa and Ligament, Left
	Hip Bursa and Ligament, Right
Transverse (cutaneous) cervical nerve	Cervical Plexus
Transverse facial artery	Temporal Artery, Right
	Temporal Artery, Left
Transverse humeral ligament	Shoulder Bursa and Ligament, Right
	Shoulder Bursa and Ligament, Left
Transverse ligament of atlas	Head and Neck Bursa and Ligament
Transverse scapular ligament	Shoulder Bursa and Ligament, Right
	Shoulder Bursa and Ligament, Left
Transverse thoracis muscle	Thorax Muscle, Right
	Thorax Muscle, Left
Transverse thoracis tendon	Thorax Tendon, Right
	Thorax Tendon, Left
Transversospinalis muscle	Trunk Muscle, Right
	Trunk Muscle, Left
Transversospinalis tendon	Trunk Tendon, Right
	Trunk Tendon, Left
Transversus abdominis muscle	Abdomen Muscle, Right
	Abdomen Muscle, Left
Transversus abdominis tendon	Abdomen Tendon, Right
	Abdomen Tendon, Left
Trapezium bone	Carpal, Left
	Carpal, Right

Anatomical Term	PCS Description
Trapezius muscle	Trunk Muscle, Right
	Trunk Muscle, Left
Trapezius tendon	Trunk Tendon, Right
	Trunk Tendon, Left
Trapezoid bone	Carpal, Left
	Carpal, Right
Triceps brachii muscle	Upper Arm Muscle, Right
	Upper Arm Muscle, Left
Triceps brachii tendon	Upper Arm Tendon, Right
	Upper Arm Tendon, Left
Tricuspid annulus	Tricuspid Valve
Trifacial nerve	Trigeminal Nerve
Trigone of bladder	Bladder
Triquetral bone	Carpal, Left
	Carpal, Right
Trochanteric bursa	Hip Bursa and Ligament, Right
	Hip Bursa and Ligament, Left
Twelfth cranial nerve	Hypoglossal Nerve
Tympanic cavity	Middle Ear, Right
	Middle Ear, Left
Tympanic nerve	Glossopharyngeal Nerve
Tympanic part of temoporal bone	Temporal Bone, Right
	Temporal Bone, Left
Ulnar collateral ligament	Elbow Bursa and Ligament, Right
	Elbow Bursa and Ligament, Left
Ulnar collateral carpal ligament	Wrist Bursa and Ligament, Right
	Wrist Bursa and Ligament, Left
Ulnar notch	Radius, Left
	Radius, Right
Ulnar vein	Brachial Vein, Right
	Brachial Vein, Left
Umbilical artery	Internal Iliac Artery, Right
	Internal Iliac Artery, Left
Ureteral orifice	Ureter
	Ureter, Left
	Ureter, Right
	Ureters, Bilateral
Ureteropelvic junction (UPJ)	Kidney Pelvis, Right
	Kidney Pelvis, Left
Ureterovesical orifice	Ureter, Left
	Ureter, Right
Uterine artery	Internal Iliac Artery, Right
	Internal Iliac Artery, Left
Uterine cornu	Uterus
Uterine tube	Fallopian Tube, Right
	Fallopian Tube, Left
Uterine vein	Hypogastric Vein, Right
	Hypogastric Vein, Left
Vaginal artery	Internal Iliac Artery, Right
	Internal Iliac Artery, Left

Anatomical Term	PCS Description
Vaginal vein	Hypogastric Vein, Right
	Hypogastric Vein, Left
Vastus intermedius muscle	Upper Leg Muscle, Right
	Upper Leg Muscle, Left
Vastus intermedius tendon	Upper Leg Tendon, Right
	Upper Leg Tendon, Left
Vastus lateralis muscle	Upper Leg Muscle, Right
	Upper Leg Muscle, Left
Vastus lateralis tendon	Upper Leg Tendon, Right
	Upper Leg Tendon, Left
Vastus medialis muscle	Upper Leg Muscle, Right
	Upper Leg Muscle, Left
Vastus medialis tendon	Upper Leg Tendon, Right
	Upper Leg Tendon, Left
Ventricular fold	Larynx
Vermiform appendix	Appendix
Vermilion border	Lower Lip
	Upper Lip
Vertebral arch	Cervical Vertebra
	Lumbar Vertebra
	Thoracic Vertebra
Vertebral canal	Spinal Canal
Vertebral foramen	Cervical Vertebra
	Lumbar Vertebra
	Thoracic Vertebra
Vertebral lamina	Cervical Vertebra
	Lumbar Vertebra
	Thoracic Vertebra
Vertebral pedicle	Cervical Vertebra
	Lumbar Vertebra
	Thoracic Vertebra
Vesical vein	Hypogastric Vein, Right
	Hypogastric Vein, Left
Vestibular (Scarpa's) ganglion	Acoustic Nerve
Vestibular nerve	Acoustic Nerve
Vestibulocochlear nerve	Acoustic Nerve
Virchow's (supraclavicular) lymph node	Lymphatic, Left Neck
	Lymphatic, Right Neck
Vitreous body	Vitreous, Left
	Vitreous, Right
Vocal fold (syn)	Vocal Cord, Right
	Vocal Cord, Left
Volar (palmar) digital vein	Hand Vein, Left
	Hand Vein, Right
Volar (palmar) metacarpal vein	Hand Vein, Left
	Hand Vein, Right
Vomer	Nasal Bone
	Nasal Septum
Xiphoid process	Sternum

Anatomical Term	PCS Description
Zonule of Zinn	Lens, Left
	Lens, Right
Zygomatic process of frontal bone	Frontal Bone, Right
	Frontal Bone, Left
Zygomatic process of temporal bone	Temporal Bone, Right
	Temporal Bone, Left
Zygomaticus muscle	Facial Muscle

Draft (2011)

Appendix D: Type and Type Qualifier Definitions Sections B–H

Section B–Imaging

Type (Character 3)	Definition
Computerized Tomography (CT Scan) (2)	Computer reformatted digital display of multiplanar images developed from the capture of multiple exposures of external ionizing radiation
Fluoroscopy (1)	Single plane or bi-plane real time display of an image developed from the capture of external ionizing radiation on a fluorescent screen. The image may also be stored by either digital or analog means
Magnetic Resonance Imaging (MRI) (3)	Computer reformatted digital display of multiplanar images developed from the capture of radiofrequency signals emitted by nuclei in a body site excited within a magnetic field
Plain Radiography (Ø)	Planar display of an image developed from the capture of external ionizing radiation on photographic or photoconductive plate
Ultrasonography (4)	Real time display of images of anatomy or flow information developed from the capture of reflected and attenuated high frequency sound waves

Section C–Nuclear Medicine

Type (Character 3)	Definition
Nonimaging Nuclear Medicine Assay (6)	Introduction of radioactive materials into the body for the study of body fluids and blood elements, by the detection of radioactive emissions
Nonimaging Nuclear Medicine Probe (5)	Introduction of radioactive materials into the body for the study of distribution and fate of certain substances by the detection of radioactive emissions; or, alternatively, measurement of absorption of radioactive emissions from an external source
Nonimaging Nuclear Medicine Uptake (4)	Introduction of radioactive materials into the body for measurements of organ function, from the detection of radioactive emissions
Planar Nuclear Medicine Imaging (1)	Introduction of radioactive materials into the body for single plane display of images developed from the capture of radioactive emissions
Positron Emission Tomographic (PET) Imaging (3)	Introduction of radioactive materials into the body for three dimensional display of images developed from the simultaneous capture, 18Ø degrees apart, of radioactive emissions
Systemic Nuclear Medicine Therapy (7)	Introduction of unsealed radioactive materials into the body for treatment
Tomographic (Tomo) Nuclear Medicine Imaging (2)	Introduction of radioactive materials into the body for three dimensional display of images developed from the capture of radioactive emissions

Section F–Physical Rehabilitation and Diagnostic Audiology

Type (Character 3)	Definition
Activities of Daily Living Assessment (2)	Measurement of functional level for activities of daily living
Activities of Daily Living Treatment (8)	Exercise or activities to facilitate functional competence for activities of daily living
Caregiver Training (F)	Training in activities to support patient's optimal level of function
Cochlear Implant Treatment (B)	Application of techniques to improve the communication abilities of individuals with cochlear implant
Device Fitting (D)	Fitting of a device designed to facilitate or support achievement of a higher level of function
Hearing Aid Assessment (4)	Measurement of the appropriateness and/or effectiveness of a hearing device
Hearing Assessment (3)	Measurement of hearing and related functions

Continued on next page

Section F–Physical Rehabilitation and Diagnostic Audiology   *Continued from previous page*

Type (Character 3)	Definition
Hearing Treatment (9)	Application of techniques to improve, augment, or compensate for hearing and related functional impairment
Motor Function Assessment/Nerve Function Assessment (1)	Measurement of motor, nerve, and related functions
Motor Treatment (7)	Exercise or activities to increase or facilitate motor function
Speech Assessment (Ø)	Measurement of speech and related functions
Speech Treatment (6)	Application of techniques to improve, augment, or compensate for speech and related functional impairment
Vestibular Assessment (5)	Measurement of the vestibular system and related functions
Vestibular Treatment (C)	Application of techniques to improve, augment, or compensate for vestibular and related functional impairment

Section F–Physical Rehabilitation and Diagnostic Audiology

Type Qualifier (Character 5)	Definition
Acoustic Reflex Decay (J)	Measures reduction in size/strength of acoustic reflex over time Includes/Examples: Includes site of lesion test
Acoustic Reflex Patterns (G)	Defines site of lesion based upon presence/absence of acoustic reflexes with ipsilateral vs. contralateral stimulation
Acoustic Reflex Threshold (H)	Determines minimal intensity that acoustic reflex occurs with ipsilateral and/or contralateral stimulation
Aerobic Capacity and Endurance (7)	Measures autonomic responses to positional changes; perceived exertion, dyspnea or angina during activity; performance during exercise protocols; standard vital signs; and blood gas analysis or oxygen consumption
Alternate Binaural or Monaural Loudness Balance (7)	Determines auditory stimulus parameter that yields the same objective sensation Includes/Examples: Sound intensities that yield same loudness perception
Anthropometric Characteristics (B)	Measures edema, body fat composition, height, weight, length and girth
Aphasia (Assessment) (C)	Measures expressive and receptive speech and language function including reading and writing
Aphasia (Treatment) (3)	Applying techniques to improve, augment, or compensate for receptive/ expressive language impairments
Articulation/Phonology (Assessment) (9)	Measures speech production
Articulation/Phonology (Treatment) (4)	Applying techniques to correct, improve, or compensate for speech productive impairment
Assistive Listening Device (5)	Assists in use of effective and appropriate assistive listening device/system
Assistive Listening System Device Selection (4)	Measures the effectiveness and appropriateness of assistive listening systems/devices
Assistive, Adaptive, Supportive or Protective Devices (9)	Explanation: Devices to facilitate or support achievement of a higher level of function in wheelchair mobility; bed mobility; transfer or ambulation ability; bath and showering ability; dressing; grooming; personal hygiene; play or leisure
Auditory Evoked Potentials (L)	Measures electric responses produced by the VIIIth cranial nerve and brainstem following auditory stimulation
Auditory Processing (Assessment) (Q)	Evaluates ability to receive and process auditory information and comprehension of spoken language
Auditory Processing (Treatment) (2)	Applying techniques to improve the receiving and processing of auditory information and comprehension of spoken language
Augmentative/Alternative Communication System (Assessment) (L)	Determines the appropriateness of aids, techniques, symbols, and/or strategies to augment or replace speech and enhance communication Includes/Examples: Includes the use of telephones, writing equipment, emergency equipment, and TDD

Continued on next page

Section F–Physical Rehabilitation and Diagnostic Audiology   *Continued from previous page*

Type Qualifier (Character 5)	Definition
Augmentative/Alternative Communication System (Treatment) (3)	Includes/Examples: Includes augmentative communication devices and aids
Aural Rehabilitation (5)	Applying techniques to improve the communication abilities associated with hearing loss
Aural Rehabilitation Status (P)	Measures impact of a hearing loss including evaluation of receptive and expressive communication skills
Bathing/Showering Techniques (Ø)	Activities to facilitate obtaining and using supplies, soaping, rinsing and drying body parts, maintaining bathing position, and transferring to and from bathing positions
Bathing/Showering (Ø)	Includes/Examples: Includes obtaining and using supplies; soaping, rinsing, and drying body parts; maintaining bathing position; and transferring to and from bathing positions
Bed Mobility (Assessment) (B)	Transitional movement within bed
Bed Mobility (Treatment) (5)	Exercise or activities to facilitate transitional movements within bed
Bedside Swallowing and Oral Function (H)	Includes/Examples: Bedside swallowing includes assessment of sucking, masticating, coughing, and swallowing. Oral function includes assessment of musculature for controlled movements, structures, and functions to determine coordination and phonation
Bekesy Audiometry (3)	Uses an instrument that provides a choice of discrete or continuously varying pure tones; choice of pulsed or continuous signal
Binaural Electroacoustic Hearing Aid Check (6)	Determines mechanical and electroacoustic function of bilateral hearing aids using hearing aid test box
Binaural Hearing Aid (Assessment) (3)	Measures the candidacy, effectiveness, and appropriateness of a hearing aid Explanation: Measures bilateral fit
Binaural Hearing Aid (Treatment) (2)	Explanation: Assists in achieving maximum understanding and performance
Bithermal, Binaural Caloric Irrigation (Ø)	Measures the rhythmic eye movements stimulated by changing the temperature of the vestibular system
Bithermal, Monaural Caloric Irrigation (1)	Measures the rhythmic eye movements stimulated by changing the temperature of the vestibular system in one ear
Brief Tone Stimuli (R)	Measures specific central auditory process
Cerumen Management (3)	Includes examination of external auditory canal and tympanic membrane and removal of cerumen from external ear canal
Cochlear Implant (Ø)	Measures candidacy for cochlear implant
Cochlear Implant Rehabilitation (Ø)	Applying techniques to improve the communication abilities of individuals with cochlear implant; includes programming the device, providing patients/families with information
Communicative/Cognitive Integration Skills (Assessment) (G)	Measures ability to use higher cortical functions Includes/Examples: Includes orientation, recognition, attention span, initiation and termination of activity, memory, sequencing, categorizing, concept formation, spatial operations, judgment, problem solving, generalization and pragmatic communication
Communicative/Cognitive Integration Skills (Treatment) (6)	Activities to facilitate the use of higher cortical functions Includes/Examples: Includes level of arousal, orientation, recognition, attention span, initiation and termination of activity, memory sequencing, judgment and problem solving, learning and generalization, and pragmatic communication
Computerized Dynamic Posturography (6)	Measures the status of the peripheral and central vestibular system and the sensory/motor component of balance; evaluates the efficacy of vestibular rehabilitation
Conditioned Play Audiometry (4)	Behavioral measures using nonspeech and speech stimuli to obtain frequency-specific and ear-specific information on auditory status from the patient Explanation: Obtains speech reception threshold by having patient point to pictures of spondaic words
Coordination/Dexterity (Assessment) (3)	Measures large and small muscle groups for controlled goal- directed movements Explanation: Dexterity includes object manipulation

Continued on next page

Section F–Physical Rehabilitation and Diagnostic Audiology

Continued from previous page

Type Qualifier (Character 5)	Definition
Coordination/Dexterity (Treatment) (2)	Exercise or activities to facilitate gross coordination and fine coordination
Cranial Nerve Integrity (9)	Measures cranial nerve sensory and motor functions, including tastes, smell and facial expression
Dichotic Stimuli (T)	Measures specific central auditory process
Distorted Speech (S)	Measures specific central auditory process
Dix-Hallpike Dynamic (5)	Measures nystagmus following Dix-Hallpike maneuver
Dressing (1)	Includes/Examples: Includes selecting clothing and accessories, obtaining clothing from storage, dressing, fastening and adjusting clothing and shoes, and applying and removing personal devices, prosthesis or orthosis
Dressing Techniques (1)	Activities to facilitate selecting clothing and accessories, dressing and undressing, adjusting clothing and shoes, applying and removing devices, prostheses or orthoses
Dynamic Orthosis (6)	Includes/Examples: Includes customized and prefabricated splints, inhibitory casts, spinal and other braces, and protective devices; allows motion through transfer of movement from other body parts or by use of outside forces
Ear Canal Probe Microphone (1)	Real ear measures
Ear Protector Attentuation (7)	Measures ear protector fit and effectiveness
Electrocochleography (K)	Measures the VIIIth cranial nerve action potential
Environmental, Home, Work Barriers (B)	Measures current and potential barriers to optimal function, including safety hazards, access problems and home or office design
Ergonomics and Body Mechanics (C)	Ergonomic measurement of job tasks, work hardening or work conditioning needs; functional capacity; and body mechanics
Eustachian Tube Function (F)	Measures eustachian tube function and patency of eustachian tube
Evoked Otoacoustic Emissions, Diagnostic (N)	Measures auditory evoked potentials in a diagnostic format
Evoked Otoacoustic Emissions, Screening (M)	Measures auditory evoked potentials in a screening format
Facial Nerve Function (7)	Measures electrical activity of the VIIth cranial nerve (facial nerve)
Feeding/Eating (Assessment) (2)	Includes/Examples: Includes setting up food, selecting and using utensils and tableware, bringing food or drink to mouth, cleaning face, hands, and clothing, and management of alternative methods of nourishment
Feeding/Eating (Treatment) (3)	Exercise or activities to facilitate setting up food, selecting and using utensils and tableware, bringing food or drink to mouth, cleaning face, hands, and clothing, and management of alternative methods of nourishment
Filtered Speech (0)	Uses high or low pass filtered speech stimuli to assess central auditory processing disorders, site of lesion testing
Fluency (Assessment) (D)	Measures speech fluency or stuttering
Fluency (Treatment) (7)	Applying techniques to improve and augment fluent speech
Gait Training/Functional Ambulation (9)	Exercise or activities to facilitate ambulation on a variety of surfaces and in a variety of environments
Gait/Balance (D)	Measures biomechanical, arthrokinematic and other spatial and temporal characteristics of gait and balance
Grooming/Personal Hygiene (Assessment) (3)	Includes/Examples: Includes ability to obtain and use supplies in a sequential fashion, general grooming, oral hygiene, toilet hygiene, personal care devices, including care for artificial airways

Continued on next page

Section F–Physical Rehabilitation and Diagnostic Audiology

Continued from previous page

Type Qualifier (Character 5)	Definition
Grooming/Personal Hygiene (Treatment) (2)	Activities to facilitate obtaining and using supplies in a sequential fashion: general grooming, oral hygiene, toilet hygiene, cleaning body, and personal care devices, including artificial airways
Hearing and Related Disorders Counseling (Ø)	Provides patients/families/caregivers with information, support, referrals to facilitate recovery from a communication disorder Includes/Examples: Includes strategies for psychosocial adjustment to hearing loss for clients and families/caregivers
Hearing and Related Disorders Prevention (1)	Provides patients/families/caregivers with information and support to prevent communication disorders
Hearing Screening (Ø)	Pass/refer measures designed to identify need for further audiologic assessment
Home Management (Assessment) (4)	Obtaining and maintaining personal and household possessions and environment Includes/Examples: Includes clothing care, cleaning, meal preparation and cleanup, shopping, money management, household maintenance, safety procedures, and childcare/parenting
Home Management (Treatment) (4)	Activities to facilitate obtaining and maintaining personal household possessions and environment Includes/Examples: Includes clothing care, cleaning, meal preparation and clean-up, shopping, money management, household maintenance, safety procedures, childcare/parenting
Instrumental Swallowing and Oral Function (J)	Definition: Measures swallowing function using instrumental diagnostic procedures Explanation: Methods include videofluoroscopy, ultrasound, manometry, endoscopy
Integumentary Integrity (1)	Includes/Examples: Includes burns, skin conditions, ecchymosis, bleeding, blisters, scar tissue, wounds and other traumas, tissue mobility, turgor and texture
Manual Therapy Techniques (7)	Techniques in which the therapist uses his/her hands to administer skilled movements Includes/Examples: Includes connective tissue massage, joint mobilization and manipulation, manual lymph drainage, manual traction, soft tissue mobilization and manipulation
Masking Patterns (W)	Measures central auditory processing status
Monaural Electroacoustic Hearing Aid Check (8)	Determines mechanical and electroacoustic function of one hearing aid using hearing aid test box
Monaural Hearing Aid (Assessment) (2)	Measures the candidacy, effectiveness, and appropriateness of a hearing aid Explanation: Measures unilateral fit
Monaural Hearing Aid (Treatment) (1)	Explanation: Assists in achieving maximum understanding and performance
Motor Function (Assessment) (4)	Measures the body's functional and versatile movement patterns Includes/Examples: Includes motor assessment scales, analysis of head, trunk and limb movement, and assessment of motor learning
Motor Function (Treatment) (3)	Exercise or activities to facilitate crossing midline, laterality, bilateral integration, praxis, neuromuscular relaxation, inhibition, facilitation, motor function and motor learning
Motor Speech (Assessment) (B)	Measures neurological motor aspects of speech production
Motor Speech (Treatment) (B)	Applying techniques to improve and augment the impaired neurological motor aspects of speech production
Muscle Performance (Assessment) (Ø)	Measures muscle strength, power and endurance using manual testing, dynamometry or computer-assisted electromechanical muscle test; functional muscle strength, power and endurance; muscle pain, tone, or soreness; or pelvic-floor musculature Explanation: Muscle endurance refers to the ability to contract a muscle repeatedly over time
Muscle Performance (Treatment) (1)	Exercise or activities to increase the capacity of a muscle to do work in terms of strength, power, and/or endurance Explanation: Muscle strength is the force exerted to overcome resistance in one maximal effort. Muscle power is work produced per unit of time, or the product of strength and speed. Muscle endurance is the ability to contract a muscle repeatedly over time
Neuromotor Development (D)	Measures motor development, righting and equilibrium reactions, and reflex and equilibrium reactions
Neurophysiologic Intraoperative (8)	Monitors neural status during surgery

Continued on next page

Section F–Physical Rehabilitation and Diagnostic Audiology

Continued from previous page

Type Qualifier (Character 5)	Definition
Non-invasive Instrumental Status (N)	Instrumental measures of oral, nasal, vocal, and velopharyngeal functions as they pertain to speech production
Nonspoken Language (Assessment) (7)	Measures nonspoken language (print, sign, symbols) for communication
Nonspoken Language (Treatment) (Ø)	Applying techniques that improve, augment, or compensate spoken communication
Oral Peripheral Mechanism (P)	Structural measures of face, jaw, lips, tongue, teeth, hard and soft palate, pharynx as related to speech production
Orofacial Myofunctional (Assessment) (K)	Measures orofacial myofunctional patterns for speech and related functions
Orofacial Myofunctional (Treatment) (9)	Applying techniques to improve, alter, or augment impaired orofacial myofunctional patterns and related speech production errors
Oscillating Tracking (3)	Measures ability to visually track
Pain (F)	Measures muscle soreness, pain and soreness with joint movement, and pain perception Includes/Examples: Includes questionnaires, graphs, symptom magnification scales or visual analog scales
Perceptual Processing (Assessment) (5)	Measures stereognosis, kinesthesia, body schema, right-left discrimination, form constancy, position in space, visual closure, figure-ground, depth perception, spatial relations and topographical orientation
Perceptual Processing (Treatment) (1)	Exercise and activities to facilitate perceptual processing Explanation: Includes stereognosis, kinesthesia, body schema, right-left discrimination, form constancy, position in space, visual closure, figure-ground, depth perception, spatial relations, and topographical orientation Includes/Examples: Includes stereognosis, kinesthesia, body schema, right-left discrimination, form constancy, position in space, visual closure, figure-ground, depth perception, spatial relations, and topographical orientation
Performance Intensity Phonetically Balanced Speech Discrimination (Q)	Measures word recognition over varying intensity levels
Postural Control (3)	Exercise or activities to increase postural alignment and control
Prosthesis (8)	Explanation: Artificial substitutes for missing body parts that augment performance or function
Psychosocial Skills (Assessment) (6)	The ability to interact in society and to process emotions Includes/Examples: Includes psychological (values, interests, self-concept); social (role performance, social conduct, interpersonal skills, self expression); self-management (coping skills, time management, self-control)
Psychosocial Skills (Treatment) (6)	The ability to interact in society and to process emotions Includes/Examples: Includes psychological (values, interests, self-concept); social (role performance, social conduct, interpersonal skills, self expression); self-management (coping skills, time management, self-control)
Pure Tone Audiometry, Air (1)	Air-conduction pure tone threshold measures with appropriate masking
Pure Tone Audiometry, Air and Bone (2)	Air-conduction and bone-conduction pure tone threshold measures with appropriate masking
Pure Tone Stenger (C)	Measures unilateral nonorganic hearing loss based on simultaneous presentation of pure tones of differing volume
Range of Motion and Joint Integrity (5)	Measures quantity, quality, grade, and classification of joint movement and/or mobility Explanation: Range of Motion is the space, distance or angle through which movement occurs at a joint or series of joints. Joint integrity is the conformance of joints to expected anatomic, biomechanical and kinematic norms
Range of Motion and Joint Mobility (Ø)	Exercise or activities to increase muscle length and joint mobility
Receptive/Expressive Language (Assessment) (8)	Measures receptive and expressive language

Continued on next page

Section F–Physical Rehabilitation and Diagnostic Audiology

Continued from previous page

Type Qualifier (Character 5)	Definition
Receptive/Expressive Language (Treatment) (B)	Applying techniques to improve and augment receptive/expressive language
Reflex Integrity (G)	Measures the presence, absence, or exaggeration of developmentally appropriate, pathologic or normal reflexes
Select Picture Audiometry (5)	Establishes hearing threshold levels for speech using pictures
Sensorineural Acuity Level (4)	Measures sensorineural acuity masking presented via bone conduction
Sensory Aids (5)	Determines the appropriateness of a sensory prosthetic device, other than a hearing aid or assistive listening system/device
Sensory Awareness/ Processing/ Integrity (6)	Includes/Examples: Includes light touch, pressure, temperature, pain, sharp/dull, proprioception, vestibular, visual, auditory, gustatory, and olfactory
Short Increment Sensitivity Index (9)	Measures the ear's ability to detect small intensity changes; site of lesion test requiring a behavioral response
Sinusoidal Vertical Axis Rotational (4)	Measures nystagmus following rotation
Somatosensory Evoked Potentials (9)	Measures neural activity from sites throughout the body
Speech/Word Recognition (2)	Measures ability to repeat/identify single syllable words; scores given as a percentage; includes word recognition/speech discrimination
Speech/Language Screening (6)	Identifies need for further speech and/or language evaluation
Speech Threshold (1)	Measures minimal intensity needed to repeat spondaic words
Speech-Language Pathology and Related Disorders Counseling (1)	Provides patients/families with information, support, referrals to facilitate recovery from a communication disorder
Speech-Language Pathology and Related Disorders Prevention (2)	Applying techniques to avoid or minimize onset and/or development of a communication disorder
Staggered Spondaic Word (3)	Measures central auditory processing site of lesion based upon dichotic presentation of spondaic words
Static Orthosis (7)	Includes/Examples: Includes customized and prefabricated splints, inhibitory casts, spinal and other braces, and protective devices; has no moving parts, maintains joint(s) in desired position
Stenger (B)	Measures unilateral nonorganic hearing loss based on simultaneous presentation of signals of differing volume
Swallowing Dysfunction (D)	Activities to improve swallowing function in coordination with respiratory function Includes/Examples: Includes function and coordination of sucking, mastication, coughing, swallowing
Synthetic Sentence Identification (5)	Measures central auditory dysfunction using identification of third order approximations of sentences and competing messages
Temporal Ordering of Stimuli (V)	Measures specific central auditory process
Therapeutic Exercise (7)	Exercise or activities to facilitate sensory awareness, sensory processing, sensory integration, balance training, conditioning, reconditioning Includes/Examples: Includes developmental activities, breathing exercises, aerobic endurance activities, aquatic exercises, stretching and ventilatory muscle training
Tinnitus Masker (Assessment) (7)	Determines candidacy for tinnitus masker
Tinnitus Masker (Treatment) (Ø)	Explanation: Used to verify physical fit, acoustic appropriateness, and benefit; assists in achieving maximum benefit
Tone Decay (B)	Measures decrease in hearing sensitivity to a tone; site of lesion test requiring a behavioral response
Transfer (5)	Transitional movement from one surface to another

Continued on next page

Section F–Physical Rehabilitation and Diagnostic Audiology

Continued from previous page

Type Qualifier (Character 5)	Definition
Transfer Training (8)	Exercise or activities to facilitate movement from one surface to another
Tympanometry (D)	Measures the integrity of the middle ear; measures ease at which sound flows through the tympanic membrane while air pressure against the membrane is varied
Unithermal Binaural Screen (2)	Measures the rhythmic eye movements stimulated by changing the temperature of the vestibular system in both ears using warm water, screening format
Ventilation/Respiration/Circulation (G)	Measures ventilatory muscle strength, power and endurance, pulmonary function and ventilatory mechanics Includes/Examples: Includes ability to clear airway, activities that aggravate or relieve edema, pain, dyspnea or other symptoms, chest wall mobility, cardiopulmonary response to performance of ADL and IAD, cough and sputum, standard vital signs
Vestibular (Ø)	Applying techniques to compensate for balance disorders; includes habituation, exercise therapy, and balance retraining
Visual Motor Integration (Assessment) (2)	Coordinating the interaction of information from the eyes with body movement during activity
Visual Motor Integration (Treatment) (2)	Exercise or activities to facilitate coordinating the interaction of information from eyes with body movement during activity
Visual Reinforcement Audiometry (6)	Behavioral measures using nonspeech and speech stimuli to obtain frequency/ear-specific information on auditory status Includes/Examples: Includes a conditioned response of looking toward a visual reinforcer (e.g., lights, animated toy) every time auditory stimuli are heard
Vocational Activities and Functional Community or Work Reintegration Skills (Assessment) (H)	Measures environmental, home, work (job/school/play) barriers that keep patients from functioning optimally in their environment Includes/Examples: Includes assessment of vocational skills and interests, environment of work (job/school/play), injury potential and injury prevention or reduction, ergonomic stressors, transportation skills, and ability to access and use community resources
Vocational Activities/Functional Community Skills/Work Reintegration Skills (Treatment) (7)	Activities to facilitate vocational exploration, body mechanics training, job acquisition, and environmental or work (job/school/play) task adaptation Includes/Examples: Includes injury prevention and reduction, ergonomic stressor reduction, job coaching and simulation, work hardening and conditioning, driving training, transportation skills, and use of community resources
Voice (Assessment) (F)	Measures vocal structure, function and production
Voice (Treatment) (C)	Applying techniques to improve voice and vocal function
Voice Prosthetic (Assessment) (M)	Determines the appropriateness of voice prosthetic/adaptive device to enhance or facilitate communication
Voice Prosthetic (Treatment) (4)	Includes/Examples: Includes electrolarynx, and other assistive, adaptive, supportive devices
Wheelchair Mobility (Assessment) (F)	Measures fit and functional abilities within wheelchair in a variety of environments
Wheelchair Mobility (Treatment) (4)	Management, maintenance and controlled operation of a wheelchair, scooter or other device, in and on a variety of surfaces and environments
Wound Management (5)	Includes/Examples: Includes non-selective and selective debridement (enzymes, autolysis, sharp debridement), dressings (wound coverings, hydrogel, vacuum-assisted closure), topical agents, etc.

Draft (2011)

Section G–Mental Health

Type (Character 3)	Definition
Biofeedback (C)	Provision of information from the monitoring and regulating of physiological processes in conjunction with cognitive-behavioral techniques to improve patient functioning or well-being Includes/Examples: Includes EEG, blood pressure, skin temperature or peripheral blood flow, ECG, electrooculogram, EMG, respirometry or capnometry, GSR/EDR, perineometry to monitor/regulate bowel/bladder activity, electrogastrogram to monitor/regulate gastric motility
Counseling (6)	The application of psychological methods to treat an individual with normal developmental issues and psychological problems in order to increase function, improve well-being, alleviate distress, maladjustment or resolve crises
Crisis Intervention (2)	Treatment of a traumatized, acutely disturbed or distressed individual for the purpose of short-term stabilization Includes/Examples: Includes defusing, debriefing, counseling, psychotherapy and/or coordination of care with other providers or agencies
Electroconvulsive Therapy (B)	The application of controlled electrical voltages to treat a mental health disorder Includes/Examples: Includes appropriate sedation and other preparation of the individual
Family Psychotherapy (7)	Treatment that includes one or more family members of an individual with a mental health disorder by behavioral, cognitive, psychoanalytic, psychodynamic or psychophysiological means to improve functioning or well-being Explanation: Remediation of emotional or behavioral problems presented by one or more family members in cases where psychotherapy with more than one family member is indicated
Group Psychotherapy (H)	Treatment of two or more individuals with a mental health disorder by behavioral, cognitive, psychoanalytic, psychodynamic or psychophysiological means to improve functioning or well-being
Hypnosis (F)	Induction of a state of heightened suggestibility by auditory, visual and tactile techniques to elicit an emotional or behavioral response
Individual Psychotherapy (5)	Treatment of an individual with a mental health disorder by behavioral, cognitive, psychoanalytic, psychodynamic or psychophysiological means to improve functioning or well-being
Light Therapy (J)	Application of specialized light treatments to improve functioning or well-being
Medication Management (3)	Monitoring and adjusting the use of medications for the treatment of a mental health disorder
Narcosynthesis (G)	Administration of intravenous barbiturates in order to release suppressed or repressed thoughts
Psychological Tests (1)	The administration and interpretation of standardized psychological tests and measurement instruments for the assessment of psychological function

Section G–Mental Health

Type Qualifier (Character 4)	Definition
Behavioral (1)	Primarily to modify behavior Includes/Examples: Includes modeling and role playing, positive reinforcement of target behaviors, response cost, and training of self-management skills
Cognitive (2)	Primarily to correct cognitive distortions and errors
Cognitive-Behavioral (8)	Combining cognitive and behavioral treatment strategies to improve functioning Explanation: Maladaptive responses are examined to determine how cognitions relate to behavior patterns in response to an event. Uses learning principles and information-processing models
Developmental (0)	Age-normed developmental status of cognitive, social and adaptive behavior skills
Intellectual and Psychoeducational (2)	Intellectual abilities, academic achievement and learning capabilities (including behaviors and emotional factors affecting learning)

Continued on next page

Section G–Mental Health

Continued from previous page

Type Qualifier (Character 4)	Definition
Interactive (0)	Uses primarily physical aids and other forms of non-oral interaction with a patient who is physically, psychologically or developmentally unable to use ordinary language for communication Includes/Examples: Includes the use of toys in symbolic play
Interpersonal (3)	Helps an individual make changes in interpersonal behaviors to reduce psychological dysfunction Includes/Examples: Includes exploratory techniques, encouragement of affective expression, clarification of patient statements, analysis of communication patterns, use of therapy relationship and behavior change techniques
Neurobehavioral Status/Cognitive Status (4)	Includes neurobehavioral status exam, interview(s), and observation for the clinical assessment of thinking, reasoning and judgment, acquired knowledge, attention, memory, visual spatial abilities, language functions, and planning
Neuropsychological (3)	Thinking, reasoning and judgment, acquired knowledge, attention, memory, visual spatial abilities, language functions, planning
Personality and Behavioral (1)	Mood, emotion, behavior, social functioning, psychopathological conditions, personality traits and characteristics
Psychoanalysis (4)	Methods of obtaining a detailed account of past and present mental and emotional experiences to determine the source and eliminate or diminish the undesirable effects of unconscious conflicts Explanation: Accomplished by making the individual aware of their existence, origin, and inappropriate expression in emotions and behavior
Psychodynamic (5)	Exploration of past and present emotional experiences to understand motives and drives using insight-oriented techniques to reduce the undesirable effects of internal conflicts on emotions and behavior Explanation: Techniques include empathetic listening, clarifying self-defeating behavior patterns, and exploring adaptive alternatives
Psychophysiological (9)	Monitoring and alteration of physiological processes to help the individual associate physiological reactions combined with cognitive and behavioral strategies to gain improved control of these processes to help the individual cope more effectively
Supportive (6)	Formation of therapeutic relationship primarily for providing emotional support to prevent further deterioration in functioning during periods of particular stress Explanation: Often used in conjunction with other therapeutic approaches
Vocational (1)	Exploration of vocational interests, aptitudes and required adaptive behavior skills to develop and carry out a plan for achieving a successful vocational placement Includes/Examples: Includes enhancing work related adjustment and/or pursuing viable options in training education or preparation

Section H - Substance Abuse Treatment

Type (Character 3)	Definition
Detoxification Services (2)	Detoxification from alcohol and/or drugs Explanation: Not a treatment modality, but helps the patient stabilize physically and psychologically until the body becomes free of drugs and the effects of alcohol
Family Counseling (6)	The application of psychological methods that includes one or more family members to treat an individual with addictive behavior Explanation: Provides support and education for family members of addicted individuals. Family member participation is seen as a critical area of substance abuse treatment
Group Counseling (4)	The application of psychological methods to treat two or more individuals with addictive behavior Explanation: Provides structured group counseling sessions and healing power through the connection with others
Individual Counseling (3)	The application of psychological methods to treat an individual with addictive behavior Explanation: Comprised of several different techniques, which apply various strategies to address drug addiction
Individual Psychotherapy (5)	Treatment of an individual with addictive behavior by behavioral, cognitive, psychoanalytic, psychodynamic or psychophysiological means
Medication Management (8)	Monitoring and adjusting the use of replacement medications for the treatment of addiction
Pharmacotherapy (9)	The use of replacement medications for the treatment of addiction

Appendix E: Components of the Medical and Surgical Approach Definitions

Approach	Definition	Access Location	Method	Type of Instrumentation	Example
Open (Ø)	Cutting through the skin or mucous membrane and any other body layers necessary to expose the site of the procedure.	Skin or mucous membraneany other body layers	Cutting	None	Abdominal hysterectomy
Percutaneous (3)	Entry, by puncture or minor incision, of instrumentation through the skin or mucous membrane and/or any other body layers necessary to reach the site of the procedure	Skin or mucous membrane, any other body layers	Puncture or minor incision	Without visualization	Needle biopsy of liver, Liposuction
Percutaneous endoscopic (4)	Entry, by puncture or minor incision, of instrumentation through the skin or mucous membrane and/or any other body layers necessary to reach and visualize the site of the procedure	Skin or mucous membrane, any other body layers	Puncture or minor incision	With visualization	Arthroscopy, Laparoscopic cholecystectomy
Via natural or artificial opening (7)	Entry of instrumentation through a natural or artificial external opening to reach the site of the procedure	Natural or artificial external opening	Direct entry	Without visualization	Endotracheal tube insertion, Foley catheter placement
Via natural or artificial opening endoscopic (8)	Entry of instrumentation through a natural or artificial external opening to reach and visualize the site of the procedure	Natural or artificial external opening	Direct entry with puncture or minor incision for instrumentation only	With visualization	Sigmoidoscopy, EGD, ERCP
Via natural or artificial opening with percutaneous endoscopic assistance (F)	Entry of instrumentation through a natural or artificial external opening to reach and visualize the site of the procedure, and entry, by puncture or minor incision, of instrumentation through the skin or mucous membrane and any other body layers necessary to aid in the performance of the procedure	Skin or mucous membrane, any other body layers	Cutting	With visualization	Laparoscopic-assisted vaginal hysterectomy
External (X)	Procedures performed directly on the skin or mucous membrane and procedures performed indirectly by the application of external force through the skin or mucous membrane	Skin or mucous membrane	Direct or indirect application	None	Closed fracture reduction, Resection of tonsils

Appendix F: Character Meanings

Ø: Medical and Surgical
Ø: Central Nervous System

Operation–Character 3		Body Part–Character 4		Approach–Character 5		Device–Character 6		Qualifier–Character 7	
1	Bypass	Ø	Brain	Ø	Open	Ø	Drainage Device	Ø	Nasopharynx
2	Change	1	Cerebral Meninges	3	Percutaneous	2	Monitoring Device	1	Mastoid Sinus
5	Destruction	2	Dura Mater	4	Percutaneous Endoscopic	3	Infusion Device	2	Atrium
8	Division	3	Epidural Space	X	External	7	Autologous Tissue Substitute	3	Blood Vessel
9	Drainage	4	Subdural Space			J	Synthetic Substitute	4	Pleural Cavity
B	Excision	5	Subarachnoid Space			K	Nonautologous Tissue Substitute	5	Intestine
C	Extirpation	6	Cerebral Ventricle			M	Electrode	6	Peritoneal Cavity
D	Extraction	7	Cerebral Hemisphere			Y	Other Device	7	Urinary Tract
F	Fragmentation	8	Basal Ganglia			Z	No Device	8	Bone Marrow
H	Insertion	9	Thalamus					9	Fallopian Tube
J	Inspection	A	Hypothalamus					B	Cerebral Cisterns
K	Map	B	Pons					F	Olfactory Nerve
N	Release	C	Cerebellum					G	Optic Nerve
P	Removal	D	Medulla Oblongata					H	Oculomotor Nerve
Q	Repair	E	Cranial Nerve					J	Trochlear Nerve
S	Reposition	F	Olfactory Nerve					K	Trigeminal Nerve
T	Resection	G	Optic Nerve					L	Abducens Nerve
U	Supplement	H	Oculomotor Nerve					M	Facial Nerve
W	Revision	J	Trochlear Nerve					N	Acoustic Nerve
X	Transfer	K	Trigeminal Nerve					P	Glossopharyngeal Nerve
		L	Abducens Nerve					Q	Vagus Nerve
		M	Facial Nerve					R	Accessory Nerve
		N	Acoustic Nerve					S	Hypoglossal Nerve
		P	Glossopharyngeal Nerve					X	Diagnostic
		Q	Vagus Nerve					Z	No Qualifier
		R	Accessory Nerve						
		S	Hypoglossal Nerve						
		T	Spinal Meninges						
		U	Spinal Canal						
		V	Spinal Cord						
		W	Cervical Spinal Cord						
		X	Thoracic Spinal Cord						
		Y	Lumbar Spinal Cord						

Ø: Medical and Surgical
1: Peripheral Nervous System

Operation–Character 3	Body Part–Character 4	Approach–Character 5	Device–Character 6	Qualifier–Character 7
2 Change	Ø Cervical Plexus	Ø Open	Ø Drainage Device	1 Cervical Nerve
5 Destruction	1 Cervical Nerve	3 Percutaneous	2 Monitoring Device	2 Phrenic Nerve
8 Division	2 Phrenic Nerve	4 Percutaneous Endoscopic	7 Autologous Tissue Substitute	4 Ulnar Nerve
9 Drainage	3 Brachial Plexus	X External	M Neurostimulator Lead	5 Median Nerve
B Excision	4 Ulnar Nerve		Y Other Device	6 Radial Nerve
C Extirpation	5 Median Nerve		Z No Device	8 Thoracic Nerve
D Extraction	6 Radial Nerve			B Lumbar Nerve
H Insertion	8 Thoracic Nerve			C Perineal Nerve
J Inspection	9 Lumbar Plexus			D Femoral Nerve
N Release	A Lumbosacral Plexus			F Sciatic Nerve
P Removal	B Lumbar Nerve			G Tibial Nerve
Q Repair	C Pudendal Nerve			H Peroneal Nerve
S Reposition	D Femoral Nerve			X Diagnostic
U Supplement	F Sciatic Nerve			Z No Qualifier
W Revision	G Tibial Nerve			
X Transfer	H Peroneal Nerve			
	K Head and Neck Sympathetic Nerve			
	L Thoracic Sympathetic Nerve			
	M Abdominal Sympathetic Nerve			
	N Lumbar Sympathetic Nerve			
	P Sacral Sympathetic Nerve			
	Q Sacral Plexus			
	R Sacral Nerve			
	Y Peripheral Nerve			

Ø: Medical and Surgical
2: Heart and Great Vessels

Operation–Character 3	Body Part–Character 4	Approach–Character 5	Device–Character 6	Qualifier–Character 7
1 Bypass	Ø Coronary Artery, One Site	Ø Open	2 Monitoring Device	Ø Allogeneic
5 Destruction	1 Coronary Artery, Two Sites	3 Percutaneous	3 Infusion Device	1 Syngeneic
7 Dilation	2 Coronary Artery, Three Sites	4 Percutaneous Endoscopic	4 Drug-eluting Intraluminal Device	2 Zooplastic
8 Division	3 Coronary Artery, Four or More Sites	X External	7 Autologous Tissue Substitute	3 Coronary Artery
B Excision	4 Coronary Vein		8 Zooplastic Tissue	4 Coronary Vein
C Extirpation	5 Atrial Septum		9 Autologous Venous Tissue	5 Coronary Circulation
F Fragmentation	6 Atrium, Right		A Autologous Arterial Tissue	6 Bifurcation
H Insertion	7 Atrium, Left		C Extraluminal Device	7 Atrium, Left
J Inspection	8 Conduction Mechanism		D Intraluminal Device	8 Internal Mammary, Right
K Map	9 Chordae Tendineae		J Synthetic Substitute	9 Internal Mammary, Left
L Occlusion	A Heart		K Nonautologous Tissue Substitute	A Pacemaker Lead
N Release	B Heart, Right		M Cardiac Lead	B Subclavian
P Removal	C Heart, Left		Q Implantable Heart Assist System	C Thoracic Artery
Q Repair	D Papillary Muscle		R External Heart Assist System	D Carotid
R Replacement	F Aortic Valve		T Radioactive Intraluminal Device	E Defibrillator Lead
S Reposition	G Mitral Valve		Z No Device	F Abdominal Artery
T Resection	H Pulmonary Valve			G Pressure Sensor
U Supplement	J Tricuspid Valve			P Pulmonary Trunk
V Restriction	K Ventricle, Right			Q Pulmonary Artery, Right
W Revision	L Ventricle, Left			R Pulmonary Artery, Left
Y Transplantation	M Ventricular Septum			S Biventricular
	N Pericardium			T Ductus Arteriosus
	P Pulmonary Trunk			W Aorta
	Q Pulmonary Artery, Right			X Diagnostic
	R Pulmonary Artery, Left			Z No Qualifier
	S Pulmonary Vein, Right			
	T Pulmonary Vein, Left			
	V Superior Vena Cava			
	W Thoracic Aorta			
	Y Great Vessel			

0: Medical and Surgical
3: Upper Arteries

Operation–Character 3	Body Part–Character 4	Approach–Character 5	Device–Character 6	Qualifier–Character 7
1 Bypass	0 Internal Mammary Artery, Right	0 Open	0 Drainage Device	0 Upper Arm Artery, Right
5 Destruction	1 Internal Mammary Artery, Left	3 Percutaneous	2 Monitoring Device	1 Upper Arm Artery, Left
7 Dilation	2 Innominate Artery	4 Percutaneous Endoscopic	3 Infusion Device	2 Upper Arm Artery, Bilateral
9 Drainage	3 Subclavian Artery, Right	X External	4 Drug-eluting Intraluminal Device	3 Lower Arm Artery, Right
B Excision	4 Subclavian Artery, Left		7 Autologous Tissue Substitute	4 Lower Arm Artery, Left
C Extirpation	5 Axillary Artery, Right		9 Autologous Venous Tissue	5 Lower Arm Artery, Bilateral
H Insertion	6 Axillary Artery, Left		A Autologous Arterial Tissue	6 Upper Leg Artery, Right
J Inspection	7 Brachial Artery, Right		B Bioactive Intraluminal Device	7 Upper Leg Artery, Left
L Occlusion	8 Brachial Artery, Left		C Extraluminal Device	8 Upper Leg Artery, Bilateral
N Release	9 Ulnar Artery, Right		D Intraluminal Device	9 Lower Leg Artery, Right
P Removal	A Ulnar Artery, Left		J Synthetic Substitute	B Lower Leg Artery, Left
Q Repair	B Radial Artery, Right		K Nonautologous Tissue Substitute	C Lower Leg Artery, Bilateral
R Replacement	C Radial Artery, Left		M Stimulator Lead	D Upper Arm Vein
S Reposition	D Hand Artery, Right		Z No Device	F Lower Arm Vein
U Supplement	F Hand Artery, Left			G Intracranial Artery
V Restriction	G Intracranial Artery			J Extracranial Artery, Right
W Revision	H Common Carotid Artery, Right			K Extracranial Artery, Left
	J Common Carotid Artery, Left			M Pulmonary Artery, Right
	K Internal Carotid Artery, Right			N Pulmonary Artery, Left
	L Internal Carotid Artery, Left			X Diagnostic
	M External Carotid Artery, Right			Z No Qualifier
	N External Carotid Artery, Left			
	P Vertebral Artery, Right			
	Q Vertebral Artery, Left			
	R Face Artery			
	S Temporal Artery, Right			
	T Temporal Artery, Left			
	U Thyroid Artery, Right			
	V Thyroid Artery, Left			
	Y Upper Artery			

Ø: Medical and Surgical
4: Lower Arteries

Operation–Character 3	Body Part–Character 4	Approach–Character 5	Device–Character 6	Qualifier–Character 7
1 Bypass	Ø Abdominal Aorta	Ø Open	Ø Drainage Device	Ø Abdominal Aorta
5 Destruction	1 Celiac Artery	3 Percutaneous	1 Radioactive Element	1 Celiac Artery
7 Dilation	2 Gastric Artery	4 Percutaneous Endoscopic	2 Monitoring Device	2 Mesenteric Artery
9 Drainage	3 Hepatic Artery	X External	3 Infusion Device	3 Renal Artery, Right
B Excision	4 Splenic Artery		4 Drug-eluting Intraluminal Device	4 Renal Artery, Left
C Extirpation	5 Superior Mesenteric Artery		7 Autologous Tissue Substitute	5 Renal Artery, Bilateral
H Insertion	6 Colic Artery, Right		9 Autologous Venous Tissue	6 Common Iliac Artery, Right
J Inspection	7 Colic Artery, Left		A Autologous Arterial Tissue	7 Common Iliac Artery, Left
L Occlusion	8 Colic Artery, Middle		C Extraluminal Device	8 Common Iliac Arteries, Bilateral
N Release	9 Renal Artery, Right		D Intraluminal Device	9 Internal Iliac Artery, Right
P Removal	A Renal Artery, Left		J Synthetic Substitute	B Internal Iliac Artery, Left
Q Repair	B Inferior Mesenteric Artery		K Nonautologous Tissue Substitute	C Internal Iliac Arteries, Bilateral
R Replacement	C Common Iliac Artery, Right		Z No Device	D External Iliac Artery, Right
S Reposition	D Common Iliac Artery, Left			F External Iliac Artery, Left
U Supplement	E Internal Iliac Artery, Right			G External Iliac Arteries, Bilateral
V Restriction	F Internal Iliac Artery, Left			H Femoral Artery, Right
W Revision	H External Iliac Artery, Right			J Femoral Artery, Left
	J External Iliac Artery, Left			K Femoral Arteries, Bilateral
	K Femoral Artery, Right			L Popliteal Artery
	L Femoral Artery, Left			M Peroneal Artery
	M Popliteal Artery, Right			N Posterior Tibial Artery
	N Popliteal Artery, Left			P Foot Artery
	P Anterior Tibial Artery, Right			Q Lower Extremity Artery
	Q Anterior Tibial Artery, Left			R Lower Artery
	R Posterior Tibial Artery, Right			S Lower Extremity Vein
	S Posterior Tibial Artery, Left			X Diagnostic
	T Peroneal Artery, Right			Z No Qualifier
	U Peroneal Artery, Left			
	V Foot Artery, Right			
	W Foot Artery, Left			
	Y Lower Artery			

0: Medical and Surgical

5: Upper Veins

Operation–Character 3	Body Part–Character 4	Approach–Character 5	Device–Character 6	Qualifier–Character 7
1 Bypass	0 Azygos Vein	0 Open	0 Drainage Device	X Diagnostic
5 Destruction	1 Hemiazygos Vein	3 Percutaneous	2 Monitoring Device	Y Upper Vein
7 Dilation	3 Innominate Vein, Right	4 Percutaneous Endoscopic	3 Infusion Device	Z No Qualifier
9 Drainage	4 Innominate Vein, Left	X External	7 Autologous Tissue Substitute	
B Excision	5 Subclavian Vein, Right		9 Autologous Venous Tissue	
C Extirpation	6 Subclavian Vein, Left		A Autologous Arterial Tissue	
D Extraction	7 Axillary Vein, Right		C Extraluminal Device	
H Insertion	8 Axillary Vein, Left		D Intraluminal Device	
J Inspection	9 Brachial Vein, Right		J Synthetic Substitute	
L Occlusion	A Brachial Vein, Left		K Nonautologous Tissue Substitute	
N Release	B Basilic Vein, Right		Z No Device	
P Removal	C Basilic Vein, Left			
Q Repair	D Cephalic Vein, Right			
R Replacement	F Cephalic Vein, Left			
S Reposition	G Hand Vein, Right			
U Supplement	H Hand Vein, Left			
V Restriction	L Intracranial Vein			
W Revision	M Internal Jugular Vein, Right			
	N Internal Jugular Vein, Left			
	P External Jugular Vein, Right			
	Q External Jugular Vein, Left			
	R Vertebral Vein, Right			
	S Vertebral Vein, Left			
	T Face Vein, Right			
	V Face Vein, Left			
	Y Upper Vein			

Ø: Medical and Surgical

6: Lower Veins

Operation–Character 3	Body Part–Character 4	Approach–Character 5	Device–Character 6	Qualifier–Character 7
1 Bypass	Ø Inferior Vena Cava	Ø Open	Ø Drainage Device	5 Superior Mesenteric Vein
5 Destruction	1 Splenic Vein	3 Percutaneous	2 Monitoring Device	6 Inferior Mesenteric Vein
7 Dilation	2 Gastric Vein	4 Percutaneous Endoscopic	3 Infusion Device	9 Renal Vein, Right
9 Drainage	3 Esophageal Vein	X External	7 Autologous Tissue Substitute	B Renal Vein, Left
B Excision	4 Hepatic Vein		9 Autologous Venous Tissue	C Hemorrhoidal Plexus
C Extirpation	5 Superior Mesenteric Vein		A Autologous Arterial Tissue	T Via Umbilical Vein
D Extraction	6 Inferior Mesenteric Vein		C Extraluminal Device	X Diagnostic
H Insertion	7 Colic Vein		D Intraluminal Device	Y Lower Vein
J Inspection	8 Portal Vein		J Synthetic Substitute	Z No Qualifier
L Occlusion	9 Renal Vein, Right		K Nonautologous Tissue Substitute	
N Release	B Renal Vein, Left		Z No Device	
P Removal	C Common Iliac Vein, Right			
Q Repair	D Common Iliac Vein, Left			
R Replacement	F External Iliac Vein, Right			
S Reposition	G External Iliac Vein, Left			
U Supplement	H Hypogastric Vein, Right			
V Restriction	J Hypogastric Vein, Left			
W Revision	M Femoral Vein, Right			
	N Femoral Vein, Left			
	P Greater Saphenous Vein, Right			
	Q Greater Saphenous Vein, Left			
	R Lesser Saphenous Vein, Right			
	S Lesser Saphenous Vein, Left			
	T Foot Vein, Right			
	V Foot Vein, Left			
	Y Lower Vein			

Ø: Medical and Surgical

7: Lymphatic and Hemic Systems

Operation–Character 3	Body Part–Character 4	Approach–Character 5	Device–Character 6	Qualifier–Character 7
2 Change	Ø Lymphatic, Head	Ø Open	Ø Drainage Device	Ø Allogeneic
5 Destruction	1 Lymphatic, Right Neck	3 Percutaneous	3 Infusion Device	1 Syngeneic
9 Drainage	2 Lymphatic, Left Neck	4 Percutaneous Endoscopic	7 Autologous Tissue Substitute	2 Zooplastic
B Excision	3 Lymphatic, Right Upper Extremity	X External	C Extraluminal Device	X Diagnostic
C Extirpation	4 Lymphatic, Left Upper Extremity		D Intraluminal Device	Z No Qualifier
D Extraction	5 Lymphatic, Right Axillary		J Synthetic Substitute	
H Insertion	6 Lymphatic, Left Axillary		K Nonautologous Tissue Substitute	
J Inspection	7 Lymphatic, Thorax		Y Other Device	
L Occlusion	8 Lymphatic, Internal Mammary, Right		Z No Device	
N Release	9 Lymphatic, Internal Mammary, Left			
P Removal	B Lymphatic, Mesenteric			
Q Repair	C Lymphatic, Pelvis			
S Reposition	D Lymphatic, Aortic			
T Resection	F Lymphatic, Right Lower Extremity			
U Supplement	G Lymphatic, Left Lower Extremity			
V Restriction	H Lymphatic, Right Inguinal			
W Revision	J Lymphatic, Left Inguinal			
Y Transplantation	K Thoracic Duct			
	L Cisterna Chyli			
	M Thymus			
	N Lymphatic			
	P Spleen			
	Q Bone Marrow, Sternum			
	R Bone Marrow, Iliac			
	S Bone Marrow, Vertebral			
	T Bone Marrow			

* Includes lymph vessels and lymph nodes.

Ø: Medical and Surgical
8: Eye

Operation–Character 3	Body Part–Character 4	Approach–Character 5	Device–Character 6	Qualifier–Character 7
Ø Alteration	Ø Eye, Right	Ø Open	Ø Drainage Device	3 Nasal Cavity
1 Bypass	1 Eye, Left	3 Percutaneous	1 Radioactive Element	4 Sclera
2 Change	2 Anterior Chamber, Right	7 Via Natural or Artificial Opening	3 Infusion Device	5 Intraocular Telescope
5 Destruction	3 Anterior Chamber, Left	8 Via Natural or Artificial Opening Endoscopic	7 Autologous Tissue Substitute	X Diagnostic
7 Dilation	4 Vitreous, Right	X External	C Extraluminal Device	Z No Qualifier
9 Drainage	5 Vitreous, Left		D Intraluminal Device	
B Excision	6 Sclera, Right		J Synthetic Substitute	
C Extirpation	7 Sclera, Left		K Nonautologous Tissue Substitute	
D Extraction	8 Cornea, Right		Y Other Device	
F Fragmentation	9 Cornea, Left		Z No Device	
H Insertion	A Choroid, Right			
J Inspection	B Choroid, Left			
L Occlusion	C Iris, Right			
M Reattachment	D Iris, Left			
N Release	E Retina, Right			
P Removal	F Retina, Left			
Q Repair	G Retinal Vessel, Right			
R Replacement	H Retinal Vessel, Left			
S Reposition	J Lens, Right			
T Resection	K Lens, Left			
U Supplement	L Extraocular Muscle, Right			
V Restriction	M Extraocular Muscle, Left			
W Revision	N Upper Eyelid, Right			
X Transfer	P Upper Eyelid, Left			
	Q Lower Eyelid, Right			
	R Lower Eyelid, Left			
	S Conjunctiva, Right			
	T Conjunctiva, Left			
	V Lacrimal Gland, Right			
	W Lacrimal Gland, Left			
	X Lacrimal Duct, Right			
	Y Lacrimal Duct, Left			

Ø: Medical and Surgical
9: Ear, Nose, Sinus

Operation–Character 3	Body Part–Character 4	Approach–Character 5	Device–Character 6	Qualifier–Character 7
Ø Alteration	Ø External Ear, Right	Ø Open	Ø Drainage Device	Ø Endolymphatic
1 Bypass	1 External Ear, Left	3 Percutaneous	7 Autologous Tissue Substitute	1 Bone Conduction
2 Change	2 External Ear, Bilateral	4 Percutaneous Endoscopic	B Airway	2 Cochlear Prosthesis, Single Channel
5 Destruction	3 External Auditory Canal, Right	7 Via Natural or Artificial Opening	D Intraluminal Device	3 Cochlear Prosthesis, Multiple Channel
7 Dilation	4 External Auditory Canal, Left	8 Via Natural or Artificial Opening Endoscopic	J Synthetic Substitute	X Diagnostic
8 Division	5 Middle Ear, Right	X External	K Nonautologous Tissue Substitute	Y Other Hearing Device
9 Drainage	6 Middle Ear, Left		S Hearing Device	Z No Qualifier
B Excision	7 Tympanic Membrane, Right		Y Other Device	
C Extirpation	8 Tympanic Membrane, Left		Z No Device	
D Extraction	9 Auditory Ossicle, Right			
H Insertion	A Auditory Ossicle, Left			
J Inspection	B Mastoid Sinus, Right			
M Reattachment	C Mastoid Sinus, Left			
N Release	D Inner Ear, Right			
P Removal	E Inner Ear, Left			
Q Repair	F Eustachian Tube, Right			
R Replacement	G Eustachian Tube, Left			
S Reposition	H Ear, Right			
T Resection	J Ear, Left			
U Supplement	K Nose			
W Revision	L Nasal Turbinate			
	M Nasal Septum			
	N Nasopharynx			
	P Accessory Sinus			
	Q Maxillary Sinus, Right			
	R Maxillary Sinus, Left			
	S Frontal Sinus, Right			
	T Frontal Sinus, Left			
	U Ethmoid Sinus, Right			
	V Ethmoid Sinus, Left			
	W Sphenoid Sinus, Right			
	X Sphenoid Sinus, Left			
	Y Sinus			

* Includes sinus ducts.

Ø: Medical and Surgical

B: Respiratory System

Operation–Character 3	Body Part–Character 4	Approach–Character 5	Device–Character 6	Qualifier–Character 7
1 Bypass	Ø Tracheobronchial Tree	Ø Open	Ø Drainage Device	Ø Allogeneic
2 Change	1 Trachea	3 Percutaneous	1 Radioactive Element	1 Syngeneic
5 Destruction	2 Carina	4 Percutaneous Endoscopic	2 Monitoring Device	2 Zooplastic
7 Dilation	3 Main Bronchus, Right	7 Via Natural or Artificial Opening	3 Infusion Device	4 Cutaneous
9 Drainage	4 Upper Lobe Bronchus, Right	8 Via Natural or Artificial Opening Endoscopic	7 Autologous Tissue Substitute	6 Esophagus
B Excision	5 Middle Lobe Bronchus, Right	X External	C Extraluminal Device	X Diagnostic
C Extirpation	6 Lower Lobe Bronchus, Right		D Intraluminal Device	Z No Qualifier
D Extraction	7 Main Bronchus, Left		E Endotracheal Device	
F Fragmentation	8 Upper Lobe Bronchus, Left		F Tracheostomy Device	
H Insertion	9 Lingula Bronchus		G Endobronchial Device	
J Inspection	B Lower Lobe Bronchus, Left		J Synthetic Substitute	
L Occlusion	C Upper Lung Lobe, Right		K Nonautologous Tissue Substitute	
M Reattachment	D Middle Lung Lobe, Right		M Diaphragmatic Pacemaker Lead	
N Release	F Lower Lung Lobe, Right		Y Other Device	
P Removal	G Upper Lung Lobe, Left		Z No Device	
Q Repair	H Lung Lingula			
S Reposition	J Lower Lung Lobe, Left			
T Resection	K Lung, Right			
U Supplement	L Lung, Left			
V Restriction	M Lungs, Bilateral			
W Revision	N Pleura, Right			
Y Transplantation	P Pleura, Left			
	Q Pleura			
	R Diaphragm, Right			
	S Diaphragm, Left			
	T Diaphragm			

Ø: Medical and Surgical

C: Mouth and Throat

Operation–Character 3	Body Part–Character 4	Approach–Character 5	Device–Character 6	Qualifier–Character 7
Ø Alteration	Ø Upper Lip	Ø Open	Ø Drainage Device	Ø Single
2 Change	1 Lower Lip	3 Percutaneous	1 Radioactive Element	1 Multiple
5 Destruction	2 Hard Palate	4 Percutaneous Endoscopic	5 External Fixation Device	2 All
7 Dilation	3 Soft Palate	7 Via Natural or Artificial Opening	7 Autologous Tissue Substitute	X Diagnostic
9 Drainage	4 Buccal Mucosa	8 Via Natural or Artificial Opening Endoscopic	B Airway	Z No Qualifier
B Excision	5 Upper Gingiva	X External	C Extraluminal Device	
C Extirpation	6 Lower Gingiva		D Intraluminal Device	
D Extraction	7 Tongue		J Synthetic Substitute	
F Fragmentation	8 Parotid Gland, Right		K Nonautologous Tissue Substitute	
H Insertion	9 Parotid Gland, Left		Y Other Device	
J Inspection	A Salivary Gland		Z No Device	
L Occlusion	B Parotid Duct, Right			
M Reattachment	C Parotid Duct, Left			
N Release	D Sublingual Gland, Right			
P Removal	F Sublingual Gland, Left			
Q Repair	G Submaxillary Gland, Right			
R Replacement	H Submaxillary Gland, Left			
S Reposition	J Minor Salivary Gland			
T Resection	M Pharynx			
U Supplement	N Uvula			
V Restriction	P Tonsils			
W Revision	Q Adenoids			
X Transfer	R Epiglottis			
	S Larynx			
	T Vocal Cord, Right			
	V Vocal Cord, Left			
	W Upper Tooth			
	X Lower Tooth			
	Y Mouth and Throat			

Ø: Medical and Surgical
D: Gastrointestinal System

Operation–Character 3	Body Part–Character 4	Approach–Character 5	Device–Character 6	Qualifier–Character 7
1 Bypass	Ø Upper Intestinal Tract	Ø Open	Ø Drainage Device	Ø Allogeneic
2 Change	1 Esophagus, Upper	3 Percutaneous	1 Radioactive Element	1 Syngeneic
5 Destruction	2 Esophagus, Middle	4 Percutaneous Endoscopic	2 Monitoring Device	2 Zooplastic
7 Dilation	3 Esophagus, Lower	7 Via Natural or Artificial Opening	3 Infusion Device	4 Cutaneous
8 Division	4 Esophagogastric Junction	8 Via Natural or Artificial Opening Endoscopic	7 Autologous Tissue Substitute	5 Esophagus
9 Drainage	5 Esophagus	X External	B Airway	6 Stomach
B Excision	6 Stomach		C Extraluminal Device	9 Duodenum
C Extirpation	7 Stomach, Pylorus		D Intraluminal Device	A Jejunum
F Fragmentation	8 Small Intestine		J Synthetic Substitute	B Ileum
H Insertion	9 Duodenum		K Nonautologous Tissue Substitute	H Cecum
J Inspection	A Jejunum		L Artificial Sphincter	K Ascending Colon
L Occlusion	B Ileum		M Stimulator Lead	L Transverse Colon
M Reattachment	C Ileocecal Valve		U Feeding Device	M Descending Colon
N Release	D Lower Intestinal Tract		Y Other Device	N Sigmoid Colon
P Removal	E Large Intestine		Z No Device	P Rectum
Q Repair	F Large Intestine, Right			Q Anus
R Replacement	G Large Intestine, Left			X Diagnostic
S Reposition	H Cecum			Z No Qualifier
T Resection	J Appendix			
U Supplement	K Ascending Colon			
V Restriction	L Transverse Colon			
W Revision	M Descending Colon			
X Transfer	N Sigmoid Colon			
Y Transplantation	P Rectum			
	Q Anus			
	R Anal Sphincter			
	S Greater Omentum			
	T Lesser Omentum			
	U Omentum			
	V Mesentery			
	W Peritoneum			

Ø: Medical and Surgical

F: Hepatobiliary System and Pancreas

Operation–Character 3	Body Part–Character 4	Approach–Character 5	Device–Character 6	Qualifier–Character 7
1 Bypass	Ø Liver	Ø Open	Ø Drainage Device	Ø Allogeneic
2 Change	1 Liver, Right Lobe	3 Percutaneous	1 Radioactive Element	1 Syngeneic
5 Destruction	2 Liver, Left Lobe	4 Percutaneous Endoscopic	2 Monitoring Device	2 Zooplastic
7 Dilation	4 Gallbladder	7 Via Natural or Artificial Opening	3 Infusion Device	3 Duodenum
8 Division	5 Hepatic Duct, Right	8 Via Natural or Artificial Opening Endoscopic	7 Autologous Tissue Substitute	4 Stomach
9 Drainage	6 Hepatic Duct, Left	X External	C Extraluminal Device	5 Hepatic Duct, Right
B Excision	8 Cystic Duct		D Intraluminal Device	6 Hepatic Duct, Left
C Extirpation	9 Common Bile Duct		J Synthetic Substitute	7 Hepatic Duct, Caudate
F Fragmentation	B Hepatobiliary Duct		K Nonautologous Tissue Substitute	8 Cystic Duct
H Insertion	C Ampulla of Vater		Y Other Device	9 Common Bile Duct
J Inspection	D Pancreatic Duct		Z No Device	B Small Intestine
L Occlusion	F Pancreatic Duct, Accessory			C Large Intestine
M Reattachment	G Pancreas			X Diagnostic
N Release				Z No Qualifier
P Removal				
Q Repair				
R Replacement				
S Reposition				
T Resection				
U Supplement				
V Restriction				
W Revision				
Y Transplantation				

Ø: Medical and Surgical

G: Endocrine System

Operation–Character 3	Body Part–Character 4	Approach–Character 5	Device–Character 6	Qualifier–Character 7
2 Change	Ø Pituitary Gland	Ø Open	Ø Drainage Device	X Diagnostic
5 Destruction	1 Pineal Body	3 Percutaneous	2 Monitoring Device	Z No Qualifier
8 Division	2 Adrenal Gland, Left	4 Percutaneous Endoscopic	3 Infusion Device	
9 Drainage	3 Adrenal Gland, Right	X External	Y Other Device	
B Excision	4 Adrenal Glands, Bilateral		Z No Device	
C Extirpation	5 Adrenal Gland			
H Insertion	6 Carotid Body, Left			
J Inspection	7 Carotid Body, Right			
M Reattachment	8 Carotid Bodies, Bilateral			
N Release	9 Para-aortic Body			
P Removal	B Coccygeal Glomus			
Q Repair	C Glomus Jugulare			
S Reposition	D Aortic Body			
T Resection	F Paraganglion Extremity			
W Revision	G Thyroid Gland Lobe, Left			
	H Thyroid Gland Lobe, Right			
	J Thyroid Gland Isthmus			
	K Thyroid Gland			
	L Superior Parathyroid Gland, Right			
	M Superior Parathyroid Gland, Left			
	N Inferior Parathyroid Gland, Right			
	P Inferior Parathyroid Gland, Left			
	Q Parathyroid Glands, Multiple			
	R Parathyroid Gland			
	S Endocrine Gland			

Ø: Medical and Surgical

H: Skin and Breast

Operation–Character 3	Body Part–Character 4	Approach–Character 5	Device–Character 6	Qualifier–Character 7
Ø Alteration	Ø Skin, Scalp	Ø Open	Ø Drainage Device	3 Full Thickness
2 Change	1 Skin, Face	3 Percutaneous	1 Radioactive Element	4 Partial Thickness
5 Destruction	2 Skin, Right Ear	7 Via Natural or Artificial Opening	7 Autologous Tissue Substitute	5 Latissimus Dorsi Myocutaneous Flap
8 Division	3 Skin, Left Ear	8 Via Natural or Artificial Opening Endoscopic	J Synthetic Substitute	6 Transverse Rectus Abdominis Myocutaneous Flap
9 Drainage	4 Skin, Neck	X External	K Nonautologous Tissue Substitute	7 Deep Inferior Epigastric Artery Perforator Flap
B Excision	5 Skin, Chest		N Tissue Expander	8 Superficial Inferior Epigastric Artery Flap
C Extirpation	6 Skin, Back		Y Other Device	9 Gluteal Artery Perforator Flap
D Extraction	7 Skin, Abdomen		Z No Device	D Multiple
H Insertion	8 Skin, Buttock			X Diagnostic
J Inspection	9 Skin, Perineum			Z No Qualifier
M Reattachment	A Skin, Genitalia			
N Release	B Skin, Right Upper Arm			
P Removal	C Skin, Left Upper Arm			
Q Repair	D Skin, Right Lower Arm			
R Replacement	E Skin, Left Lower Arm			
S Reposition	F Skin, Right Hand			
T Resection	G Skin, Left Hand			
U Supplement	H Skin, Right Upper Leg			
W Revision	J Skin, Left Upper Leg			
X Transfer	K Skin, Right Lower Leg			
	L Skin, Left Lower Leg			
	M Skin, Right Foot			
	N Skin, Left Foot			
	P Skin			
	Q Finger Nail			
	R Toe Nail			
	S Hair			
	T Breast, Right			
	U Breast, Left			
	V Breast, Bilateral			
	W Nipple, Right			
	X Nipple, Left			
	Y Supernumerary Breast			

* Includes skin and breast glands and ducts.

Ø: Medical and Surgical
J: Subcutaneous Tissue and Fascia

Operation–Character 3	Body Part–Character 4	Approach–Character 5	Device–Character 6	Qualifier–Character 7
Ø Alteration	Ø Subcutaneous Tissue and Fascia, Scalp	Ø Open	Ø Drainage Device	Ø Pacemaker, Single Chamber
2 Change	1 Subcutaneous Tissue and Fascia, Face	3 Percutaneous	1 Radioactive Element	1 Pacemaker, Single Chamber Rate Responsive
5 Destruction	4 Subcutaneous Tissue and Fascia, Anterior Neck	X External	2 Monitoring Device	2 Pacemaker, Dual Chamber
8 Division	5 Subcutaneous Tissue and Fascia, Posterior Neck		3 Infusion Device	3 Cardiac Resynchronization Pacemaker Pulse Generator
9 Drainage	6 Subcutaneous Tissue and Fascia, Chest		7 Autologous Tissue Substitute	4 Defibrillator Generator
B Excision	7 Subcutaneous Tissue and Fascia, Back		H Contraceptive Device	5 Cardiac Resynchronization Defibrillator Pulse Generator
C Extirpation	8 Subcutaneous Tissue and Fascia, Abdomen		J Synthetic Substitute	6 Single Array
D Extraction	9 Subcutaneous Tissue and Fascia, Buttock		K Nonautologous Tissue Substitute	7 Dual Array
H Insertion	B Subcutaneous Tissue and Fascia, Perineum		M Stimulator Generator	8 Single Array Rechargeable
J Inspection	C Subcutaneous Tissue and Fascia, Pelvic Region		N Tissue Expander	9 Dual Array Rechargeable
N Release	D Subcutaneous Tissue and Fascia, Right Upper Arm		P Cardiac Rhythm Related Device	A Contractility Modulation Device
P Removal	F Subcutaneous Tissue and Fascia, Left Upper Arm		V Infusion Pump	B Skin and Subcutaneous Tissue
Q Repair	G Subcutaneous Tissue and Fascia, Right Lower Arm		W Reservoir	C Skin, Subcutaneous Tissue and Fascia
R Replacement	H Subcutaneous Tissue and Fascia, Left Lower Arm		X Vascular Access Device	D Hemodynamic
W Revision	J Subcutaneous Tissue and Fascia, Right Hand		Y Other Device	X Diagnostic
X Transfer	K Subcutaneous Tissue and Fascia, Left Hand		Z No Device	Y Other Cardiac Rhythm Related Device
	L Subcutaneous Tissue and Fascia, Right Upper Leg			Z No Qualifier
	M Subcutaneous Tissue and Fascia, Left Upper Leg			
	N Subcutaneous Tissue and Fascia, Right Lower Leg			
	P Subcutaneous Tissue and Fascia, Left Lower Leg			
	Q Subcutaneous Tissue and Fascia, Right Foot			
	R Subcutaneous Tissue and Fascia, Left Foot			
	S Subcutaneous Tissue and Fascia, Head and Neck			
	T Subcutaneous Tissue and Fascia, Trunk			
	V Subcutaneous Tissue and Fascia, Upper Extremity			
	W Subcutaneous Tissue and Fascia, Lower Extremity			

Ø: Medical and Surgical

K: Muscles

Operation–Character 3	Body Part–Character 4	Approach–Character 5	Device–Character 6	Qualifier–Character 7
2 Change	Ø Head Muscle	Ø Open	Ø Drainage Device	Ø Skin
5 Destruction	1 Facial Muscle	3 Percutaneous	7 Autologous Tissue Substitute	1 Subcutaneous Tissue
8 Division	2 Neck Muscle, Right	4 Percutaneous Endoscopic	J Synthetic Substitute	2 Skin and Subcutaneous Tissue
9 Drainage	3 Neck Muscle, Left	X External	K Nonautologous Tissue Substitute	6 Transverse Rectus Abdominis Myocutaneous Flap
B Excision	4 Tongue, Palate, Pharynx Muscle		M Stimulator Lead	X Diagnostic
C Extirpation	5 Shoulder Muscle, Right		Y Other Device	Z No Qualifier
H Insertion	6 Shoulder Muscle, Left		Z No Device	
J Inspection	7 Upper Arm Muscle, Right			
M Reattachment	8 Upper Arm Muscle, Left			
N Release	9 Lower Arm and Wrist Muscle, Right			
P Removal	B Lower Arm and Wrist Muscle, Left			
Q Repair	C Hand Muscle, Right			
S Reposition	D Hand Muscle, Left			
T Resection	F Trunk Muscle, Right			
U Supplement	G Trunk Muscle, Left			
W Revision	H Thorax Muscle, Right			
X Transfer	J Thorax Muscle, Left			
	K Abdomen Muscle, Right			
	L Abdomen Muscle, Left			
	M Perineum Muscle			
	N Hip Muscle, Right			
	P Hip Muscle, Left			
	Q Upper Leg Muscle, Right			
	R Upper Leg Muscle, Left			
	S Lower Leg Muscle, Right			
	T Lower Leg Muscle, Left			
	V Foot Muscle, Right			
	W Foot Muscle, Left			
	X Upper Muscle			
	Y Lower Muscle			

Draft (2011)

Ø: Medical and Surgical

L: Tendons

Operation–Character 3	Body Part–Character 4	Approach–Character 5	Device–Character 6	Qualifier–Character 7
2 Change	Ø Head and Neck Tendon	Ø Open	Ø Drainage Device	X Diagnostic
5 Destruction	1 Shoulder Tendon, Right	3 Percutaneous	7 Autologous Tissue Substitute	Z No Qualifier
8 Division	2 Shoulder Tendon, Left	4 Percutaneous Endoscopic	J Synthetic Substitute	
9 Drainage	3 Upper Arm Tendon, Right	X External	K Nonautologous Tissue Substitute	
B Excision	4 Upper Arm Tendon, Left		Y Other Device	
C Extirpation	5 Lower Arm and Wrist Tendon, Right		Z No Device	
J Inspection	6 Lower Arm and Wrist Tendon, Left			
M Reattachment	7 Hand Tendon, Right			
N Release	8 Hand Tendon, Left			
P Removal	9 Trunk Tendon, Right			
Q Repair	B Trunk Tendon, Left			
R Replacement	C Thorax Tendon, Right			
S Reposition	D Thorax Tendon, Left			
T Resection	F Abdomen Tendon, Right			
U Supplement	G Abdomen Tendon, Left			
W Revision	H Perineum Tendon			
X Transfer	J Hip Tendon, Right			
	K Hip Tendon, Left			
	L Upper Leg Tendon, Right			
	M Upper Leg Tendon, Left			
	N Lower Leg Tendon, Right			
	P Lower Leg Tendon, Left			
	Q Knee Tendon, Right			
	R Knee Tendon, Left			
	S Ankle Tendon, Right			
	T Ankle Tendon, Left			
	V Foot Tendon, Right			
	W Foot Tendon, Left			
	X Upper Tendon			
	Y Lower Tendon			

* Includes synovial membrane.

Ø: Medical and Surgical

M: Bursae and Ligaments

Operation–Character 3	Body Part–Character 4	Approach–Character 5	Device–Character 6	Qualifier–Character 7
2 Change	Ø Head and Neck Bursa and Ligament	Ø Open	Ø Drainage Device	X Diagnostic
5 Destruction	1 Shoulder Bursa and Ligament, Right	3 Percutaneous	7 Autologous Tissue Substitute	Z No Qualifier
8 Division	2 Shoulder Bursa and Ligament, Left	4 Percutaneous Endoscopic	J Synthetic Substitute	
9 Drainage	3 Elbow Bursa and Ligament, Right	X External	K Nonautologous Tissue Substitute	
B Excision	4 Elbow Bursa and Ligament, Left		Y Other Device	
C Extirpation	5 Wrist Bursa and Ligament, Right		Z No Device	
D Extraction	6 Wrist Bursa and Ligament, Left			
J Inspection	7 Hand Bursa and Ligament, Right			
M Reattachment	8 Hand Bursa and Ligament, Left			
N Release	9 Upper Extremity Bursa and Ligament, Right			
P Removal	B Upper Extremity Bursa and Ligament, Left			
Q Repair	C Trunk Bursa and Ligament, Right			
S Reposition	D Trunk Bursa and Ligament, Left			
T Resection	F Thorax Bursa and Ligament, Right			
U Supplement	G Thorax Bursa and Ligament, Left			
W Revision	H Abdomen Bursa and Ligament, Right			
X Transfer	J Abdomen Bursa and Ligament, Left			
	K Perineum Bursa and Ligament			
	L Hip Bursa and Ligament, Right			
	M Hip Bursa and Ligament, Left			
	N Knee Bursa and Ligament, Right			
	P Knee Bursa and Ligament, Left			
	Q Ankle Bursa and Ligament, Right			
	R Ankle Bursa and Ligament, Left			
	S Foot Bursa and Ligament, Right			
	T Foot Bursa and Ligament, Left			
	V Lower Extremity Bursa and Ligament, Right			
	W Lower Extremity Bursa and Ligament, Left			
	X Upper Bursa and Ligament			
	Y Lower Bursa and Ligament			

* Includes synovial membrane.

0: Medical and Surgical
N: Head and Facial Bones

Operation–Character 3	Body Part–Character 4	Approach–Character 5	Device–Character 6	Qualifier–Character 7
2 Change	0 Skull	0 Open	0 Drainage Device	X Diagnostic
5 Destruction	1 Frontal Bone, Right	3 Percutaneous	4 Internal Fixation Device	Z No Qualifier
8 Division	2 Frontal Bone, Left	4 Percutaneous Endoscopic	5 External Fixation Device	
9 Drainage	3 Parietal Bone, Right	X External	7 Autologous Tissue Substitute	
B Excision	4 Parietal Bone, Left		J Synthetic Substitute	
C Extirpation	5 Temporal Bone, Right		K Nonautologous Tissue Substitute	
H Insertion	6 Temporal Bone, Left		M Bone Growth Stimulator	
J Inspection	7 Occipital Bone, Right		N Neurostimulator Generator	
N Release	8 Occipital Bone, Left		S Hearing Device	
P Removal	B Nasal Bone		Y Other Device	
Q Repair	C Sphenoid Bone, Right		Z No Device	
R Replacement	D Sphenoid Bone, Left			
S Reposition	F Ethmoid Bone, Right			
T Resection	G Ethmoid Bone, Left			
U Supplement	H Lacrimal Bone, Right			
W Revision	J Lacrimal Bone, Left			
	K Palatine Bone, Right			
	L Palatine Bone, Left			
	M Zygomatic Bone, Right			
	N Zygomatic Bone, Left			
	P Orbit, Right			
	Q Orbit, Left			
	R Maxilla, Right			
	S Maxilla, Left			
	T Mandible, Right			
	V Mandible, Left			
	W Facial Bone			
	X Hyoid Bone			

Ø: Medical and Surgical

P: Upper Bones

Operation–Character 3	Body Part–Character 4	Approach–Character 5	Device–Character 6	Qualifier–Character 7
2 Change	Ø Sternum	Ø Open	Ø Drainage Device	3 Monoplanar
5 Destruction	1 Rib, Right	3 Percutaneous	4 Internal Fixation Device	4 Ring
8 Division	2 Rib, Left	4 Percutaneous Endoscopic	5 External Fixation Device	5 Hybrid
9 Drainage	3 Cervical Vertebra	X External	6 Intramedullary Fixation Device	8 Rigid Plate
B Excision	4 Thoracic Vertebra		7 Autologous Tissue Substitute	9 Limb Lengthening Device
C Extirpation	5 Scapula, Right		J Synthetic Substitute	X Diagnostic
H Insertion	6 Scapula, Left		K Nonautologous Tissue Substitute	Z No Qualifier
J Inspection	7 Glenoid Cavity, Right		M Bone Growth Stimulator	
N Release	8 Glenoid Cavity, Left		Y Other Device	
P Removal	9 Clavicle, Right		Z No Device	
Q Repair	B Clavicle, Left			
R Replacement	C Humeral Head, Right			
S Reposition	D Humeral Head, Left			
T Resection	F Humeral Shaft, Right			
U Supplement	G Humeral Shaft, Left			
W Revision	H Radius, Right			
	J Radius, Left			
	K Ulna, Right			
	L Ulna, Left			
	M Carpal, Right			
	N Carpal, Left			
	P Metacarpal, Right			
	Q Metacarpal, Left			
	R Thumb Phalanx, Right			
	S Thumb Phalanx, Left			
	T Finger Phalanx, Right			
	V Finger Phalanx, Left			
	Y Upper Bone			

Ø: Medical and Surgical
Q: Lower Bones

Operation–Character 3	Body Part–Character 4	Approach–Character 5	Device–Character 6	Qualifier–Character 7
2 Change	Ø Lumbar Vertebra	Ø Open	Ø Drainage Device	3 Monoplanar
5 Destruction	1 Sacrum	3 Percutaneous	4 Internal Fixation Device	4 Ring
8 Division	2 Pelvic Bone, Right	4 Percutaneous Endoscopic	5 External Fixation Device	5 Hybrid
9 Drainage	3 Pelvic Bone, Left	X External	6 Intramedullary Fixation Device	9 Limb Lengthening Device
B Excision	4 Acetabulum, Right		7 Autologous Tissue Substitute	X Diagnostic
C Extirpation	5 Acetabulum, Left		J Synthetic Substitute	Z No Qualifier
H Insertion	6 Upper Femur, Right		K Nonautologous Tissue Substitute	
J Inspection	7 Upper Femur, Left		M Bone Growth Stimulator	
N Release	8 Femoral Shaft, Right		Y Other Device	
P Removal	9 Femoral Shaft, Left		Z No Device	
Q Repair	B Lower Femur, Right			
R Replacement	C Lower Femur, Left			
S Reposition	D Patella, Right			
T Resection	F Patella, Left			
U Supplement	G Tibia, Right			
W Revision	H Tibia, Left			
	J Fibula, Right			
	K Fibula, Left			
	L Tarsal, Right			
	M Tarsal, Left			
	N Metatarsal, Right			
	P Metatarsal, Left			
	Q Toe Phalanx, Right			
	R Toe Phalanx, Left			
	S Coccyx			
	Y Lower Bone			

Ø: Medical and Surgical
R: Upper Joints

Operation–Character 3	Body Part–Character 4	Approach–Character 5	Device–Character 6	Qualifier–Character 7
2 Change	Ø Occipital-cervical Joint	Ø Open	Ø Drainage Device	Ø Anterior Approach, Anterior Column
5 Destruction	1 Cervical Vertebral Joint	3 Percutaneous	3 Infusion Device OR Interbody Internal Fixation (for root operation FUSION only)	1 Posterior Approach, Posterior Column
9 Drainage	2 Cervical Vertebral Joint, 2 or more	4 Percutaneous Endoscopic	4 Internal Fixation Device	2 Interspinous Process
B Excision	3 Cervical Vertebral Disc	X External	5 External Fixation Device	3 Pedicle-based Dynamic Stabilization
C Extirpation	4 Cervicothoracic Vertebral Joint		7 Autologous Tissue Substitute	4 Facet
G Fusion	5 Cervicothoracic Vertebral Disc		8 Spacer	5 Reverse Ballard Socket
H Insertion	6 Thoracic Vertebral Joint		J Synthetic Substitute	6 Humeral Surface
J Inspection	7 Thoracic Vertebral Joint, 2 to 7		K Nonautologous Tissue Substitute	7 Glenoid Surface
N Release	8 Thoracic Vertebral Joint, 8 or more		Y Other Device	J Posterior Approach, Anterior Column
P Removal	9 Thoracic Vertebral Disc		Z No Device	X Diagnostic
Q Repair	A Thoracolumbar Vertebral Joint			Z No Qualifier
R Replacement	B Thoracolumbar Vertebral Disc			
S Reposition	C Temporomandibular Joint, Right			
T Resection	D Temporomandibular Joint, Left			
U Supplement	E Sternoclavicular Joint, Right			
W Revision	F Sternoclavicular Joint, Left			
	G Acromioclavicular Joint, Right			
	H Acromioclavicular Joint, Left			
	J Shoulder Joint, Right			
	K Shoulder Joint, Left			
	L Elbow Joint, Right			
	M Elbow Joint, Left			
	N Wrist Joint, Right			
	P Wrist Joint, Left			
	Q Carpal Joint, Right			
	R Carpal Joint, Left			
	S Metacarpocarpal Joint, Right			
	T Metacarpocarpal Joint, Left			
	U Metacarpophalangeal Joint, Right			
	V Metacarpophalangeal Joint, Left			
	W Finger Phalangeal Joint, Right			
	X Finger Phalangeal Joint, Left			
	Y Upper Joint			

* Includes synovial membrane.

Ø: Medical and Surgical

S: Lower Joints

Operation–Character 3	Body Part–Character 4	Approach–Character 5	Device–Character 6	Qualifier–Character 7
2 Change	Ø Lumbar Vertebral Joint	Ø Open	Ø Drainage Device	Ø Anterior Approach, Anterior Column
5 Destruction	1 Lumbar Vertebral Joint, 2 or more	3 Percutaneous	3 Infusion Device OR Interbody Internal Fixation (for root operation FUSION only)	1 Approach, Posterior Posterior Column
9 Drainage	2 Lumbar Vertebral Disc	4 Percutaneous Endoscopic	4 Internal Fixation Device	2 Interspinous Process
B Excision	3 Lumbosacral Joint	X External	5 External Fixation Device	3 Pedicle-based Dynamic Stabilization
C Extirpation	4 Lumbosacral Disc		7 Autologous Tissue Substitute	4 Facet
G Fusion	5 Sacrococcygeal Joint		8 Spacer	5 Metal on Polyethylene
H Insertion	6 Coccygeal Joint		9 Liner	6 Metal on Metal
J Inspection	7 Sacroiliac Joint, Right		B Resurfacing Device	7 Ceramic on Ceramic
N Release	8 Sacroiliac Joint, Left		J Synthetic Substitute	8 Ceramic on Polyethylene
P Removal	9 Hip Joint, Right		K Nonautologous Tissue Substitute	C Patellar Surface
Q Repair	B Hip Joint, Left		Y Other Device	F Metal
R Replacement	C Knee Joint, Right		Z No Device	G Ceramic
S Reposition	D Knee Joint, Left			H Polyethylene
T Resection	F Ankle Joint, Right			J Posterior Approach, Anterior Column
U Supplement	G Ankle Joint, Left			X Diagnostic
W Revision	H Tarsal Joint, Right			Z No Qualifier
	J Tarsal Joint, Left			
	K Metatarsal-Tarsal Joint, Right			
	L Metatarsal-Tarsal Joint, Left			
	M Metatarsal-Phalangeal Joint, Right			
	N Metatarsal-Phalangeal Joint, Left			
	P Toe Phalangeal Joint, Right			
	Q Toe Phalangeal Joint, Left			
	Y Lower Joint			

* Includes synovial membrane.

Ø: Medical and Surgical

T: Urinary System

Operation–Character 3	Body Part–Character 4	Approach–Character 5	Device–Character 6	Qualifier–Character 7
1 Bypass	Ø Kidney, Right	Ø Open	Ø Drainage Device	Ø Allogeneic
2 Change	1 Kidney, Left	3 Percutaneous	2 Monitoring Device	1 Syngeneic
5 Destruction	2 Kidneys, Bilateral	4 Percutaneous Endoscopic	3 Infusion Device	2 Zooplastic
7 Dilation	3 Kidney Pelvis, Right	7 Via Natural or Artificial Opening	7 Autologous Tissue Substitute	3 Kidney Pelvis, Right
8 Division	4 Kidney Pelvis, Left	8 Via Natural or Artificial Opening Endoscopic	C Extraluminal Device	4 Kidney Pelvis, Left
9 Drainage	5 Kidney	X External	D Intraluminal Device	6 Ureter, Right
B Excision	6 Ureter, Right		J Synthetic Substitute	7 Ureter, Left
C Extirpation	7 Ureter, Left		K Nonautologous Tissue Substitute	8 Colon
D Extraction	8 Ureters, Bilateral		L Artificial Sphincter	9 Colocutaneous
F Fragmentation	9 Ureter		M Stimulator Lead	A Ileum
H Insertion	B Bladder		Y Other Device	B Bladder
J Inspection	C Bladder Neck		Z No Device	C Ileocutaneous
L Occlusion	D Urethra			D Cutaneous
M Reattachment				X Diagnostic
N Release				Z No Qualifier
P Removal				
Q Repair				
R Replacement				
S Reposition				
T Resection				
U Supplement				
V Restriction				
W Revision				
X Transfer				
Y Transplantation				

0: Medical and Surgical
U: Female Reproductive System

Operation–Character 3	Body Part–Character 4	Approach–Character 5	Device–Character 6	Qualifier–Character 7
1 Bypass	0 Ovary, Right	0 Open	0 Drainage Device	0 Allogeneic
2 Change	1 Ovary, Left	3 Percutaneous	1 Radioactive Element	1 Syngeneic
5 Destruction	2 Ovaries, Bilateral	4 Percutaneous Endoscopic	3 Infusion Device	2 Zooplastic
7 Dilation	3 Ovary	7 Via Natural or Artificial Opening	7 Autologous Tissue Substitute	5 Fallopian Tube, Right
8 Division	4 Uterine Supporting Structure	8 Via Natural or Artificial Opening Endoscopic	C Extraluminal Device	6 Fallopian Tube, Left
9 Drainage	5 Fallopian Tube, Right	F Via Natural or Artificial Opening With Percutaneous Endoscopic Assistance	D Intraluminal Device	9 Uterus
B Excision	6 Fallopian Tube, Left	X External	G Pessary	X Diagnostic
C Extirpation	7 Fallopian Tubes, Bilateral		H Contraceptive Device	Z No Qualifier
D Extraction	8 Fallopian Tube		J Synthetic Substitute	
F Fragmentation	9 Uterus		K Nonautologous Tissue Substitute	
H Insertion	B Endometrium		Y Other Device	
J Inspection	C Cervix		Z No Device	
L Occlusion	D Uterus and Cervix			
M Reattachment	F Cul-de-sac			
N Release	G Vagina			
P Removal	H Vagina and Cul-de-sac			
Q Repair	J Clitoris			
S Reposition	K Hymen			
T Resection	L Vestibular Gland			
U Supplement	M Vulva			
V Restriction	N Ova			
W Revision				
X Transfer				
Y Transplantation				

Ø: Medical and Surgical

V: Male Reproductive System

Operation–Character 3	Body Part–Character 4	Approach–Character 5	Device–Character 6	Qualifier–Character 7
1 Bypass	Ø Prostate	Ø Open	Ø Drainage Device	J Epididymis, Right
2 Change	1 Seminal Vesicle, Right	3 Percutaneous	1 Radioactive Element	K Epididymis, Left
5 Destruction	2 Seminal Vesicle, Left	4 Percutaneous Endoscopic	3 Infusion Device	N Vas Deferens, Right
7 Dilation	3 Seminal Vesicles, Bilateral	7 Via Natural or Artificial Opening	7 Autologous Tissue Substitute	P Vas Deferens, Left
9 Drainage	4 Prostate and Seminal Vesicles	8 Via Natural or Artificial Opening Endoscopic	C Extraluminal Device	X Diagnostic
B Excision	5 Scrotum	X External	D Intraluminal Device	Z No Qualifier
C Extirpation	6 Tunica Vaginalis, Right		J Synthetic Substitute	
H Insertion	7 Tunica Vaginalis, Left		K Nonautologous Tissue Substitute	
J Inspection	8 Scrotum and Tunica Vaginalis		Y Other Device	
L Occlusion	9 Testis, Right		Z No Device	
M Reattachment	B Testis, Left			
N Release	C Testes, Bilateral			
P Removal	D Testis			
Q Repair	F Spermatic Cord, Right			
R Replacement	G Spermatic Cord, Left			
S Reposition	H Spermatic Cords, Bilateral			
T Resection	J Epididymis, Right			
U Supplement	K Epididymis, Left			
W Revision	L Epididymis, Bilateral			
	M Epididymis and Spermatic Cord			
	N Vas Deferens, Right			
	P Vas Deferens, Left			
	Q Vas Deferens, Bilateral			
	R Vas Deferens			
	S Penis			
	T Prepuce			
	V Male External Genitalia			

Ø: Medical and Surgical
W: Anatomical Regions, General

Operation–Character 3	Body Region–Character 4	Approach–Character 5	Device–Character 6	Qualifier–Character 7
Ø Alteration	Ø Head	Ø Open	Ø Drainage Device	Ø Vagina
1 Bypass	1 Cranial Cavity	3 Percutaneous	1 Radioactive Element	1 Penis
2 Change	2 Face	4 Percutaneous Endoscopic	3 Infusion Device	2 Stoma
3 Control	3 Oral Cavity and Throat	7 Via Natural or Artificial Opening	7 Autologous Tissue Substitute	4 Cutaneous
4 Creation	4 Upper Jaw	8 Via Natural or Artificial Opening Endoscopic	J Synthetic Substitute	9 Pleural Cavity, Right
8 Division	5 Lower Jaw	X External	K Nonautologous Tissue Substitute	B Pleural Cavity, Left
9 Drainage	6 Neck		Y Other Device	G Peritoneal Cavity
B Excision	8 Chest Wall		Z No Device	J Pelvic Cavity
C Extirpation	9 Pleural Cavity, Right			X Diagnostic
F Fragmentation	B Pleural Cavity, Left			Y Lower Vein
H Insertion	C Mediastinum			Z No Qualifier
J Inspection	D Pericardial Cavity			
M Reattachment	F Abdominal Wall			
P Removal	G Peritoneal Cavity			
Q Repair	H Retroperitoneum			
U Supplement	J Pelvic Cavity			
W Revision	K Upper Back			
	L Lower Back			
	M Perineum, Male			
	N Perineum, Female			
	P Gastrointestinal Tract			
	Q Respiratory Tract			
	R Genitourinary Tract			

0: Medical and Surgical
X: Anatomical Regions, Upper Extremities

Operation–Character 3	Body Part–Character 4	Approach–Character 5	Device–Character 6	Qualifier–Character 7
Ø Alteration	Ø Forequarter, Right	Ø Open	Ø Drainage Device	Ø Complete
2 Change	1 Forequarter, Left	3 Percutaneous	1 Radioactive Element	1 High
3 Control	2 Shoulder Region, Right	4 Percutaneous Endoscopic	3 Infusion Device	2 Mid
6 Detachment	3 Shoulder Region, Left	X External	7 Autologous Tissue Substitute	3 Low
9 Drainage	4 Axilla, Right		J Synthetic Substitute	4 Complete 1st Ray
B Excision	5 Axilla, Left		K Nonautologous Tissue Substitute	5 Complete 2nd Ray
H Insertion	6 Upper Extremity, Right		Y Other Device	6 Complete 3rd Ray
J Inspection	7 Upper Extremity, Left		Z No Device	7 Complete 4th Ray
M Reattachment	8 Upper Arm, Right			8 Complete 5th Ray
P Removal	9 Upper Arm, Left			9 Partial 1st Ray
Q Repair	B Elbow Region, Right			B Partial 2nd Ray
R Replacement	C Elbow Region, Left			C Partial 3rd Ray
U Supplement	D Lower Arm, Right			D Partial 4th Ray
W Revision	F Lower Arm, Left			F Partial 5th Ray
X Transfer	G Wrist Region, Right			L Thumb, Right
	H Wrist Region, Left			M Thumb, Left
	J Hand, Right			N Toe, Right
	K Hand, Left			P Toe, Left
	L Thumb, Right			X Diagnostic
	M Thumb, Left			Z No Qualifier
	N Index Finger, Right			
	P Index Finger, Left			
	Q Middle Finger, Right			
	R Middle Finger, Left			
	S Ring Finger, Right			
	T Ring Finger, Left			
	V Little Finger, Right			
	W Little Finger, Left			

Ø: Medical and Surgical

Y: Anatomical Regions, Lower Extremities

Operation–Character 3	Body Part–Character 4	Approach–Character 5	Device–Character 6	Qualifier–Character 7
Ø Alteration	Ø Buttock, Right	Ø Open	Ø Drainage Device	Ø Complete
2 Change	1 Buttock, Left	3 Percutaneous	1 Radioactive Element	1 High
3 Control	2 Hindquarter, Right	4 Percutaneous Endoscopic	3 Infusion Device	2 Mid
6 Detachment	3 Hindquarter, Left	X External	7 Autologous Tissue Substitute	3 Low
9 Drainage	4 Hindquarter, Bilateral		J Synthetic Substitute	4 Complete 1st Ray
B Excision	5 Inguinal Region, Right		K Nonautologous Tissue Substitute	5 Complete 2nd Ray
H Insertion	6 Inguinal Region, Left		Y Other Device	6 Complete 3rd Ray
J Inspection	7 Femoral Region, Right		Z No Device	7 Complete 4th Ray
M Reattachment	8 Femoral Region, Left			8 Complete 5th Ray
P Removal	9 Lower Extremity, Right			9 Partial 1st Ray
Q Repair	A Inguinal Region, Bilateral			B Partial 2nd Ray
U Supplement	B Lower Extremity, Left			C Partial 3rd Ray
W Revision	C Upper Leg, Right			D Partial 4th Ray
	D Upper Leg, Left			F Partial 5th Ray
	E Femoral Region, Bilateral			X Diagnostic
	F Knee Region, Right			Z No Qualifier
	G Knee Region, Left			
	H Lower Leg, Right			
	J Lower Leg, Left			
	K Ankle Region, Right			
	L Ankle Region, Left			
	M Foot, Right			
	N Foot, Left			
	P 1st Toe, Right			
	Q 1st Toe, Left			
	R 2nd Toe, Right			
	S 2nd Toe, Left			
	T 3rd Toe, Right			
	U 3rd Toe, Left			
	V 4th Toe, Right			
	W 4th Toe, Left			
	X 5th Toe, Right			
	Y 5th Toe, Left			

1: Obstetrics

Ø: Pregnancy

Operation–Character 3	Body Part–Character 4	Approach–Character 5	Device–Character 6	Qualifier–Character 7
2 Change	Ø Products of Conception	Ø Open	3 Monitoring Electrode	Ø Classical
9 Drainage	1 Products of Conception, Retained	3 Percutaneous	Y Other Device	1 Low Cervical
A Abortion	2 Products of Conception, Ectopic	4 Percutaneous Endoscopic	Z No Device	2 Extraperitoneal
D Extraction		7 Via Natural or Artificial Opening		3 Low Forceps
E Delivery		8 Via Natural or Artificial Opening Endoscopic		4 Mid Forceps
H Insertion		X External		5 High Forceps
J Inspection				6 Vacuum
P Removal				7 Internal Version
Q Repair				8 Other
S Reposition				9 Fetal Blood
T Resection				A Fetal Cerebrospinal Fluid
Y Transplantation				B Fetal Fluid, Other
				C Amniotic Fluid, Therapeutic
				D Fluid, Other
				E Nervous System
				F Cardiovascular System
				G Lymphatics & Hemic
				H Eye
				J Ear, Nose & Sinus
				K Respiratory System
				L Mouth & Throat
				M Gastrointestinal System
				N Hepatobiliary & Pancreas
				P Endocrine System
				Q Skin
				R Musculoskeletal System
				S Urinary System
				T Female Reproductive System
				U Amniotic Fluid, Diagnostic
				V Male Reproductive System
				W Laminaria
				X Abortifacient
				Y Other Body Systems
				Z No Qualifier

2: Placement
W: Anatomical Regions

Operation–Character 3	Body Region Character 4	Approach–Character 5	Device–Character 6	Qualifier–Character 7
Ø Change	Ø Head	X External	Ø Traction Apparatus	Z No Qualifier
1 Compression	1 Face		1 Splint	
2 Dressing	2 Neck		2 Cast	
3 Immobilization	3 Abdominal Wall		3 Brace	
4 Packing	4 Chest Wall		4 Bandage	
5 Removal	5 Back		5 Packing Material	
6 Traction	6 Inguinal Region, Right		6 Pressure Dressing	
	7 Inguinal Region, Left		7 Intermittent Pressure Device	
	8 Upper Extremity, Right		8 Stereotatic Apparatus	
	9 Upper Extremity, Left		9 Wire	
	A Upper Arm, Right		Y Other Device	
	B Upper Arm, Left		Z No Device	
	C Lower Arm, Right			
	D Lower Arm, Left			
	E Hand, Right			
	F Hand, Left			
	G Thumb, Right			
	H Thumb, Left			
	J Finger, Right			
	K Finger, Left			
	L Lower Extremity, Right			
	M Lower Extremity, Left			
	N Upper Leg, Right			
	P Upper Leg, Left			
	Q Lower Leg, Right			
	R Lower Leg, Left			
	S Foot, Right			
	T Foot, Left			
	U Toe, Right			
	V Toe, Left			

2: Placement
Y: Anatomical Orifices

Operation–Character 3	Body Orifice–Character 4	Approach Character–5	Device Character–6	Qualifier Character–7
Ø Change	Ø Mouth and Pharynx	X External	5 Packing Material	Z No Qualifier
4 Packing	1 Nasal			
5 Removal	2 Ear			
	3 Anorectal			
	4 Female Genital Tract			
	5 Urethra			

3: Administration
Ø: Circulatory

Operation–Character 3	Body System/Region Character 4	Approach–Character 5	Substance–Character 6	Qualifier–Character 7
2 Transfusion	3 Peripheral Vein	Ø Open	A Stem Cells, Embryonic	Ø Autologous
	4 Central Vein	3 Percutaneous	G Bone Marrow	1 Nonautologous
	5 Peripheral Artery	7 Via Natural or Artificial Opening	H Whole Blood	Z No Qualifier
	6 Central Artery		J Serum Albumin	
	7 Products of Conception, Circulatory		K Frozen Plasma	
			L Fresh Plasma	
			M Plasma Cryoprecipitate	
			N Red Blood Cells	
			P Frozen Red Cells	
			Q White Cells	
			R Platelets	
			S Globulin	
			T Fibrinogen	
			V Antihemophilic Factors	
			W Factor IX	
			X Stem Cells, Cord Blood	
			Y Stem Cells, Hematopoietic	

3: Administration
C: Indwelling Device

Operation–Character 3	Body System/Region Character 4	Approach–Character 5	Substance–Character 6	Qualifier–Character 7
1 Irrigation	Z None	X External	8 Irrigating Substance	Z No Qualifier

3: Administration
E: Physiological Systems and Anatomical Regions

Operation–Character 3	Body System/Region–Character 4	Approach–Character 5	Substance–Character 6	Qualifier–Character 7
Ø Introduction	Ø Skin and Mucous Membranes	Ø Open	Ø Antineoplastic	Ø Autologous
1 Irrigation	1 Subcutaneous Tissue	3 Percutaneous	1 Thrombolytic	1 Nonautologous
	2 Muscle	7 Via Natural or Artificial Opening	2 Anti-infective	2 High-dose Interleukin-2
	3 Peripheral Vein	8 Via Natural or Artificial Opening Endoscopic	3 Anti-inflammatory	3 Low-dose Interleukin-2
	4 Central Vein	X External	4 Serum, Toxoid and Vaccine	4 Liquid Brachytherapy Radioisotope
	5 Peripheral Artery		5 Adhesion Barrier	5 Other Antineoplastic
	6 Central Artery		6 Nutritional Substance	6 Recombinant Human-activated Protein C
	7 Coronary Artery		7 Electrolytic and Water Balance Substance	7 Other Thrombolytic
	8 Heart		8 Irrigating Substance	8 Oxazolidinones
	9 Nose		9 Dialysate	9 Other Anti-infective
	A Bone Marrow		A Stem Cells, Embryonic	B Recombinant Bone Morphogenetic Protein
	B Ear		B Local Anesthetic	C Other Substance
	C Eye		C Regional Anesthetic	D Nitric Oxide
	D Mouth and Pharynx		D Inhalation Anesthetic	F Other Gas
	E Products of Conception		E Stem Cells, Somatic	G Insulin
	F Respiratory Tract		F Intracirculatory Anesthetic	H Human B-type Natriuretic Peptide
	G Upper GI		G Other Therapeutic Substance	J Other Hormone
	H Lower GI		H Radioactive Substance	K Immunostimulator
	J Biliary and Pancreatic Tract		J Contrast Agent	L Immunosuppressive
	K Genitourinary Tract		K Other Diagnostic Substance	M Monoclonal Antibody
	L Pleural Cavity		L Sperm	N Blood Brain Barrier Disruption
	M Peritoneal Cavity		M Pigment	P Clofarabine
	N Male Reproductive		N Analgesics, Hypnotics, Sedatives	X Diagnostic
	P Female Reproductive		P Platelet Inhibitor	Z No Qualifier
	Q Cranial Cavity and Brain		Q Fertilized Ovum	
	R Spinal Canal		R Antiarrhythmic	
	S Epidural Space		S Gas	
	T Peripheral Nerves and Plexi		T Destructive Agent	
	U Joints		U Pancreatic Islet Cells	
	V Bones		V Hormone	
	W Lymphatics		W Immunotherapeutic	
	X Cranial Nerves		X Vasopressor	
	Y Pericardial Cavity			

4: Measurement and Monitoring
A: Physiological Systems

Operation–Character 3	Body System–Character 4	Approach–Character 5	Function/Device–Character 6	Qualifier–Character 7
Ø Measurement	Ø Central Nervous	Ø Open	Ø Acuity	Ø Central
1 Monitoring	1 Peripheral Nervous	3 Percutaneous	1 Capacity	1 Peripheral
	2 Cardiac	4 Percutaneous Endoscopic	2 Conductivity	2 Portal
	3 Arterial	7 Via Natural or Artificial Opening	3 Contractility	3 Pulmonary
	4 Venous	8 Via Natural or Artificial Opening Endoscopic	4 Electrical Activity	4 Stress
	5 Circulatory	X External	5 Flow	5 Ambulatory
	6 Lymphatic		6 Metabolism	6 Right Heart
	7 Visual		7 Mobility	7 Left Heart
	8 Olfactory		8 Motility	8 Bilateral
	9 Respiratory		9 Output	9 Sensory
	B Gastrointestinal		B Pressure	A Guidance
	C Biliary		C Rate	B Motor
	D Urinary		D Resistance	C Coronary
	F Musculoskeletal		F Rhythm	D Intracranial
	H Products of Conception, Cardiac		G Secretion	F Other Thoracic
	J Products of Conception, Nervous		H Sound	G Intraoperative
	Z None		J Pulse	Z No Qualifier
			K Temperature	
			L Volume	
			M Total Activity	
			N Sampling and Pressure	
			P Action Currents	
			Q Sleep	
			R Saturation	

4: Measurement and Monitoring
B: Physiological Devices

Operation–Character 3	Body System–Character 4	Approach–Character 5	Function/Device–Character 6	Qualifier–Character 7
Ø Measurement	Ø Central Nervous	X External	S Pacemaker	Z No Qualifier
	1 Peripheral Nervous		T Defibrillator	
	2 Cardiac		V Stimulator	
	9 Respiratory			
	F Musculoskeletal			

5: Extracorporeal Assistance and Performance
A: Physiological Systems

Operation–Character 3	Body System–Character 4	Duration–Character 5	Function–Character 6	Qualifier–Character 7
Ø Assistance	2 Cardiac	Ø Single	Ø Filtration	Ø Balloon Pump
1 Performance	5 Circulatory	1 Intermittent	1 Output	1 Hyperbaric
2 Restoration	9 Respiratory	2 Continuous	2 Oxygenation	2 Manual
	C Biliary	3 Less than 24 Consecutive Hours	3 Pacing	3 Membrane
	D Urinary	4 24-96 Consecutive Hours	4 Rhythm	4 Nonmechanical
		5 Greater than 96 Consecutive Hours	5 Ventilation	5 Pulsatile Compression
		6 Multiple		6 Other Pump
				7 Continuous Positive Airway Pressure
				8 Intermittent Positive Airway Pressure
				9 Continuous Negative Airway Pressure
				B Intermittent Negative Airway Pressure
				C Supersaturated
				D Impeller Pump
				Z No Qualifier

6: Extracorporeal Therapies
A: Physiological Systems

Operation–Character 3	Body System–Character 4	Duration–Character 5	Qualifier–Character 6	Qualifier–Character 7
Ø Atmospheric Control	Ø Skin	Ø Single	Z No Qualifier	Ø Erythrocytes
1 Decompression	1 Urinary	1 Multiple		1 Leukocytes
2 Electromagnetic Therapy	2 Central Nervous			2 Platelets
3 Hyperthermia	3 Musculoskeletal			3 Plasma
4 Hypothermia	5 Circulatory			4 Head and Neck Vessels
5 Pheresis	Z None			5 Heart
6 Phototherapy				6 Peripheral Vessels
7 Ultrasound Therapy				7 Other Vessels
8 Ultraviolet Light Therapy				T Stem Cells, Cord Blood
9 Shock Wave Therapy				V Stem Cells, Hematopoietic
				Z No Qualifier

7: Osteopathic
W: Anatomical Regions

Operation–Character 3	Body Region–Character 4	Approach–Character 5	Method–Character 6	Qualifier–Character 7
Ø Treatment	Ø Head	X External	Ø Articulatory-Raising	Z None
	1 Cervical		1 Fascial Release	
	2 Thoracic		2 General Mobilization	
	3 Lumbar		3 High Velocity-Low Amplitude	
	4 Sacrum		4 Indirect	
	5 Pelvis		5 Low Velocity-High Amplitude	
	6 Lower Extremities		6 Lymphatic Pump	
	7 Upper Extremities		7 Muscle Energy-Isometric	
	8 Rib Cage		8 Muscle Energy-Isotonic	
	9 Abdomen		9 Other Method	

8: Other Procedures
C: Indwelling Devices

Operation–Character 3	Body Region–Character 4	Approach–Character 5	Method–Character 6	Qualifier–Character 7
Ø Other procedures	1 Nervous System	X External	6 Collection	J Cerebrospinal Fluid
	2 Circulatory System			K Blood
				L Other Fluid

8: Other Procedures
E: Physiological Systems and Anatomical Regions

Operation–Character 3	Body Region–Character 4	Approach–Character 5	Method–Character 6	Qualifier–Character 7
Ø Other Procedures	1 Nervous System	Ø Open	Ø Acupuncture	Ø Anesthesia
	2 Circulatory System	3 Percutaneous	1 Therapeutic Massage	1 In Vitro Fertilization
	9 Head and Neck Region	4 Percutaneous Endoscopic	6 Collection	2 Breast Milk
	H Integumentary System and Breast	7 Via Natural or Artificial Opening	B Computer Assisted Procedure	3 Sperm
	K Musculoskeletal System	8 Via Natural or Artificial Opening Endoscopic	C Robotic Assisted Procedure	4 Yoga Therapy
	U Female Reproductive System	X External	D Near Infrared Spectroscopy	5 Meditation
	V Male Reproductive System		Y Other Method	6 Isolation
	W Trunk Region			7 Examination
	X Upper Extremity			8 Suture Removal
	Y Lower Extremity			9 Piercing
	Z None			C Prostate
				D Rectum
				F With Fluoroscopy
				G With Computerized Tomography
				H With Magnetic Resonance Imaging
				Z No Qualifier

9: Chiropractic
W: Anatomical Regions

Operation–Character 3	Body Region–Character 4	Approach–Character 5	Method–Character 6	Qualifier–Character 7
B Manipulation	Ø Head	X External	B Non-Manual	Z None
	1 Cervical		C Indirect Visceral	
	2 Thoracic		D Extra-Articular	
	3 Lumbar		F Direct Visceral	
	4 Sacrum		G Long Lever Specific Contact	
	5 Pelvis		H Short Lever Specific Contact	
	6 Lower Extremities		J Long and Short Lever Specific Contact	
	7 Upper Extremities		K Mechanically Assisted	
	8 Rib Cage		L Other Method	
	9 Abdomen			

B: Imaging

Body System–Character 2	Type–Character 3	Meanings–Character 4	Contrast–Character 5	Qualifier–Character 6	Qualifier–Character 7
Ø Central Nervous System	Ø Plain Radiography	See next page	Ø High Osmolar	Ø Unenhanced and Enhanced	Ø Intraoperative
2 Heart	1 Fluoroscopy		1 Low Osmolar	1 Laser	1 Densitometry
3 Upper Arteries	2 Computerized Tomography (CT Scan)		Y Other Contrast	2 Intravascular Optical Coherence	3 Intravascular
4 Lower Arteries	3 Magnetic Resonance Imaging (MRI)		Z None	Z None	4 Transesophageal
5 Veins	4 Ultrasonography				A Guidance
7 Lymphatic System					Z None
8 Eye					
9 Ear, Nose, Mouth and Throat					
B Respiratory System					
D Gastrointestinal System					
F Hepatobiliary System and Pancreas					
G Endocrine System					
H Skin, Subcutaneous Tissue and Breast					
L Connective Tissue					
N Skull and Facial Bones					
P Non-Axial Upper Bones					
Q Non-Axial Lower Bones					
R Axial Skeleton, Except Skull and Facial Bones					
T Urinary System					
U Female Reproductive System					
V Male Reproductive System					
W Anatomical Regions					
Y Fetus and Obstetrical					

B: Imaging

Body Part—Character 4 Meanings

Body System–Character 2		Body Part–Character 4	
Ø	Central Nervous System	Ø	Brain
		7	Cisterna
		8	Cerebral Ventricle(s)
		9	Sella Turcica/Pituitary Gland
		B	Spinal Cord
		C	Acoustic Nerves
2	Heart	Ø	Coronary Artery, Single
		1	Coronary Arteries, Multiple
		2	Coronary Artery Bypass Graft, Single
		3	Coronary Artery Bypass Grafts, Multiple
		4	Heart, Right
		5	Heart, Left
		6	Heart, Right and Left
		7	Internal Mammary Bypass Graft, Right
		8	Internal Mammary Bypass Graft, Left
		B	Heart with Aorta
		C	Pericardium
		D	Pediatric Heart
		F	Bypass Graft, Other
3	Upper Arteries	Ø	Thoracic Aorta
		1	Brachiocephalic-Subclavian Artery, Right
		2	Subclavian Artery, Left
		3	Common Carotid Artery, Right
		4	Common Carotid Artery, Left
		5	Common Carotid Arteries, Bilateral
		6	Internal Carotid Artery, Right
		7	Internal Carotid Artery, Left
		8	Internal Carotid Arteries, Bilateral
		9	External Carotid Artery, Right
		B	External Carotid Artery, Left
		C	External Carotid Arteries, Bilateral
		D	Vertebral Artery, Right
		F	Vertebral Artery, Left
		G	Vertebral Arteries, Bilateral
		H	Upper Extremity Arteries, Right
		J	Upper Extremity Arteries, Left
		K	Upper Extremity Arteries, Bilateral
		L	Intercostal and Bronchial Arteries
		M	Spinal Arteries
		N	Upper Arteries, Other
		P	Thoraco-Abdominal Aorta
		Q	Cervico-Cerebral Arch
		R	Intracranial Arteries
		S	Pulmonary Artery, Right
		T	Pulmonary Artery, Left
		V	Ophthalmic Arteries

Continued on next page

B: Imaging
Body Part—Character 4 Meanings

Continued from previous page

Body System–Character 2	Body Part–Character 4	
4 Lower Arteries	0	Abdominal Aorta
	1	Celiac Artery
	2	Hepatic Artery
	3	Splenic Arteries
	4	Superior Mesenteric Artery
	5	Inferior Mesenteric Artery
	6	Renal Artery, Right
	7	Renal Artery, Left
	8	Renal Arteries, Bilateral
	9	Lumbar Arteries
	B	Intra-Abdominal Arteries, Other
	C	Pelvic Arteries
	D	Aorta and Bilateral Lower Extremity Arteries
	F	Lower Extremity Arteries, Right
	G	Lower Extremity Arteries, Left
	H	Lower Extremity Arteries, Bilateral
	J	Lower Arteries, Other
	K	Celiac and Mesenteric Arteries
	L	Femoral Artery
	M	Renal Artery Transplant
	N	Penile Arteries
5 Veins	0	Epidural Veins
	1	Cerebral and Cerebellar Veins
	2	Intracranial Sinuses
	3	Jugular Veins, Right
	4	Jugular Veins, Left
	5	Jugular Veins, Bilateral
	6	Subclavian Vein, Right
	7	Subclavian Vein, Left
	8	Superior Vena Cava
	9	Inferior Vena Cava
	B	Lower Extremity Veins, Right
	C	Lower Extremity Veins, Left
	D	Lower Extremity Veins, Bilateral
	F	Pelvic (Iliac) Veins, Right
	G	Pelvic (Iliac) Veins, Left
	H	Pelvic (Iliac) Veins, Bilateral
	J	Renal Vein, Right
	K	Renal Vein, Left
	L	Renal Veins, Bilateral
	M	Upper Extremity Veins, Right
	N	Upper Extremity Veins, Left
	P	Upper Extremity Veins, Bilateral
	Q	Pulmonary Vein, Right
	R	Pulmonary Vein, Left
	S	Pulmonary Veins, Bilateral
	T	Portal and Splanchnic Veins
	V	Veins, Other
	W	Dialysis Shunt/Fistula
7 Lymphatic System	0	Abdominal/Retroperitoneal Lymphatics, Unilateral
	1	Abdominal/Retroperitoneal Lymphatics, Bilateral
	4	Lymphatics, Head and Neck
	5	Upper Extremity Lymphatics, Right
	6	Upper Extremity Lymphatics, Left
	7	Upper Extremity Lymphatics, Bilateral
	8	Lower Extremity Lymphatics, Right
	9	Lower Extremity Lymphatics, Left
	B	Lower Extremity Lymphatics, Bilateral
	C	Lymphatics, Pelvic

Continued on next page

B: Imaging

Body Part—Character 4 Meanings

Continued from previous page

Body System–Character 2		Body Part–Character 4	
8	Eye	Ø	Lacrimal Duct, Right
		1	Lacrimal Duct, Left
		2	Lacrimal Ducts, Bilateral
		3	Optic Foramina, Right
		4	Optic Foramina, Left
		5	Eye, Right
		6	Eye, Left
		7	Eyes, Bilateral
9	Ear, Nose, Mouth and Throat	Ø	Ear
		2	Paranasal Sinuses
		4	Parotid Gland, Right
		5	Parotid Gland, Left
		6	Parotid Glands, Bilateral
		7	Submandibular Gland, Right
		8	Submandibular Gland, Left
		9	Submandibular Glands, Bilateral
		B	Salivary Gland, Right
		C	Salivary Gland, Left
		D	Salivary Glands, Bilateral
		F	Nasopharynx/Oropharynx
		G	Pharynx and Epiglottis
		H	Mastoids
		J	Larynx
B	Respiratory System	2	Lung, Right
		3	Lung, Left
		4	Lungs, Bilateral
		6	Diaphragm
		7	Tracheobronchial Tree, Right
		8	Tracheobronchial Tree, Left
		9	Tracheobronchial Trees, Bilateral
		B	Pleura
		C	Mediastinum
		D	Upper Airways
		F	Trachea/Airways
		G	Lung Apices
D	Gastrointestinal System	1	Esophagus
		2	Stomach
		3	Small Bowel
		4	Colon
		5	Upper GI
		6	Upper GI and Small Bowel
		7	Gastrointestinal Tract
		8	Appendix
		9	Duodenum
		B	Mouth/Oropharynx
		C	Rectum
F	Hepatobiliary System and Pancreas	Ø	Bile Ducts
		1	Biliary and Pancreatic Ducts
		2	Gallbladder
		3	Gallbladder and Bile Ducts
		4	Gallbladder, Bile Ducts and Pancreatic Ducts
		5	Liver
		6	Liver and Spleen
		7	Pancreas
		8	Pancreatic Ducts
		C	Hepatobiliary System, All
G	Endocrine System	Ø	Adrenal Gland, Right
		1	Adrenal Gland, Left
		2	Adrenal Glands, Bilateral
		3	Parathyroid Glands
		4	Thyroid Gland

Continued on next page

B: Imaging

Body Part—Character 4 Meanings

Continued from previous page

Body System–Character 2	Body Part–Character 4	
H	Skin, Subcutaneous Tissue and Breast	Ø	Breast, Right
		1	Breast, Left
		2	Breasts, Bilateral
		3	Single Mammary Duct, Right
		4	Single Mammary Duct, Left
		5	Multiple Mammary Ducts, Right
		6	Multiple Mammary Ducts, Left
		7	Extremity, Upper
		8	Extremity, Lower
		9	Abdominal Wall
		B	Chest Wall
		C	Head and Neck
		D	Subcutaneous Tissue, Head/Neck
		F	Subcutaneous Tissue, Upper Extremity
		G	Subcutaneous Tissue, Thorax
		H	Subcutaneous Tissue, Abdomen and Pelvis
		J	Subcutaneous Tissue, Lower Extremity
L	Connective Tissue	Ø	Connective Tissue, Upper Extremity
		1	Connective Tissue, Lower Extremity
		2	Tendons, Upper Extremity
		3	Tendons, Lower Extremity
N	Skull and Facial Bones	Ø	Skull
		1	Orbit, Right
		2	Orbit, Left
		3	Orbits, Bilateral
		4	Nasal Bones
		5	Facial Bones
		6	Mandible
		7	Temporomandibular Joint, Right
		8	Temporomandibular Joint, Left
		9	Temporomandibular Joints, Bilateral
		B	Zygomatic Arch, Right
		C	Zygomatic Arch, Left
		D	Zygomatic Arches, Bilateral
		F	Temporal Bones
		G	Tooth, Single
		H	Teeth, Multiple
		J	Teeth, All
P	Non-Axial Upper Bones	Ø	Sternoclavicular Joint, Right
		1	Sternoclavicular Joint, Left
		2	Sternoclavicular Joints, Bilateral
		3	Acromioclavicular Joints, Bilateral
		4	Clavicle, Right
		5	Clavicle, Left
		6	Scapula, Right
		7	Scapula, Left
		8	Shoulder, Right
		9	Shoulder, Left
		A	Humerus, Right
		B	Humerus, Left
		C	Hand/Finger Joint, Right
		D	Hand/Finger Joint, Left
		E	Upper Arm, Right
		F	Upper Arm, Left
		G	Elbow, Right
		H	Elbow, Left
		J	Forearm, Right
		K	Forearm, Left

Continued on next page

B: Imaging

Body Part—Character 4 Meanings

Continued from previous page

Body System–Character 2	Body Part–Character 4	
P Non-Axial Upper Bones	L	Wrist, Right
	M	Wrist, Left
	N	Hand, Right
	P	Hand, Left
	Q	Hands and Wrists, Bilateral
	R	Finger(s), Right
	S	Finger(s), Left
	T	Upper Extremity, Right
	U	Upper Extremity, Left
	V	Upper Extremities, Bilateral
	W	Thorax
	X	Ribs, Right
	Y	Ribs, Left
Q Non-Axial Lower Bones	Ø	Hip, Right
	1	Hip, Left
	2	Hips, Bilateral
	3	Femur, Right
	4	Femur, Left
	7	Knee, Right
	8	Knee, Left
	9	Knees, Bilateral
	B	Tibia/Fibula, Right
	C	Tibia/Fibula, Left
	D	Lower Leg, Right
	F	Lower Leg, Left
	G	Ankle, Right
	H	Ankle, Left
	J	Calcaneus, Right
	K	Calcaneus, Left
	L	Foot, Right
	M	Foot, Left
	P	Toe(s), Right
	Q	Toe(s), Left
	R	Lower Extremity, Right
	S	Lower Extremity, Left
	V	Patella, Right
	W	Patella, Left
	X	Foot/Toe Joint, Right
	Y	Foot/Toe Joint, Left

Continued on next page

B: Imaging

Body Part—Character 4 Meanings

Continued from previous page

Body System–Character 2	Body Part–Character 4	
R	Axial Skeleton, Except Skull and Facial Bones	Ø	Cervical Spine
		1	Cervical Disc(s)
		2	Thoracic Disc(s)
		3	Lumbar Disc(s)
		4	Cervical Facet Joint(s)
		5	Thoracic Facet Joint(s)
		6	Lumbar Facet Joint(s)
		7	Thoracic Spine
		8	Thoracolumbar Joint
		9	Lumbar Spine
		B	Lumbosacral Joint
		C	Pelvis
		D	Sacroiliac Joints
		F	Sacrum and Coccyx
		G	Whole Spine
		H	Sternum
T	Urinary System	Ø	Bladder
		1	Kidney, Right
		2	Kidney, Left
		3	Kidneys, Bilateral
		4	Kidneys, Ureters and Bladder
		5	Urethra
		6	Ureter, Right
		7	Ureter, Left
		8	Ureters, Bilateral
		9	Kidney Transplant
		B	Bladder and Urethra
		C	Ileal Diversion Loop
		D	Kidney, Ureter and Bladder, Right
		F	Kidney, Ureter and Bladder, Left
		G	Ileal Loop, Ureters and Kidneys
		J	Kidneys and Bladder
U	Female Reproductive System	Ø	Fallopian Tube, Right
		1	Fallopian Tube, Left
		2	Fallopian Tubes, Bilateral
		3	Ovary, Right
		4	Ovary, Left
		5	Ovaries, Bilateral
		6	Uterus
		8	Uterus and Fallopian Tubes
		9	Vagina
		B	Pregnant Uterus
		C	Uterus and Ovaries
V	Male Reproductive System	Ø	Corpora Cavernosa
		1	Epididymis, Right
		2	Epididymis, Left
		3	Prostate
		4	Scrotum
		5	Testicle, Right
		6	Testicle, Left
		7	Testicles, Bilateral
		8	Vasa Vasorum
		9	Prostate and Seminal Vesicles
		B	Penis

Continued on next page

B: Imaging
Body Part—Character 4 Meanings

Continued from previous page

Body System–Character 2	Body Part–Character 4
W Anatomical Regions	Ø Abdomen
	1 Abdomen and Pelvis
	3 Chest
	4 Chest and Abdomen
	5 Chest, Abdomen and Pelvis
	8 Head
	9 Head and Neck
	B Long Bones, All
	C Lower Extremity
	F Neck
	G Pelvic Region
	H Retroperitoneum
	J Upper Extremity
	K Whole Body
	L Whole Skeleton
	M Whole Body, Infant
	P Brachial Plexus
Y Fetus and Obstetrical	Ø Fetal Head
	1 Fetal Heart
	2 Fetal Thorax
	3 Fetal Abdomen
	4 Fetal Spine
	5 Fetal Extremities
	6 Whole Fetus
	7 Fetal Umbilical Cord
	8 Placenta
	9 First Trimester, Single Fetus
	B First Trimester, Multiple Gestation
	C Second Trimester, Single Fetus
	D Second Trimester, Multiple Gestation
	F Third Trimester, Single Fetus
	G Third Trimester, Multiple Gestation

Draft (2011)

C: Nuclear Medicine

Body System– Character 2	Type– Character 3	Meanings– Character 4	Radionuclide– Character 5	Qualifier– Character 6	Qualifier– Character 7
0 Central Nervous System	1 Planar Nuclear Medicine Imaging	See next Page	1 Technetium 99m (Tc-99m)	Z None	Z None
2 Heart	2 Tomographic (Tomo) Nuclear Medicine Imaging		7 Cobalt 58 (Co-58)		
5 Veins	3 Positron Emission Tomographic (PET) Imaging		8 Samarium 153 (Sm-153)		
7 Lymphatic and Hematologic System	4 Nonimaging Nuclear Medicine Uptake		9 Krypton (Kr-81m)		
8 Eye	5 Nonimaging Nuclear Medicine Probe		B Carbon 11 (C-11)		
9 Ear, Nose, Mouth and Throat	6 Nonimaging Nuclear Medicine Assay		C Cobalt 57 (Co-57)		
B Respiratory System	7 Systemic Nuclear Medicine Therapy		D Indium 111 (In-111)		
D Gastrointestinal System			F Iodine 123 (I-123)		
F Hepatobiliary System and Pancreas			G Iodine 131 (I-131)		
G Endocrine System			H Iodine 125 (I-125)		
H Skin, Subcutaneous Tissue and Breast			K Fluorine 18 (F-18)		
P Musculoskeletal System			L Gallium 67 (Ga-67)		
T Urinary System			M Oxygen 15 (O-15)		
V Male Reproductive System			N Phosphorus 32 (P-32)		
W Anatomical Regions			P Strontium 89 (Sr-89)		
			Q Rubidium 82 (Rb-82)		
			R Nitrogen 13 (N-13)		
			S Thallium 201 (Tl-201)		
			T Xenon 127 (Xe-127)		
			V Xenon 133 (Xe-133)		
			W Chromium (Cr-51)		
			Y Other Radionuclide		
			Z None		

C: Nuclear Medicine

Body Part—Character 4 Meanings

Body System–Character 2		Body Part–Character 4	
Ø	Central Nervous System	Ø	Brain
		5	Cerebrospinal Fluid
		Y	Central Nervous System
2	Heart	6	Heart, Right and Left
		G	Myocardium
		Y	Heart
5	Veins	B	Lower Extremity Veins, Right
		C	Lower Extremity Veins, Left
		D	Lower Extremity Veins, Bilateral
		N	Upper Extremity Veins, Right
		P	Upper Extremity Veins, Left
		Q	Upper Extremity Veins, Bilateral
		R	Central Veins
		Y	Veins
7	Lymphatic and Hematologic System	Ø	Bone Marrow
		2	Spleen
		3	Blood
		5	Lymphatics, Head and Neck
		D	Lymphatics, Pelvic
		J	Lymphatics, Head
		K	Lymphatics, Neck
		L	Lymphatics, Upper Chest
		M	Lymphatics, Trunk
		N	Lymphatics, Upper Extremity
		P	Lymphatics, Lower Extremity
		Y	Lymphatic and Hematologic System
8	Eye	9	Lacrimal Ducts, Bilateral
		Y	Eye
9	Ear, Nose, Mouth and Throat	B	Salivary Glands, Bilateral
		Y	Ear, Nose, Mouth and Throat
B	Respiratory System	2	Lungs and Bronchi
		Y	Respiratory System
D	Gastrointestinal System	5	Upper Gastrointestinal Tract
		7	Gastrointestinal Tract
		Y	Digestive System
F	Hepatobiliary System and Pancreas	4	Gallbladder
		5	Liver
		6	Liver and Spleen
		C	Hepatobiliary System, All
		Y	Hepatobiliary System and Pancreas
G	Endocrine System	1	Parathyroid Glands
		2	Thyroid Gland
		4	Adrenal Glands, Bilateral
		Y	Endocrine System
H	Skin, Subcutaneous Tissue and Breast	Ø	Breast, Right
		1	Breast, Left
		2	Breasts, Bilateral
		Y	Skin, Subcutaneous Tissue and Breast

Continued on next page

C: Nuclear Medicine

Body Part—Character 4 Meanings

Continued from previous page

Body System–Character 2	Body Part–Character 4
P Musculoskeletal System	1 Skull
	2 Cervical Spine
	3 Skull and Cervical Spine
	4 Thorax
	5 Spine
	6 Pelvis
	7 Spine and Pelvis
	8 Upper Extremity, Right
	9 Upper Extremity, Left
	B Upper Extremities, Bilateral
	C Lower Extremity, Right
	D Lower Extremity, Left
	F Lower Extremities, Bilateral
	G Thoracic Spine
	H Lumbar Spine
	J Thoracolumbar Spine
	N Upper Extremities
	P Lower Extremities
	Y Musculoskeletal System, Other
	Z Musculoskeletal System, All
T Urinary System	3 Kidneys, Ureters and Bladder
	H Bladder and Ureters
	Y Urinary System
V Male Reproductive System	9 Testicles, Bilateral
	Y Male Reproductive System
W Anatomical Regions	Ø Abdomen
	1 Abdomen and Pelvis
	3 Chest
	4 Chest and Abdomen
	6 Chest and Neck
	B Head and Neck
	D Lower Extremity
	G Thyroid
	J Pelvic Region
	M Upper Extremity
	N Whole Body
	Y Anatomical Regions, Multiple
	Z Anatomical Region, Other

D: Radiation Oncology

Body System– Character 2		Modality– Character 3		Meanings– Character 4	Modality–Qualifier Character 5		Isotope– Character 6		Qualifier– Character 7	
Ø	Central and Peripheral Nervous System	Ø	Beam Radiation	See next Page	Ø	Photons <1 MeV	7	Cesium 137 (Cs-137)	Ø	Intraoperative
7	Lymphatic and Hematologic System	1	Brachytherapy		1	Photons 1 - 1Ø MeV	8	Iridium 192 (Ir-192)	Z	None
8	Eye	2	Stereotactic Radiosurgery		2	Photons >1Ø MeV	9	Iodine 125 (I-125)		
9	Ear, Nose, Mouth and Throat	Y	Other Radiation		3	Electrons	B	Palladium 1Ø3 (Pd-1Ø3)		
B	Respiratory System				4	Heavy Particles (Protons, Ions)	C	Californium 252 (Cf-252)		
D	Gastrointestinal System				5	Neutrons	D	Iodine 131 (I-131)		
F	Hepatobiliary System and Pancreas				6	Neutron Capture	F	Phosphorus 32 (P-32)		
G	Endocrine System				7	Contact Radiation	G	Strontium 89 (Sr-89)		
H	Skin				8	Hyperthermia	H	Strontium 9Ø (Sr-9Ø)		
M	Breast				9	High Dose Rate (HDR)	Y	Other Isotope		
P	Musculoskeletal System				B	Low Dose Rate (LDR)	Z	None		
T	Urinary System				C	Intraoperative Radiation Therapy (IORT)				
U	Female Reproductive System				D	Stereotactic Other Photon Radiosurgery				
V	Male Reproductive System				F	Plaque Radiation				
W	Anatomical Regions				G	Isotope Administration				
					H	Stereotactic Particulate Radiosurgery				
					J	Stereotactic Gamma Beam Radiosurgery				
					K	Laser Interstitial Thermal Therapy				

        Draft (2011)

D. Radiation Oncology

Treatment Site—Character 4 Meanings

Body System–Character 2		Treatment Site–Character 4	
Ø	Central and Peripheral Nervous System	Ø	Brain
		1	Brain Stem
		6	Spinal Cord
		7	Peripheral Nerve
7	Lymphatic and Hematologic System	Ø	Bone Marrow
		1	Thymus
		2	Spleen
		3	Lymphatics, Neck
		4	Lymphatics, Axillary
		5	Lymphatics, Thorax
		6	Lymphatics, Abdomen
		7	Lymphatics, Pelvis
		8	Lymphatics, Inguinal
8	Eye	Ø	Eye
9	Ear, Nose, Mouth and Throat	Ø	Ear
		1	Nose
		3	Hypopharynx
		4	Mouth
		5	Tongue
		6	Salivary Glands
		7	Sinuses
		8	Hard Palate
		9	Soft Palate
		B	Larynx
		C	Pharynx
		D	Nasopharynx
		F	Oropharynx
B	Respiratory System	Ø	Trachea
		1	Bronchus
		2	Lung
		5	Pleura
		6	Mediastinum
		7	Chest Wall
		8	Diaphragm
D	Gastrointestinal System	Ø	Esophagus
		1	Stomach
		2	Duodenum
		3	Jejunum
		4	Ileum
		5	Colon
		7	Rectum
		8	Anus
F	Hepatobiliary System and Pancreas	Ø	Liver
		1	Gallbladder
		2	Bile Ducts
		3	Pancreas
G	Endocrine System	Ø	Pituitary Gland
		1	Pineal Body
		2	Adrenal Glands
		4	Parathyroid Glands
		5	Thyroid

Continued on next page

D. Radiation Oncology

Treatment Site—Character 4 Meanings

Continued from previous page

Body System–Character 2		Treatment Site–Character 4	
H	Skin	2	Skin, Face
		3	Skin, Neck
		4	Skin, Arm
		5	Skin, Hand
		6	Skin, Chest
		7	Skin, Back
		8	Skin, Abdomen
		9	Skin, Buttock
		B	Skin, Leg
		C	Skin, Foot
M	Breast	Ø	Breast, Left
		1	Breast, Right
P	Musculoskeletal System	Ø	Skull
		2	Maxilla
		3	Mandible
		4	Sternum
		5	Rib(s)
		6	Humerus
		7	Radius/Ulna
		8	Pelvic Bones
		9	Femur
		B	Tibia/Fibula
		C	Other Bone
T	Urinary System	Ø	Kidney
		1	Ureter
		2	Bladder
		3	Urethra
U	Female Reproductive System	Ø	Ovary
		1	Cervix
		2	Uterus
V	Male Reproductive System	Ø	Prostate
		1	Testis
W	Anatomical Regions	1	Head and Neck
		2	Chest
		3	Abdomen
		4	Hemibody
		5	Whole Body
		6	Pelvic Region

F: Physical Rehabilitation and Diagnostic Audiology
Ø: Rehabilitation

See next page for Character 5 Meanings

Type–Character 3		Body System–Body Region–Character 4		Equipment –Character 6		Qualifier–Character 7	
Ø	Speech Assessment	Ø	Neurological System - Head and Neck	1	Audiometer	Z	None
1	Motor and/or Nerve Function Assessment	1	Neurological System - Upper Back / Upper Extremity	2	Sound Field / Booth		
2	Activities of Daily Living Assessment	2	Neurological System - Lower Back / Lower Extremity	4	Electroacoustic Immitance / Acoustic Reflex		
6	Speech Treatment	3	Neurological System - Whole Body	5	Hearing Aid Selection / Fitting / Test		
7	Motor Treatment	4	Circulatory System - Head and Neck	7	Electrophysiologic		
8	Activities of Daily Living Treatment	5	Circulatory System - Upper Back / Upper Extremity	8	Vestibular / Balance		
9	Hearing Treatment	6	Circulatory System - Lower Back / Lower Extremity	9	Cochlear Implant		
B	Cochlear Implant Treatment	7	Circulatory System - Whole Body	B	Physical Agents		
C	Vestibular Treatment	8	Respiratory System - Head and Neck	C	Mechanical		
D	Device Fitting	9	Respiratory System - Upper Back / Upper Extremity	D	Electrotherapeutic		
F	Caregiver Training	B	Respiratory System - Lower Back / Lower Extremity	E	Orthosis		
		C	Respiratory System - Whole Body	F	Assistive, Adaptive, Supportive or Protective		
		D	Integumentary System - Head and Neck	G	Aerobic Endurance and Conditioning		
		F	Integumentary System - Upper Back / Upper Extremity	H	Mechanical or Electromechanical		
		G	Integumentary System - Lower Back / Lower Extremity	J	Somatosensory		
		H	Integumentary System - Whole Body	K	Audiovisual		
		J	Musculoskeletal System - Head and Neck	L	Assistive Listening		
		K	Musculoskeletal System - Upper Back / Upper Extremity	M	Augmentative / Alternative Communication		
		L	Musculoskeletal System - Lower Back / Lower Extremity	N	Biosensory Feedback		
		M	Musculoskeletal System - Whole Body	P	Computer		
		N	Genitourinary System	Q	Speech Analysis		
		Z	None	S	Voice Analysis		
				T	Aerodynamic Function		
				U	Prosthesis		
				V	Speech Prosthesis		
				W	Swallowing		
				X	Cerumen Management		
				Y	Other Equipment		
				Z	None		

F: Physical Rehabilitation and Diagnostic Audiology

0: Rehabilitation

Type Qualifier—Character 5 Meanings

Type–Character 3	Type Qualifier–Character 5
Ø Speech Assessment	Ø Filtered Speech
	1 Speech Threshold
	2 Speech/Word Recognition
	3 Staggered Spondaic Word
	4 Sensorineural Acuity Level
	5 Synthetic Sentence Identification
	6 Speech and/or Language Screening
	7 Nonspoken Language
	8 Receptive/Expressive Language
	9 Articulation/Phonology
	B Motor Speech
	C Aphasia
	D Fluency
	F Voice
	G Communicative/Cognitive Integration Skills
	H Bedside Swallowing and Oral Function
	J Instrumental Swallowing and Oral Function
	K Orofacial Myofunctional
	L Augmentative/Alternative Communication System
	M Voice Prosthetic
	N Non-invasive Instrumental Status
	P Oral Peripheral Mechanism
	Q Performance Intensity Phonetically Balanced Speech Discrimination
	R Brief Tone Stimuli
	S Distorted Speech
	T Dichotic Stimuli
	V Temporal Ordering of Stimuli
	W Masking Patterns
	X Other Specified Central Auditory Processing
1 Motor and/or Nerve Function Assessment	Ø Muscle Performance
	1 Integumentary Integrity
	2 Visual Motor Integration
	3 Coordination/Dexterity
	4 Motor Function
	5 Range of Motion and Joint Integrity
	6 Sensory Awareness/Processing/Integrity
	7 Facial Nerve Function
	8 Neurophysiologic Intraoperative
	9 Somatosensory Evoked Potentials
	B Bed Mobility
	C Transfer
	D Gait and/or Balance
	F Wheelchair Mobility
	G Reflex Integrity
2 Activities of Daily Living Assessment	Ø Bathing/Showering
	1 Dressing
	2 Feeding/Eating
	3 Grooming/Personal Hygiene
	4 Home Management
	5 Perceptual Processing
	6 Psychosocial Skills
	7 Aerobic Capacity and Endurance
	8 Anthropometric Characteristics
	9 Cranial Nerve Integrity
	B Environmental, Home and Work Barriers
	C Ergonomics and Body Mechanics
	D Neuromotor Development
	F Pain
	G Ventilation, Respiration and Circulation
	H Vocational Activities and Functional Community or Work Reintegration Skills

Continued on next page

Draft (2011)

F: Physical Rehabilitation and Diagnostic Audiology
0: Rehabilitation
Type Qualifier—Character 5 Meanings   *Continued from previous page*

Type–Character 3	Type Qualifier–Character 5
6 Speech Treatment	Ø Nonspoken Language 1 Speech-Language Pathology and Related Disorders Counseling 2 Speech-Language Pathology and Related Disorders Prevention 3 Aphasia 4 Articulation/Phonology 5 Aural Rehabilitation 6 Communicative/Cognitive Integration Skills 7 Fluency 8 Motor Speech 9 Orofacial Myofunctional B Receptive/Expressive Language C Voice D Swallowing Dysfunction
7 Motor Treatment	Ø Range of Motion and Joint Mobility 1 Muscle Performance 2 Coordination/Dexterity 3 Motor Function 4 Wheelchair Mobility 5 Bed Mobility 6 Therapeutic Exercise 7 Manual Therapy Techniques 8 Transfer Training 9 Gait Training/Functional Ambulation
8 Activities of Daily Living Treatment	Ø Bathing/Showering Techniques 1 Dressing Techniques 2 Grooming/Personal Hygiene 3 Feeding/Eating 4 Home Management 5 Wound Management 6 Psychosocial Skills 7 Vocational Activities and Functional Community or Work Reintegration Skills
9 Hearing Treatment	Ø Hearing and Related Disorders Counseling 1 Hearing and Related Disorders Prevention 2 Auditory Processing 3 Cerumen Management
B Cochlear Implant Treatment	Ø Cochlear Implant Rehabilitation
C Vestibular Treatment	Ø Vestibular 1 Perceptual Processing 2 Visual Motor Integration 3 Postural Control
D Device Fitting	Ø Tinnitus Masker 1 Monaural Hearing Aid 2 Binaural Hearing Aid 3 Augmentative/Alternative Communication System 4 Voice Prosthetic 5 Assistive Listening Device 6 Dynamic Orthosis 7 Static Orthosis 8 Prosthesis 9 Assistive, Adaptive, Supportive or Protective Devices

Continued on next page

F: Physical Rehabilitation and Diagnostic Audiology

0: Rehabilitation

Type Qualifier—Character 5 Meanings

Continued from previous page

Type–Character 3	Type Qualifier–Character 5
F Caregiver Training	Ø Bathing/Showering Technique 1 Dressing 2 Feeding and Eating 3 Grooming/Personal Hygiene 4 Bed Mobility 5 Transfer 6 Wheelchair Mobility 7 Therapeutic Exercise 8 Airway Clearance Techniques 9 Wound Management B Vocational Activities and Functional Community or Work Reintegration Skills C Gait Training/Functional Ambulation D Application, Proper Use and Care of Assistive, Adaptive, Supportive or Protective Devices F Application, Proper Use and Care of Orthoses G Application, Proper Use and Care of Prosthesis H Home Management J Communication Skills

F: Physical Rehabilitation and Diagnostic Audiology

1: Diagnostic Audiology

Type–Character 3	Body System–Body Region–Character 4	Meanings–Character 5	Equipment–Character 6	Qualifer–Character 7
3 Hearing Assessment 4 Hearing Aid Assessment 5 Vestibular Assessment	Z None	See next page	Ø Occupational Hearing 1 Audiometer 2 Sound Field / Booth 3 Tympanometer 4 Electroacoustic Immitance / Acoustic Reflex 5 Hearing Aid Selection / Fitting / Test 6 Otoacoustic Emission (OAE) 7 Electrophysiologic 8 Vestibular / Balance 9 Cochlear Implant K Audiovisual L Assistive Listening P Computer Y Other Equipment Z None	Z None

F: Physical Rehabilitation and Diagnostic Audiology

1: Diagnostic Audiology

Type Qualifier—Character 5 Meanings

Type–Character 3	Type Qualifier–Character 5
3 Hearing Assessment	Ø Hearing Screening 1 Pure Tone Audiometry, Air 2 Pure Tone Audiometry, Air and Bone 3 Bekesy Audiometry 4 Conditioned Play Audiometry 5 Select Picture Audiometry 6 Visual Reinforcement Audiometry 7 Alternate Binaural or Monaural Loudness Balance 8 Tone Decay 9 Short Increment Sensitivity Index B Stenger C Pure Tone Stenger D Tympanometry F Eustachian Tube Function G Acoustic Reflex Patterns H Acoustic Reflex Threshold J Acoustic Reflex Decay K Electrocochleography L Auditory Evoked Potentials M Evoked Otoacoustic Emissions, Screening N Evoked Otoacoustic Emissions, Diagnostic P Aural Rehabilitation Status Q Auditory Processing
4 Hearing Aid Assessment	Ø Cochlear Implant 1 Ear Canal Probe Microphone 2 Monaural Hearing Aid 3 Binaural Hearing Aid 4 Assistive Listening System/Device Selection 5 Sensory Aids 6 Binaural Electroacoustic Hearing Aid Check 7 Ear Protector Attentuation 8 Monaural Electroacoustic Hearing Aid Check
5 Vestibular Assessment	Ø Bithermal, Bionaural Caloric Irrigation 1 Bithermal, Monaural Caloric Irrigation 2 Unithermal Binaural Screen 3 Oscillating Tracking 4 Sinusoidal Vertical Axis Rotational 5 Dix-Hallpike Dynamic 6 Computerized Dynamic Posturography 7 Tinnitus Masker

G: Mental Health

Z: Body System—None

Type–Character 3	Type Qualifier –Character 4	Qualifier–Character 5	Qualifier–Character 6	Qualifier–Character 7
1 Psychological Tests	Ø Developmental	Z None	Z None	Z None
	1 Personality and Behavioral			
	2 Intellectual and Psychoeducational			
	3 Neuropsychological			
	4 Neurobehavioral and Cognitive Status			
2 Crisis Intervention	Z None			
3 Medication Management	Z None			
5 Individual Psychotherapy	Ø Interactive			
	1 Behavioral			
	2 Cognitive			
	3 Interpersonal			
	4 Psychoanalysis			
	5 Psychodynamic			
	6 Supportive			
	8 Cognitive-Behavioral			
	9 Psychophysiological			
6 Counseling	Ø Educational			
	1 Vocational			
	3 Other Counseling			
7 Family Psychotherapy	2 Other Family Psychotherapy			
B Electroconvulsive Therapy	Ø Unilateral-Single Seizure			
	1 Unilateral-Multiple Seizure			
	2 Bilateral-Single Seizure			
	3 Bilateral-Multiple Seizure			
	4 Other Electroconvulsive Therapy			
C Biofeedback	9 Other Biofeedback			
F Hypnosis	Z None			
G Narcosynthesis	Z None			
H Group Psychotherapy	Z None			
J Light Therapy	Z None			

H: Substance Abuse Treatment

Z: Body System—None

Type–Character 3	Type Qualifier–Character 4	Qualifier–Character 5	Qualifier–Character 6	Qualifier–Character 7
2 Detoxification Services	Z None	Z None	Z None	Z None
3 Individual Counseling	Ø Cognitive 1 Behavioral 2 Cognitive-Behavioral 3 12-Step 4 Interpersonal 5 Vocational 6 Psychoeducation 7 Motivational Enhancement 8 Confrontational 9 Continuing Care B Spiritual C Pre/Post-Test Infectious Disease			
4 Group Counseling	Ø Cognitive 1 Behavioral 2 Cognitive-Behavioral 3 12-Step 4 Interpersonal 5 Vocational 6 Psychoeducation 7 Motivational Enhancement 8 Confrontational 9 Continuing Care B Spiritual C Pre/Post-Test Infectious Disease			
5 Individual Psychotherapy	Ø Cognitive 1 Behavioral 2 Cognitive-Behavioral 3 12-Step 4 Interpersonal 5 Interactive 6 Psychoeducation 7 Motivational Enhancement 8 Confrontational 9 Supportive B Psychoanalysis C Psychodynamic D Psychophysiological			
6 Family Counseling	3 Other Family Counseling			
8 Medication Management	Ø Nicotine Replacement 1 Methadone Maintenance 2 Levo-alpha-acetyl-methadol (LAAM) 3 Antabuse 4 Naltrexone 5 Naloxone 6 Clonidine 7 Bupropion 8 Psychiatric Medication 9 Other Replacement Medication			
9 Pharmacotherapy	Ø Nicotine Replacement 1 Methadone Maintenance 2 Levo-alpha-acetyl-methadol (LAAM) 3 Antabuse 4 Naltrexone 5 Naloxone 6 Clonidine 7 Bupropion 8 Psychiatric Medication 9 Other Replacement Medication			

Appendix G: Answers to Coding Exercises

Medical Surgical Section

Procedure	Code
Excision of malignant melanoma from skin of right ear	0HB2XZZ
Laparoscopy with excision of endometrial implant from left ovary	0UB14ZZ
Percutaneous needle core biopsy of right kidney	0TB03ZX
EGD with gastric biopsy	0DB68ZX
Open endarterectomy of left common carotid artery	03BJ0ZZ
Excision of basal cell carcinoma of lower lip	0CB1XZZ
Open excision of tail of pancreas	0FBG0ZZ
Percutaneous biopsy of right gastrocnemius muscle	0KBS3ZX
Sigmoidoscopy with sigmoid polypectomy	0DBN8ZZ
Open excision of lesion from right Achilles tendon	0LBN0ZZ
Open resection of cecum	0DTH0ZZ
Total excision of pituitary gland, open	0GT00ZZ
Explantation of left failed kidney, open	0TT10ZZ
Open left axillary total lymphadenectomy	07T60ZZ (*Resection* is coded for cutting out a chain of lymph nodes.)
Laparoscopic-assisted total vaginal hysterectomy	0UT9FZZ
Right total mastectomy, open	0HTT0ZZ
Open resection of papillary muscle	02TD0ZZ (The papillary muscle refers to the heart and is found in the *Heart and Great Vessels* body system.)
Radical retropubic prostatectomy, open	0VT00ZZ
Laparoscopic cholecystectomy	0FT44ZZ
Endoscopic bilateral total maxillary sinusectomy	09TQ4ZZ, 09TR4ZZ
Amputation at right elbow level	0X6B0ZZ
Right below-knee amputation, proximal tibia/fibula	0Y6H0Z1 (The qualifier *High* here means the portion of the tib/fib closest to the knee.)
Fifth ray carpometacarpal joint amputation, left hand	0X6K0Z8 (A *complete* ray amputation is through the carpometacarpal joint.)
Right leg and hip amputation through ischium	0Y620ZZ (The *Hindquarter* body part includes amputation along any part of the hip bone.)

Procedure	Code
DIP joint amputation of right thumb	0X6L0Z3 (The qualifier *low* here means through the distal interphalangeal joint.)
Right wrist joint amputation	0X6J0Z0 (Amputation at the wrist joint is actually complete amputation of the hand.)
Trans-metatarsal amputation of foot at left big toe	0Y6N0Z9 (A *partial* amputation is through the shaft of the metatarsal bone.)
Mid-shaft amputation, right humerus	0X680Z2
Left fourth toe amputation, mid-proximal phalanx	0Y6W0Z1 (The qualifier *High* here means anywhere along the proximal phalanx.)
Right above-knee amputation, distal femur	0Y6C0Z3
Cryotherapy of wart on left hand	0H5GXZZ
Percutaneous radiofrequency ablation of right vocal cord lesion	0C5T3ZZ
Left heart catheterization with laser destruction of arrhythmogenic focus, A-V node	02583ZZ
Cautery of nosebleed	095KXZZ
Transurethral endoscopic laser ablation of prostate	0V508ZZ
Cautery of oozing varicose vein, left calf	065Y3ZZ (The approach is coded *Percutaneous* because that is the normal route to a vein. No mention is made of approach, because likely the skin has eroded at that spot.)
Laparoscopy with destruction of endometriosis, bilateral ovaries	0U524ZZ
Laser coagulation of right retinal vessel hemorrhage, percutaneous	085G3ZZ (The *Retinal Vessel* body-part values are in the *Eye* body system.)
Talc injection pleurodesis, left side	0B5P3ZZ (See section 3, *Administration*, for applicable injection code.)
Sclerotherapy of brachial plexus lesion, alcohol injection	01533ZZ (See section 3, *Administration*, for applicable injection code.)
Forceps total mouth extraction, upper and lower teeth	0CDWXZ2, 0CDXXZ2

Procedure	Code
Removal of left thumbnail	ØHDQXZZ (No separate body-part value is given for thumbnail, so this is coded to *Fingernail*.)
Extraction of right intraocular lens without replacement, percutaneous	Ø8DJ3ZZ
Laparoscopy with needle aspiration of ova for in vitro fertilization	ØUDN4ZZ
Nonexcisional debridement of skin ulcer, right foot	ØHDMXZZ
Open stripping of abdominal fascia, right side	ØJD80ZZ
Hysteroscopy with D&C, diagnostic	ØUDB8ZX
Liposuction for medical purposes, left upper arm	ØJDF3ZZ (The *Percutaneous* approach is inherent in the liposuction technique.)
Removal of tattered right ear drum fragments with tweezers	Ø9D77ZZ
Microincisional phlebectomy of spider veins, right lower leg	Ø6DY3ZZ
Routine Foley catheter placement	ØT9B70Z
Incision and drainage of external perianal abscess	ØD9QXZZ
Percutaneous drainage of ascites	ØW9G3ZZ (This is drainage of the cavity and not the peritoneal membrane itself.)
Laparoscopy with left ovarian cystotomy and drainage	ØU914ZZ
Laparotomy with hepatotomy and drain placement for liver abscess, right lobe	ØF9100Z
Right knee arthrotomy with drain placement	ØS9C00Z
Thoracentesis of left pleural effusion	ØW9B3ZZ This is drainage of the pleural cavity
Phlebotomy of left median cubital vein for polycythemia vera	Ø59F3ZZ This median cubital vein is a branch of the cephalic vein
Percutaneous chest tube placement for right pneumothorax	ØW9930Z
Endoscopic drainage of left ethmoid sinus	Ø99V4ZZ
Removal of foreign body, right cornea	Ø8C8XZZ
Percutaneous mechanical thrombectomy, left brachial artery	Ø3C83ZZ
Esophagogastroscopy with removal of bezoar from stomach	ØDC68ZZ
Foreign body removal, skin of left thumb	ØHCGXZZ (There is no specific value for thumb skin, so the procedure is coded to *Hand*.)
Transurethral cystoscopy with removal of bladder stone	ØTCB8ZZ
Forceps removal of foreign body in right nostril	Ø9CKXZZ (Nostril is coded to the *Nose* body-part value.)
Laparoscopy with excision of old suture from mesentery	ØDCV4ZZ

Procedure	Code
Incision and removal of right lacrimal duct stone	Ø8CX0ZZ
Nonincisional removal of intraluminal foreign body from vagina	ØUCG7ZZ (The approach *External* is also a possibility. It is assumed here that since the patient went to the doctor to have the object removed, that it was not in the vaginal orifice.)
Open excision of retained sliver, subcutaneous tissue of left foot	ØJCR0ZZ
Extracorporeal shockwave lithotripsy (ESWL), bilateral ureters	ØTF6XZZ, ØTF7XZZ (The *Bilateral Ureter* body-part value is not available for the root operation *Fragmentation,* so the procedures are coded separately.)
Endoscopic Retrograde Cholangiopancreatography (ERCP) with lithotripsy of common bile duct stone	ØFF98ZZ (ERCP is performed through the mouth to the biliary system via the duodenum, so the approach value is *Via Natural or Artificial Opening Endoscopic*.)
Thoracotomy with crushing of pericardial calcifications	Ø2FN0ZZ
Transurethral cystoscopy with fragmentation of bladder calculus	ØTFB8ZZ
Hysteroscopy with intraluminal lithotripsy of left fallopian tube calcification	ØUF68ZZ
Division of right foot tendon, percutaneous	ØL8V3ZZ
Left heart catheterization with division of bundle of HIS	Ø2883ZZ
Open osteotomy of capitate, left hand	ØP8N0ZZ (The capitate is one of the carpal bones of the hand.)
EGD with esophagotomy of esophagogastric junction	ØD848ZZ
Sacral rhizotomy for pain control, percutaneous	Ø18R3ZZ
Laparotomy with exploration and adhesiolysis of right ureter	ØTN60ZZ
Incision of scar contracture, right elbow	ØHNDXZZ (The skin of the elbow region is coded to *Lower Arm*.)
Frenulotomy for treatment of tongue-tie syndrome	ØCN7XZZ (The frenulum is coded to the body-part value *Tongue*.)
Right shoulder arthroscopy with coracoacromial ligament release	ØMN14ZZ
Mitral valvulotomy for release of fused leaflets, open approach	Ø2NG0ZZ
Percutaneous left Achilles tendon release	ØLNP3ZZ
Laparoscopy with lysis of peritoneal adhesions	ØDNW4ZZ

Draft (2011)

Procedure	Code
Manual rupture of right shoulder joint adhesions under general anesthesia	ØRNJXZZ
Open posterior tarsal tunnel release	Ø1NGØZZ (The nerve released in the posterior tarsal tunnel is the tibial nerve.)
Laparoscopy with freeing of left ovary and fallopian tube	ØUN14ZZ, ØUN64ZZ
Liver transplant with donor matched liver	ØFYØØZØ
Orthotopic heart transplant using porcine heart	Ø2YAØZ2 (The donor heart comes from an animal [pig], so the qualifier value is *Zooplastic.*)
Right lung transplant, open, using organ donor match	ØBYKØZØ
Left kidney/pancreas organ bank transplant	ØFYGØZØ, ØTY1ØZØ
Replantation of avulsed scalp	ØHMØXZZ
Reattachment of severed right ear	Ø9MØXZZ
Reattachment of traumatic left gastrocnemius avulsion, open	ØKMTØZZ
Closed replantation of three avulsed teeth, lower jaw	ØCMXXZ1
Reattachment of severed left hand	ØXMKØZZ
Right hand open palmaris longus tendon transfer	ØLX7ØZZ
Endoscopic radial to median nerve transfer	Ø1X64Z5
Fasciocutaneous flap closure of left thigh, open	ØJXMØZC (The qualifier identifies the body layers in addition to fascia included in the procedure.)
Transfer left index finger to left thumb position, open	ØXXPØZM
Percutaneous fascia transfer to fill defect, anterior neck	ØJX43ZZ
Trigeminal to facial nerve transfer, percutaneous endoscopic	ØØXK4ZM
Endoscopic left leg flexor hallucis longus tendon transfer	ØLXP4ZZ
Right scalp advancement flap to right temple	ØHXØXZZ
Bilateral TRAM pedicle flap reconstruction status post mastectomy, muscle only, open	ØKXKØZ6, ØKXLØZ6 (The transverse rectus abdominus muscle (TRAM) flap is coded for each flap developed.)
Skin transfer flap closure of complex open wound, left lower back	ØHX6XZZ
Open fracture reduction, right tibia	ØQSGØZZ
Laparoscopy with gastropexy for malrotation	ØDS64ZZ
Left knee arthroscopy with reposition of anterior cruciate ligament	ØMSP4ZZ
Open transposition of ulnar nerve	Ø1S4ØZZ
Closed reduction with percutaneous internal fixation of right femoral neck fracture	ØQS634Z
Trans-vaginal intraluminal cervical cerclage	ØUVC7DZ
Cervical cerclage using Shirodkar technique	ØUVC7ZZ

Procedure	Code
Thoracotomy with banding of left pulmonary artery using extraluminal device	Ø2VRØCZ
Restriction of thoracic duct with intraluminal stent, percutaneous	Ø7VK3DZ
Craniotomy with clipping of cerebral aneurysm	Ø3VGØCZ (The clip is placed lengthwise on the outside wall of the widened portion of the vessel.)
Nonincisional, trans-nasal placement of restrictive stent in right lacrimal duct	Ø8VX7DZ
Percutaneous ligation of esophageal vein	Ø6L33ZZ
Percutaneous embolization of left internal carotid-cavernous fistula	Ø3LL3DZ
Laparoscopy with bilateral occlusion of fallopian tubes using Hulka extraluminal clips	ØUL74CZ
Open suture ligation of failed AV graft, left brachial artery	Ø3L8ØZZ
Percutaneous embolization of vascular supply, intracranial meningioma	Ø3LG3DZ
ERCP with balloon dilation of common bile duct	ØF798ZZ
PTCA of two coronary arteries, LAD with stent placement, RCA with no stent	Ø27Ø3DZ, Ø27Ø3ZZ (A separate procedure is coded for each artery dilated, since the device value differs for each artery.)
Cystoscopy with intraluminal dilation of bladder neck stricture	ØT7C8ZZ
Open dilation of old anastomosis, left femoral artery	Ø47LØZZ
Dilation of upper esophageal stricture, direct visualization, with Bougie sound	ØD717ZZ
PTA of right brachial artery stenosis	Ø3773ZZ
Transnasal dilation and stent placement in right lacrimal duct	Ø87X7DZ
Hysteroscopy with balloon dilation of bilateral fallopian tubes	ØU778ZZ
Tracheoscopy with intraluminal dilation of tracheal stenosis	ØB718ZZ
Cystoscopy with dilation of left ureteral stricture, with stent placement	ØT778DZ
Open gastric bypass with Roux-en-Y limb to jejunum	ØD16ØZA
Right temporal artery to intracranial artery bypass using Gore-Tex graft, open	Ø31SØJG
Tracheostomy formation with tracheostomy tube placement, percutaneous	ØB113F4
PICVA (percutaneous in situ coronary venous arterialization) of single coronary artery	Ø21Ø3D4
Open left femoral-popliteal artery bypass using cadaver vein graft	Ø41LØKL
Shunting of intrathecal cerebrospinal fluid to peritoneal cavity using synthetic shunt	ØØ16ØJ6
Colostomy formation, open, transverse colon to abdominal wall	ØD1LØZ4
Open urinary diversion, left ureter, using ileal conduit to skin	ØT17ØZC

Procedure	Code	Procedure	Code
CABG of LAD using left internal mammary artery, open off-bypass	0210029	Percutaneous phacoemulsification of right eye cataract with prosthetic lens insertion	08RJ3JZ
Open pleuroperitoneal shunt, right pleural cavity, using synthetic device	0W190JG	Aortic valve annuloplasty using ring, open	02UF07Z
End-of-life replacement of spinal neurostimulator generator, dual array, in lower abdomen	0JH80M7 Taking out of the old generator is coded separately to the root operation REMOVAL.	Laparoscopic repair of left inguinal hernia with marlex plug	0YU64JZ
		Autograft nerve graft to right median nerve, percutaneous endoscopic (do not code graft harvest for this exercise)	01U547Z
Percutaneous insertion of spinal neurostimulator lead, lumbar spinal cord	00HV3MZ	Exchange of liner in femoral component of previous left hip replacement, open approach	0SUB09Z
Percutaneous placement of broken pacemaker lead in left atrium	02H73MZ	Anterior colporrhaphy with polypropylene mesh reinforcement, open approach	0UUG0JZ
Open placement of dual chamber pacemaker generator in chest wall	0JH60P2	Implantation of CorCap cardiac support device, open approach	02UA0JZ
Percutaneous placement of venous central line in right internal jugular	05HM33Z	Abdominal wall herniorrhaphy, open, using synthetic mesh	0WUF0JZ
Open insertion of multiple channel cochlear implant, left ear	09HE0S3	Tendon graft to strengthen injured left shoulder using autograft, open (do not code graft harvest for this exercise)	0LU207Z
Percutaneous placement of Swan-Ganz catheter in superior vena cava	02HV32Z (The Swan-Ganz catheter is coded to the device value *Monitoring Device* because it monitors pulmonary artery output.)	Onlay lamellar keratoplasty of left cornea using autograft, external approach	08U9X7Z
		Resurfacing procedure on right femoral head, open approach	0SU90BZ
		Exchange of drainage tube from right hip joint	0S2YX0Z
Bronchoscopy with insertion of brachytherapy seeds, right main bronchus	0BH081Z	Tracheostomy tube exchange	0B21XFZ
Placement of intrathecal infusion pump for pain management, percutaneous	0JH73VZ (The device resides principally in the subcutaneous tissue of the back, so it is coded to body system *Subcutaneous Tissue and Fascia*.)	Change chest tube for left pneumothorax	0W2BX0Z
		Exchange of cerebral ventriculostomy drainage tube	0020X0Z
		Foley urinary catheter exchange	0T2BX0Z (This is coded to *Drainage Device* because urine is being drained.)
Open placement of bone growth stimulator, left femoral shaft	0QHY0MZ	Open removal of lumbar sympathetic neurostimulator	01PY0MZ
Cystoscopy with placement of brachytherapy seeds in prostate gland	0VH081Z	Nonincisional removal of Swan-Ganz catheter from right pulmonary artery	02PYX2Z
Full-thickness skin graft to right lower arm, autograft (do not code graft harvest for this exercise)	0HRDX73	Laparotomy with removal of pancreatic drain	0FPG00Z
		Extubation, endotracheal tube	0BP1XEZ
		Nonincisional PEG tube removal	0DP6XUZ
Excision of necrosed left femoral head with bone bank bone graft to fill the defect, open	0QR70KZ	Transvaginal removal of extraluminal cervical cerclage	0UPD7CZ
Penetrating keratoplasty of right cornea with donor matched cornea, percutaneous approach	08R83KZ	Incision with removal of K-wire fixation, right first metatarsal	0QPN04Z
		Cystoscopy with retrieval of left ureteral stent	0TP98DZ
Bilateral mastectomy with concomitant saline breast implants, open	0HRV0JZ	Removal of nasogastric drainage tube for decompression	0DP6X0Z
Excision of abdominal aorta with Gore-Tex graft replacement, open	04R00JZ	Removal of external fixator, left radial fracture	0PPJX5Z
Total right knee arthroplasty with insertion of total knee prosthesis	0SRC0JZ	Reposition of Swan-Ganz catheter insertion in superior vena cava	02WYX2Z
Bilateral mastectomy with free TRAM flap reconstruction	0HRV076	Open revision of right hip replacement, with readjustment of prosthesis	0SW90JZ
Tenonectomy with graft to right ankle using cadaver graft, open	0LRS0KZ	Adjustment of position, pacemaker lead in left ventricle, percutaneous	02WA3MZ
Mitral valve replacement using porcine valve, open	02RG08Z	External repositioning of Foley catheter to bladder	0TWBX0Z
		Revision of VAD reservoir placement in chest wall, causing patient discomfort, open	0JWT0WZ

Procedure	Code
Thoracotomy with exploration of right pleural cavity	0WJ90ZZ
Diagnostic laryngoscopy	0CJS8ZZ
Exploratory arthrotomy of left knee	0SJD0ZZ
Colposcopy with diagnostic hysteroscopy	0UJD8ZZ
Digital rectal exam	0DJD7ZZ
Diagnostic arthroscopy of right shoulder	0RJJ4ZZ
Endoscopy of bilateral maxillary sinus	09JY4ZZ, 09JY4ZZ
Laparotomy with palpation of liver	0FJ00ZZ
Transurethral diagnostic cystoscopy	0TJB8ZZ
Colonoscopy, discontinued at sigmoid colon	0DJD8ZZ
Percutaneous mapping of basal ganglia	00K83ZZ
Heart catheterization with cardiac mapping	02K83ZZ
Intraoperative whole brain mapping via craniotomy	00K00ZZ
Mapping of left cerebral hemisphere, percutaneous endoscopic	00K74ZZ
Intraoperative cardiac mapping during open heart surgery	02K80ZZ
Hysteroscopy with cautery of post-hysterectomy oozing and evacuation of clot	0W3R8ZZ
Open exploration and ligation of post-op arterial bleeder, left forearm	0X3F0ZZ
Control of post-operative retroperitoneal bleeding via laparotomy	0W3H0ZZ
Reopening of thoracotomy site with drainage and control of post-op hemopericardium	0W3C0ZZ
Arthroscopy with drainage of hemarthrosis at previous operative site, right knee	0Y3F4ZZ
Radiocarpal fusion of left hand with internal fixation, open	0RGP04Z
Posterior spinal fusion at L1-L3 level with BAK cage interbody fusion device, open	0SG1031
Intercarpal fusion of right hand with bone bank bone graft, open	0RGQ0KZ
Sacrococcygeal fusion with bone graft from same operative site, open	0SG507Z
Interphalangeal fusion of left great toe, percutaneous pin fixation	0SGQ34Z
Suture repair of left radial nerve laceration	01Q60ZZ (The approach value is *Open*, though the surgical exposure may have been created by the wound itself.)
Laparotomy with suture repair of blunt force duodenal laceration	0DQ90ZZ
Perineoplasty with repair of old obstetric laceration, open	0WQN0ZZ
Suture repair of right biceps tendon laceration, open	0LQ30ZZ
Closure of abdominal wall stab wound	0WQF0ZZ
Cosmetic face lift, open, no other information available	0W020ZZ
Bilateral breast augmentation with silicone implants, open	0HV0JZ

Procedure	Code
Cosmetic rhinoplasty with septal reduction and tip elevation using local tissue graft, open	090K07Z
Abdominoplasty (tummy tuck), open	0W0F0ZZ
Liposuction of bilateral thighs	0J0L3ZZ, 0J0M3ZZ
Creation of penis in female patient using tissue bank donor graft	0W4N0K1
Creation of vagina in male patient using synthetic material	0W4M0J0

Obstetrics

Procedure	Code
Abortion by dilation and evacuation following laminaria insertion	10A07ZW
Manually assisted spontaneous abortion	10E0XZZ (Since the pregnancy was not artificially terminated, this is coded to *Delivery* because it captures the procedure objective. The fact that it was an abortion will be identified in the diagnosis coding.)
Abortion by abortifacient insertion	10A07ZX
Bimanual pregnancy examination	10J07ZZ
Extraperitoneal C-section, low transverse incision	10D00Z2
Fetal spinal tap, percutaneous	10903ZA
Fetal kidney transplant, laparoscopic	10Y04ZS
Open in utero repair of congenital diaphragmatic hernia	10Q00ZK (Diaphragm is classified to the *Respiratory* body system in the *Medical and Surgical* section.)
Laparoscopy with total excision of tubal pregnancy	10T24ZZ
Transvaginal removal of fetal monitoring electrode	10P073Z

Placement

Procedure	Code
Placement of packing material, right ear	2Y42X5Z
Mechanical traction of entire left leg	2W6MX0Z
Removal of splint, right shoulder	2W5AX1Z
Placement of neck brace	2W32X3Z
Change of vaginal packing	2Y04X5Z
Packing of wound, chest wall	2W44X5Z
Sterile dressing placement to left groin region	2W27X4Z
Removal of packing material from pharynx	2Y50X5Z
Placement of intermittent pneumatic compression device, covering entire right arm	2W18X7Z
Exchange of pressure dressing to left thigh	2W0PX6Z

Administration

Procedure	Code
Peritoneal dialysis via indwelling catheter	3E1M39Z
Transvaginal artificial insemination	3E0P7LZ
Infusion of total parenteral nutrition via central venous catheter	3E0436Z
Esophagogastroscopy with Botox injection into esophageal sphincter	3E0G8GC (Botulinum toxin is a paralyzing agent with temporary effects; it does not sclerose or destroy the nerve.)
Percutaneous irrigation of knee joint	3E1U38Z
Epidural injection of mixed steroid and local anesthetic for pain control	3E0S33Z (This is coded to the substance value *Anti-inflammatory*. The anesthetic is added only to lessen the pain of the injection.)
Chemical pleurodesis using injection of tetracycline	3E0L3TZ
Transfusion of antihemophilic factor, (nonautologous) via arterial central line	30263V1
Transabdominal in vitro fertilization, implantation of donor ovum	3E0P3Q1
Autologous bone marrow transplant via central venous line	30243G0

Measurement and Monitoring

Procedure	Code
Cardiac stress test, single measurement	4A02XM4
EGD with biliary flow measurement	4A0C85Z
Temperature monitoring, rectal	4A1Z7KZ
Peripheral venous pulse, external, single measurement	4A04XJ1
Holter monitoring	4A12X45
Respiratory rate, external, single measurement	4A09XCZ
Fetal heart rate monitoring, transvaginal	4A1H7CZ
Visual mobility test, single measurement	4A07X7Z
Pulmonary artery wedge pressure monitoring from Swan-Ganz catheter	4A133B3
Olfactory acuity test, single measurement	4A08X0Z

Extracorporeal Assistance and Performance

Procedure	Code
Mechanical ventilation, 16 hours	5A1935Z
Liver dialysis, single encounter	5A1C00Z
Cardiac countershock with successful conversion to sinus rhythm	5A2204Z
IPPB (intermittent positive pressure breathing) for mobilization of secretions, 22 hours	5A09358
Renal dialysis, series of encounters	5A1D60Z
IABP (intra-aortic balloon pump) continuous	5A02210
Intra-operative cardiac pacing, continuous	5A1223Z
ECMO (extracorporeal membrane oxygenation), continuous	5A15223
Controlled mechanical ventilation (CMV), 45 hours	5A1945Z
Pulsatile compression boot with intermittent inflation	5A02115 (This is coded to the function value *Cardiac Output*, because the purpose of such compression devices is to return blood to the heart faster.)

Extracorporeal Therapies

Procedure	Code
Donor thrombocytapheresis, single encounter	6A55ØZ2
Bili-lite UV phototherapy, series treatment	6A8Ø1ZZ
Whole body hypothermia, single treatment	6A4ZØZZ
Circulatory phototherapy, single encounter	6A65ØZZ
Shock wave therapy of plantar fascia, single treatment	6A93ØZZ
Antigen-free air conditioning, series treatment	6A0Z1ZZ
TMS (transcranial magnetic stimulation), series treatment	6A221ZZ
Therapeutic ultrasound of peripheral vessels, single treatment	6A75ØZZ
Plasmapheresis, series treatment	6A551Z3
Extracorporeal electromagnetic stimulation (EMS) for urinary incontinence, single treatment	6A21ØZZ

Osteopathic

Procedures	Code
Isotonic muscle energy treatment of right leg	7WØ6X8Z
Low velocity-high amplitude osteopathic treatment of head	7WØØX5Z
Lymphatic pump osteopathic treatment of left axilla	7WØ7X6Z
Indirect osteopathic treatment of sacrum	7WØ4X4Z
Articulatory osteopathic treatment of cervical region	7WØ1XØZ

Other Procedures

Procedure	Code
Near infrared spectroscopy of leg vessels	8EØ23DZ
CT computer assisted sinus surgery	8EØ9XBG
Suture removal, abdominal wall	8EØWXY8
Isolation after infectious disease exposure	8EØZXY6
Robotic assisted open prostatectomy	8EØWØCZ

Chiropractic

Procedure	Code
Chiropractic treatment of lumbar region using long lever specific contact	9WB3XGZ
Chiropractic manipulation of abdominal region, indirect visceral	9WB9XCZ
Chiropractic extra-articular treatment of hip region	9WB6XDZ
Chiropractic treatment of sacrum using long and short lever specific contact	9WB4XJZ
Mechanically-assisted chiropractic manipulation of head	9WBØXKZ

Imaging

Procedure	Code
Noncontrast CT of abdomen and pelvis	BW21ZZZ
Ultrasound guidance for catheter placement, left subclavian artery	B342ZZZ
Chest x-ray, AP/PA and lateral views	BWØ3ZZZ
Endoluminal ultrasound of gallbladder and bile ducts	BF43ZZZ
MRI of thyroid gland, contrast unspecified	BG34YZZ
Esophageal videofluoroscopy study with oral barium contrast	BD11YZZ
Portable x-ray study of right radius/ulna shaft, standard series	BPØJZZZ
Routine fetal ultrasound, second trimester twin gestation	BY4DZZZ
CT scan of bilateral lungs, high osmolar contrast with densitometry	BB24ØZZ
Fluoroscopic guidance for percutaneous transluminal angioplasty (PTA) of left common femoral artery, low osmolar contrast	B41G1ZZ

Nuclear Medicine

Procedure	Code
Tomo scan of right and left heart, unspecified radiopharmaceutical, qualitative gated rest	C226YZZ
Technetium pentetate assay of kidneys, ureters, and bladder	CT631ZZ
Uniplanar scan of spine using technetium oxidronate, with first-pass study	CP151ZZ
Thallous chloride tomographic scan of bilateral breasts	CH22SZZ
PET scan of myocardium using rubidium	C23GQZZ
Gallium citrate scan of head and neck, single plane imaging	CW1BLZZ
Xenon gas nonimaging probe of brain	CØ5ØVZZ
Upper GI scan, radiopharmaceutical unspecified, for gastric emptying	CD15YZZ
Carbon 11 PET scan of brain with quantification	CØ3ØBZZ
Iodinated albumin nuclear medicine assay, blood plasma volume study	C763HZZ

Radiation Oncology

Procedure	Code
Plaque radiation of left eye, single port	D8YØFZZ
8 MeV photon beam radiation to brain	DØØ11ZZ
IORT of colon, 3 ports	DDY5CZZ
HDR brachytherapy of prostate using palladium-103	DV1Ø9BZ
Electron radiation treatment of right breast, with custom device	DMØ13ZZ
Hyperthermia oncology treatment of pelvic region	DWY68ZZ
Contact radiation of tongue	D9Y57ZZ
Heavy particle radiation treatment of pancreas, four risk sites	DFØ34ZZ
LDR brachytherapy to spinal cord using iodine	DØ16B9Z
Whole body Phosphorus 32 administration with risk to hematopoetic system	DWY5GFZ

Physical Rehabilitation and Diagnostic Audiology

Procedure	Code
Bekesy assessment using audiometer	F13Z31Z
Individual fitting of left eye prosthesis	FØDZ8UZ
Physical therapy for range of motion and mobility, patient right hip, no special equipment	FØ7LØZZ
Bedside swallow assessment using assessment kit	FØØZHYZ
Caregiver training in airway clearance techniques	FØFZ8ZZ
Application of short arm cast in rehabilitation setting	FØDZ7EZ (Inhibitory cast is listed in the equipment reference table under E, *Orthosis*.)
Verbal assessment of patient's pain level	FØ2ZFZZ
Caregiver training in communication skills using manual communication board	FØFZJMZ (Manual communication board is listed in the equipment reference table under M, *Augmentative/ Alternative Communication.*)
Group musculoskeletal balance training exercises, whole body, no special equipment	FØ7M6ZZ (Balance training is included in the motor treatment reference table under *Therapeutic Exercise*.)
Individual therapy for auditory processing using tape recorder	FØ9Z2KZ (Tape recorder is listed in the equipment reference table under *Audiovisual Equipment*.)

Mental Health

Procedure	Code
Cognitive-behavioral psychotherapy, individual	GZ58ZZZ
Narcosynthesis	GZGZZZZ
Light therapy	GZJZZZZ
ECT (electroconvulsive therapy), unilateral, multiple seizure	GZB1ZZZ
Crisis intervention	GZ2ZZZZ
Neuropsychological testing	GZ13ZZZ
Hypnosis	GZFZZZZ
Developmental testing	GZ1ØZZZ
Vocational counseling	GZ61ZZZ
Family psychotherapy	GZ72ZZZ

Substance Abuse Treatment

Procedure	Code
Naltrexone treatment for drug dependency	HZ94ZZZ
Substance abuse treatment family counseling	HZ63ZZZ
Medication monitoring of patient on methadone maintenance	HZ81ZZZ
Individual interpersonal psychotherapy for drug abuse	HZ54ZZZ
Patient in for alcohol detoxification treatment	HZ2ZZZZ
Group motivational counseling	HZ47ZZZ
Individual 12-step psychotherapy for substance abuse	HZ53ZZZ
Post-test infectious disease counseling for IV drug abuser	HZ3CZZZ
Psychodynamic psychotherapy for drug dependent patient	HZ5CZZZ
Group cognitive-behavioral counseling for substance abuse	HZ42ZZZ